Tylman's
THEORY AND PRACTICE OF
FIXED PROSTHODONTICS

Tylman's THEORY AND PRACTICE OF FIXED PROSTHODONTICS

William F. P. Malone
D.D.S., M.S., Ph.D., F.A.C.D

David L. Koth
D.D.S., M.S.

Consulting Editors

Edmund Cavazos, Jr., D.D.S.
David A. Kaiser, D.D.S., M.S.D.
Steven M. Morgano, D.M.D.

EIGHTH EDITION
Illustrated

Ishiyaku EuroAmerica, Inc.
St. Louis • Tokyo

Editor in Chief: Gregory Hacke, D.C.
Index Editor: Stephen Graef, M.M.

EIGHTH EDITION

Ishiyaku EuroAmerica, Inc.
716 Hanley Industrial Court, St. Louis, Missouri 63144

Library of Congress Catalogue Number 88-45369

Malone, William F.P.
    Tylman's Theory and Practice of Fixed
    Prosthodontics (Eighth Edition)

ISBN 0-912791-48-9

Ishiyaku EuroAmerica, Inc.
St. Louis • Tokyo

Composition by Graphic World, Inc.,
St. Louis, Missouri
Printed in the United States of America by
BookCrafters, Chelsea, Michigan

Contributing Authors

Robert F. Baima, B.S., D.D.S.
Director, Advanced Prosthodontics, Wadsworth Veterans Administration Hospital, Los Angeles, California; Diplomate, American Boards of Prosthodontics and Periodontics

Yvonne Balthazar-Hart, B.A., D.D.S., M.S.
Associate Professor, Department of Fixed Prosthodontics, Marquette University Dental School, Milwaukee, Wisconsin

Edmund Cavazos, Jr., B.S., D.D.S.
Associate Professor, Department of Restorative Dentistry, Division Head, Crown and Bridge, University of Texas, San Antonio, Texas; Diplomate, American Board of Prosthodontics

Gordon J. Christensen, D.D.S., M.S.D., Ph.D.
Codirector, Clinical Research Associates, Provo, Utah; Former Associate Dean, University of Colorado; Diplomate, American Board of Prosthodontics

Robert J. Crum, B.S., D.D.S.
Former Director, Prosthodontics, Hines Veterans Administration Hospital, Maywood, Illinois; Diplomate, American Board of Prosthodontics

E. Steven Duke, B.S., D.D.S., M.S.
Associate Professor, Department of Restorative Dentistry, Division of Occlusion and Biomaterial, University of Texas, San Antonio, Texas; Certification, Operative Dentistry

Ledeane Fattore-Bruno, B.S., D.D.S., M.S.
Assistant Professor and Head, Department of Prosthodontics, Zoller Clinic, University of Chicago, Chicago, Illinois

John E. Flocken, B.S., D.D.S.
Former Associate Dean, Professor, Department of Prosthodontics, University of California at Los Angeles, School of Dentistry, Los Angeles, California

Franklin Garcia-Godoy, B.S., D.D.S., M.S.
Associate Professor of Pediatric Dentistry, University of Texas, San Antonio, Texas; Editor, American Journal of Dentistry

Patrick M. Garvin, B.S., D.D.S., M.S.
Clinical Associate Professor, Department of Fixed Prosthodontics, Northwestern University Dental School, Chicago, Illinois; Illinois State Prosthodontics Specialty License

James D. Harrison, B.S., D.D.S., M.S.
Professor and Chairman, Department of Fixed Prosthodontics, Louisiana State University Dental School, New Orleans, Louisiana

Timothy O. Hart, B.S., D.D.S., M.S.
Clinical Assistant Professor, Department of Fixed Prosthodontics, Marquette University Dental School, Milwaukee, Wisconsin

Richard A. Hesby, B.S., D.D.S.
Professor and Chairman, Department of Fixed Prosthodontics, Northwestern University Dental School, Chicago, Illinois; Diplomate, American Board of Prosthodontics

Ronald Highton, B.S., D.D.S.
Guest Lecturer, Biomaterials, University of California at Los Angeles, School of Dentistry, Los Angeles, California

Maria Lopez Howell, B.S., D.D.S.
Clinical Assistant Professor, Department of Restorative Dentistry, Division of Operative Dentistry, University of Texas, San Antonio, Texas

Gaylord J. James, Jr., A.B., D.D.S.
Associate Professor, Department of Prosthodontics, Southern Illinois University, School of Dental Medicine, Alton, Illinois

Lee M. Jameson, B.S., D.D.S., M.S.

Professor and Director, Advanced Prosthodontics, Northwestern University Dental School, Chicago, Illinois; Diplomate, American Board of Prosthodontics

David A. Kaiser, B.S., D.D.S., M.S.D.

Associate Professor, Department of Restorative Dentistry, Division Head, Operative Dentistry, University of Texas, San Antonio, Texas; Diplomate, American Board of Prosthodontics

William J. Kelly, Jr., B.S., D.D.S., M.S.

Clinical Associate Professor, Department of Prosthodontics, Southern Illinois University, School of Dental Medicine, Alton, Illinois

David L. Koth, B.S., D.D.S., M.S.

Professor and Chairman, Department of Fixed Prosthodontics, University of North Carolina, Chapel Hill, North Carolina

William F.P. Malone, D.D.S., M.S., Ph.D.

Professor, Restorative Dentistry, Coordinator of Fixed and Removable Prosthodontics, Washington University School of Dental Medicine, St. Louis, Missouri

Delmo J. Maroso, B.S., D.D.S.

Professor, Department of Restorative Dentistry, Southern Illinois University, School of Dental Medicine, Alton, Illinois

Thomas D. Marshall, A.B., M.S.Ed., D.D.S.

Associate Professor, Department of Restorative Dentistry, Division of Operative Dentistry, University of Texas, San Antonio, Texas

Maury Massler, D.D.S., M.S., D.Sc.

Professor Emeritus, Tufts University, School of Dental Medicine, Boston, Massachusetts; Former Associate Dean, Postgraduate Education, University of Illinois, College of Dentistry, Chicago, Illinois

Boleslaw Mazur, B.S., D.D.S., M.S.

Professor, Department of Fixed Prosthodontics, Loyola University, School of Dentistry, Maywood, Illinois

John W. McLean, O.B.E., D.Sc., M.D.S., L.D.S., R.C.S. (England)

Eastman Dental Hospital, London, England

Steven M. Morgano, B.A., D.M.D.

Staff Prosthodontist, Edith Nourse Rogers Memorial Veterans Hospital, Bedford, Massachusetts; Assistant Professor, Department of Prosthodontics, Boston University, Boston, Massachusetts; Diplomate, American Board of Prosthodontics

Bernard W. Murray, B.S., D.D.S.

Clinical Assistant Professor, Department of Graduate Periodontics, Loyola University, School of Dentistry, Maywood, Illinois; Illinois State Periodontics Specialty License

Bernard L. Muzynski, B.S., D.D.S., M.S.

Private Practice; Former Associate Professor, Department of Fixed Prosthodontics, Northwestern University Dental School, Chicago, Illinois; Illinois State Prosthodontic Specialty License

Donald H. Newell, B.S., D.D.S., M.S.

Associate Professor, Department of Periodontics, University of Texas, San Antonio, Texas; Diplomate, American Board of Periodontics

Jerry W. Nicholson, B.S., D.D.S., M.A.

Assistant Professor, Department of Restorative Dentistry, Division of Operative Dentistry, University of Texas, San Antonio, Texas

Barry K. Norling, Ph.D.

Associate Professor, Department of Restorative Dentistry, Division Head, Biomaterials, University of Texas, San Antonio, Texas

Zigmund C. Porter, B.S., D.D.S.

Former Associate Professor, Department of Graduate Periodontics, University of Illinois, College of Dentistry, Chicago, Illinois; Illinois State Periodontics Specialty License

Gerald J. Re, B.S., D.D.S., M.A.

Associate Professor, Department of Restorative Dentistry, Division of Operative Dentistry, University of Texas, San Antonio, Texas

J. Marvin Reynolds, B.S., D.D.S.

Professor, Department of Restorative Dentistry, Chairman, Division of Occlusion, Medical College of Georgia, School of Dentistry, Augusta, Georgia; Diplomate, American Board of Prosthodontics

Joseph T. Richardson, B.S., D.D.S., M.S.

Former Associate Dean and Professor, Department of Restorative Dentistry, Division of Crown and Bridge, University of Texas, San Antonio, Texas

Edwin (Ted) Riley, B.S., D.M.D.

Clinical Assistant Professor, Department of Prosthodontics, Forsythe Dental Center, Boston, Massachusetts

Ernst Schelb, B.S., D.D.S., M.S.D.

Assistant Professor, Department of Restorative Dentistry, Division of Crown and Bridge, University of Texas, San Antonio, Texas

James R. Schmidt, B.S., D.D.S., M.S.D.

Former Section Head, Fixed Prosthodontics, Southern Illinois University, School of Dental Medicine, Alton, Illinois

John Sobieralski, B.S., D.D.S., M.S.

Assistant Professor, Department of Restorative Dentistry, University of Texas, San Antonio, Texas

Elwood H. Stade, B.S., D.D.S.

Associate Professor, Department of Prosthodontics, Southern Illinois University, School of Dental Medicine, Alton, Illinois; Diplomate, American Board of Prosthodontics

William D. Sulik, B.S., D.D.S.

Clinical Associate Professor, Department of Fixed Prosthodontics, University of North Carolina, Chapel Hill, North Carolina

David L. Tay, B.S., D.D.S., M.S.

Senior Lecturer, Department of Prosthodontics, University of Singapore Dental School, Singapore

G. Roger Troendle, B.S., D.D.S., M.S.

Clinical Associate Professor, Department of Restorative Dentistry, Division of Crown and Bridge, University of Texas, San Antonio, Texas

Karen B. Troendle, B.S., D.D.S.

Associate Professor, Department of Restorative Dentistry, Division of Crown and Bridge, University of Texas, San Antonio, Texas

Richard N. Wells, B.S., D.D.S., M.A.T.

Clinical Associate Professor, Department of Fixed Prosthodontics, Northwestern University Dental School, Chicago, Illinois

Earl L. Woerner, B.S., D.D.S.

Clinical Associate Professor, Department of Prosthodontics, Southern Illinois University, School of Dental Medicine, Alton, Illinois

Anthony T. Young, B.S., D.D.S., M.S.

Private Practice; Illinois State Prosthodontics and Orthodontics Specialty Licenses

Gerald J. Ziebert, B.S., D.D.S., M.S.

Professor and Chairman, Department of Fixed Prosthodontics, Marquette University Dental School, Milwaukee, Wisconsin; Diplomate, American Board of Prosthodontics

Contributing Artists

Steven M. Morgano, Londonderry, N.H.
Chapters 1, 3, 4, 6, 8, 11, 13, 14, 15, 19

Charles Whitehead, San Antonio, Tex.
Chapters 2, 6, 7, 10, 11

Delmo J. Maroso, Alton, Ill.
Chapters 6, 8, 13

David J. Edmonds, Chicago, Ill.
Chapter 12

L.M. Jameson, Chicago, Ill.
Chapters 5, 14

Anthony T. Young, Westchester, Ill.
Chapters 5, 6

Thomas D. Marshall, San Antonio, Tex.
Chapter 2

L. Paul Lustig, Boston, Mass.
Chapter 5

William F.P. Malone, Alton, Ill.
Chapters 5, 6

Mary Ruth Malone Pleak, San Antonio, Tex.
Chapters 5, 24

David A. Kaiser, San Antonio, Tex.
Chapter 6

Richard Wells, Chicago, Ill.
Chapter 18

Julia Allen, Chicago, Ill.
Chapters 5, 6

William D. Sulik, Chapel Hill, N.C.
Chapter 26

James R. Schmidt, Alton, Ill.
Chapters 6, 22

Consultant in Dental Technology

Yoichi Miyazawa, St. Louis, Mo.

Preface

Education and research are continual processes. Innovative biologic discoveries in related specialties have affected the practice of prosthodontics. The interrelationship of periodontics, orthodontics, removable prosthetics, and endodontics with fixed prosthodontics has provided more comprehensive patient care.

Dentistry has currently embarked upon an era of conservative microretention that is a drastic departure from the conventional. The emphasis upon acid etched surfaces for resin cements and micro-tooth preparation is extremely attractive to patients. It also presents a challenge to dental education to identify with longitudinal clinical studies and basic research the limitations of this promising therapy. Therefore, the purpose of the eighth edition is to provide a publication that stresses current treatment in fixed prosthodontics and related specialties.

Advances in therapeutics involve scholarly conflicts that are reflected as intellectual controversy. There are conflicting, if not diametrically opposed ideas, between authors of various chapters. However, innovative concepts based upon scientific data, evaluated in an academic atmosphere, produce a healthy climate for the advancement of dentistry. This implies that the dentist accepts the responsibility of familiarization with improved methods of treatment that depart from the traditional. Imaginative treatment is impossible to implement if the dentist is unaware of its existence.

To render service to the dental patient, a planned sequence of therapy is necessary for versatile oral health treatment. If prosthodontics are initiated prior to the establishment of a sound, scholarly diagnosis, or if the sequence is illogical, the desired result becomes elusive. Oral diagnosis, problem solving, and treatment planning are dealt with in the text as complementary procedures. This text accentuates a programmed, intellectual review of diagnostic data prior to the initiation of treatment. A practical treatment plan should be flexible for alternate therapy but relatively uncomplicated in overall application. We sincerely hope that this book not only presents traditional fixed prosthodontics in a comprehensive, enthusiastic manner, but also elucidates the innovative dental procedures.

There is justifiable emphasis on the interaction of periodontics, occlusion, and restorative dentistry. The step by step illustrations were designed to clarify use of improved materials and imaginative techniques. The trend to microretentive techniques is a natural development in light of effective preventive dentistry and economics. A greater focus on periodontics, esthetics and the influence of fixed-removable prosthodontics was also considered essential.

Many distinguished authors have contributed to the eighth edition and we extend our heartfelt thanks. We are also indebted to the artists, scientists, journals, and dental manufacturers who graciously assisted in furnishing material and illustrations. Research groups are too numerous to thank individually, but are gratefully acknowledged by the authors. We have attempted to perpetuate the life work of Dr. Stanley Tylman (1894-1983) whose outstanding contributions to society as an author, researcher, dentist, and a man transcend time.

This book is dedicated to the families of all the authors of the text whose patience and encouragement were essential to its completion. A special dedication is made to former consulting editor, the late Hosea F. Sawyer, B.S., D.D.S., M.S., whose vision and intellect are legendary among his former students, associates, friends, and family. We would also like to extend our sincere appreciation to Dr. Gregory Hacke for his superior editing and general resourcefulness and to acknowledge the encouragement and perceptive planning of Mr. Manuel Ponte, President of I.E.A. Publishers.

William F.P. Malone
David L. Koth

Contents

Tylman's
THEORY AND PRACTICE OF
FIXED PROSTHODONTICS

1

Steven M. Morgano, Patrick M. Garvin,
Bernard L. Muzynski, and
William F.P. Malone

DIAGNOSIS AND TREATMENT PLANNING

Diagnosis is the determination of the nature of a disease process. Treatment is any measure designed to remedy a disease. Competent treatment depends upon the careful evaluation of all available information, a definitive diagnosis, and a realistic treatment plan that offers a favorable prognosis. The treatment plan follows the diagnosis, and no treatment other than emergency care should be performed without a comprehensive treatment plan.

More than one rational treatment approach is often possible. The challenge is to determine which plan is best for the patient's needs and desires.

TERMINOLOGY

Prosthodontics

Prosthodontics is that discipline of dentistry pertaining to the restoration of oral function, comfort, appearance, and health by restoring natural teeth and replacing missing teeth and contiguous oral and maxillofacial tissues with artificial substitutes. There are three main branches of prosthodontics: fixed, removable, and maxillofacial.

Fixed prosthodontics pertains to the restoration or replacement of teeth with artificial substitutes that are attached to natural teeth, roots, or implants and that are not readily removable.

Removable prosthodontics pertains to the replacement of missing teeth and contiguous oral structures with artificial substitutes that are readily removable.

Maxillofacial prosthetics pertains to the restoration of developmental or acquired defects of the stomatognathic system and associated facial structures with artificial substitutes.

Extracoronal Restorations

Extracoronal restorations use a veneer to restore external portions of a prepared tooth to tissue-compatible contour and obtain retention and resistance to displacement primarily from the fit of the restoration to the external walls of the preparation.

Complete veneer crowns restore all surfaces of the clinical crown (Fig. 1-1). The restorative material may be all metal, all porcelain (ceramic), a metal-ceramic combination, or a metal with processed resin.

Partial veneer crowns restore only a portion of the clinical crown.

Three-quarter crowns restore the occlusal surface and three of the four axial surfaces (not including the facial surface).

Reverse three-quarter crowns restore all surfaces except the lingual surface.

Seven-eighths crowns are extensions of the three-quarter crown to include a major portion of the facial surface.

One-half crown veneers restore the occlusal and mesial surfaces, as well as portions of the facial and lingual surfaces. The one-half crown restoration is sometimes indicated as a retainer for a fixed partial denture (FPD) abutment with a pronounced mesial inclination (see section on the mesially tilted molar).

Laminates are veneer restorations that restore the facial surface of a tooth for esthetic purposes. They are fabricated from resin or dental porcelain; they bond (microretention) (Fig. 1-2) to etched enamel with a composite resin luting agent.

Resin-bonded restorations are cast metal partial veneers that are bonded to etched enamel. Resin-bonded restorations are used most often as a retainer for an FPD. This type of prosthesis is commonly referred to as a *Maryland bridge*.

Intracoronal Restorations

Intracoronal restorations obtain their retention and resistance to displacement from the intimate fit of the restoration within the confines of the coronal portion of the tooth.

An *inlay* is the classic intracoronal restoration.

The *onlay* is a modification of the inlay to restore the occlusal surface of the tooth.

Pinledge refers to the modification of an anterior three-quarter crown preparation to obtain primary retention and resistance from long parallel pins (Fig. 1-3).

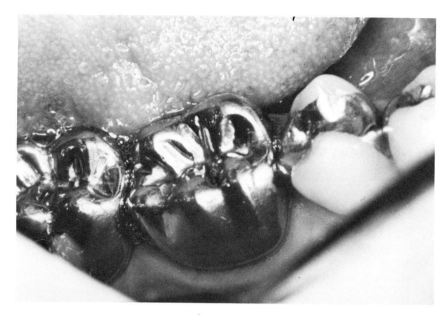

Fig. 1-1. Complete veneer crowns for mandibular molars.

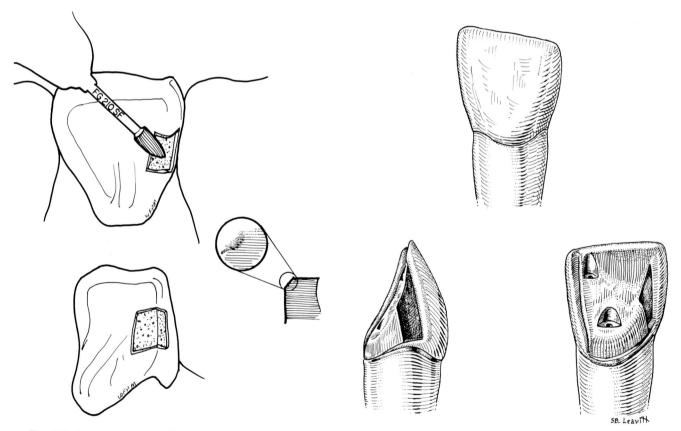

Fig. 1-2. Contemporary bonding techniques establish microretention with etched enamel.

Fig. 1-3. A pinlege retainer with a mesial box modification. From McElroy, D.L., and Malone, W.F.P.: Oral diagnosis. Philadelphia, Williams and Wilkins, 1969.

Radicular Retained Restorations

Radicular retained restorations consist of a post or dowel with an attached core that obtains its retention and resistance to displacement from the prepared root portion of an endodontically treated tooth. While the root preparation retains the post, the core establishes retention and resistance for a complete veneer crown that restores the pulpless tooth to normal form and function (Fig. 1-4). This *post and core* (dowel and core) may be *custom cast*, where the radicular retainer is fabricated to fit the root preparation, or *prefabricated*, where the root preparation is designed to fit a stock post, and a core is built up with silver amalgam or, rarely, composite resin.

Fixed Partial Dentures

Fixed partial dentures (FPD's) replace one or more missing teeth and are attached definitively to the remaining teeth. The replacement tooth is a *pontic*. The teeth that support the FPD are the *abutments*. The restorations that are cemented to the abutments and retain the FPD in place are the *retainers*. The retainers are joined to the pontic by *connectors* (Figs. 1-5 and 1-6). Generally, a pontic is supported by a mesial and distal abutment. If a pontic is supported on one side only (mesial or distal), it is referred to as a *cantilever pontic*.

DIAGNOSIS

Scholarly diagnosis is the basis for a rational treatment plan and competent dental care is only possible with effective planning. Diagnosis involves the collection of facts obtained from a comprehensive patient history (medical and dental), a patient interview, thorough clinical examination, critical evaluation of mounted diagnostic casts, and a radiographic interpretation.

Patient History

The value of a thorough medical history cannot be overstated. The medical history will reveal systemic conditions (e.g., diabetes mellitus) that not only contribute to existing dental disease, but also affect the prognosis of dental treatment. The medical history will alert the practitioner to any disorders (e.g., rheumatic heart disease) that require antibiotic prophylaxis, as well as carrier states of infectious diseases such as hepatitis B and acquired immune deficiency syndrome (AIDS).

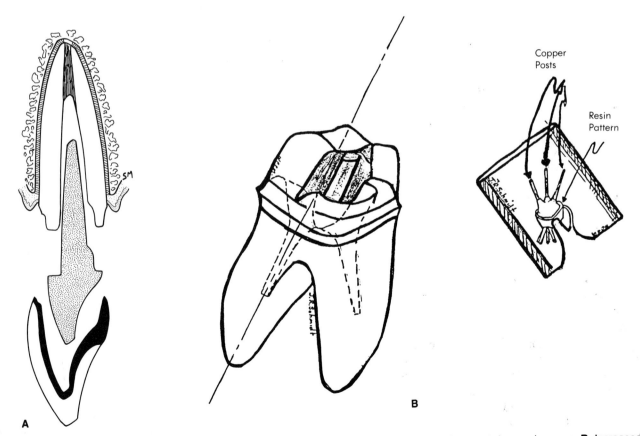

Fig. 1-4. A, Cast metal post and core for an anterior tooth provides retention and resistance for a metal ceramic crown. **B,** Increased patient concern has sponsored imaginative techniques for radicular restorations. The interlocking cast metal post and core is used for a severely damaged pulpless molar.

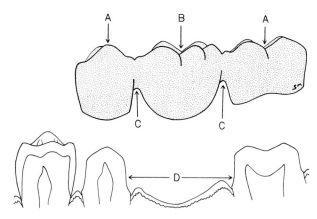

Fig. 1-5. A mandibular FPD. The retainers (A) are attached to the pontic (B) by rigid connectors (C). The FPD is supported by the abutments (D).

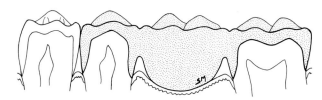

Fig. 1-6. A cross-sectional view of the FPD in Fig. 1-5 seated on the abutments.

A history of allergies, adverse drug reactions, hypertension, cardiac disease, emotional disorders, seizures, oral trauma, prosthetic joint replacements, head and neck malignancies, and many other medical conditions influence dental treatment. The presence of a pacemaker contraindicates electrosurgical soft tissue dilation for impression procedures. Previous radiation therapy for neoplastic disease of the head and neck region can have a profound effect on the oral cavity.

A review of the patient's past and current medications may reveal illnesses that were overlooked on the written health questionnaire and may explain any adverse side effects to drug therapy. A myriad of commonly prescribed drugs can induce moderate-to-severe xerostomia (Table 1-1). Cervical dental caries and periodontitis are serious sequelae to chronic xerostomia and will contribute to early failure of fixed restorations.

The dental history is an adjunct to the medical history and provides information about the patient's past dental experiences, including prior dental treatment (when, by whom, and what kind), when and why missing teeth were removed, previous problems with dental treatment, pernicious habits such as clenching and bruxism, temporomandibular joint (TMJ) symptoms, dental phobias, and any abnormal gag reflexes.

Patient Interview

A candid interview with the patient is invaluable. During the interview the medical and dental histories are reviewed, and a chief complaint is determined. Frank communication is established and patient attitudes are assessed.

Are the patient's expectations realistic? Is the patient aware of the time and finances that must be invested? Is the patient physically and emotionally prepared for the long arduous appointments routinely required for fixed prosthodontics? Are there any emotional conditions that are contributing to dysfunction of the TMJ or muscles of mastication? Is the patient motivated to maintain a healthy oral environment after treatment is completed?

Not all problems can be solved with our state-of-the-art restorative dentistry. Sometimes the complications of treatment are worse than the initial problem. For some patients, the best treatment plan is no treatment. Every patient should be fully aware of the limitations of treatment, especially esthetic limitations.

Clinical Examination

Head and neck examination. A regional examination of the head and neck should include an evaluation of the size, shape, and symmetry of the head and neck, including the overall profile (retrognathic, mesiognathic, or prognathic). The skin and hair are examined. Special attention should be given to abnormalities such as lymph node enlargements, cutaneous ulcerations, scars, exophytic growths, or anomalous pigmentations. The TMJs and the muscles of mastication are evaluated for dysfunction. (Chapter 23 provides a comprehensive review of the TMJ examination.)

Oral examination. The oral examination begins with a screening for malignancy, and the patient is referred to an appropriate specialist if any suspicious lesions are discovered.

General oral assessment. An oral assessment includes an evaluation of the oral hygiene, overall caries activity, general periodontal status, and the quality and quantity of saliva. Poor hygiene is an ominous sign and will contribute to carious and periodontal breakdown after prosthodontic care. A high caries rate may be due to frequent sucrose intake, xerostomia, or both. Xerostomia may be the result of medication (Table 1-1), radiotherapy to the head and neck region, or a systemic disorder.

Examination of teeth. Inspection of visible tooth surfaces should coincide with review of the radiographs. Each tooth is examined for dental caries, decalcifications, erosion, abrasion, occlusal attrition, hypersensitive exposed root surfaces, or fractures. The restorations are scrutinized for defects or recurrent

Table 1-1. Medications with xerostomia as a side effect*

Drug	Description	Drug	Description
Actifed	Decongestant/antihistamine	Librax	Tranquilizer/antispasmodic
Actifed-C	Decongestant/antihistamine	Limbitrol	Antidepressant
Aldomet	Antihypertensive	Marax	Antiasthmatic/tranquilizer
Aldoril	Antihypertensive/diuretic	Mellaril	Tranquilizer/antipsychotic
Antivert	Antihistamine/sedative	Minipress	Antihypertensive
Artane	Antispasmodic	Naldecon	Decongestant/antihistamine
Atarax	Tranquilizer/antihistamine	Navane	Tranquilizer
Benadryl	Antihistamine	Norgesic-Forte	Muscle relaxant/analgesic
Bentyl	Antispasmodic	Norpace	Antiarrhythmic
Benylin	Antihistamine	Periactin	Antihistamine/antipiuritic
Catapres	Antihypertensive	Phenergan	Antihistamine/decongestant
Chlor-trimeton	Decongestant/antihistamine	w/Codeine	Antihistamine/decongestant
Combid	Antispasmodic	VC w/Codeine	Antihistamine/decongestant
Compazine	Tranquilizer	Regroton	Diuretic/antihypertensive
Dalmane	Tranquilizer	SER-AP-ES	Tranquilizer/diuretic antihypertensive
Dimetapp	Antihistamine/decongestant	Sinemet	Antispasmodic
Donnatal	Antispasmodic/sedative	Sinequan	Tranquilizer
Dyazide	Diuretic	Stelazine	Tranquilizer
Elavil	Antidepressant	Tenuat	Anorexiant
Fastin	Anorexiant	Thorazine	Tranquilizer
Flagyl	Antitrichomonacidal	Tofranil	Antidepressant
Flexeril	Antispasmodic	Tranxene	Tranquilizer
Haldol	Tranquilizer	Triavil	Tranquilizer/antidepressant
Hydropress	Antihypertensive/diuretic	Tuss-Ornade	Antidepressant/antitussive
Imodium	Antispasmodic	Vistaril	Tranquilizer
		Zaroxoyl	Diuretic/antihypertensive

From Bangston 1984 (Lecture: U. of Chicago Zoller Clinic)
*Many drugs affect the amount and consistency of saliva. Drugs that cause xerostomia include anorexiants, antidepressants, antihistamines, antihypertensives, antineoplastics, antipsychotics, antispasmodics, decongestants, diuretics, and tranquilizers. This table lists the most frequently prescribed drugs that are accompanied by xerostomia.

caries, and abnormalities in crown height, contour, or alignment are recorded.

Occlusal examination. The nature of the patient's occlusion is evaluated according to the Angle classification: vertical and horizontal overlap of the anterior teeth; occlusal plane; vertical dimension of occlusion; any missing, supraerupted, rotated, or malaligned teeth; interceptive occlusal contacts; and evidence of bruxism. A more detailed occlusal examination is possible with mounted diagnostic casts (see section on diagnostic casts).

Periodontal examination. The gingiva is observed for any abnormalities in color, size, shape, consistency, or texture, as well as areas of recession. The periodontal probe scrutinizes the crevicular space for periodontal pockets, furcation invasions (see Chapter 4), and mucogingival defects. The mobility patterns of the teeth are evaluated and correlated with areas of bone loss determined from radiographs or interceptive occlusal contacts.

Any periodontal pathosis is identified along with associated cofactors in the disease process, including overcontoured and overhanging restorations. Chapter 3 includes a more detailed discussion of the periodontal examination.

Diagnostic Casts

Diagnostic casts are made from impressions of the dental arches. These casts are used to evaluate soft tissue contours, vestibular morphology and frenum attachments, bony contours (e.g., tori), crown length and morphology, tooth alignment and paths of insertion, available pontic space, existing restorations, esthetic factors, and the occlusion.

Diagnostic impression material. Diagnostic impressions are commonly made with irreversible hydrocolloid (alginate). This material is inexpensive, accurate, and easily manipulated. It does not require a custom tray and is readily retrieved from undercuts.

Making impressions. Perforated rim-lock stock metal trays that allow a uniform thickness of 3 to 5 mm of impression material are desirable. The trays must also be large enough to cover the hamular notches in the maxillary arch and the retromolar pads in the mandible. If the flanges of the trays do not extend to the mucobuccal folds, "periphery wax" can be added to the borders. The lingual flanges of the mandibular tray must extend to the functional reflection of the floor of the mouth (below the mylohyoid crest) without constricting tongue movements.

The trays are evaluated with a practice insertion to

verify that they seat completely without binding or patient discomfort. The mandibular impression is made first, with the dentist positioned at the 8 o'clock position and the patient seated at a 45-degree angle to the floor.

The mouth is gently dried. Accurately proportioned alginate is added to measured water (approximately 72 degrees F) in a flexible bowl. The material is vigorously spatulated for 45 seconds. The impression tray is loaded without entrapping air. Excess impression material is wiped into critical areas such as the occlusal surfaces, and the impression tray is centered over the dental arch and seated.

While the tray is being inserted, the patient is instructed to bring the tongue up and forward. The tray must be held completely still while the alginate sets. The final set of the impression material occurs 3½ minutes after the beginning of the mix. The tray is removed with a quick snap.

The impression is rinsed, gently dried, and stored in a damp paper towel while the maxillary impression is being made. Before the maxillary impression is made, excess mucinous saliva is wiped from the palate with a gauze sponge. The impression is made with the patient in an upright position and the dentist at the 11 o'clock position.

The completed impressions are inspected for defects, bubbles, voids, or tears. There should be a smooth surface to the alginate with well-rounded borders and adequate coverage and detail of all anatomic landmarks—including the hamular notches and retromolar pads.

The impressions are poured as soon as possible with vacuum-mixed, proportioned cast stone. A water-powder ratio of 30 ml water/100 g stone is recommended. The stone is added slowly under vibration with a No. 7 wax spatula. Air entrapment at the cusp tips and incisal edges must be avoided (Fig. 1-7).

After the stone has set, the casts are retrieved. Small nodules are removed with a sharp instrument. The bases are trimmed to preserve all anatomic landmarks and all vestibular areas (Figs. 1-8 and 1-9).

Mounted diagnostic casts. The casts are mounted on a semiadjustable articulator with a facebow transfer (Fig. 1-10). This mounting is a fundamental record of the patient's pretreatment occlusal relationships and aids in presenting the finalized treatment plan to the patient (Fig. 1-11). A diagnostic waxing of the proposed FPD on duplicate diagnostic casts gives a preview of the anticipated occlusal scheme and esthetic form (Fig. 1-12).

Radiographic Interpretation

A well-defined, complete mouth radiographic series (14 periapical and 4 bitewing radiographs) is essential.

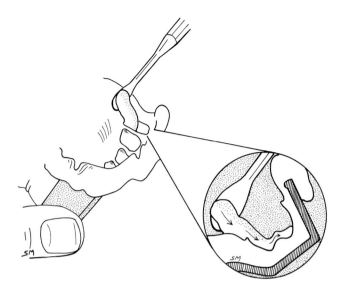

Fig. 1-7. Stone is added to the impression *slowly* under vibration to avoid air entrapment.

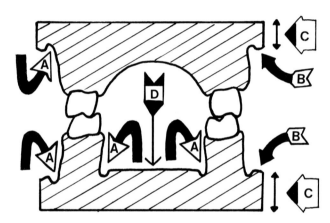

Fig. 1-8. Acceptable diagnostic casts include: (A), mucobuccal, mucolabial, and mucolingual folds, (B), a land area of 2 to 3 mm, (C), a cast base approximately ¾ inch thick, and (D), a flat lingual area.

TMJ radiographs may be indicated for patients with joint dysfunction (See Chapter 23), and a panoramic radiograph can also be helpful.

Radiographs provide information that cannot be determined clinically; they are an adjunct, however, and not the sole or primary source of diagnostic information. The radiographic interpretation is combined with all other available findings when making a definitive diagnosis and developing a treatment plan.

An intraoral radiographic examination reveals:
1. Remaining bone support.
2. Root number and morphology (short, long, slender, broad, bifurcated, fused, dilacerated, etc.) and root proximity.
3. Quality of supporting bone, trabecular patterns, and reactions to functional changes.

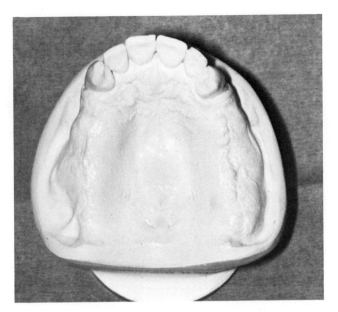

Fig. 1-9. A, An acceptable maxillary diagnostic cast.

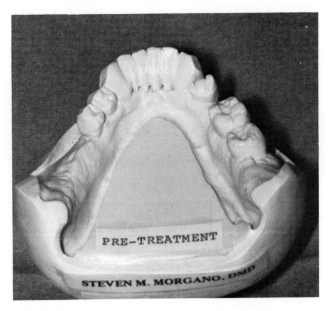

Fig. 1-9. B, An acceptable mandibular diagnostic cast.

4. Width of the periodontal ligament spaces and evidence of trauma from occlusion.
5. Areas of vertical and horizontal osseous resorption and furcation invasions.
6. Axial inclination of teeth (degree of nonparallelism if present).
7. Continuity and integrity of the lamina dura.
8. Pulpal morphology and previous endodontic treatment with or without post and cores.
9. Presence of apical disease, root resorption, or root fractures.
10. Retained root fragments, radiolucent areas, calcifications, foreign bodies, or impacted teeth.
11. Presence of carious lesions, the condition of existing restorations, and the proximity of caries and restorations to the dental pulp.
12. Proximity of carious lesions and restorations to the alveolar crest.
13. Calculus deposits.
14. Oral roentgenographic manifestations of systemic disease.

The Definitive Diagnosis

After a careful review of all available information, a definitive diagnosis is made. The dental diagnosis commonly includes a determination of the periodontal health, occlusal relationships, TMJ function, condition of edentulous areas, anatomic abnormalities, serviceability of existing prostheses, and status of the remaining dentition—including previous dental treatment, dental caries, defective restorations, and pulpal disease. Treatment options follow logically from the diagnoses.

CONSIDERATIONS IN TREATMENT PLANNING
Patient's Desires, Expectations, and Needs

When planning treatment for the "entire patient," the desires of the patient take priority; yet the dentist should not deliver substandard care, claiming "the patient wanted it." The patient's expectations must also be realistic. Disappointment with the outcome of prosthodontic care is often the result of poor communication and lack of understanding of the limitations of treatment.

Systemic and Emotional Health

The patient's systemic and emotional condition will influence treatment. Elderly or debilitated patients, unable to tolerate the long appointments routinely required for extensive fixed prosthodontics, may be better served with more conservative care, removable prostheses, or both. Patients requiring antibiotic prophylaxis should have as much treatment performed per appointment as possible to reduce the frequency of dentist-induced bacteremias.

Many medications commonly prescribed for a number of systemic and emotional disorders can result in significant xerostomia, which, as previously stated, will unfavorably affect the outcome of treatment. Bruxism, common in emotionally tense individuals, taxes the reparative capacities of the periodontium and the serviceability of restorative dentistry. Carrier states of infectious diseases such as hepatitis B and AIDS require special precautions in the dental operatory and laboratory to prevent cross-contamination. An overnight soak of impressions (vinyl polysiloxane material is recommended) in fresh, activated glutar-

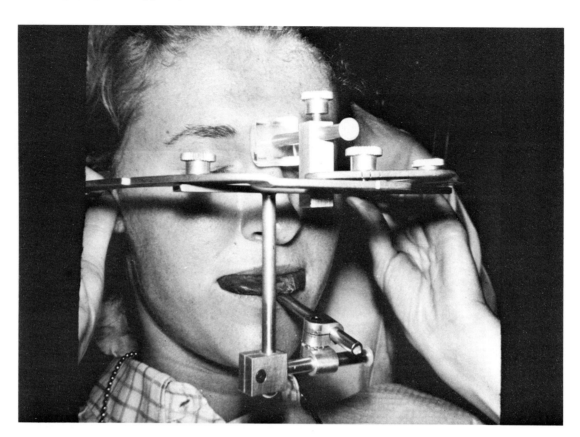

Fig. 1-10. A, A face bow record is obtained.

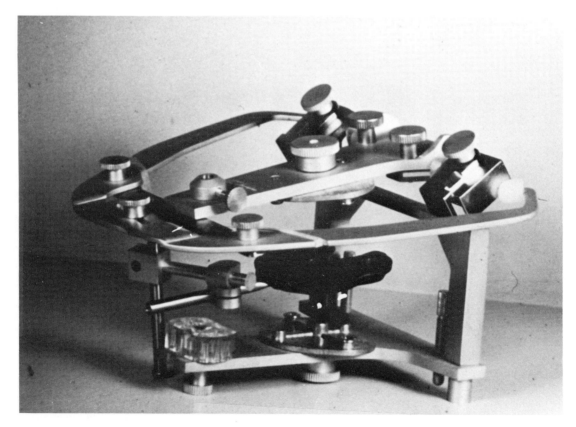

Fig. 1-10. B, The maxillary cast is mounted with a face bow record to relate the patient's hinge axis to the axis on the articulator. (Courtesy Dr. Anda Solarski, Chicago, Ill.)

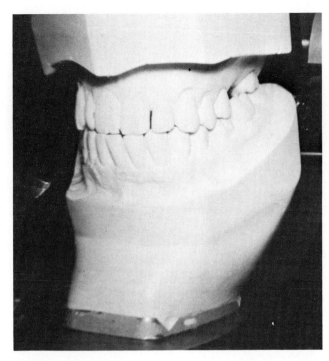

Fig. 1-11. Mounted diagnostic casts are a fundamental record of the patient's pretreatment occlusal relationships and aids in presenting the treatment plan.

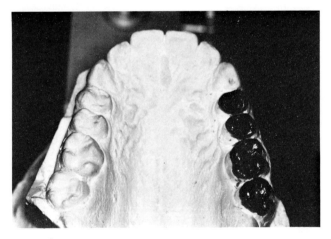

Fig. 1-12. The diagnostic waxing gives a preview of the occlusal scheme.

aldehyde solution is advised for high-risk patients. Forthcoming research will clarify the solution's effect on impression materials and tray plastics.[1]

Periodontal Factors

Inflammation. A diagnosis of periodontitis is not uncommon for the patient requiring prosthodontics because one or more teeth may already have been lost to periodontal disease.

The goals of periodontal therapy for the prosthodontic patient are: to resolve the inflammation; con-

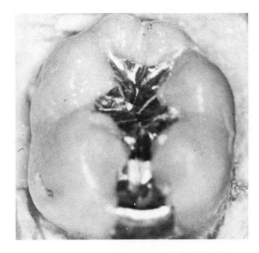

Fig. 1-13. Broad extension of cavity preparations to develop margins in "caries immune" areas is not universally advocated.

vert periodontal pocket depths to clinically normal sulcular depths; establish physiologic gingival architecture; and provide an adequate zone of attached gingiva. Adequate oral hygiene is fundamental to the maintenance of a healthy periodontium.

If surgical intervention is required to achieve therapeutic goals, approximately six to eight weeks of healing is recommended before the gingival termination of the tooth preparations is completed.

Furcation invasions. Teeth with furcation invasions require special consideration. The section on periodontally compromised dentitions in Chapter 4 discusses diagnosis and treatment planning for the tooth with a furcation involvement.

Margin placement. G.V. Black's original concepts of "extension for prevention"[2] have been modified. Broad extension of cavity preparations to place margins in "caries immune" areas is not universally advocated (Fig. 1-13). The recommendation that all gingival finish lines be developed within the gingival crevice has been challenged.[3-15]

The gingivae are healthiest when margins are placed well above (i.e., 1 to 2 mm) the gingival crest[16] (Fig. 1-14), and intracrevicular margin placement is not the universal solution to dental caries. Nevertheless, there are still indications for the intracrevicular gingival margin. Often esthetics, retention requirements, the location of caries or preexisting restorations, root sensitivity, and areas of cervical erosion or root fracture will make placement of supragingival margins impractical. The supragingival margin may also be more susceptible to cement dissolution.[17]

Biologic width. Histologic studies by Gargiulo, et al.[18] have demonstrated a band of soft tissue attachment between the base of the gingival sulcus and the alveolar crest that is composed of approximately 1 mm of junctional epithelium (attachment epithelium) and

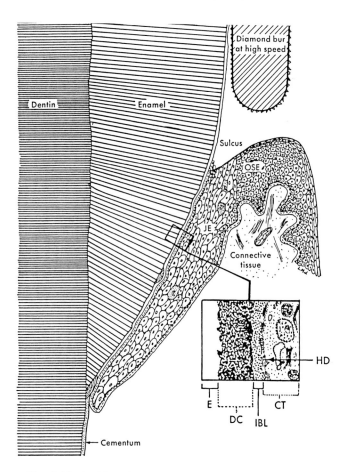

Fig. 1-14. Avoiding the intracrevicular space (the Bermuda triangle of dentistry) is fundamental for uncomplicated, predictable restorative dentistry.

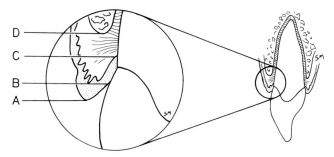

Fig. 1-15. The dentogingival junction includes the gingival sulcus (A-B) approximately 0.8 mm; the junctional epithelium (B-C) 0.7 to 1.3 mm (average 1 mm); the connective tissue attachment (C-D) 1.07 mm. The biologic width (B-D) averages 2 mm in occlusogingival height.

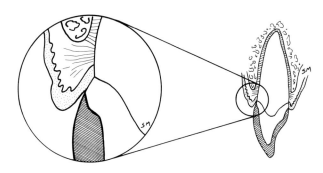

Fig. 1-16. The gingival termination of a tooth preparation must be at least 2 mm coronal to the alveolar crest, i.e., the intracrevicular margin.

1 mm of connective tissue fibers. This dentogingival attachment, referred to as the "biologic width"[19,20] (Fig. 1-15), has significant implications in treatment planning.

In the past, the gingival termination of a complete veneer crown was commonly prepared "as far subgingivally as possible" to "prevent" caries, maximize retention, and hide the "unesthetic" margins. The contemporary approach to placing a margin beneath the gingival crest (when such extension is indicated) is to confine the finish line to the gingival crevice, i.e., the intracrevicular margin. To avoid encroaching on the biologic width, the tooth preparation must terminate at least 2 mm coronal to the alveolar crest (Fig. 1-16).

The presence of caries, fractured root structure, or previous restorations apical to the gingival crest may predispose to violation of the biologic width during tooth preparation. A short clinical crown may induce the dentist to overextend the preparation apically in an attempt to enhance retention.

Severing the natural dentogingival attachment will produce chronic gingival inflammation, pocket formation, and osseous defects as the bone, fibrous connective tissue, and epithelium remodel in an attempt to reestablish a physiologic attachment (Fig. 1-17). Elective crown lengthening with controlled ostectomy and apically positioned flaps is more desirable (Fig. 1-18). While the surgical crown lengthening technique is a viable alternative to impingement on the biologic width, it is not a panacea.

The removal of tooth-supporting bone on a questionable abutment may adversely affect the crown-to-root ratio or expose furcations, root concavities, or both on the abutment tooth as well as the contiguous teeth! Elective extraction or root resection/hemisection for the proposed abutment may be preferable to decreasing the bone support and exposing furcations on contiguous teeth.

OCCLUSION

Every fixed restoration affects occlusion. Our aim is to "do no harm" when restoring the occlusal surfaces of teeth (Fig. 1-19). Occlusal restoration with fixed prosthodontics should result in:

1. Simultaneous equalized contact of all teeth (anterior and posterior) in maximum intercuspation

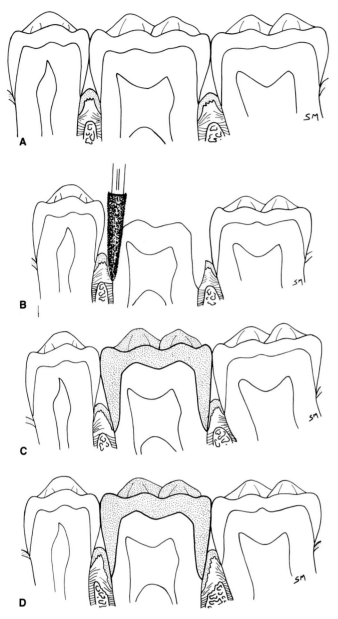

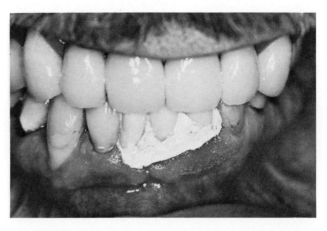

Fig. 1-18. A, Crown lengthening procedures have become routine for restorative dentistry. Note the three-unit heat-polymerized acrylic resin splint with a surgical pack.

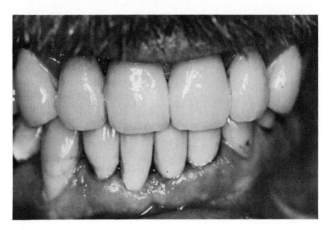

Fig. 1-18. B, Postsurgical tissue (2 weeks) response to crown lengthening.

Fig. 1-17. A, Healthy dento-gingival attachment. **B,** The diamond is extended apically beyond the gingival crevice into the attachment zone during tooth preparation. **C,** The biologic width has been violated, and the completed restoration prevents reattachment. **D,** Despite the fit of the restoration, remodeling of the alveolar crest occurs and a new dentogingival attachment is established apical to the restoration.

(centric occlusion) at a physiologic vertical dimension of occlusion.*

2. A physiologic plane of occlusion.
3. A functional anterior guidance (vertical and horizontal overlap of the anterior teeth) that will protect the posterior teeth from interceptive occlusal contacts in eccentric positions.*
4. A comfortable, unlocked arrangement of cusps, fossae, grooves, and ridges that will not restrict functional jaw movements.
5. Axial loading of all posterior teeth.
6. An anatomic form to the cusps, fossae, marginal ridges, and sluiceways that will minimize interdental food impaction and contribute to efficient comminution of food.
7. Occlusal and proximal tooth contacts that will lend long-term stability to the occlusal scheme.
8. An aesthetic and phonetic relationship of the anterior teeth.
9. Occlusal surfaces fabricated of a material that wears like natural enamel.

A programmed evaluation of the patient's occlusion with these goals in mind will result in a sensible approach to treatment planning. Mounted diagnostic casts will commonly reveal problems that are not

---

*The objectives of the anterior tooth arrangement are modified when mandibular fixed restorations occlude with a maxillary complete denture (see Chapter 14).

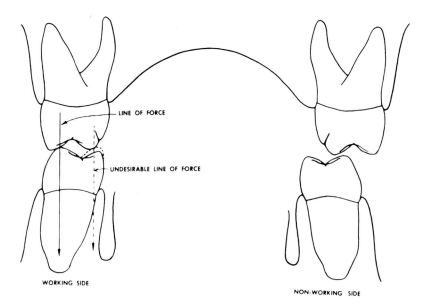

Fig. 1-19. Our aim is to do no harm when restoring the occlusal surfaces of teeth.

readily apparent clinically, and a systematic review of radiographs may also disclose troublesome situations such as a widened periodontal ligament space, indicating trauma from occlusion.

Aberrations in the occlusal plane, gross interceptive occlusal contacts, malalignment of teeth, abnormal jaw relationships (Class II or III), marked occlusal attrition, bruxism habits, previous occlusal reconstructive therapy, and TMJ dysfunction symptoms may create numerous obstacles to achieving our goals.[21] Unfortunately, protracted partial edentulism can produce an occlusal scheme that is virtually impossible to restore (Fig. 1-20) without selective extractions.

Specific recommendations for restoring an occlusion with fixed restorations—including procedures for combined fixed-removable prostheses—are discussed in detail in Chapter 14. It must be emphasized, however, that the diagnostic waxing on mounted diagnostic casts is our fundamental guide or blueprint for fixed restorative care and is the most valuable aid to planning our occlusal reconstructions. What seems impossible may indeed be realizeable and vice versa. The diagnostic waxing will clearly delineate the limits of what can be achieved with a prosthetic occlusion.

Esthetics

A multitude of factors affecting esthetics may have motivated the patient to seek dental care. The patient's concern with esthetics should not be underestimated.

While the restoration of maxillary anterior teeth can tax the ingenuity of the dentist, any dental procedure can have esthetic repercussions. An unfavorable anterior guidance or plane of occlusion will not only

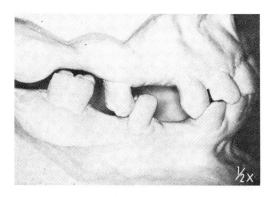

Fig. 1-20. An occlusal scheme that is virtually impossible to restore without selective extractions.

adversely affect occlusal function but will also produce an unnatural appearance.

Drifting of teeth into edentulous areas may reduce the available pontic space; whereas a diastema before extraction may result in excessive mesiodistal width to the pontic space (Fig. 1-21). Thin, friable, translucent gingiva combined with a high lip line can defy inconspicuous finish lines for maxillary anterior esthetic veneer crowns. The long clinical crowns that commonly result from surgical periodontics are particularly troublesome to restore esthetically (Fig. 1-22).

A defect in an anterior edentulous ridge as a result of trauma, developmental abnormality, or severe periodontal disease will require special attention to esthetics. The defective ridge area can often be restored surgically with some form of ridge augmentation followed by a conventional FPD. Prosthetic restoration

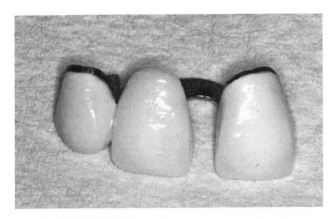

Fig. 1-21. A, A maxillary right central incisor is replaced with loop connector FPD for a patient who had a natural central diastema. The palatal loop connector reproduces the diastema.

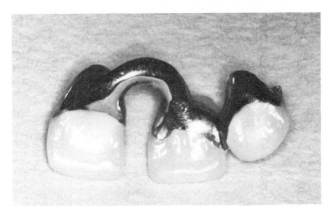

Fig. 1-21. B, Lingual view of the FPD.

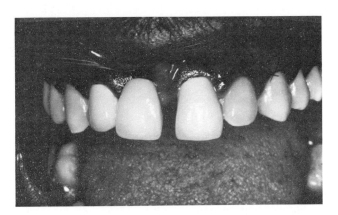

Fig. 1-21. C, Clinical view of the FPD. The patient is pleased with the esthetic result. Exceptional oral hygiene is mandatory.

may be employed using an FPD (i.e., with gingival colored porcelain) or, more commonly, with a removable partial denture (RPD).

A maxillary canine or premolar that must serve as an abutment to an RPD will often display an esthetically objectionable clasp. A precision attachment retainer is a viable alternative to the extracoronal clasp retainer when esthetic requirements are paramount.

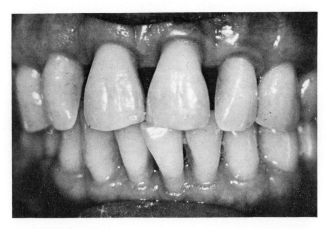

Fig. 1-22. Extended clinical crowns after surgical periodontics create esthetic problems.

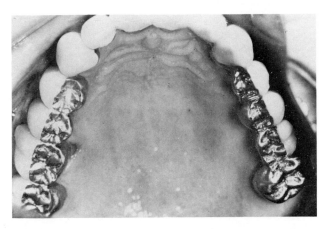

Fig. 1-23. The occlusal surfaces of maxillary posterior teeth are not part of the esthetic zone. A cast metal occlusal surface is preferred.

Precision attachments are discussed in the seventh edition of *Tylman's Theory and Practice of Fixed Prosthodontics.*[22]

Bonded laminate veneers can be a conservative alternative to esthetic veneer crowns. Laminates are recommended to restore esthetics to blemished but sound anterior teeth and are particularly useful with tetracycline-stained teeth. Bonded composite resin can be employed to close diastemas and repair small fractures. Esthetic bonding is comprehensively reviewed in Chapter 7.

Every effort should be made to produce an esthetic result—without compromising functional requirements. Porcelain has captured the attention of the dentist and the patient because of its outstanding esthetic potential; however, dental porcelain is not the ideal restorative material for the occlusal surfaces of posterior teeth. Whenever esthetics will permit, a cast metal occlusal surface is greatly preferred (Fig. 1-23). There is little justification for placing a complete por-

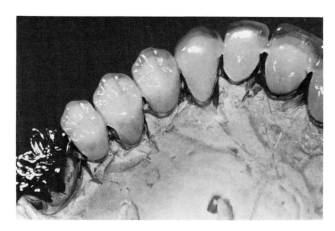

Fig. 1-24. A, Porcelain occlusal surface is required when the teeth in the opposing arch are restored with a porcelain occlusion. Note that the terminal molar (which occludes with natural enamel) is maintained in metal.

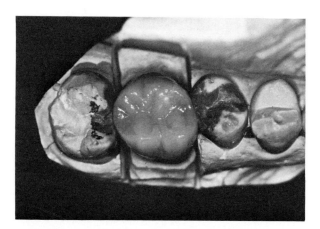

Fig. 1-24. B, Maxillary artificial crown is in occlusion with a mandibular artificial crown with a porcelain occlusal surface.

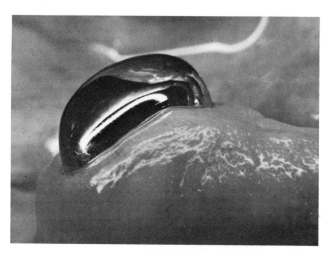

Fig. 1-25. A, Mandibular, endodontically treated canine restored with a cast metal post-coping to support an overdenture. Long parallel pins can be used to retain the coping if the canal cannot be negotiated.

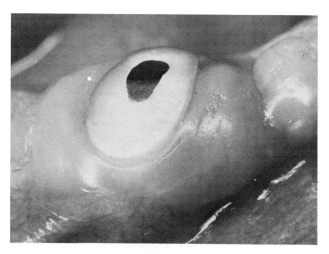

Fig. 1-25. B, Sound tooth structure does not require a cast coping.

celain occlusal surface on maxillary second molars or mandibular molars unless the occluding tooth has a porcelain occlusal surface (Fig. 1-24).

Endodontic Considerations

The endodontically treated tooth. An endodontically treated tooth is commonly restored with conservative tooth preparation and a cast restoration. When there is insufficient remaining tooth structure to support an extracoronal restoration, coronoradicular stabilization with a post and core is indicated.

Pulpless teeth can successfully function as abutments to an FPD or RPD. However, it must be appreciated that these teeth are weakened by the loss of significant supporting dentin, and a post and core is usually required. The endodontically treated tooth that supports an extension base RPD is particularly subject to fracture, and double abutting with splinted retainers is indicated.

The prognosis is poor for a pulpless tooth with an extremely short root or with a canal that cannot be negotiated to place a post as an abutment to an FPD or RPD; such a tooth is better suited to support a complete or partial overdenture (Fig. 1-25) (see also Chapter 19). A pulpless tooth is contraindicated as an abutment to a cantilever FPD.[23]

Elective endodontic therapy. Endodontic treatment may be necessary for a supraerupted or malaligned tooth to improve the arch relationship with a post and core while facilitating fabrication of a cast restoration with a more favorable arch position and occlusion. A tooth that has lost most or all of the coronal tooth structure is often treated endodontically to permit placement of a post and core for retaining a complete veneer crown.

While elective endodontic therapy can improve the prognosis of a badly damaged tooth, it may present more problems than it resolves. Teeth with aberrant

Table 1-2. Dimensions of root surface areas

Type of tooth	1 Average area (mm²)	2 Standard deviation	3 Coefficient of variation	4 Number of measurements	5 Relative sizes	6 Boyd (1958)
Maxilla						
Central	204	31.4	15.4	19	6	204.5
Lateral	179	24.9	13.9	25	7	177.3
Cuspid	273	43.9	16.1	26	3	266.5
First bicuspid	234	33.7	14.4	20	4	219.7
Second bicuspid	220	39.0	17.7	19	5	216.7
First molar	433	40.9	9.4	15	1	454.8
Second molar	431	62.5	14.5	10	2	416.9
Mandible						
Central	154	26.5	17.2	10	7	162.2
Lateral	168	21.5	12.8	10	6	174.8
Cuspid	268	42.2	15.7	18	3	272.2
First bicuspid	180	27.2	15.1	24	5	196.9
Second bicuspid	207	26.6	12.9	17	4	204.3
First molar	431	59.5	13.8	15	1	450.3
Second molar	426	69.7	16.4	10	2	399.7

From Jepsen, A.: Acta Odont. Scand. **21**:35, 1963.

Table 1-3. Factors modifying Ante's law

Condition existing	Probable modification in Ante's law
1. Bone loss from periodontal disease	Increase the number of abutments used for support
2. Mesial or distal tipping or changes in axial inclination	Increase the number of abutments used for support
3. Migration (bodily movement) of abutment teeth decreasing mesiodistal length of edentulous area	Decrease the number of abutments used (less pericemental support required)
4. Less than favorable opposing arch relationships producing increased occlusal load	Increase the number of abutments used for support
5. Endodontically restored abutment teeth with root resections	Increase the number of abutments used for support
6. Arch-form situations creating greater leverage factors	Increase the number of abutments used for support
7. Tooth mobility created after osseous surgery	Increase the number of abutments used for support (splinting procedure)

root canal morphology do not offer a favorable endodontic prognosis, and intentional devitalization of these teeth should be avoided whenever practical. Techniques for the restoration of endodontically treated teeth are discussed in Chapter 22.

Abutment Selection

Bone support. Ante[24] states that "the abutment teeth should have a combined pericemental area equal to or greater in pericemental area than the tooth or teeth to be replaced," and this recommendation has been referred to as "Ante's law".[25] Jespen[26] has reported average measurements of root surface areas that can be used to calculate the abutment-to-pontic ratio (Table 1-2). A ratio of 1:1 or greater would satisfy "Ante's law".

The dentist must, however, not depend exclusively on a calculated ratio based upon a recommendation made in 1926![27] Individual crown-to-root ratios, root morphology, and occlusal conditions are equally important parameters.

A favorable crown-to-root ratio is 1:1 or greater. Teeth with short, conical, or blunted roots offer the poorest support, whereas teeth with long, irregularly shaped roots or with divergent multiple roots offer the best prognosis. Teeth with moderate periodontal osseous resorption may be less desirable as abutments because of the reduced bone support and the exposed furcations and root concavities that complicate oral hygiene procedures.

The occlusal scheme is an additional consideration. Unfavorable forces can be mitigated with narrowed occlusal tables, an occlusal plane and vertical dimension of occlusion that are physiologic, and a programmed canine disclusion. An FPD that occludes with a removable prosthesis is subjected to reduced occlusal loading.

Table 1-3 summarizes factors that influence abutment tooth selection and that can result in modifications to Ante's Law.

Root proximities. There must be adequate clearance between the roots of proposed abutments to permit the development of physiologic embrasures in the completed prosthesis. Malpositioned anterior teeth and the mesiobuccal roots of maxillary molars often present unfavorable root proximities where desired embrasure form is not possible. Selective extraction or root resection procedures (see Chapter 4, preparation of periodontally compromised dentition) may be the only solution to the root proximity.

Common path of insertion. Abutment teeth to an FPD must be prepared with a common path of insertion for all retainers when a rigid design is employed. Evaluation of the diagnostic casts with the dental surveyor coincides with the radiographic evaluation to determine the most favorable path of insertion. If the long axes of the teeth diverge or converge from parallelism by more than 25 degrees, tooth preparation becomes more difficult.[28]

Mesially titled molar. The mesiolingually titled molar is commonly encountered.[29] The mesial one-half crown preparation (Fig. 1-26), the nonrigid attachment (semiprecision or stress-breaker attachment Fig. 1-27), and the telescopic prosthesis (Fig. 1-28) have been suggested as solutions to the problem. With extreme malalignment, orthodontic therapy may be the only logical approach.[30]

The mesial one-half crown requires an unblemished distal surface on the molar abutment (Fig. 1-26). The nonrigid attachment must not be used indiscriminantly. Because of the mesial component of force, the female portion of the attachment is usually placed on the distal surface of the mesial abutment. The cantilever effect of the nonrigid design can place additional lateral stresses on the abutment with the rigid connector[23]; therefore, the rigid connector is only placed on a strong abutment, and the nonrigid design is avoided altogether with long-span pontics (Fig. 1-27). Telescopic prostheses require radical tooth preparation to provide adequate space for the telescopic coping and the overcasting (Fig. 1-28).

Clinical guidelines for establishing parallelism. Developing a mutual path of insertion on multiple abutments without overtapering the preparations or exposing the pulp is a fundamental skill that can be mastered. While there is no mystique to the biomechanics of this process, malpositioned, tilted, rotated, and supraerupted teeth increase the need for planning the path of insertion with a dental surveyor. Once the path of insertion has been established, the base of the cast is scribed with multiple lines parallel to this path to aid in planning tooth preparations. The following clinical guidelines are suggested:

1. Select rotary instruments with a standard (2 to 3 degree) taper. Diamond stones without a taper

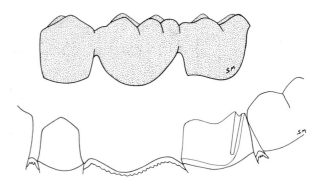

Fig. 1-26. The mesial one-half crown preparation on a mesially tilted mandibular molar. An unblemished distal surface is required.

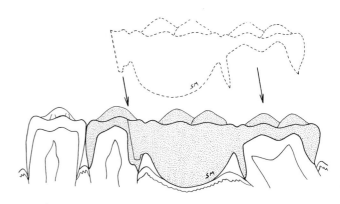

Fig. 1-27. Nonrigid (semiprecision) attachment. Additional tooth reduction in the premolar is required to house the attachment in order to prevent overcontouring.

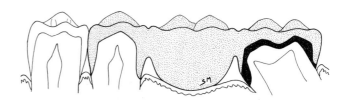

Fig. 1-28. The telescopic coping on the molar can be milled parallel to the premolar preparation to produce a common path of insertion for the FPD. Additional tooth reduction is required for the molar abutment to prevent overcontouring.

must be tilted freehand to avoid undercuts. Freehand tipping of the diamond commonly overtapers the preparations, causing a loss of retentive form and increasing the risk of pulpal irritation or exposure.

2. Occlusal or incisal reduction is accomplished first. The occlusal or incisal surfaces are reduced **parallel** to the planned occlusal plane.

3. Depth guides are placed on the buccal and lingual surfaces of all abutment teeth. These depth guides are prepared parallel to the planned path of insertion, as indicated by the scribe lines on the base of the diagnostic cast.

4. With the diamond stone held **parallel to the planned path** of insertion (depth guides), the most inaccessible surface of the most inaccessible abutment is reduced first.
5. Tooth reduction is continued with the diamond stone held parallel to the prepared depth guides; the distal, lingual, facial, and mesial surfaces are reduced systematically. The most accessible surfaces are reduced last. Pay strict attention to parallelism between the mesial and distal surfaces of posterior teeth and the facial surfaces of incisors.
6. After bulk reduction, parallelism is verified with large intraoral mirrors. If there is any doubt about undercuts, an alginate impression is made and poured in impression plaster. The plaster cast is evaluated on the dental surveyor, and any undercuts are corrected intraorally.
7. The preparations are refined (i.e., two-plane reductions, elimination of external sharp line angles, development of discernable finish lines, etc.), taking care not to create new undercuts.

Abutment selection for the cantilever. A cantilever pontic can be successfully employed if the principles of leverage are understood and provisions are made to control deleterious forces. A classic FPD design is the lateral incisor cantilever pontic supported by a strong canine (Fig. 1-29 A). A cantilever first premolar pontic can occasionally eliminate the need to prepare the canine—thus preserving the natural canine function (Fig. 1-29 B). An imaginative approach to the cantilever pontic can be the difference between an RPD (an inherently bulky restoration) and restoring the arch entirely with fixed prosthodontics (Figs. 1-30 to 1-33).

Because of the lever action that occurs with a cantilever, a disciplined approach to treatment planning is essential. The abutments must offer better than average support; tooth preparations must be extremely retentive; and the occlusal scheme must be as close to ideal as possible. Endodontically treated teeth are avoided as proximal abutments to the cantilever pontic. A small, narrow, premolar pontic is preferred to the molar pontic, which would produce more torque; immediate canine disclusion of the cantilever pontic is established whenever practical.

Pier abutments. A pier (intermediate) abutment has the potential to produce unfavorable leverage and an unseating effect on terminal retainers.[31] Fracture of the cement seal and cement washout is a distinct possibility (Fig. 1-34).

The nonrigid connector has been suggested as a solution to this problem.[32] The female portion of the nonrigid connector is commonly placed within the confines of normal tooth contours on the distal surface of the intermediate abutment (Fig. 1-34).

Splinting. Splinting was once widely accepted in

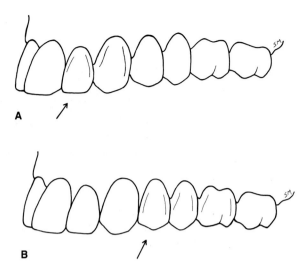

Fig. 1-29. A, Lateral incisor cantilever pontic *(arrow)* supported by a strong canine abutment. **B,** First premolar cantilever pontic *(arrow)* supported by the second premolar and first molar abutments eliminates the need to prepare the canine and preserves the natural canine function.

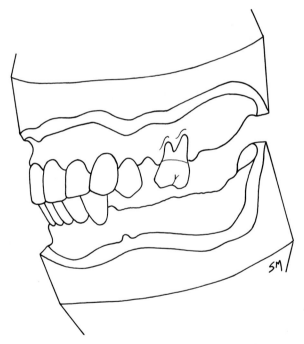

Fig. 1-30. Mounted, diagnostic casts. Mandibular arch requires an RPD reducing the occlusal force transmitted to the maxillary posterior segment. Mesiobuccal and distobuccal roots on the maxillary molar are nontreatable.

prosthodontics. Immobilization of teeth by joining them together with soldered retainers was thought to prevent the periodontal breakdown of healthy teeth and to arrest bone loss in compromised teeth.[33]

Experience has shown that splinting can create more problems than it solves.[34] Splinting is arduous, expensive, and time consuming; the completed restoration is difficult for the patient to clean. Long-term

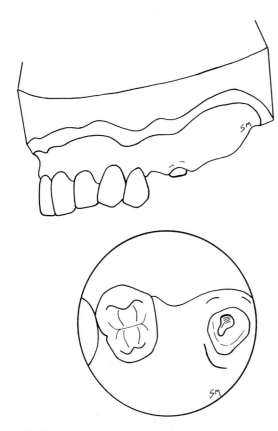

Fig. 1-31. The mesiobuccal and distobuccal roots are extracted, and the palatal root maintained to support a cantilever pontic. The palatal root is prepared for an overdenture post-coping (see Chapter 19).

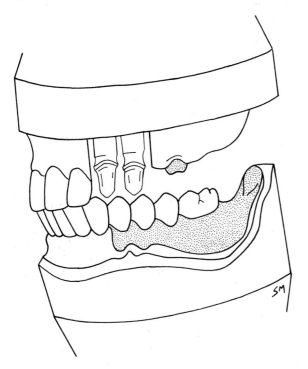

Fig. 1-32. The cast gold coping is cemented on the palatal root. The canine and first premolar are prepared for metal ceramic retainers. The master cast is mounted with a mandibular trial setup for the RPD.

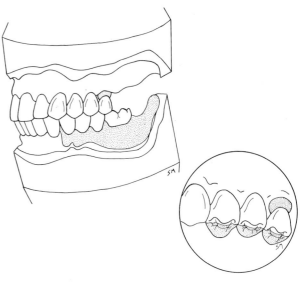

Fig. 1-33. The completed metal ceramic FPD with two cantilever pontics eliminates the need for a maxillary RPD. The retained palatal molar root supports the pontics. Planning of the occlusal scheme is essential.

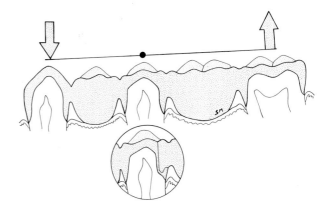

Fig. 1-34. The pier abutment acts as a fulcrum and produces unseating forces on terminal retainers. The nonrigid attachment (inset) has been suggested as a solution.

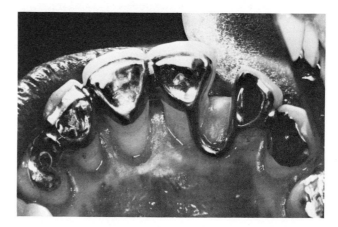

Fig. 1-35. A six-unit pinledge splint. Failure of a single retainer or abutment jeopardizes the entire prosthesis. Note the loop connector maintaining the diastema is a liability for oral hygiene.

serviceability is a significant disadvantage of splinting, and the failure of a single abutment or retainer can jeopardize the *entire* prosthesis (Fig. 1-35).

When in doubt, do not splint! Hypermobility is not necessarily an indication for splinting, since the mobility can often be reduced or resolved with an occlusal adjustment.[35] Splinting will not prevent periodontitis and may actually increase the chances of inflammatory disease, since home care will be inhibited. A questionable tooth should not be splinted to a healthy tooth in an attempt to strengthen the weakened tooth. The result is often accelerated periodontal deterioration of both teeth.

Available Tooth Structure and Crown Morphology

The amount of remaining sound tooth structure for a proposed abutment will influence treatment options. Teeth with extensive defective restorations, carious lesions, or fractures may require intentional endodontic therapy and post and core fabrication to provide a sufficiently retentive and resistant form to the preparations.[36] Crown lengthening may be indicated to expose sound tooth structure coronal to the biologic width when caries, restorations, or fractures are in proximity to the alveolar crest.

The crown morphology and quantity of sound enamel and dentin also influence retainer design, i.e., partial veneer retainer designs. Partial veneer retainers are often preferable to complete veneer crowns if retentive and esthetic requirements are satisfied (see Section C in Chapter 6). A resin-bonded prosthesis (Maryland bridge) depends upon a sufficient quantity of intact enamel that can be etched to provide microretention. Treatment planning for the resin-bonded prosthesis is described in Chapter 8.

Combining Fixed and Removable Prosthodontics

As more patients retain their teeth into the latter decades of life, the need for innovative approaches to treatment planning intensifies.[36-38] The combined fixed-removable prosthesis is fabricated far more frequently today (Figs. 1-36 to 1-39) and yet this topic has received cursory coverage in many texts. An entire chapter in this text has been devoted to the fixed-removable prosthesis (Chapter 19); it includes a comprehensive review of treatment planning. In addition, a major portion of the occlusion chapter (Chapter 14) discusses the management of the occlusion when fixed and removable prosthodontics are integrated.

TMJ and Muscles of Mastication

The status of the patient's muscles of mastication and TMJ's must be assessed. A quiescent TMJ problem may become painfully apparent after fixed prosthodontic care—with the dental treatment seemingly the cause.

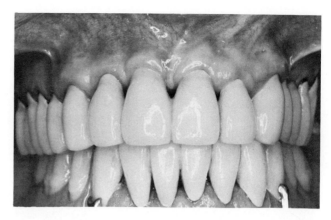

Fig. 1-36. Combined fixed-removable prostheses are more commonly used today, but meticulous planning is fundamental. Note the excellent embrasure form. (Courtesy Dr. Paul Tischler and Dr. Toby Boyd, Alton, Ill.)

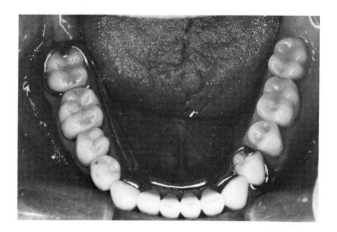

Fig. 1-37. A combined fixed-removable prosthesis. RPD's are suitable when perceptive tooth preparation is followed by appropriate contours. (Courtesy Dr. Paul Tischler and Dr. Toby Boyd, Alton, Ill.)

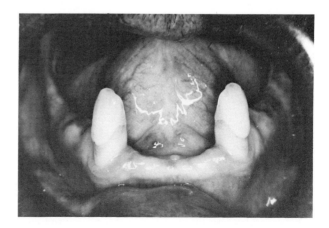

Fig. 1-38. Indication for a tooth-supported denture.

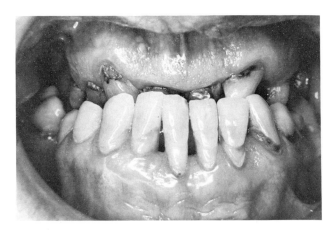

Fig. 1-39. Class III malocclusions are particularly arduous to restore. Fixed-removable prostheses are indicated.

Any evidence of dysfunction (see Chapter 23) must be addressed before any definitive prosthodontic care.

Comprehensive Planning

A comprehensive, sequential approach to treatment planning is essential. Planning for fixed prosthodontics must not be independent of other disciplines of dentistry. Hasty, segmented planning that ignores major aspects of needed treatment defies modern concepts of treating "the whole patient" rather than individual teeth.

Fig. 1-40 demonstrates a hypothetical patient who requires comprehensive care. The patient's chief complaint is a loose upper denture.

The diagnostic casts are mounted at the desired vertical dimension of occlusion. The mandibular anterior teeth have obviously supraerupted. There is severe ridge resorption in the anterior portion of the maxillary arch, and the tuberosities are elongated well below the planned occlusal plane.

The mandibular incisors have a 2+ mobility with periodontal pockets, and there is more than 50 percent loss of osseous support. The canines are firm with 10 to 15 percent bone loss. The right and left first premolars have extensive amalgam restorations with recurrent caries, but there is no radiographically detectable osseous resorption. Clinically, there is generalized gingival inflammation, but sulcus depths on the canines and premolars are within normal limits. The mandibular second premolars and all molars are missing bilaterally with a pronounced resorption of the mandibular edentulous ridge bilaterally. The TMJ's and muscles of mastication show no evidence of dysfunction.

Fig. 1-41 represents a diagnostic waxing with a trial setup for a maxillary complete denture and a mandibular removable partial denture on duplicate diagnostic casts. The hyperplastic tuberosities have been altered

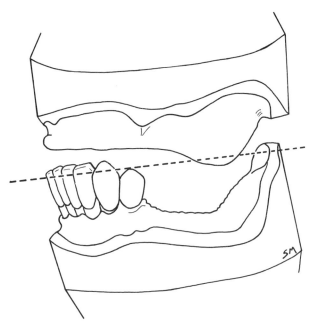

Fig. 1-40. There is supraeruption of the mandibular anterior teeth combined with elongation of the maxillary tuberosities. Failure to reduce the height of the anterior teeth and/or surgically correct the tuberosities prevents a favorable occlusal plane. The dotted line represents the desired plane.

on the stone cast to permit favorable location of the occlusal plane and to serve as a guide to surgical correction. Fig. 1-42 demonstrates the proposed design of the mandibular RPD framework on a stone duplicate of the diagnostic waxing.

After a thorough evaluation of all diagnostic information, our definitive diagnosis is:

1. Severe periodontitis about Nos. 23 to 26 (mandibular incisors).
2. Slight-to-moderate periodontitis about Nos. 22 and 27 (mandibular canines).
3. Moderate gingivitis about Nos. 21 and 28 (mandibular first premolars).
4. Supraeruption of the mandibular anterior teeth above the occlusal plane.*
5. Advanced resorption of the maxillary anterior and mandibular posterior edentulous ridges.*
6. Hyperplasia of the maxillary tuberosities bilaterally.*
7. Recurrent dental caries about amalgam restorations on Nos. 21 and 28 with insufficient remaining tooth structure to support an RPD.
8. Totally edentulous maxillary arch with an ill fitting, maloccluded complete denture.
9. Partially edentulous mandibular arch with an ill fitting maloccluded RPD.

---

*Diagnoses 4, 5, and 6 suggest a "combination syndrome" described by Kelley.[39,40]

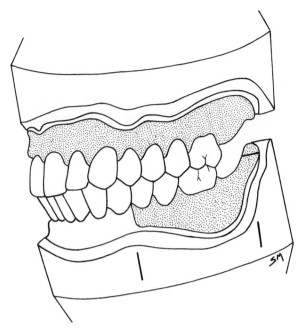

Fig. 1-41. A diagnostic waxing of the mandibular FPD and a trial setup for the maxillary complete denture and mandibular RPD. Note the ideal location of the occlusal plane (posterior height is two-thirds the height of the retromolar pads). Scribed lines on the base of the mandibular cast represent the planned path of insertion for the RPD.

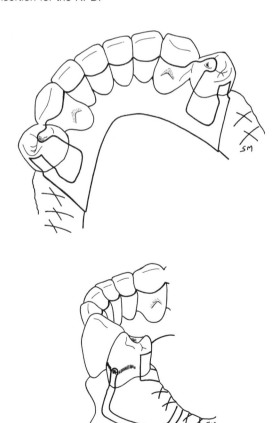

Fig. 1-42. A stone duplicate of the diagnostic waxing with the proposed RPD framework completely outlined. This cast is a guide to the technician when fabricating the FPD.

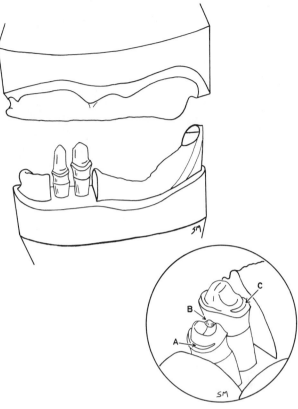

Fig. 1-43. The mounted mandibular master cast for the FPD. The FPD is fabricated to receive the planned RPD and to occlude with the trial denture setup. Inset: Distolingual view of master dies. (A), The facial shoulder on the premolar has been carried lingually to allow the development of a flat guiding plane. (B), Recess on the mesiocclusal surface for a mesial rest seat. (C), Lingual ledge on the canine cingulum for a cingulum rest seat.

Our definitive treatment plan follows logically from our diagnoses. Because of the aberrant occlusal relationship, relining the existing removable prostheses is contraindicated[41] even though the chief complaint is "looseness" of the maxillary denture! A reasonable treatment plan is:

1. Surgical reduction of the maxillary tuberosities bilaterally.
2. Caries control on Nos. 21 and 28.
3. Dental scaling and root planning followed by oral hygiene instructions.
4. Intentional endodontic therapy for Nos. 21 and 28 followed by cast metal post and cores.
5. Extraction of Nos. 23, 24, 25, 26, and fabrication of an immediate provisional FPD that extends from Nos. 21 to 28. Tooth preparations are accomplished with the definitive design of the RPD (see Chapter 19) and with the planned reduction in the height of the mandibular anterior teeth in mind (Fig. 1-43).
6. Fabrication of a definitive metal ceramic FPD extending from Nos. 21 to 28 that is surveyed

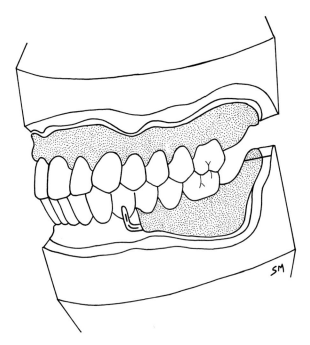

Fig. 1-44. The definitive metal ceramic FPD is seated. The premolars are splinted to the canine retainers since they are endodontically treated with post and cores. Fabrication of the maxillary complete denture and mandibular RPD is accomplished uneventfully because of the programmed planning.

and designed to receive the planned RPD framework *and* that occludes favorably with the maxillary diagnostic setup (see Chapter 14).

7. Fabrication of a maxillary complete denture and mandibular RPD (Fig. 1-44).

PROGNOSIS

The dentist should propose a treatment plan that offers a favorable prognosis. While strategic teeth may be salvaged at considerable cost, not every tooth is of equal importance to the long-term maintenance of dental health. It is unfair to include a nonessential tooth with a poor prognosis in a long-span fixed prosthesis—despite patient insistence. While dentistry is dedicated to saving teeth, the concept of maintaining teeth that are assets, not liabilities, prevails.

The less disease present at the onset and the less complex the treatment, the more favorable the prognosis. The approach to treatment planning should be meticulous, flexible, and scholarly.

SELECTED REFERENCES

1. Johansen, R.E., and Stackhouse, J.A.: Dimensional changes of elastomers during cold sterilization, J. Prosthet. Dent. **57**:233-236, 1987.
2. Blackwell, R.E.: G.V. Black's Operative Dentistry, Vol. 11, ed. 9, South Milwaukee, 1955, Medico-Dental Publishing Co., pp. 110-111.
3. Romanelli, J.H.: Periodontal considerations in tooth preparation for crowns and bridges, Dent. Clin. North Am. **24**:2, 271-283, 1980.
4. Waerhaug, J.: Temporary restorations: advantages and disadvantages, Dent. Clin. North Am. **24**:2, 305-316, 1980.
5. Silness, J.: Fixed prosthodontics and periodontal health, Dent. Clin. North Am. **24**:2, 317-329, 1980.
6. Waerhaug, J.: Histologic considerations which govern where the margins of restorations should be located in relation to the gingiva, Dent. Clin. North Am. **4**:161-176, Mar. 1960.
7. Silness, J.: Periodontal conditions in patients treated with dental bridges. III. The relationship between the location of the crown margin and the periodontal condition, J. Periodont. Res. **5**:225-229, 1970.
8. Karlsen, K.: Gingival reactions to dental restorations, Acta Odontol. Scand. **28**:895, 1970.
9. Keszthelyi, G., and Szabo, I.: Influence of Class II amalgam fillings on attachment loss, J. Clin. Periodontol. **11**:81, 1984.
10. Lang, N., Kiel, R., and Anderhalden, K.: Clinical and microbiological effects of subgingival restorations with overhanging or clinically perfect margins, J. Clin. Periodontol. **10**:563, 1983.
11. Newcomb, G.: The relationship between the location of subgingival crown margins and gingival inflammation, J. Periodontol. **45**:151, 1974.
12. Renggli, H., and Regolati, B.: Gingival inflammation and plaque accumulation by well-adapted supragingival and subgingival proximal restorations, Helv. Odontol. Acta. **16**:99, 1972.
13. Waerhaug, J.: Tissue reactions around artificial crowns, J. Periodontol. **24**:172, 1953.
14. Sachs, R.I.: Restorative dentistry and the periodontium, Dent. Clin. North Am. **29**:2, 261-278, 1985.
15. Marcum, J.S.: The effect of crown marginal depth upon gingival tissue, J. Prosthet. Dent. **17**:479, 1967.
16. Glickman, I.: Clinical Periodontology, ed. 4, Philadelphia, 1972, W.B. Saunders Co., pp. 897-898.
17. Miller, L.: A clinician's interpretation of tooth preparation and design of metal substructures for metal-ceramic restorations. In McLean, J.W., editor: Dental Ceramics: Proceedings of the First International Symposium on Ceramics, Chicago, 1983, Quintessence Publishing Co., Inc., pp. 169-170.
18. Gargiulo, A.W., Wentz, F,M., and Orban, B.: Dimensions and relations of the dentogingival junction in humans, J. Periodontol. **32**:261, 1961.
19. Ingber, J.S., Rose, L.F., Coslet, J.G.: The "biologic width"— a concept in periodontics and restorative dentistry, Alpha Omegan. **10**:62, 1977.
20. Nevins, M., and Skurow, H.: The intracrevicular restorative margin, the biologic width, and the maintenance of the gingival margin, Int. J. Periodontol. Rest. Dent. **4**:31, 1984.
21. Brecker, S.C.: Practical oral rehabilitation, J. Prosthet. Dent. **10**:1001, 1959.
22. Boitel, R.H.: Precision attachments: an overview. In Tylman, S.D., and Malone, W.F.P.: Tylman's Theory and Practice of Fixed Prosthodontics, ed. 7, St. Louis, 1978, The C.V. Mosby Co., pp. 501-568.
23. Schweitzer, J.M., Schweitzer, R.D., and Schweitzer, J.: Free-end pontics used on fixed partial dentures, J. Prosthet. Dent. **20**:120, 1968.
24. Ante, I.H.: The fundamental principles of abutments, Mich. State Dent. Soc. Bul. **8**:14, 1926.
25. Johnston, J.F., Phillips, R.W., and Dykema, R.W.: Modern Practice in Crown and Bridge Prosthodontics, ed. 3, Philadelphia, 1971, W.B. Saunders Co., p. 11.
26. Jespen, A.: Root surface measurement and a method for x-ray determination of root surface area, Acta Odontol. Scand. **21**:35, 1963.
27. Moulton, P.S.: Selection of abutment teeth. In Clark, J.W.,

ed.: Clinical Dentistry, Vol. 4, Chap. 33, Philadelphia, 1986, Harper & Row.

28. Reynolds, J.M.: Abutment selection for fixed prosthodontics, J. Prosthet. Dent. **19:**483, 1968.
29. Picton, D.C.A.: Tilting movements of teeth during biting, Arch. Oral Biol. **7:**151, 1962.
30. Khouw, F.E., and Norton, L.A.: The mechanism of fixed molar uprighting appliances, J. Prosthet. Dent. **27:**381, 1972.
31. Shillingburg, H.T., and Fisher, D.W.: Nonrigid connectors for fixed partial dentures, J.A.D.A. **87:**1195, 1973.
32. Kornfeld, M.: Mouth Rehabilitation Clinical and Laboratory Procedures, ed. 2, St. Louis, 1974, The C.V. Mosby Co., p. 268.
33. Waerhaug, J.: Justification for splinting in periodontal therapy, J. Prosthet. Dent. **22:**201, 1969.
34. Fischman, B.M.: The influence of fixed splints on mandibular flexure, J. Prosthet. Dent. **35:**643, 1976.
35. Dawson, P.E.: Evaluation, diagnosis, and treatment of occlusal problems, St. Louis, 1974, The C.V. Mosby Co., p. 372.
36. Shillingburg, H.T., Jacobi, R., and Brackett, S.E.: Preparation modifications for damaged vital posterior teeth, Dent. Clin. North Am. **29:**305, 1985.
37. Culpepper, W.D., and Moulton, P.: Considerations in fixed prosthodontics, Dent. Clin. North Am. **23:**21, 1979.
38. Behrend, D.A.: Posterior fixed partial dentures, J. Prosthet. Dent. **37:**622, 1977.
39. Kelly, E.: Changes caused by a mandibular removable partial denture opposing a maxillary complete denture, J. Prosthet. Dent. **27:**140, 1972.
40. Schmitt, S.M.: Combination syndrome: A treatment approach, J. Prosthet. Dent. **54:**664, 1985.
41. Saunders, T.R., Gillis, Jr., R.E., and Desjardins, R.P.: Maxillary complete denture opposing the mandibular bilateral distal-extension partial denture: treatment considerations, J. Prosthet. Dent. **41:**124, 1979.

2

CARIES MANAGEMENT

**Maury Massler, Thomas D. Marshall, and
William F.P. Malone**

Dental caries is of bacterial origin; it is an insidious infection that attacks the hard tissues of the teeth. Caries cannot be produced in germ-free animals. A carious lesion can only occur when a mass of cariogenic microorganisms colonize on the tooth surface and form a plaque. These bacteria then produce acids to demineralize the underlying mineralized tooth tissues of enamel, dentin, or cementum. The residual organic matrix is then digested, resulting in cavitation.

There are three classes of carious lesions, produced by three different classes of cariogenic microorganisms in three different locations on the tooth and at three different age periods (Fig. 2-1). Pit and fissure caries occur primarily in newly erupted teeth and are usually initiated by cariogenic *Lactobacillus acidophilus* organisms. Smooth-surface (enamel) caries occur primarily in adolescents in newly erupted teeth, while the enamel and dentin remain permeable and immature (Fig. 2-2). The organism responsible for almost all carious lesions in adults is the destructive group of *Streptococcus mutans*. Cemental caries in the patient past age 50 is produced primarily by the *Odontomyces viscoses*.

Lactobacilli cannot form dextrans (bacterial glue) from sucrose as streptococci do and therefore do not form plaques on smooth surfaces. Instead, they invade retention sites such as pits and fissures and the leaky margins of restorations. Pits and fissures in newly erupted teeth contain biodegradable glycoproteins upon which these organisms can grow and produce acids (Fig. 2-1). With age, the contents of pits and fissures acquire sulfydryl groups from the saliva and become hard, leathery, and dark brown (Fig. 2-3). This material becomes the nonbiodegradable, leathery, salivary pellicle.

The lesions produced by dental caries can also be divided into active and arrested types, which can be distinguished by clinical appraisal of the texture, color of the surface of the lesion, and by the pain response. The surface of the active carious lesion is soft, cheesy, and friable, with a light brown color, and is painful upon probing and application of cold (Fig. 2-4). The surface of the arrested lesion is hard and leathery or eburnated with a dark brown to black color (Figs. 2-5 and 2-6). The patient suffers minimal pain upon probing or thermal applications.[1] The active lesion is found more frequently in children and proceeds at a faster rate.[2] The progress of arrested carious lesions is slower and more obvious in patients past 40 years of age.

S. mutans appears in the oral environment at any time from infancy to advanced age. It is a destructive organism and deeply invasive in the young. It acts more slowly and intermittently in older age groups, probably because enamel and dentin become more resistant with age. Enamel caries is less frequent after age 35 because the enamel becomes more dense and acquires a higher fluoride content.

CARIES IN THE AGED

O. viscoses is common in the elderly. The oral flora, like the pharyngeal, gastrointestinal, and skin floras, changes with every decade of life. The reasons are unclear, but the indigenous bacterial flora in the mouth does change. Dry mouth due to general dehydration increases the numbers of odontomyces in the oral cavity.

In the person past age 70, *Monilia albicans* infests the oral cavity, while *O. viscoses* tends to be insignificant. Monilia grow in moist, stagnant areas, e.g., under dentures. They form a white, cheesy colony under which the mucosal tissue becomes raw, red, and painful.

The normal habitat of the *O. viscoses* is among the filiform papillae of the tongue with a white, nonadherent material. This coating can be easily removed using a soft toothbrush or a dry gauze pad for the bedridden. The coating can also be removed by "detergent" foods such as hard bread, dry cereal, uncooked vegetables, and fibrous meats. In some countries, the elderly use a tongue scraper to remove the white, slimy odontomyces coating.

The tongue should be cleansed twice daily; in the morning upon arising, and in the evening on retiring. Oral hygiene in the elderly is essential to prevent *O. viscoses* from proliferating and forming a critical mass.

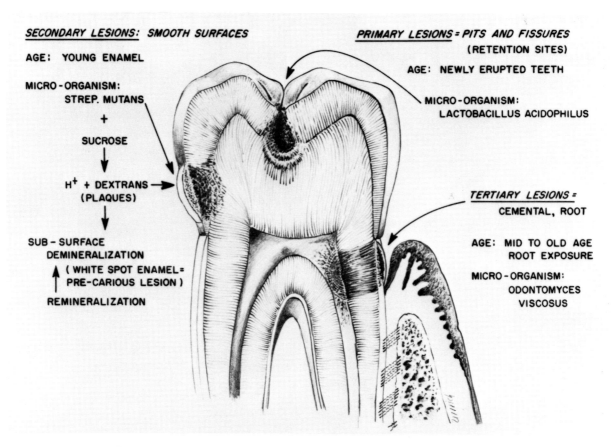

Fig. 2-1. Three types of carious lesions by age and associated microorganisms.

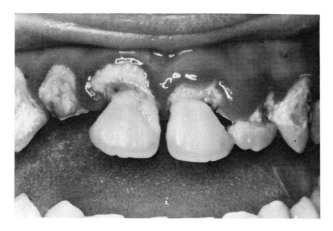

Fig. 2-2. Adolescent, active caries displaying *Streptococcus mutans* sucrose and plaques. (Malone, W.F.P., and Sarlas, C.: D. Clin. N. Amer. **13:**461, 1969.)

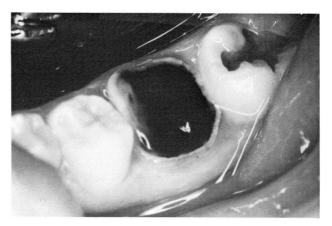

Fig. 2-3. Arrested dentinal lesion on a young patient with a high DMF rate.

The organisms then spread to the exposed cementum and are particularly prone to invade and grow within the gingival pockets, where they can form a bacterial plaque. Under this plaque, a carious lesion is produced through the cementum and into the dentin. When exposed to view, the lesion is shallow and deeply pigmented, i.e., dark brown (Figs. 2-7 to 2-9).

Cavitation is deeper, as under a streptococcal plaque. The dentin is softened and discolored. The radiograph shows the lesion in the dentin as a vague, radiolucent streak. Progress is generally slow. Conversely, in irradiated patients with xerostomia and friable tissues, the cemental lesion is rapid and highly destructive (Figs. 2-10 and 2-11).

The enamel and dentin defense against the bacte-

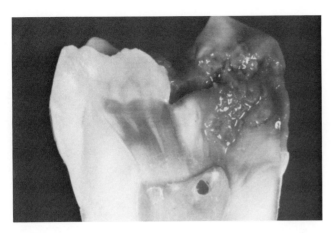

Fig. 2-4. Active carious lesion that is soft, friable, and light brown. (Malone, W.F.P., and Manning, J.L.: Ill. State Dent. J. **36:**724, 1968.)

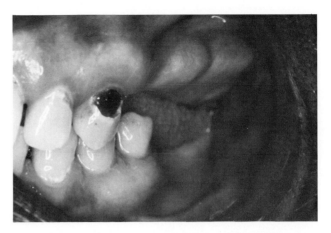

Fig. 2-6. Arrested lesion of aged patient with high DMF rate.

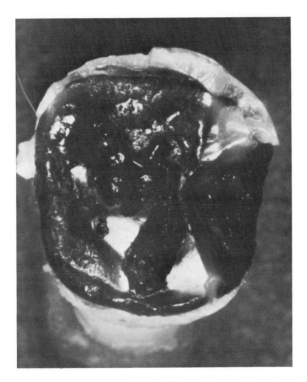

Fig. 2-5. Arrested carious lesion with hard eburnated surface but with active caries at DE junction. (Malone, W.F.P., and Manning, J.L.: Ill. State Dent. J. **36:**724, 1968.)

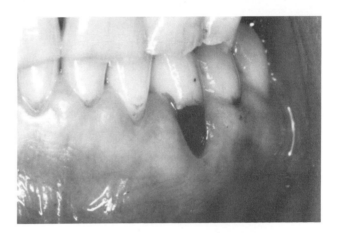

Fig. 2-7. Arrested, shallow cemental dark brown lesion.

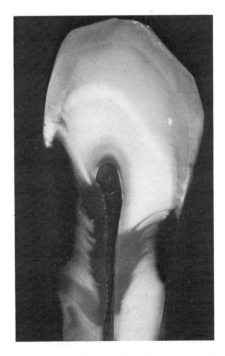

Fig. 2-8. Root caries with a shallow lesion on right and older lesion on left.

riologically initiated disease depends upon the response of its cellular components and its degree of mineralization. In enamel (Fig. 2-12), resistance to decay depends upon a highly mineralized surface (50 to 15 μm) that is less soluble and permeable to acids and other ions from the oral environment.[3,4] The defensive response in dentin is different and is characterized by a progressive sclerotic calcification within the tubules and the formation of reparative dentin by the pulpal cells.

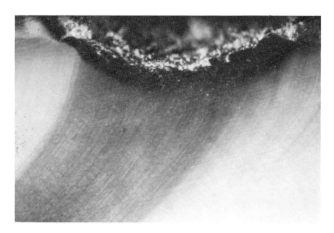

Fig. 2-9. Higher magnification of a deeper cemented lesion. A bacterial colony (plaque) is on surface, with leathery pigmented dentin toward pulp.

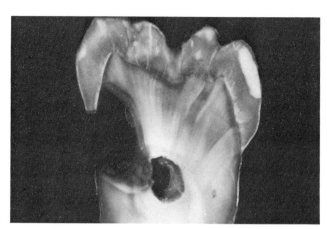

Fig. 2-11. Deep cemental lesion requiring endodontic treatment and a cast restoration.

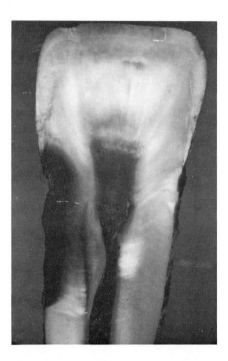

Fig. 2-10. Broad lesion with remineralization in progress and repaired dentin near the pulp.

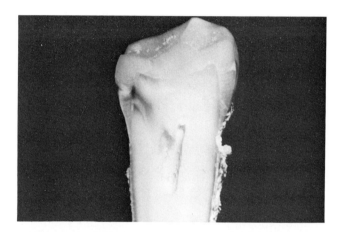

Fig. 2-12. Caries in enamel and dentinal surfaces on the left; the right proximal surface has an enamel carious white spot.

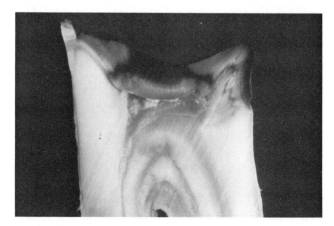

Fig. 2-13. Arrested lesion with hypermineralized reparative dentin above the pulp. The cavosurface angles of the lesion remain active and must be removed.

A defense observed in both enamel and dentin is the arrest of the carious process. The two most notable clinical differences between arrested and active carious dentinal lesions are increased hardness and pigmentation of the arrested lesion. The harder surface of the arrested dentinal lesion suggests increased mineralization (Fig. 2-13). Variations in the mineral content of different carious lesions have been confirmed by histologic specimens, physical studies, and chemical analyses.[5]

Caries Control

Caries control must be instituted if radiographic evidence indicates that carious lesions may threaten the dental pulp. Regardless of the proposed treatment plan, the actively carious material is removed from the involved teeth, beginning with the tooth most seriously affected. This last point is determined by three factors:

1. Indication by the patient that a specific tooth is painful.
2. The dentist's judgment.
3. The terminal molars and canines commonly receive preferential treatment because of strategic arch position *after* the patient discomfort and esthetics are addressed.

Generally, all actively carious teeth are treated and restored in amalgam before placement of castings (Figs. 2-14, A and B). However, there are exceptions to this guideline.

The sequence in a caries control program is:

1. Removal of infected carious material[6]
2. Protection of the pulp
3. Reconstructive measures for compromised teeth
4. Restoration of destroyed tooth structure

Removal of Infected Carious Material

It has been demonstrated that not all decalcified dentin is infected; this is especially true of the dentin closest to the pulp! Subject to the discretion of the dentist, exposure of the pulp is avoided unless the symptoms indicate acute pulpal involvement. The symptoms are not considered here since they are not well known and acute pulpitis can be reversible.

Whenever feasible, the rubber dam is placed before removing deep caries (Fig. 2-15). The cavity outline is commonly obtained using high-speed instrumentation with a water coolant before dam placement. The sequence is directed toward maintaining the vitality of the pulp and conserving tooth structure. When pulpal involvement is anticipated, aseptic conditions are provided. The most effective medium to accomplish this is the rubber dam.[7]

Two techniques have limited use in the excavation of caries. One is ultrahigh speed; the other is a spoon excavator. The method of choice is a round bur of suitable size, i.e., a No. 6 to No. 10, which rotates slowly. The carious tooth structure is removed by a round bur with special attention to the D-E junction under cusps.[6] Undue pressure is avoided, and the excavation terminates short of actual exposure. If soft dentin remains in the deepest penetration, it is considered sterile if the cavity remains aseptic. The carious process will not advance if sealed, but the caries is always active in the dentinoenamel junction. Stained or carious material at or near the dentino-

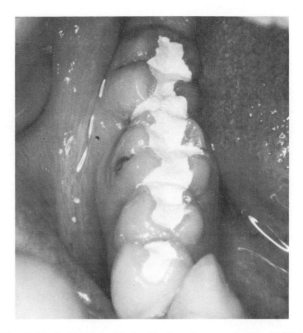

Fig. 2-14. A, Caries control with glass ionomer and/or "I.R.M." and appropriate liners to eliminate caries as an infectious disease prior to cast restorations. (Malone, W.F.P., Sarlas, C.: Dent. Clin. N. Amer. **13**:461, 1969.)

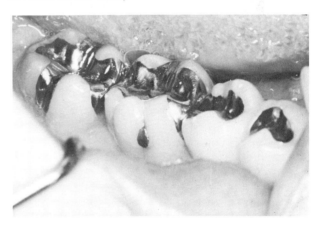

Fig. 2-14. B, Cast restorations (from Fig. 2-14.A).

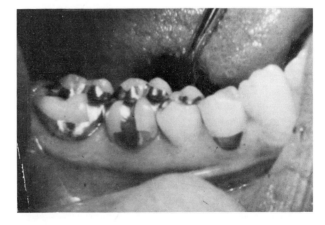

Fig. 2-14. C, Caries control program with amalgam restorations. (Malone, W.F.P., Sarlas, C.: Dent. Clin. N. Amer. **13**:461, 1969.)

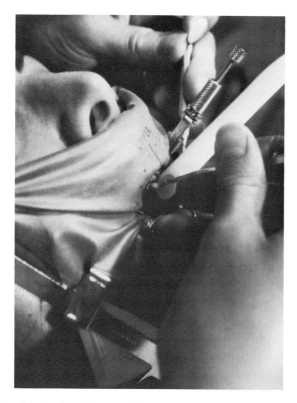

Fig. 2-15. Rubberdam provides an isolated, clean area that is similar to the surgical drape of patients having surgery.

enamel junction must be removed even at the expense of undermining the cusps. This situation can be treated later by flexibility in cavity preparation and with retentive pins. Special attention is devoted to reconstructive pins because individual artificial crowns are rarely placed on healthy teeth. Most teeth requiring crowns have been severely compromised by caries or fractures.

PROTECTION OF THE PULP

After the removal of infected carious material, the next procedure is pulp protection and odontoblastic stimulation to promote secondary dentin formation. Under normal metabolic conditions, a sufficient layer of secondary dentin is deposited to protect the pulp in 8 to 12 weeks.

A $Ca(OH)_2$ preparation is the base routinely used to encourage the odontoblastic activity. $Ca(OH)_2$ is available in a paste or in commercial products such as Dy-Cal and Life. The results usually depend upon the dentist's experience and knowledge, not product superiority claimed by the manufacturer.

Another crucial consideration is the capability of repair inherent in the pulp. The material is applied without pressure over the area of deepest penetration. Commercial products with accelerating ingredients, visible light activation, or both, harden the base in minutes to form a stiff protective layer. This is followed

by the application of a cavity varnish over the entire internal surface and margins of the cavity.

RECONSTRUCTIVE MEASURES FOR COMPROMISED TEETH

The reconstruction of severely compromised teeth demands skill, ingenuity, and dedication. Unlike the typical restoration, which derives primary retention from opposing walls, the compromised tooth requires the dentist to establish substitute retention. Widely used retentive substitutes are the pin, the horizontal slot, and the dentinal chamber. Each is locked into or prepared in the dentin to fasten restorative materials to sound tooth structure.

Retentive Pins

Since 1958, when Markley[8] first reported the cemented pin technique for the retention of amalgam foundations, the use of pins has become commonplace. There are three types of pin systems: cemented pins, friction-locked pins, and self-threading pins. The research of Dilts et al. (1968)[9], and Moffa et al. (1969)[10] clearly demonstrates that the self-threading pin is the most retentive pin both in dentin and amalgam. The procedure involves preparing a pin channel in dentin and placing a slightly larger-diameter, self-threading stainless steel or titanium pin approximately 2 mm into the channel with 2 mm of the pin free to retain the amalgam restoration. Self-threading pins are available in several sizes to accommmodate the patient's tooth. Some recent worthwhile changes have occurred in the design of self-threading pins. Self-shearing points have been engineered for reliability, pins are attached to contra-angle shanks for easier and faster pin placement, and pins are available in titanium as well as stainless steel.

Twist Drills

Two basic types of twist drills are available for preparing pin channels: the 4 to 5 mm long twist drill and the limited-depth twist drill. The limited-depth twist drill has matching pins and is recommended for preparing channels for self-threading pins.

Horizontal Slots and Dentinal Chambers

Investigators report favorable results following laboratory and clinical studies comparing dentinal slot retention with metallic pin retention.[11,12] Others also report favorable results from their studies comparing dentinal chamber "amalgapins" retention with that obtained from self-threading stainless steel pins.[13-16] Horizontal slots (Figs. 2-16, A through D) and dentinal chamber "amalapins" (Fig. 2-17) are now popular alternatives to the use of retentive pins for reconstructive procedures. Either or both of these retentive substitutes can be used when dentin is scarce, cracks are

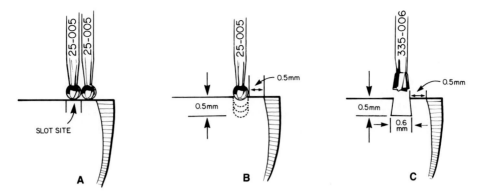

Fig. 2-16. A through **C** show a recommended measurement procedure for slot preparation within the D-E junction.

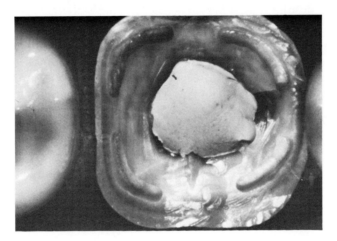

Fig. 2-16. D, Horizontal slots placed 1½-2 mm within dentin.

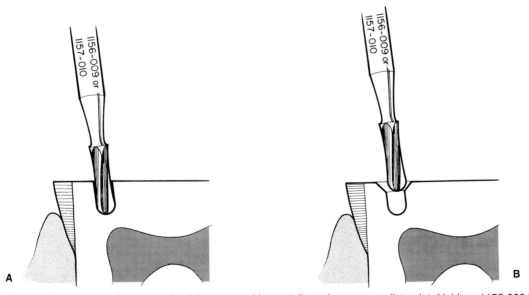

Fig. 2-17. A, Measure two to three diameters of a 0.5 mm round bur axially and prepare a pilot point. Hold an 1156-009/1157-010 bur parallel to the nearest external surface over the pilot point and prepare a chamber 2 mm deep. Each chamber so prepared will be non-parallel to each other and therefore retentive. **B,** Bevel the chamber entrance with the end of the 1156-009/1157-010 bur. Restore when ready.

present in dentin or enamel or both, or the dentist chooses not to use pins. Both involve preparing undercuts in dentin to lock the restorative material to tooth structure.

Supplemental Retention Grooves

Horizontal and vertical retention grooves, illustrated in Fig. 2-18 can be used to supplement any of the three retentive substitutes.

Recommended Reconstructive Procedures

Steps 1 through 7, illustrated in Fig. 2-19, outline procedures to follow for the treatment of a cariously compromised mandibular right first molar, from the rough outline form, caries removal, and pulp protection to the finish of the enamel walls.

1. Establish outline form as if caries or existing restorations did not exist (Fig. 2-19, B).
2. Caries removal with a slowly revolving No. 6-8 round bur (Fig. 2-19, C).
3. Spoon excavator used to check texture of dentin following caries removal, stain permitted (Fig. 2-19, D).
4. Caries removal from D-E junction using small round bur, no stain permitted to remain (Fig. 2-19, E).
5. Caries removal complete. D-E junction stain free and firm-textured. Thin layer of calcium hydroxide placed in deepest recess only and covered with glass ionomer lining cement (Fig. 2-19, F).
6. Proximal walls and cavo-surface angles trimmed with an enamel hatchet (Fig. 2-19, G).
7. Gingival cavo-surface angle trimmed with a gingival margin trimmer, thus completing the outline (Fig. 2-19, H).

Pin Channel Location

The usual method for locating pin channels axially is to place them half-way between the pulp and the D-E junction (external surface if no enamel) parallel to the nearest external surface. A recommended method for locating pin channels axially is illustrated in Fig. 2-20. The following information should be reviewed before using pins or other substitute retentive methods:

1. Tooth anatomy, internal and external
2. Pulpal biology
3. Roentgenograms
4. Comparisons of teeth and roentgenograms

Steps 8 to 10 are for teeth with limited available dentin:

8. With a 0.5 mm round bur, measure two diameters axially from the D-E junction (external surface if no enamel) and the pulp (Fig. 2-20, A).
9. Holding the 0.5 mm round bur at the second placement, prepare a pilot point for twist drill guidance, one bur radius deep (Fig. 2-20, B).
10. 0.5 mm of dentin remains between the D-E junction and the edge of the pin channel (Fig. 2-20, C).

Steps 11 to 13 are for teeth with more available dentin:

11. Measure three diameters of a 0.5 mm round bur axially from the D-E junction. Prepare a slight cove in the axial wall if necessary (Fig. 2-20, D).
12. Holding the 0.5 mm round bur at the third placement, prepare a pilot point, one bur radius deep (Fig. 2-20, E).
13. 1.0 mm of dentin remains between the D-E

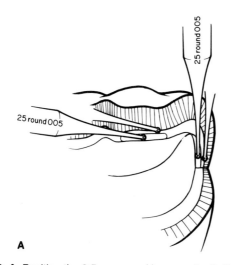

A

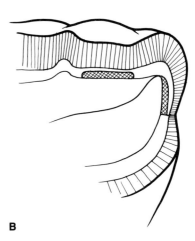

B

Fig. 2-18. A, Position the 0.5 mm round bur over the D-E junction, half on enamel and half on dentin, then move the bur one diameter axially or pulpally, whichever is the case, and prepare the groove approximately parallel to the D-E junction and one bur radius deep. **B,** Vertical and horizontal retention grooves.

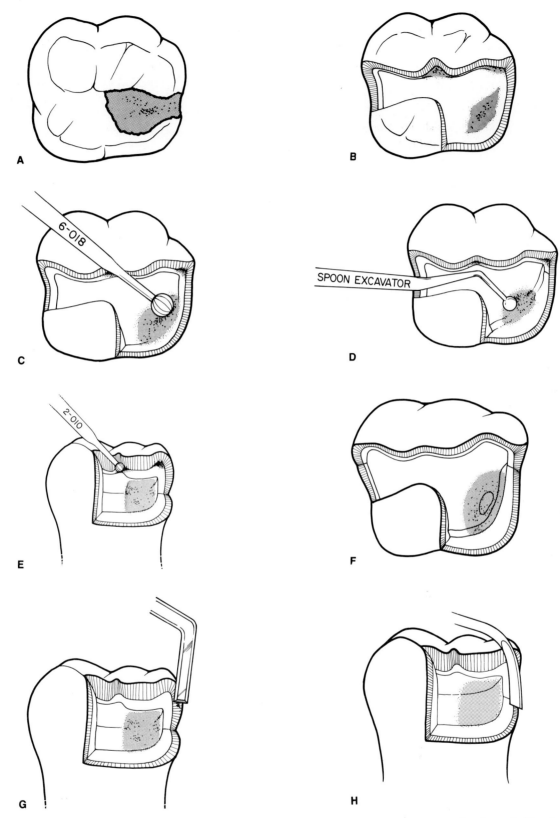

Fig. 2-19. A, Disto-lingual cusp of the mandibular right molar, undermined by caries. **B,** Step 1, the outline form. **C,** Step 2, caries removal with slowly revolving round bur. **D,** Step 3, spoon excavator used to check texture of dentin following caries removal. **E,** Step 4, caries removal from D-E junction with a small round bur. **F,** Step 5, caries removal complete. D-E junction stain free and firm textured. Thin layer of calcium hydroxide placed in deepest recess and covered with glass ionomer cement. **G,** Step 6, proximal walls and cavo-surface angles trimmed with an enamel hatchet. **H,** Step 7, gingival cavo-surface angle trimmed with a gingival margin trimmer.

junction and the edge of the pin channel (Fig. 2-20, F).

The distal lingual cusp of the mandibular first molar usually is an ideal site for a pin because the pulpal tissue is not usually in this area.

Supplemental Retention Grooves

Steps 14 and 15, illustrated in Fig. 2-18, detail a procedure for the safe placement of vertical or horizontal supplemental retention grooves (Marshall, unpublished).[17]

14. Position the 0.5 mm round bur over the D-E junction, as shown in Fig. 2-18, A, half on the enamel and half on the dentin; then move the bur one diameter axially or pulpally and prepare the groove approximately parallel to the D-E junction and one bur radius deep.

15. Vertical and horizontal retention grooves for use in conjunction with pins, horizontal slots, and dentinal chambers (Fig. 2-18, B).

Pin Channel Preparation

Steps 16 to 18, shown in Fig. 2-21, detail the procedures to follow when preparing pin channels. Mar-

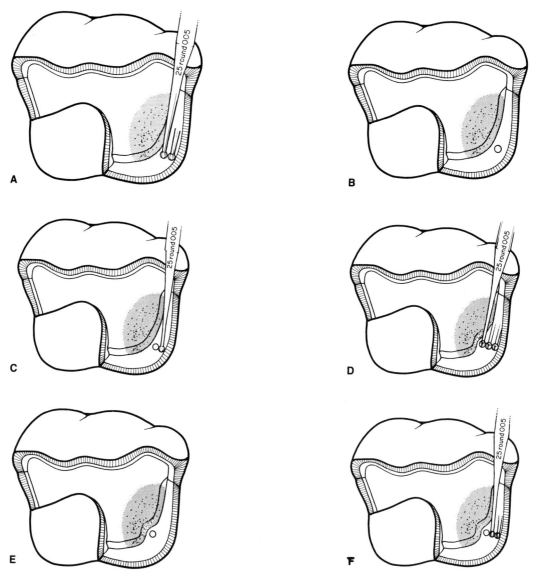

Fig. 2-20. A, Step 8, for limited available dentin. With a 0.5 mm round bur, measure two diameters axially from the D-E junction (external surface if no enamel). **B,** Step 9, holding the 0.5 mm round bur at the second placement, prepare a pilot point for twist drill guidance, one radius in depth. **C,** Step 10, 0.5 mm of dentin remains between the D-E junction and the edge of the pin channel. **D,** Step 11, when more dentin is available, measure three diameters of a 0.5 mm round bur axially from the D-E junction. Prepare a slight cove in the axial wall if necessary. **E,** Step 12, holding the 0.5 mm round bur at the third placement, prepare a pilot point, one radius deep. **F,** Step 13, 1.0 mm of dentin remains between the D-E junction (external surface if no enamel) and the edge of the pin channel.

shall et al. demonstrated that the conventional speed contra angle handpiece can be successfully used to prepare pin channels and seat self-threading and self-shearing pins.[18] Caution is necessary because the speed for channel preparation and pin placement must only be enough to prevent stalling of the twist drill or pin. When insufficient rotational speed causes the twist drill to stall, frequent fractures of the drill occur when a restart is attempted. When the speed for pin placement is insufficient, the pin stalls and shears upon restart. Excess twist drill speeds can cause heat buildup, crazes, cracks, and oversized channels; excess speed during pin placement can cause crazes, cracks, stripping of channel threads, and increased stress at the end of the channel. Speed reduction contra angles are available for channel preparation and pin placement.

16. Holding a limited depth twist drill in a conventional speed contra angle handpiece, orient the drill parallel to the nearest external surface over the pilot point without touching it. With a stream of air directed at the drill, bring the drill to a clockwise rotational speed of approximately 750 to 1000 rpm, and with a firm pressure, contact the pilot point and begin to prepare the channel (Fig. 2-21, A).

17. Penetrate to half the length of the drill, and without stopping the rotation, remove the drill from the channel, clear the flutes, and re-enter the channel (Fig. 2-21, B).

18. Penetrate to the full length of the limited depth twist drill (Fig. 2-21, C) and, again without slowing or stopping, remove the drill from the channel. Do not make more than two drill passes. Only use twist drills 10 to 12 times, and then discard.

Pin Placement

Steps 19 through 21 illustrate threaded pins (Figs. 2-22, A and B) that were attached to plastic or metal shanks for insertion into conventional-speed contra angle handpieces for easy placement.

19. To place pin, insert shank with pin into contra angle handpiece, position the pin over and parallel to the channel, but not touching; then bring clockwise speed to approximately 750 to 1000 rpm, and with slight pressure contact the channel entrance. The pin should seat and shear with ease.

20. Pins can be easily cut to the desired length, (Fig. 2-22, C), with a 0.5 mm round carbide bur if an ultraspeed contra angle with water spray is used and the bur is held at right angles to the pin.

21. Pins can be easily bent using a specifically designed bending tool (Fig. 2-22, D).

This self-threading, self-shearing pin type is available in stainless steel and titanium from Whaledent International and Fairfax Dental, Inc. This same pin type is available in titanium only from Vivadent.

22. The threaded pin displayed in (Fig. 2-22, B) was placed using the same technique as the pins in step 19 and comes with a metal shank designed to fit into a special speed reduction contra angle. The part of the pin that engages the restorative material has a different design. This pin type is available in titanium from Brasseler Inc., USA.

Horizontal Slots

Steps 23 to 25, Fig. 2-23, A through D, detail the recommended procedure for placing a horizontal slot in the pulpal or gingival floor.

23. With a 0.5 mm round bur (Fig. 2-23, A), mea-

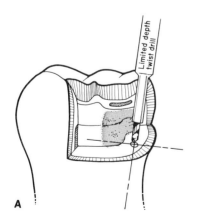
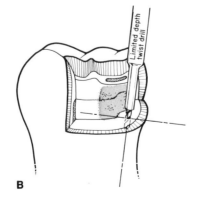
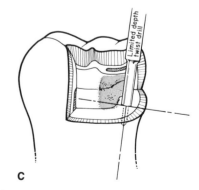

Fig. 2-21. A, Step 16, holding a limited depth twist drill in a contra angle handpiece, orient the drill parallel to the nearest external surface over the pilot point without touching it. With a clockwise rotational speed of approx. 750-1000 rpm, enter the pilot point. **B,** Step 17, with a stream of air directed at the drill, penetrate to half the length of the drill, never stopping the rotation, remove drill from channel, clear flutes, re-enter the channel and **C,** Step 18, penetrate to the full length of the limited depth twist drill and again without slowing or stopping, remove the drill from the channel. Never make more than two drill passes.

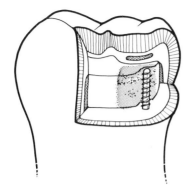 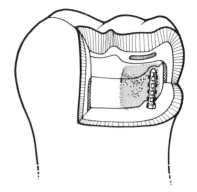

Fig. 2-22. A, Diagram of a self-threading, single self-shearing, stainless steel/titanium pin, with threads for engaging the restorative material. This pin type is available in stainless steel or titanium from Whaledent International and Fairfax Dental Inc. This same pin type is available in titanium only from Vivadent. Limited depth twist drills are available and are recommended for channel preparation. **B,** Diagram of a self-threading, single self-shearing, titanium Microdontic Pin by Brasseler Inc. USA. Step 19, matching twist drills accompany these pins.

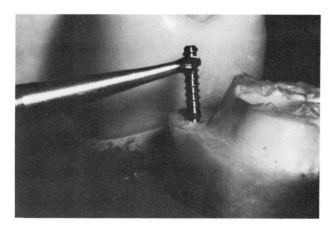 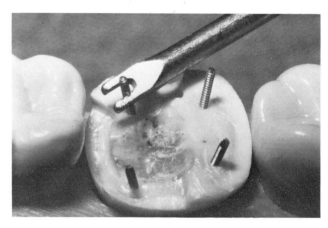

Fig. 2-22. C, Step 20, the bur/pin orientation for cutting a pin.

Fig. 2-22. D, Step 21, the pin/bending tool. Step 22 displays different pin designs.

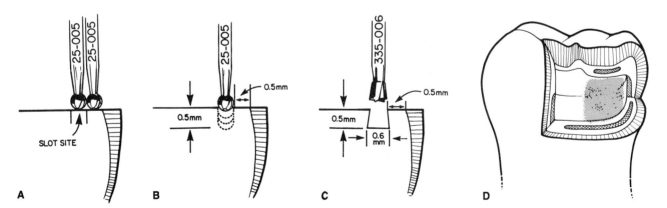

Fig. 2-23. A, Step 23, using a 0.5 mm round bur, measure two diameters axially from the D-E junction (or the external surface if no enamel). **B,** Step 24, holding the 0.5 mm round bur at the second placement, prepare a groove parallel to the D-E junction, to desired slot length and to the depth of the bur. **C,** Step 25, replace the 0.5 mm round bur with a 0.6 mm inverted cone bur (33.5) and finish preparing the inverted slot. **D,** Finished slot preparation ready for an amalgam reconstruction prior to a cast restoration. Vertical and horizontal grooves are also exhibited.

sure two diameters axially from the D-E junction or the external surface if no enamel is present.

24. Holding the 0.5 mm round bur at the second placement (Fig. 2-23, B) prepare a groove parallel to the D-E junction to the desired slot length and the diameter of the bur.

25. Replace the 0.5 mm bur with a 0.6 mm inverted cone bur (33.5) and finish preparing the inverted slot (Fig. 2-23, C).

The diagrams in Fig. 2-22, A and B, and Fig. 2-23, D, illustrate a compromised tooth prepared and ready to receive extensive amalgams. Notice that Fig. 2-22, A and B, shows one pin each plus two vertical grooves and one horizontal groove; the tooth has received a thin calcium hydroxide liner covered with a glass io-

nomer cement base. Fig. 2-23, D, illustrates a compromised tooth with a horizontal slot instead of a pin, plus two vertical grooves and one horizontal groove (as in Fig. 2-22), and a thin layer of calcium hydroxide covered with a glass ionomer base. Fig. 2-23, E and F, demonstrates two views of the same tooth with four horizontal slots.

Dentinal Chambers

Steps 26, 27, and Fig. 2-24 illustrate the preparation of dentinal chambers used to form "amalgapins."[13,14]

26. Measure two or three diameters of a 0.5 mm round bur and place a pilot point at the second or third placement. Holding a 1156-009/1157-010 bur parallel to the external surface, prepare a chamber approximately 2 mm deep (Fig. 2-

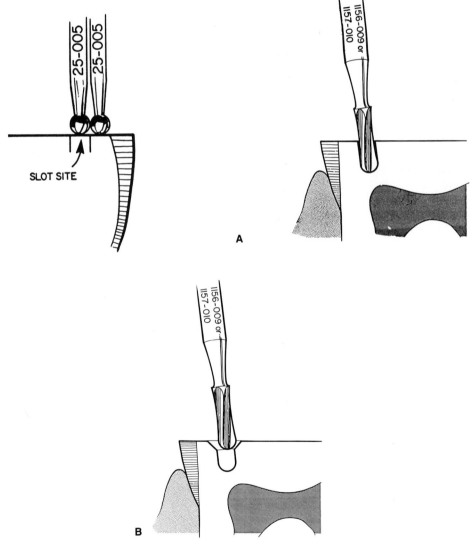

Fig. 2-24. A and **B** detail the recommended procedure for preparing dentinal chambers. **A,** Step 26, measure two to three diameters of a 0.5 mm round bur axially and prepare a pilot point. Hold an 1156-009/1157-010 bur parallel to the nearest external surface over the pilot point and prepare a chamber 2 mm deep. Each chamber so prepared will be non-parallel to each other and therefore retentive. **B,** Step 27, bevel the chamber entrance with the end of the 1156-009/1157-010 bur. Restore when ready.

24, A). Prepare approximately one chamber for each missing cusp. When finished, the chambers should be nonparallel to each other and thus retentive.

27. Bevel the circular chamber entrance using the end of the 1156-009/1157-010 bur (Fig. 2-24, B).[14]

Custom Matrices

Compound supported custom matrices are recommended for all teeth prepared for reconstructive procedures. One example of this matrix is the welded stainless steel matrix shown in (Fig. 2-25).

28. Stainless steel matrix material is cut and contoured with the Unitek contouring plier No. 113 (Figs. 2-25, A and B).

29. Adapt, remove, weld, and readapt the matrix, making sure that it is in direct contact with the adjacent tooth. Next wedge and support the matrix with compound (Fig. 2-25, C). Reburnish the contact area of the matrix band using a warm spoon excavator to assure metal-to-tooth contact (Fig. 2-25, D).

30. Reconstruct the prepared and matrixed tooth with amalgam (Fig. 2-25, E).

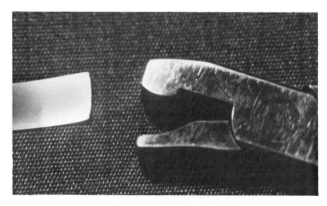

Fig. 2-25. A, Restoration of a compromised tooth, Step 28.

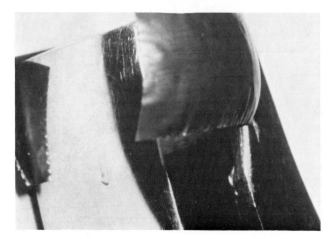

Fig. 2-25. B, Restoration of a compromised tooth, Step 28. Matrix material cut and contoured with Unitek plier #113.

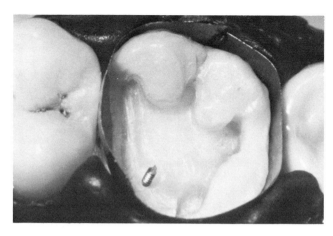

Fig. 2-25. C, Restoration of a compromised tooth, Step 29. Custom matrix adapted and supported with compound.

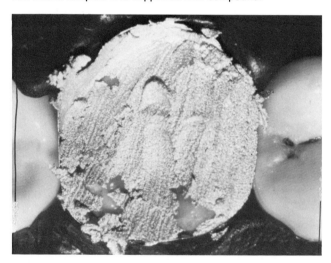

Fig. 2-25. D, Restoration of a compromised tooth, Step 29. The contact is re-established by burnishing with a warm spoon to assure metal to tooth contact.

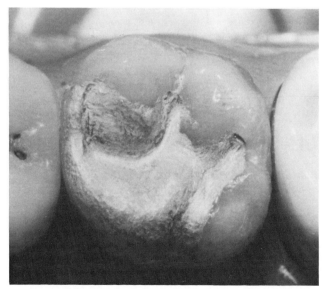

Fig. 2-25. E, Restoration of a compromised tooth, Step 30. The prepared and matrixed tooth is reconstructed with amalgam.

Reconstructed Tooth, completed

A finished and polished reconstructed tooth is shown in Fig. 2-26.

Summary

A summary of the reconstructive management of a compromised tooth is presented in Fig. 2-27, A through D. This information is in the form of diagnostic/decision-making/treatment procedural flow

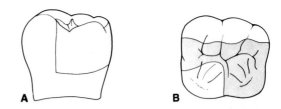

Fig. 2-26. A and **B,** Diagrams of a finished and polished reconstruction of a compromised tooth.

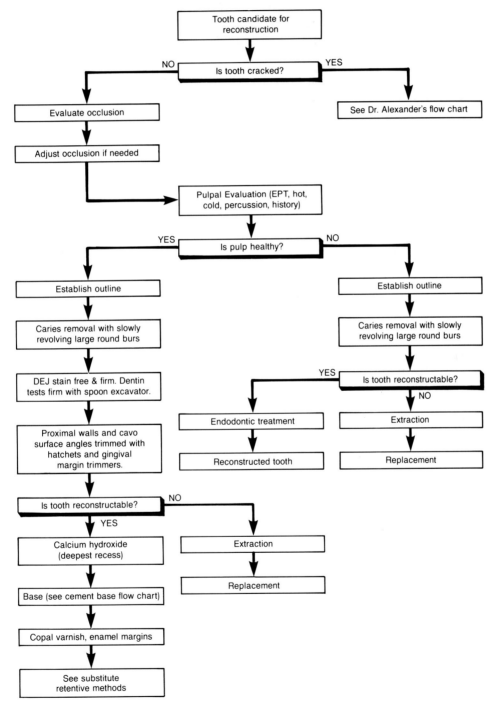

Fig. 2-27. A, Procedural flow chart for diagnosis and treatment of a compromised tooth. (Courtesy Dr. Thomas D. Marshall.)

Continued.

charts. The first two flow charts (Fig. 2-27, A and B) are designed to summarize the main yes/no decisions and necessary treatment when considering a compromised tooth for reconstruction. The yes/no decisions can lead to the following:

1. Reconstruction of a vital tooth using substitute retentive methods.
2. Endodontics and reconstruction of a nonvital tooth.
3. Extraction and replacement.

Fig. 2-27, C, is a treatment flow chart and a continuation of Fig. 2-27, A. It offers three substitute retentive methods for reconstructing a compromised tooth. One or more can be used in the same tooth, depending on available dentin. Fig. 2-27, D, is a treatment flow chart for cemented pins and self-threading and self-shearing pins. Fig. 2-27, E, is a procedural flow chart for each of the four main types of dental cements.

Untold numbers of teeth have been returned to function using the reconstructive procedures presented in this chapter.

RESTORATION OF DESTROYED TOOTH STRUCTURE

The sedative material commonly used for caries control is a zinc oxide eugenol base (IRM) cement. This material has a relatively low crushing strength and <u>cannot</u> be depended upon for an extended period of time; therefore, more substantial dental materials should be placed. Glass ionomers have been successfully placed as an interim restoration and have the added attraction of gradual fluoride release. Glass ionomers have a history of belated sensitivity as a luting agent, but they are innocuous and have distinct advantages as a base (Fig. 17-1-8). However, it is just as expedient to restore posterior teeth with a calcium hydroxide liner/glass ionomer base and silver amalgam as to continually change zinc oxide eugenol or monitor the attrition of a glass ionomer restoration (Fig. 2-28).

Freshly placed silver amalgams are subject to initial microleakage, which diminishes as the alloy matures and produces a suitable seal. Nevertheless, cavity varnish is applied over the margins to prevent leakage.

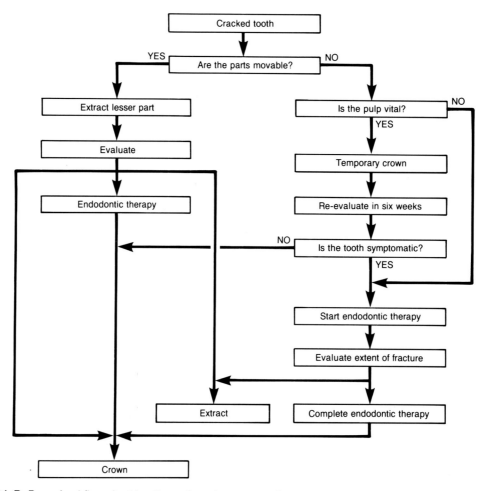

Fig. 2-27, cont'd. B, Procedural flow chart for diagnosis and treatment of a cracked tooth. (Courtesy Dr. Joel Alexander.)

Current research has confirmed that this procedure has minimized microleakage until the seal is created.[19]

Caries control is performed primarily to eliminate caries as a disease, because it has been demonstrated that a drop in *Lactobacillus* counts occurs only after the last carious lesion is treated.[20] A caries control program is a beneficial service that should be followed by more definitive treatment within an acceptable time frame. Failure to implement a timely, definitive treatment plan defeats the entire rationale and ultimately gives a "bad name" to a worthwhile procedure. Based upon the caries control program, scholarly diagnosis can also be formulated to reduce the subjective aspects of treatment planning.

PREVENTION OF CARIES

Dental investigators have identified fluoride as the naturally occurring element in water that protects teeth against caries. Research has determined that fluoride concentrations from 0.7 mm to 1.2 ppm in drinking water could preserve teeth without causing dental fluorosis, tooth discoloration, or both. Fluoridation has reduced the incidence of dental caries in selected areas by approximately 70 percent.[21]

Community dentistry programs have demonstrated that effective, inexpensive caries prevention can be introduced in municipalities and rural areas. The commercial emphasis on fluoride-containing dentifrices has also gained popularity, so that the majority of tooth pastes now contain fluoride. The "decayed-missing-filled" (DMF) rate is now approximately 32 percent lower than before fluoride introduction, but even more impressive is the increased number of caries-free children.

Despite these statistics, investigators are expanding present caries prevention programs through more innovative measures. The optimal levels for water fluoridation have been known for nearly 40 years, but more than 70 million people still live in communities without fluorided water.

Prevention through Restorative Dentistry

Fluoridation has reduced caries, but does not eliminate the disease. People still require restorative dentistry. Because many areas lack fluoridation and do not enjoy a communal water supply, only a segment of the population can benefit from fluoridation. Many people rely on early restorative dentistry to preserve their teeth. In addition, fluoride programs have con-

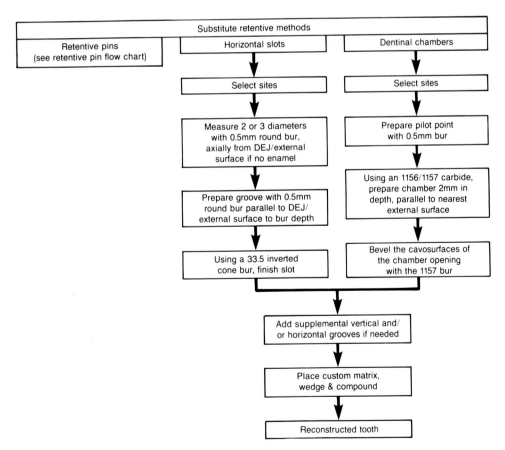

Fig. 2-27, cont'd. C, Continuation of flow chart 2-27A showing substitute retentive methods and treatment. (Courtesy Dr. Thomas D. Marshall.)

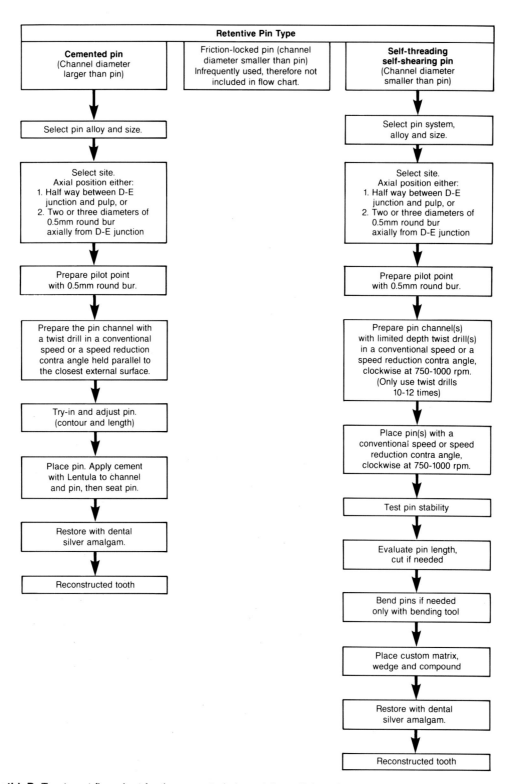

Fig. 2-27, cont'd. D, Treatment flow chart for the cemented pin and the self-threading and self-shearing pin. (Courtesy Dr. Thomas D. Marshall.)

Continued.

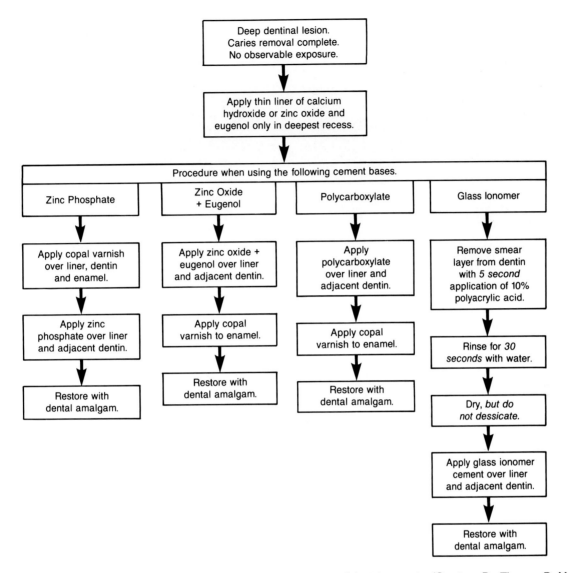

Fig. 2-27, cont'd. E, Procedural flow chart for each of the four main types of dental cements. (Courtesy Dr. Thomas D. Marshall.)

sistently demonstrated effectiveness mainly in preventing dental caries on smooth surfaces. While pit and fissure regions represent only 12.5 percent of the coronal surfaces of teeth, they account for over 50 percent of the carious lesions. Recognition of this specific problem led to the development of adhesive fissure sealants (Fig. 2-29).

Sealants

Early evidence suggested that the incidence of occlusal caries was reduced by sealing the pits and fissures with low-viscosity resins. However, success of sealants depends upon obtaining and maintaining an effective seal. Incomplete adaptation of the resin to the tooth can permit oral fluids with microorganisms to penetrate the sealant, placing the tooth in jeopardy.[22] Although the last 10 years have evidenced a decided improvement in the acid etchants and composite resins, sealants remain controversial. Glass io-

nomer cements with fluoride release have also interested the profession and have been effectively employed as an occlusal sealant, caries control material, and for preventive restorations.

Diet

Despite encouraging data, preventive dentistry through fluoride and sealants is not a cure-all. Decay-causing bacteria can overcome resistance to caries when a constant source of fermentable foods is present. Although the need for alterations in the American diet has long been recognized by the health professions and the public, the per capita consumption of convenience foods, which are high in sucrose, increases. Adolescents have a legendary appetite for sweet snacks consumed at irregular hours. Unfortunately, many secondary schools do not participate in institutional fluoride programs or provide oral health education. A combination of sealants, fluoride, diet,

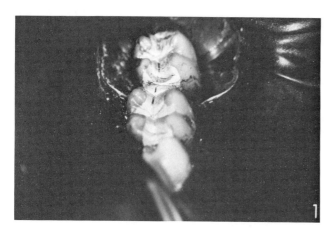

Fig. 2-28. A, Caries control in amalgam prior to cast restorations. Redundant interproximal tissue may require electrosurgical tissue management.

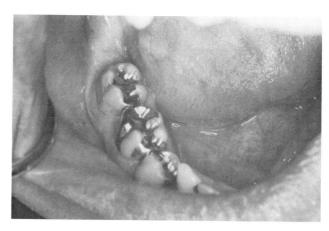

Fig. 2-28. B, Polished interim amalgam restorations prior to cast restorations.

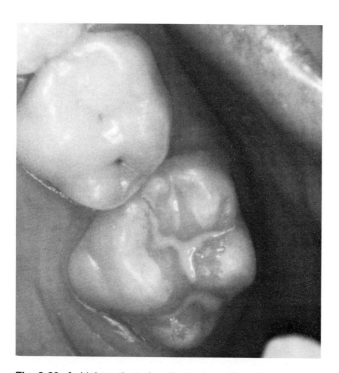

Fig. 2-29. A, Light-activated sealant on maxillary 1st molar in a mixed dentition.

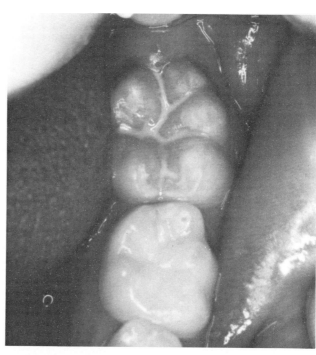

Fig. 2-29. B, Sealant on acid-etched grooves of mandibular 1st molar. The cusp-fossa relationship of the opposing molar will not be jeopardized. (Courtesy of Dr. Lawrence Lenz; Palos Park, Ill.)

counseling, restorative dentistry, and periodic dental examinations is required for effective ephebodontic programs. Although the victims of extensive dental caries have traditionally been teenagers, the elderly are now displaying an inordinately high caries rate, particularly in the form of root caries (Figs. 2-30, A-C). The elevated DMF rate for adults over 40 is particularly important because fixed prosthodontics is commonly performed for this age group.

Prevention of Root Caries

The practice of regular tongue brushing should be initiated as soon as the tongue shows signs of developing a thick, white mucoid coat that appears after rising before breakfast. Tongue hygiene is a crucial part of oral hygiene in the mature adult to control the growth of *O. viscoses*.

Topical applications of stannous fluoride solutions to the decalcified enamel, cementum, and dentin re-mineralizes the tissue and increases its resistance to further chelation after removal of the surface bacterial plaque. Cementum absorbs the fluoride more rapidly and in higher concentration than enamel and dentin. Stannous fluoride, 4 percent, is preferred, although scientific evidence is not yet available to compare its effectiveness with sodium fluoride or the acidulated fluorophosphate.

Elimination of gingival pockets is encouraged. Gingival pockets are predilection sites for cemental caries caused by *O. viscoses*. These organisms are anaerobes and prefer deep pockets for growth. Exposure of the cementum to the washing action of the saliva and the cleaning action of detergent foods will cause even active cemental lesions to become arrested. The hard tissue will become partially remineralized, hard and leathery, and deeply pigmented. These arrested lesions can remain static for years without restorations if the area is smoothed, kept cleaned by brushing, and subjected to periodic fluoride treatment. If the cavitation is deep, restoration of contour to support the gingivae is indicated after treatment with a stannous fluoride solution.

FUTURE CONSIDERATIONS

Research has established that fluoride, adhesive sealants, and improved oral hygiene with diet management prevents tooth decay in healthy patients. The treatment and prevention of root caries and topical remineralization are the challenges for future investigators. Studies are also needed to identify the role of antimicrobials, fluoride-releasing dental restorative materials, and medications to combat xerostomia in medically compromised patients.

The effects of antimicrobials that control the number of microorganisms in contact with the teeth is encouraging but requires guidelines for patient safety and reliability. The ideal antimicrobial should 1) reduce plaque, 2) eliminate only pathogenic bacteria without encouraging the development of resistant strains, 3) be without adverse effects (tooth staining, etc.), and 4) be easy to administer.

Currently, plaque-inhibiting activity is identified with chlorhexidine. Presumably, this plaque reduction is attained by three modes:

1. Blocking acidic groups on salivary glycoproteins, which reduces the protein absorption to tooth surfaces.
2. Binding to the surface of the salivary bacteria.
3. Precipitating the acid agglutination factors in saliva and displacing calcium, which is involved in "gluing" the plaque.[24]

Approximately 30 percent of the chlorhexidine is retained intraorally by reversible interactions with phosphate sulfate and carboxyl on the soft tissue. The remaining 60 percent is expectorated, and 10 percent is swallowed. The chief objection to chlorhexidine is

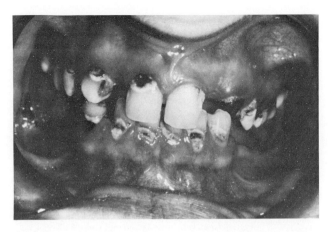

Fig. 2-30. A, Prohibitive DMF ratio of a patient reduces treatment alternatives. Tooth-supported complete denture service is indicated.

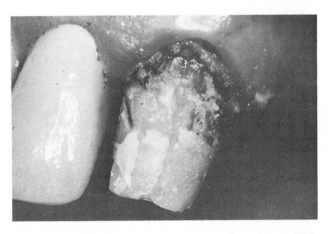

Fig. 2-30. B, Extensive root caries surrounding a former RPD abutment. Endodontic therapy is a common solution, including a double abuted cast restoration with broad embrasures.

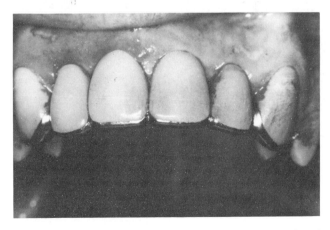

Fig. 2-30. C, Disclosing solution demonstrates the tenacity of plaque on abutments of a 6 unit FPD.

discoloration of the teeth and tooth-colored restorations. It has also been suggested as an additional ingredient for luting agents with promising results.[25]

The Keyes method of exposing the gingival sulcus to a 1 percent solution of hydrogen peroxide followed by a sodium bicarbonate-chloride rinse has also been suggested as a caries control method, but it is more effective in controlling organisms associated with periodontal disease than with caries.[26,27]

Biochemical and electron microscopic evaluations have also been conducted to explore the mechanism of N-mono-chloroglycine. It is the active ingredient of GK-101 E, which is used in caries removal of large lesions.[28] This method (Caridex) of caries removal has tremendous patient appeal because carious lesions can be excavated without "numbing," but detailed refined tooth preparation still requires anesthesia.

Vaccines

Vaccines have become a provocative issue because they may be less effective, although more expensive, than fluoride therapy, and may present greater risk of side effects to the patient. Nevertheless, a vaccine would be a distinct advantage when public water fluoridation is impractical and the patient has an inordinately high DMF rate.

Before vaccines become widely used, the safety of immunization, cost, and specific indications require clarification. Crevicular and salivary leukocytes have been demonstrated as active in phagocytosis of *S. mutans;* however, crevicular polymorpholeukocytes can be functional phagocytes, but the effectiveness of salivary polymorpholeukocytes is limited.[29,30]

The ability of the host to gradually arrest the carious process raises questions concerning the amount and type of carious tooth structure to be removed and the degree of faith placed by the dentist in this remarkable healing process. One cardinal sin of omission to be avoided is leaving caries in the DE junction under cusps. The entire carious lesion can appear arrested, but it is always active in the DE junction.

Extensive root caries can present an almost insurmountable problem for the restorative dentist.[31-39] The problem is further magnified by medically compromised patients with xerostomia resulting from chemotherapy and/or medication.

Caries control is a practical restorative procedure to eliminate the infectious process of dental caries as a disease entity. Caries management programs also facilitate the implementation of a flexible, logical sequence in a treatment plan and can be performed concomitantly with periodontal therapy. Until established preventive measures exhibit greater effectiveness, or more comprehensive information on the carious process is available, excavation of carious material remains a practical approach.

The age groups that benefit most from a caries management program are the 12 to 18 year-olds in an active growth period, medically compromised patients, and the aged.

The dentist is a unique therapist because he or she replaces lost tissue with metal and tooth-colored biologic materials. The environment of the oral cavity must be free of infection, however, or the restoration will fail despite its quality. Prevention and control of dental caries is the foremost objective of restorative dentistry. Within the past 20 years, preventive programs have been extremely successful in improving the dental health of millions of people; but the entire population should be receiving the benefits of caries research and dental educational programs.

SELECTED REFERENCES

1. Miller, W.A., and Massler, Maury: Permeability and staining of active and arrested lesions in dentine, Br. Dent. J., **112**:187, 1962.
2. Massler, Maury: Teenage caries, J. Dent. Res. **12**:57, 1945.
3. Koulourides, T., et al.: Rehardening of softened enamel surfaces of teeth by solutions of calcium phosphates, Nature, **189**:226, 1961.
4. Wei, S.H.Y., and Wefel, J.S.: In vitro interactions between surfaces of enamel white spots and calcifying solutions, J. Dent. Res. **55**(1):135, 1976.
5. Malone, W.F.P., Bell, Charles, and Massler, Maury: Physicochemical characteristics of active and arrested carious lesions of dentine, J. Dent. Res. **45**:16, 1966.
6. Malone, W.F.P., and Manning, J.L.: Caries control, Illinois State Dent. J. **36**:724, 1967.
7. Malone, W.F.P., and Balaty, Jerry: The rubber dam dilemma, Ill. State Dent. J. **37**:138, 1968.
8. Markley, Miles R.: Pin reinforcement and retention of amalgam foundations and restorations, J.A.D.A. **56**:675-679, 1958.
9. Dilts, Walter E., et al.: Retentive properties of pin materials in pin-retained silver amalgam restorations, J.A.D.A. **77**:1085-1089, 1968.
10. Moffa, Joseph P., et al.: Pins—a comparison of their retentive properties, J.A.D.A. **78**:529-535, 1969.
11. Outhwaite, William C., Garman, Thomas A., and Pashley, David H.: Pin vs. slot retention in extensive amalgam restorations, J. Prosth. Dent. **41**(4):396-400, 1979.
12. Garman, Thomas A., et al.: A clinical comparison of dentinal slot retention with metallic pin retention, J.A.D.A. **107**:762-763, 1983.
13. Shavell, H.M.: The amalgapin technique for complex amalgam restorations, J. Cal. Dent. Assoc. **8**(4):48, 1980.
14. Shavell, H.M.: Updating the amalgapin technique for complex amalgam restorations, Int. J. Periodont. Restor. Dent. Vol. 5, 1986.
15. Seng, George F., et al.: Placement of retentive amalgam inserts in tooth structure for supplemental retention, Gen. Dent., November-December 1980.
16. Davis, Samuel P., et al.: Self-threading pins and amalgapins compared in resistance form for complex amalgams, Oper. Dent. **8**:88-93, 1983.
17. Marshall, Thomas D.: Unpublished.
18. Marshall, T.D., Porter, K.H., and Re, G.J.: In vitro evaluation of the shoulder stop in a self-threading pin, J. Prosth. Dent. **56**(4):428, 1986.
19. Going, R.E., and Massler, M.: Influence of cavity liners under

amalgam restorations on penetration of radioactive isotopes, J. Prosth. Dent. **11**:298, 1961.

20. Sklair, A., Englander, Stein, and Kesel, R.: Preliminary report on the effect of complete mouth rehabilitation on oral lactobacilli counts, J.A.D.A. **53**:155, 1966.

21. Ast, D.B.: Effectiveness of water fluoridation, J.A.D.A. **65**:581, 1962.

22. Wilkins, J.S., Swartz, M.L., and Philips, R.W.: Testing of pit and fissure sealants in the monkey, J. Prosth. Dent. **37**:666, 1977.

23. Ripa, L.W.: The current status of pit and fissure sealants, Can. Dent. Assoc. J. **51**:367, 1985.

24. Rolla, G., and Nelson, B.: On the mechanism of the plaque inhibition of chlorhexidine, J. Dent. Res. **54**:57, 1975.

25. Schwartzman, B., Caputo, A., and Schein, B.: Dental cements, J. Prosthet. Dent. **43**:309, 1980.

26. Gjermo, Per: Some aspects of drug dynamics as related to soft tissue, J. Dent. Res. **54**:44, 1975.

27. Fletcher, R.D., Brostins, E.D., Albers, A.C., and Conway, J.: The effect of Keyes procedure in vitro on microbial agents associated with periodontal disease, Chicago, Quintessence International, March 1984, p. 329.

28. Schutzbank, S.G., Galaini, J., Goldman, M., and Clark, R.E.: A comparative in vitro study of G.K.-101 and G.K.-101 E in caries removal, J. Dent. Res. **57**:861, 1978.

29. Scully, C.: Phagocytic and killing activity of human blood, gingival crevicular, and salivary polymorphonuclear leukocytic for oral streptococci, J. Dent. Res. **61**:636, 1982.

30. Mukherjie, A.: Significance of crevicular fluid, The Compendium of Continuing Education, Vol: VI:611, Sept. 1985.

31. Muzynski, B.L., Greener, E., Jameson, L.M., Malone, W.F.P.: Fluoride release from glass ionomers used as luting agents, J. Prosthet. Dent., in Press 1986.

32. Hazen, S.P., Chilton, N.W., and Mumma, R.D., J.R.: The problem of root caries. Literature review and clinical description, J.A.D.A. **86**:137-144, 1973.

33. Sumney, D.L., Jordan, J.V., and Englander, H.R.: The prevalence of root surface caries in selected populations, J. Periodontol. **44**:500-504, 1973.

34. Syed, S.A., Loesche, W.J., Pape, H.L., and Grenier, E.: Predominant cultivable flora isolated from human root surface plaque, Infect. Immun. **11**:727-731, 1975.

35. Banting, D.W., and Ellen, R.P.: Carious lesions on the roots of teeth, a review for the general practitioner, J. Can. Dent. Assoc. **42**:496-502, 1976.

36. Levy, M.S.: Expansion of the proper use of systemic fluoride supplements, J.A.D.A. Vol. 112:30, January 1986.

37. Maryniuk, G.A., Kaplan, S.H.: Longevity of restorations: survey results of dentist's estimates and attitudes, J.A.D.A. Vol. 112:39, January 1986.

38. Lustig, L.P.: A precisely controllable atraumatic microdontic retention pin system, Quintessence International Vol. 17:391, July 1986.

39. Marzouk, M.A., Simonton, A.L., Gross, R.D.: Operative Dentistry Modern Theory and Practice. St. Louis-Tokyo, 1985, Ishiyaku EuroAmerica, Inc.

BIBLIOGRAPHY

Addy, M., Moran, J., Griffiths, A.A., and Wils-Wood, N.J.: Extrinsic tooth discoloration by metals and chlorhexidine. I. Surface protein denaturation or dietary precipitation? Br. Dent. J. **159**:281-285, 1985.

Bahn, Arthur N., Quillman, Paul D., and Kendrick, Francis J.: Intraoral localization of micro-organisms, J. Dent. Res. **41**:715, 1962.

Baum, Lloyd, et al.: Textbook of Operative Dentistry, ed. 2, Philadelphia, 1985, W.B. Saunders Co., Chapter 13.

Baum, Lloyd, and McCoy, Richard B.: Advanced Restorative Dentistry, Philadelphia, 1984, W.B. Saunders Co., Chapter 1.

Beck, J.D., Hunt, R.J., Hand, J.S., and Field, H.M.: Prevalence of root canal coronal caries in a noninstitutionalized older population, J.A.D.A. **11**:964, 1985.

Beck, J.D., Hunt, R., Hand, J., Field, H., and Kohout, F.: Prevalence of root caries in ambulatory elderly, Caries Res. **19**:165, 1985.

Bibby, B.G., Mundorff, S.A., Zero, D.T., and Almekinder, K.J.: Oral food clearance and the pH of plaque and saliva, J.A.D.A. **112**:333-337, 1986.

Bohannan, H.M., Stamm, J.W., Graves, R.C., Disney, J.A., and Bader, J.D.: Fluoride mouth rinse programs in fluoridated communities, J.A.D.A. **111**:783, 1985.

Bowen, W.H., Amsbaugh, S.M., Torrens-Monell, S., et al.: A method to assess cariogenic potential of foodstuffs, J.A.D.A. **100**:677, 1980.

Boyd, M.A., and Richardson, A.S.: Frequency of amalgam replacement in general dental practice, Can. Dent. Assoc. J. **51**:763, 1985.

Branorstrom, M., et al.: Invasion of micro organisms and some structural changes in incipient enamel caries, Caries Res. **14**:276, 1980.

Burt, B.A.: The future of the caries decline, J. Public Health Dent. **45**:261, 1985.

Caputo, A.A., and Standlee, J.P.: Biomechanics in clinical dentistry, Chicago, 1987, Quintessence Publishing Co., Inc., pp. 117-120.

DePaola, D.P., Alfano, M.D., and Modraw, C.L.: Assessing the nutritional status of the dental patient: a triphasic analysis, Am. Diet Assoc., Cassette-A-Month Series, June (CAM6) 1978.

Evans, Joseph R., and Wetz, Jon H.: Atlas of Operative Dentistry, Chicago, 1985, Quintessence Publishing Co., Inc., Chapter 2.

Firestone, A.F.: Human interdental plaque pH data and rat caries tests; results with the same substances, J. Dent. Res. **61**(10):1130-1136, 1982.

Firestone, A.R., Schmid, R., and Muhlemann, H.R.: Effect of the length and number of intervals between meals on caries in rats, Caries Res. **18**:128-133, 1984.

Garcia-Godoy, F.: The preventive glass ionomer restoration, Quintessence International, October 1986.

Garcia-Gody, F.: Retention of a light cured fissure sealant (Helioseal R) in a tropical environment after 12 months, Clin. Preven. Dent. **8**:11, May-June, 1986.

Garcia-Godoy, F., and Malone, W.F.P.: The effect of acid etching on two glass ionomer lining cements, Quintessence International, **17**:621, October 1986.

Graves, R.C., and Stamm, J.W.: Decline of dental caries. What occurred and will it continue? Can. Dent. Assoc. J. **51**:693, 1985.

Hagan, P.P., Roxier, R.C., and Bawden, J.W.: The caries-preventive effects of full and half strength topical acidulated phosphate fluoride, Pediatr. Dent. **7**:185, 1985.

Herrin, H.K., and Shen, C.: Microleakage of root caries restorations, Gerodontics **1**:156-159, 1985.

Jensen, O.E., Handelman, S.L., and Perez-Diez, F.: Occlusal wear of four pit and fissure sealants over two years, Pediatr. Dent. **7**:23, 1985.

Katz, R.V.: Root caries—is it the problem of the future? Can. Dent. Assoc. J. **51**:511, 1985.

Katz, R.V., Newitter, D.A., and Clive, J.M.: Root caries prevalence in adult dental patients, J. Dent. Res. **64**:293, 1985 (Abstr. No. 1069).

Levy, S.M., Rozier, R.G., and Bawden, J.W.: Determinants of requests for water fluoride assay among North Carolina dentists, J. Dent. Res. **65**:71-74, 1986.

Mandel, I.D.: Changing patterns of dental caries, Quintessence International **16**:81, 1985.

Marzouk, M.A., et al.: Operative Dentistry, Modern Theory and Practice, St. Louis-Tokyo, 1985, Ishiyaku EuroAmerica, Inc., Chapter 11.

Massler, Maury: Geriatric nutrition, IV. The role of fiber in the diet, J. Prosthet. Dent. **50:**5, 1983.

Massler, Maury: Geriatric nutrition, II. Dehydration of the elderly, U. Prosthet. Dent. **42:**489, 1979.

Mejare, I., and Brannstrom, M.: Deep bacterial penetration of early proximal caries lesions in young molars, ASDC J. Dent. Child. **52:**103, 1985.

Mellberg, J.R., and Chomicki, W.G.: Effect of soluble calcium on fluoride uptake by artificial caries lesions in vivo, Caries Res. **19:**122, 1985.

Mellberg, J.R., Chomicki, W.G., Mallon, D.E., and Castrovina, L.A.: Remineralization in vivo of artificial caries lesions by a monofluorophosphate dentifrice, Caries Res. **19:**126, 1985.

Moffa, Joseph P., Razzano, Michael R., and Folio, John: Influence of cavity varnish on microleakage and retention of various pin-retaining devices, J. Prosth. Dent. **20:**541, 1968.

Reintsema, H., and Arends, J.: An in vivo study of the fluoride uptake in demineralized enamel from dentifrices, Caries Res. **19:**170, 1985.

Ripa, L.W.: The current status of pit and fissure sealants, Can. Dent. Assoc. J. **51:**367, 1985.

Ripa, L.W., Leske, G.S., and Sposato, A.: The surface-specific caries pattern of participants in a school-based fluoride mouth rinsing program with implications for the use of sealants, J. Public Health Dent. **45:**90, 1985.

Schutzban, S.F., et al.: In vitro study of the effect of GK-101 on the removal of carious material, J. Dent. Res. **54:**907, 1975.

Seppa, L.: A scanning electron microscopic study of early subsurface bacterial penetration of fissureenamel, Caries Res. **19:**186, 1985.

Shannon, I.L., Trodahi, J.N., and Strcke, E.N.: Remineralization of enamel by a saliva substitute designed for use by irradiated patients, Cancer **41:**1746, 1978.

Soremark, Rune, Wing, Kenneth, Olsson, Kurt, and Goldin, Joel: Penetration of metallic ions from restorations into teeth, J. Prosth. Dent. **20:**531, 1968.

Steinman, R.R., and Leonora, J.: Relationship of fluid transport through the dentin to the incidence of caries, J. Dent. Res. **50:**1536, 1971.

Straffon, L.H., Dennison, J.B., and More, F.G.: Three-year evaluation of sealant. Effect of isolation of efficacy, J.A.D.A. **110:**714, 1985.

Sturdevant, Clifford M.: The Art and Science of Operative Dentistry, St. Louis, 1985, The C.V. Mosby Co., Chapter 13.

Titus, Harry W.: The use of the rubber dam to control the operating field, U.T.H.S.C.S.A. Press 1984.

Zickert, I., Emilson, C.G., and Krasse, B.: Prediction of caries incidence based on salivary S. mutans and Lactobacillus counts, J. Dent. Res. **64:**346, 1985 (Abstr. No. 1545).

3

Zigmund C. Porter and
Bernard W. Murray

PERIODONTAL CONSIDERATIONS FOR FIXED PROSTHODONTICS

The goal of every dentist is to maintain a healthy dentition for their patients. With advances in restorative dentistry, it is possible to reconstruct an entire mouth decayed to the root; but it is an almost insurmountable task to maintain the mouth after advanced periodontal disease. The best way to serve patients for continued dental health is through early recognition and prevention (Table 3-1).

PERIODONTAL DISEASE

Attachment Unit

When discussing a diseased state, it is imperative to understand the normal relationship of the tooth to the supporting structure (Fig. 3-1). Understanding the deviation from normal facilitates comprehension of the disease. Fig. 3-2 demonstrates a normal relationship of the gingival margin to the tooth, the epithelial attachment, and the fibers attached from the cementum to the gingiva.

The clinical gingival sulcus depth normally measures 1 to 2 mm, whereas the epithelial attachment is 1 mm and the connective tissue attachment 1 mm. The alveolar crest is therefore located approximately 2 mm apical to the base of the sulcus.[1] In a normal healthy patient, there is no visible flow of sulcular fluid,[2] but as the disease progresses, the crevicular fluid flow increases.[3]

Periodontal Ligament

The periodontal ligament is composed of collagen fibers arranged in bundles that are attached from the cementum of the tooth to the alveolar bone of the jaw. It is subject to the constant flux of change attributable to disease and masticatory forces. The healthy periodontal ligament in functional occlusion is about 0.25 ± 0.1 mm wide; it is widest at the margin and apex, while narrowest in the middle one third.

Understanding the normal attachment of a tooth to the alveolar process increases the usefulness of dif-

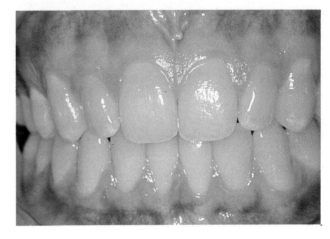

Fig. 3-1. Normal gingiva in young adult.

ferent measurements obtained when a periodontal probe is used to establish the difference between health and disease. The two basic forms of periodontal disease are gingivitis and periodontitis.

Gingivitis

Gingivitis is defined as inflammation of the gingiva. Microscopically, gingivitis is characterized by the presence of an inflammatory cellular exudate, edema in the gingival lamina propria, destruction of gingival fibers, ulceration, and proliferation of the sulcular epithelium.[4]

Periodontitis

Periodontitis is an inflammatory disease of the gingiva or the deeper tissues of the periodontium and is characterized by pocket formation and bone destruction. Periodontitis is considered a direct extension of neglected gingivitis. Periodontitis is caused by extrinsic irritating factors and is complicated by intrinsic disease, endocrine disturbances, nutritional deficiencies, periodontal traumatism, and other factors.[5]

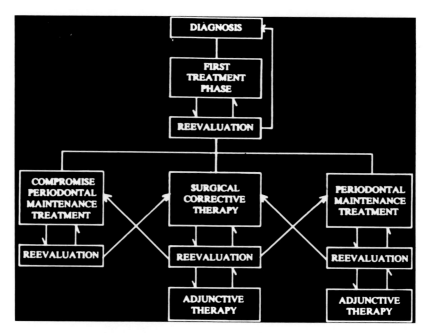

Table 3-1. Flow chart for periodontal therapy

Microbiologic Aspect of Periodontal Disease

There are at least five bacteriologically distinct periodontal diseases. Studies conducted between 1976 and the present have made this last statement possible. Although the amount of microorganisms is a factor in certain forms of periodontal disease, the type of microorganism involved is the most important factor in the disease process. This is complicated by the fact that the microflora in a diseased state is <u>not</u> a specific microorganism but a complex mixture. In addition, the disease repeatedly alternates from an active to an inactive disease state. This periodicity reflects the true state of periodontal disease progress; the process is not continuous and ongoing. It is possible to identify a "dirty mouth" by clinical and microbial means. We can also, by microbial means, describe the difference between a "healthy" and a "nonhealthy" periodontal pocket. It is difficult, however, to distinguish microbiologically whether a disease is progressing or quiescent.

Socransky, Tanner, and Goodson (1984) attempted to monitor patients for active and recent alveolar bone loss. They compared their findings with those from sites that had probing depths of more than 5 mm but that did not exhibit any progression during the monitoring period. They also compared the microflora of patients with active disease to that of comparable patients without active disease. They discovered similar organisms in both groups of patients. They did not observe proportional differences in the sites that had active disease, which would have indicated a distinct microflora that predisposes to an active period of disease; this indicates that an alteration of the ecology is

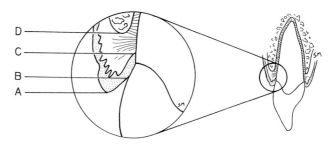

Fig. 3-2. A-B, Gingival crevice, B-C, Junctional epithelium, C-D, Connective tissue attachments, B-D, Biologic width.

<u>not</u> always necessary to initiate an active disease period.

Marginal Lesion

The initial stages of the disease can be identified histologically before clinical manifestations appear, but it is impossible to perform a biopsy on each suspect papilla (Fig. 3-3). Clinical examinations are therefore necessary. Early recognition is the decisive factor in preventing periodontal disease. The dentist examines clinical changes in the interdental papilla that are characterized by redness, swelling, tenderness, and bleeding and should inform the patient about these subtle changes to enable them to recognize symptoms when they first appear. A patient can be in a gingivally diseased state for many years and be unaware of the signs. Once patients have been returned to health by treatment and education, they are subsequently more aware of signs of disease such as swollen and bleeding areas.

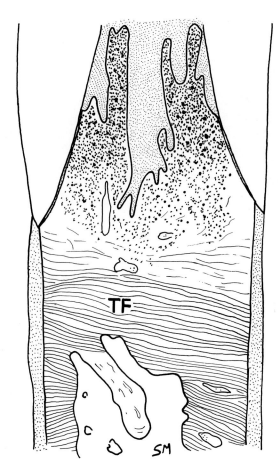

Fig. 3-3. Gingivitis in the beginning stages of the disease with local infiltration of inflammatory cells. Transseptal fibers, are still intact and there is no apparent resorption of alveolar crest.

Disease begins with the formation of plaque. A tooth can appear clean and healthy, but a pellicle may have formed from the saliva.[6] Plaque is invisible at this stage, but when it mineralizes, it becomes calculus. Bacterial substances attach to the tooth, irritate the gingiva, and initiate inflammation. At this point, clinical signs of redness and swelling are visible. The inflammation then spreads from the lamina propria of the connective tissue to the alveolar bone. There is a positive relationship between the presence of bacterial plaque and the existence of periodontal disease. The classic studies proving this were performed by Löe[7] in 1965 and Theilade et al.[8] in 1966. A group of dental students thoroughly cleaned their teeth before the study began and then stopped oral hygiene procedures. Gingivitis was noted in most of the subjects in a 10-day to 2-week period. They then initiated oral hygiene procedures, and the gingivitis disappeared.

Löe then described the three phases of plaque maturation. The first phase occurs within a 2-day period during which there is proliferation of gram-positive cocci and rods and a 30 percent gram-negative balance

of cocci and rods. During the second phase, which is between 1 and 4 days, *Fusobacterium* and filamentous organisms appear; spirilla and spirochetes appear during phase 3—within 9 days. At the time of infiltration by the polymorphonuclear leukocytes into the sulcular epithelium, the area begins to widen, encouraging the ingress of further antigens into the connective tissue. If the retention of plaque around the tooth continues, the acute inflammatory lesion advances to a chronic inflammatory lesion by the ingress of mast cells, plasma cells, lymphocytes, and other mononuclear cells. It is these cells that demonstrate the breakdown of the deeper connective tissue through immediate[9] or delayed hypersensitivities.[10]

Through the study of immunology, dentists are beginning to understand the etiology of periodontal disease. There is still considerable research needed to elucidate the differences between immunologic reactions.[11,11a] One clearly emerging factor is that the removal of plaque before development of the acute lesion prevents periodontal disease. Once the inflammatory lesion forms, all the other factors enhance the lesion; i.e., diabetes,[12] hormonal disturbances,[13] stress,[14] and altered nutrition.[15] Stress is unavoidable in today's society, and the Selye studies[16] have proven the influence of stress on pathologic lesions.

Advanced Lesions

Once the marginal lesion has developed to the point of chronic inflammation, the deeper layers of the connective tissues become involved with the ingress of the inflammatory cells (lymphocytes) that enhance osteoclastic activity, resulting in the breakdown of the alveolar process[17] (Fig. 3-4). If, at the same time, the tooth is under occlusal trauma, this area will change. There can be a concomitant lesion of periodontal disease, with the occlusal traumatic lesion enhancing the loss of bone around the tooth. The teeth become mobile and are eventually removed. The tooth can withstand forces along the long axis because of the arrangement of its fibers. Teeth only meet briefly during mastication and this is not enough force to create trauma to the supporting structure.[18] The trauma can only be instituted at times other than during mastication.

Occlusal Traumatism

Occlusal traumatism is defined as a force originating by movement of the maxillary and mandibular teeth in a way that creates a pathologic lesion.

Primary occlusal trauma. Primary occlusal trauma is a pathologic lesion that has been created by a force strong enough to disturb a normal intact periodontium.

Secondary occlusal trauma. Secondary occlusal trauma is a lesion created by a normal function on a

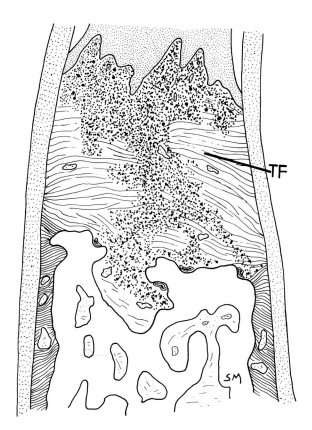

Fig. 3-4. Periodontitis. Local inflammatory cells have spread gingivally into transseptal fiber area. Note the beginning stages of resorption of alveolar crest.

weakened periodontium because of periodontal disease. This noninflammatory lesion is caused by trauma in the form of pressure atrophy; there is eventual necrosis of the affected area. Factors that enhance occlusal traumatism are clenching, grinding (bruxism), tongue thrusting, and nail biting. Of these, the one that appears to have the greatest effect is grinding. Some misconceptions are that 1) if an occlusal adjustment has been performed correctly, a patient will stop grinding and 2) that grinding is attributable to emotional distress and an individual grinds despite harmonious occlusion. A practical guideline to treatment lies between these approaches.

PERIODONTAL POCKET

A periodontal pocket is defined as a diseased periodontal attachment unit. The pocket may result from the enlargement of the gingival tissue. It is caused by the apical migration of the epithelial attachment with the loss of connective tissue attachment and, eventually, of osseous support. The clinical significance of a pocket is that if it extends beyond 3 to 4 mm, the patient has increasing difficulty maintaining normal brushing and flossing techniques. If an area cannot be maintained and mature plaque is allowed adjacent to the epithelium, the disease con-

tinues. The ideal situation is for the entire mouth to be free of pockets.

EXAMINATION

Visual Examination

It is important during the examination to evaluate the color, consistency, texture, and shape of the gingival unit. It is also critical to recognize the initial stages of a marginal lesion through the change of color and consistency. An adequate light source is essential to differentiate between normal and diseased tissue; a fiberoptic unit is used to examine inaccessible areas.

Attached Gingiva

The width of attached gingiva necessary to maintain gingival health has remained controversial. Studies that suggest minimal or no attached tissue to preserve health used animal models, nonrestored teeth, or were abbreviated studies. A 6-year report on humans using a split-mouth design reported nongrafted sites had no additional loss of attachment in patients with good plaque control and regular maintenance recalls. However, patients who abandoned the study received no maintenance recalls and had poor plaque control, exhibiting continual recession of the nongrafted sites as opposed to the grafted sites. The authors speculated that a free gingival graft acts as a barrier to prolong the tissue from further recession.

Crown margins can be gingival irritants and plaque traps, so enhancing the attached gingiva is advised for restorations. Keratinized tissue is often present and mistakenly restored, after which the dentist and patient are disappointed when recession continues. It must be realized that clinically, the first 2 mm of keratinized tissue represents 1 mm of sulcus and 1 mm of epithelial attachment, therefore, only keratinized tissue in excess of 2 mm can be considered attached by connective tissue.

Probing

There are periodontal instruments designed for probing (Fig. 3-5, A to D). The thinnest probe is desired, this permits probing the depth of a pocket without patient discomfort and allows the greatest dexterity in differentiating the dimensions of the pocket. These probes are generally calibrated in millimeters. Probing can be one of the most arduous aspects of examination, yet it is mistakenly taken for granted because it appears simple. The dentist should probe six areas around the tooth, paying specific attention to root anatomy. Evaluation should include bifurcation and trifurcation areas on the maxillary and mandibular molars and on the maxillary first premolars.

The mouth of a patient with poor oral hygiene habits will be difficult to accurately probe. Once oral hygiene has been established, the patient's mouth may be probed accurately (Fig. 3-6). During the probing pro-

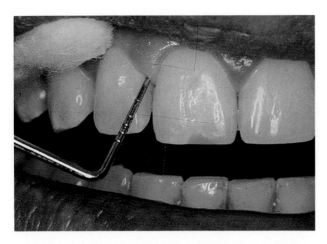

Fig. 3-5. A, Periodontal probe with markings are in millimeters.

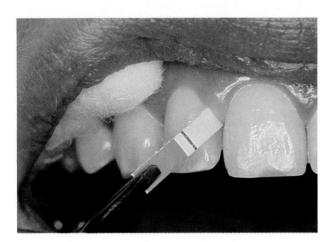

Fig. 3-5. B, Specially treated paper to monitor the intracrevicular fluid.

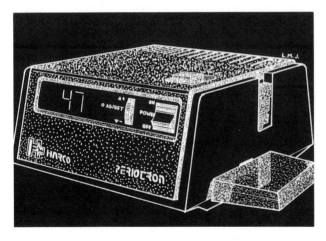

Fig. 3-5. C, Periotron used to (digitally) record volume of fluid in the sulcus by measuring "wetness" of special paper. Elevated volume indicates increased inflammation.

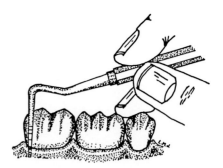

Fig. 3-5. D, Glickman periodontal Probe #26G for measuring the entire perimeter of the tooth before placing subgingival margins.

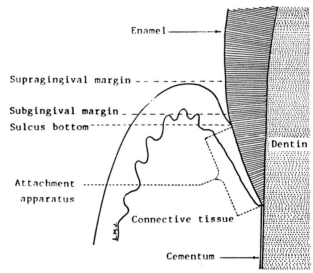

Fig. 3-6. Gingival termination in relationship to periodontal structures. The intracrevicular space is the "Bermuda Triangle" for the dentist. Supragingival margins are preferred; vertical retention, esthetics, caries, extension of former restorations, and patient pain indicate subgingival margins, but the biologic width is preserved.

cedure, the dentist should also check for bleeding or exudation, these are also signs of periodontal disease. Clinically, the bleeding of the gingiva during probing is the sign of ulceration of the sulcular epithelium.

Local anesthesia is recommended when the bony contours are probed to establish whether surgery is necessary. This is generally performed at the time of surgery before deciding the type of procedure to be performed. There are also special probes that can be used in the bifurcation or trifurcation areas.

Mobility

Mobility can be determined with the handle of the probe, also, with the handle end of the mirror, placed on the buccal and lingual surfaces and applying pressure to the tooth with the hand. The extent of mobility is then evaluated when pressure is applied. A classification of 1 to 3 is used, with 1 representing the early stage of mobility and 3 representing a tooth mobile in all directions and depressible in its socket. Mobility is an indication of the loss of the tooth's attachment

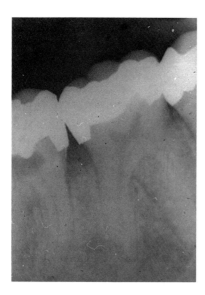

Fig. 3-7. Resorption of the alveolar crest, furcation involvement, and periapical lesion on the terminal molar. The rationale for *concomitant* caries control and interceptive periodontics is evident. Insidious diseases can be disguised in youthful patients.

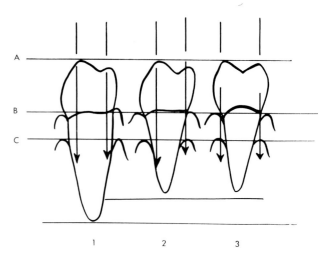

Fig. 3-8. Unfavorable distribution of functional forces associated with variations in crown-root relationship as accentuated in cases of reduced periodontal support. 1, Normal premolar. Vertical forces of occlusion fall within confines of root when support is at cementoenamel junction, B, and also when height of periodontium is reduced, C. In the first instance, the clinical crown is A-B and in the second instance A-C. 2, Premolar with normal crown and short root when periodontium is at cementoenamel line, A. However, when periodontium is reduced (C), vertical forces of occlusion fall outside root. 3, Premolar with abnormally wide crown and short root. Vertical forces of occlusion are directed beyond periphery of root when periodontium is at cementoenamel line, B, and also when level of periodontium is reduced, C. (From Glickman, I: Clinical Periodontology, ed. 4, Philadelphia, 1972, W.B. Saunders Co.)

to the jaw. This can be seen radiographically as a widened periodontal ligament space caused by occlusal trauma or orthodontic movement. It can also be caused by periodontal disease when the amount of the support has diminished sufficiently to loosen the tooth or by overloading of a tooth with restorative work. It must be emphasized that *because a tooth is mobile does not mean that the tooth will be lost*. The entire dentition can exhibit a class I mobility and sustain this form for many years without splinting. However, if the tooth is under secondary occlusal trauma, a number of teeth are splinted for the required support.

Radiographs

Radiographs are essential for diagnosis, treatment, and maintenance in periodontics. Although the radiograph is limited by being two dimensional, if it is accompanied by a three-dimensional image it can be visualized. The major consideration in examining radiographs is that the appropriate radiograph be taken. The most useful type in evaluating the tooth-to-bone relationship is the long cone technique.[19] A film positioning holder should be employed. The advantage of a holder is the ability to achieve a reproducible image that encourages comparisons.

An appropriate length of cone is necessary in obtaining radiographs to ensure their reliability as a diagnostic aid. The areas to be reviewed on the radiographs are:

1. Alveolar crest resorption (Fig. 3-7)
2. Integrity of thickness of the lamina dura
3. Evidence of generalized horizontal bone loss
4. Evidence of vertical bone loss
5. Widened periodontal ligament space
6. Density of the trabeculae of both arches
7. Size and shape of the roots compared to the crown to determine crown-to-root ratio

The radiograph can determine the area of root embedded in bone; this is crucial in determining the patient's prognosis. Often a patient with short conical roots will display minimal bone loss but maximal mobility, and the prognosis is thus guarded to poor (Fig. 3-8). Other patients can lose 50 percent of the bone but not exhibit mobility, and yet have an encouraging prognosis because they have normal-shaped roots.

Habits

The major habit to consider is bruxism (Fig. 3-9, A to D). Visual examination of wear facet patterns and x-ray interpretation of thickened laminae durae and widened periodontal ligament spaces determines whether a patient grinds during sleep. It is important to inform the patient of the condition and then reevaluate this factor later.

One condition that indicates bruxism is a complete arch that exhibits mobility despite adequate osseous support. The teeth may not have been worn from the pressure of grinding, but may have become mobile while resisting this force. Wear facets are noted in areas where a person does not normally chew, making it difficult to diagnose bruxism.

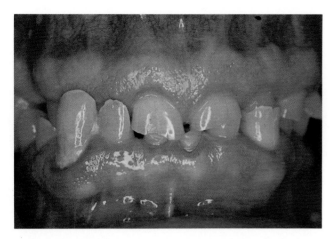

Fig. 3-9. A, Fifty-year-old male exhibiting abrasion due to prolonged exposure to commercial abrasives. (Courtesy Dr. John Graneto, St. Louis, Mo.)

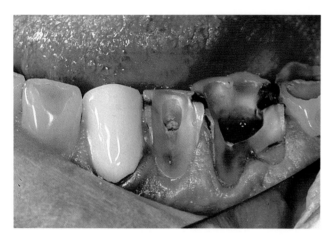

Fig. 3-9. B, Fifty-five-year-old male with dental attrition—erosion and surprisingly healthy gingiva. (Courtesy Dr. Eric Langenwalter, Alton, Ill.)

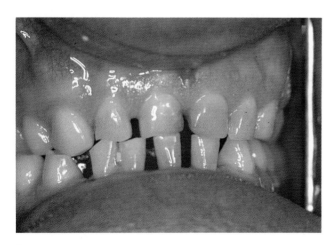

Fig. 3-9. C, Preoperative view of a forty-five-year-old male with considerable wear in the anteriors due to loss of posterior support and bruxism. (Dr. W.F.P. Malone, Alton, Ill.)

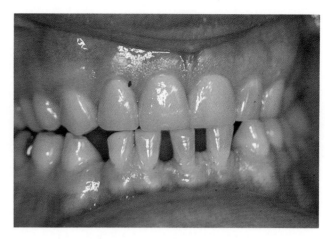

Fig. 3-9. D, Post-operative view after placement of maxillary right lateral, right central, and left central incisors with P.F.M. crowns after mandibular enameloplasty. (Dr. W.F.P. Malone, Alton, Ill.)

Preparation of Tissues

It is important from a periodontal standpoint for the patient to be informed of a problem and to be educated in the methods necessary to correct it. Ideally, this should be accomplished through a combination of audiovisual aids and reading material. After the patient has been examined and the diagnosis and prognosis established, the final course of treatment is discussed with the patient.

Treatment objectives outlined by Goldman and Cohen[20] are:

1. Pocket elimination and obviation of the inflammatory lesion.
2. Establishment of physiologic tissue contours necessary for self-cleansing and physiotherapeutic management.
   a. Thin, parabolically curved gingival margins.
   b. Pyramidal interdental papillae that conform architecturally and adapt tightly to tooth contours while permitting the free egress of food and debris from the interproximal areas. (Once surgical intervention is dictated because of existing disease, it is appropriate to eliminate the "col" form of gingiva interdentally and to substitute an occlusally convex tissue form short of the contact areas between adjacent teeth.)
   c. Rigid zone of keratinizing attached gingiva (rigidity implies density and firm attachment to tooth and bone).
   d. Sufficient depth of the vestibular fornix to allow food to escape from the vestibular and gingival area. (The musculature of the fornix, also the lips and cheeks, requires additionally the freedom of activity adequate to permit evulsion of food.)
3. Placement and modification of tooth morphology to protect the periodontium from insults.

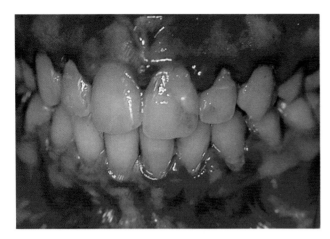

Fig. 3-10. A, Periodontitis of young adult. Professional periodontal cleaning using disclosing solutions to emphasize effective plaque control is fundamental.

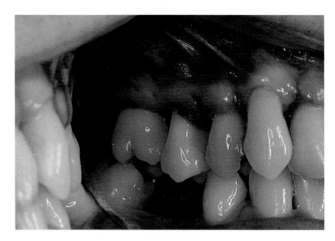

Fig. 3-10. C, Excellent post-surgical results for a young adult with osseous ramping. The patient requires orthodontic treatment prior to restorative dentistry.

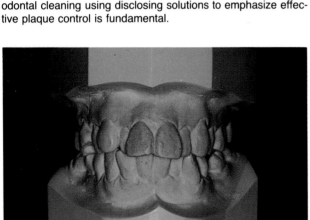

Fig. 3-10. B, Diagnostic casts are essential in demonstrating occlusal discrepancies, root proximity and esthetics.

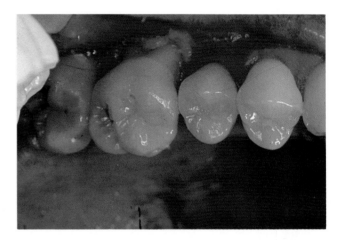

Fig. 3-10. D, Extreme bone loss of a "caries-free" adolescent. Caries free adolescents with bone loss are more numerous due to the concomitant benefits of fluoride.

4. Eradication of dysfunctional occlusal habits.
5. Tooth stabilization to protect the attaching tissues and to encourage healing.
6. Patient cooperation in the performance of preventive physiotherapeutics.

Teeth can function despite the loss of considerable investing and supporting tissues.[20]

Although these are treatment objectives, it is mandatory for the dentist to understand the patient's objectives. Consultations should be arranged with patients so they can explain their expectations.

TREATMENT PLANNING
Initial Preparation

Oral physiotherapy. The initial preparation is the teaching of oral physiotherapeutics; preparing the patient for maintaining the mouth in a healthy state. The patient must comprehend the implications of plaque, an area neglected by patients that causes most dentists to become discouraged. Full use of auxiliary personnel

will increase opportunities for patient education and make effective dental hygiene more likely.

The plaque control record by O'Leary[21] effectively demonstrates the efficiency of plaque removal on four surfaces of the tooth and allows the patient to visualize progress in a percentage form (Figs. 3-10, A to D). The patient ordinarily reaches a level of 20 to 10 percent plaque retention before surgery is performed. The average periodontal patient before hygiene instruction, starts at 90 to 80 percent.

Preparation of Oral Tissues

The second most important aspect is to have patients restore gingival tissues to a healthy condition that can then be maintained with proper instruction. The first step is scaling and curettage of the root structures, which accomplishes the following:

1. Eliminates the irritants around the attachments.
2. Smooths the root surfaces to facilitate brushing and flossing.

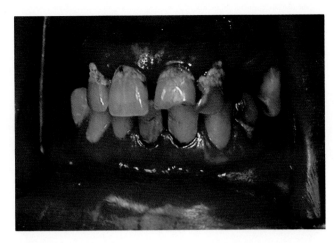

Fig. 3-11. A, Pre-treatment condition of forty-five-year-old male patient.

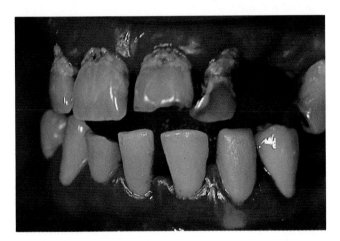

Fig. 3-11. B, Post treatment results with astringent oral hygiene instructions and repeated sealings and curettage. A maxillary complete denture was anticipated.

3. Reduces swollen tissue so it is manageable for surgery, if indicated; this may require more appointments, depending on the state of the disease (Fig. 3-11, A and B).

Scaling and curettage must be followed by:
1. Removal of hopelessly involved teeth.
2. Excavation and temporization of caries.
3. Evaluation of teeth for possible endodontic involvement. This area of periodontal diagnosis is not emphasized enough; a necrotic pulp can hinder periodontal healing.
4. Initiation of orthodontic tooth movement for selective cases.
5. Occlusal adjustment.
6. Fabrication of an acrylic occlusal night guard in cases of bruxism.
7. Reevaluation.

The entire mouth is then reevaluated with the periodontal probe to record pocket depth and to determine the necessity of surgery. If the patient has not demonstrated willingness to cooperate in oral physiotherapy, it is best to discontinue therapy and reconsider a conservative approach to maintaining the patient's teeth. When the patient is maintaining the mouth properly, the dentist may proceed to surgical correction.

Surgery

General principles. Pocket elimination and establishment of physiologic tissue contours are the prime goals. If scaling and curettage have not attained these objectives, surgery is required. To restore the patient's mouth, it is important to differentiate between different surgical techniques such as gingivectomy, mucogingival procedure, and mucoperiosteal flap entry with osseous recontouring. Ideally, the lost osseous tissue is rebuilt along with the attachment lost because of periodontal disease. In most patients we are basically reestablishing the physiologic architecture of the bone as it existed before the disease, but in an apical location.

Advanced surgical techniques. Many times heroic periodontal procedures are necessary to save a part of a tooth for restoration.
1. The mandibular molar can have one root removed as a hemisection.
2. On maxillary molars it is possible to remove the distobuccal root or the mesiobuccal root and then to restore this tooth to function, with the tooth splinted to the adjacent tooth (Fig. 3-12).
3. Bone transplantation. Since 1960[22] dentists have been attempting to add bone to osseous defects. There are many ways of accomplishing this:
   a. Swage procedures[23]
   b. Osseous coagulum procedures[24] (Fig. 3-13)
   c. Bone from recent extraction sites[25] or trephine autografts
   d. Bone from the posterior iliac crest[26] that has been removed by an orthopedic surgeon or hematologist

These procedures are only performed in selected cases where it is absolutely necessary to save the tooth. Many times, however, it is more appropriate to sacrifice the tooth if the results are not certain rather than jeopardize the restorative effort.

Final preparation of tissues
1. A final scaling, curettage, and polishing of the entire dentition to smooth the surfaces and allow the patient to maintain this area with plaque control.
2. An occlusal adjustment to eliminate interferences after surgery.
3. Relieving tooth sensitivity. Root sensitivity is a problem for the periodontal patient. Even though patients are told that more than 50 percent of the sensitivity is attributable to accumulation of bacterial products on the tooth, they

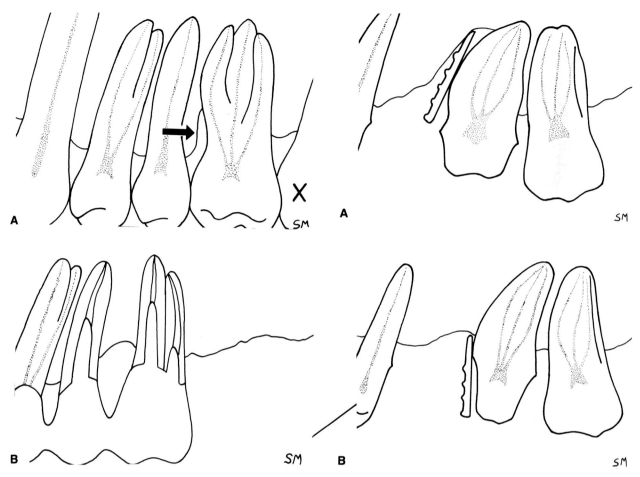

Fig. 3-12. A, Forty-two-year-old male patient with a class III furcation involvement around mesiobuccal root. Arrow, Radiolucency in this area. X marks tooth that was hopelessly involved and later extracted. **B,** Same areas but with mesiobuccal root removed and restoration in place 5 years later.

Fig. 3-13. A, Radiograph (graphic) of infraosseous defect with a Hirschfeld point in place to show apical defect. **B,** Infraosseous three-wall defect was filled with osseous coagulum, and radiograph graphic shows the fill after 8 months.

may discontinue brushing because of severe sensitivity. The areas checked are caries, traumatic occlusion, bruxism, plaque retention, and degeneration of pulpal tissue. One of the best methods of correcting sensitivity is by using an 8 percent fluoride solution with calcium phosphate burnished into the root. If this is ineffective, endodontic therapy may be indicated.

4. Reevaluation of the patient for restorative recommendations.
5. A review of oral physiotherapy techniques, which becomes necessary because of the improved condition of the patient's mouth. The patient is now ready for the restorative treatment.

PERIODONTAL ASPECT OF FIXED OCCLUSION
Occlusion and Its Effect on Periodontium

When there is an increased functional demand upon the periodontium, it commonly accommodates these forces. This adaptive capacity varies between persons

and, in the same person, varies with circumstances. The effect of occlusal forces upon the periodontium is influenced by their severity, direction, duration, and frequency.[27] When severity increases, the periodontal fibers thicken and increase and the alveolar bone becomes denser. Changing the direction of the occlusal forces changes the orientation of the periodontal ligament fibers.[20] These fibers are oriented to withstand forces in the long axis of the tooth. Horizontal or lateral forces are usually located in balancing side interferences and are deleterious to the periodontium (Fig. 3-14, A to C). Lateral forces initiate bone resorption in areas of pressure and bone formation in areas of tension[28] (Fig. 3-15).

Rotational forces cause tension and pressure on the periodontium and are the most injurious forces. The duration and frequency affect the response of the alveolar bone to occlusal forces because constant pressure on bone causes resorption, but intermittent forces promote bone formation.[29,30] Recurrent forces over short intervals have essentially the same resorb-

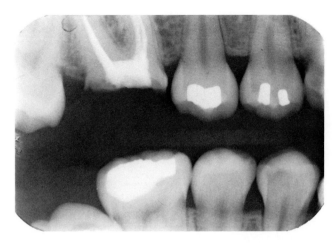

Fig. 3-14. A, Supraeruption of a maxillary first molar eventually creates mediotrusive and laterotrusive destructive contacts. Crown lengthening, osseous recontouring and coronal-radicular stabilization with non parallel posts are necessary if the mandibular tooth is retained. Complete gold veneer crowns are indicated for maxillary and mandibular molars. Restricted interocclusal space is an insurmountable problem for the restorative dentist without assistance from a periodontist and/or endodontist.

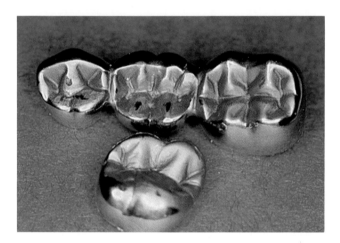

Fig. 3-14. B, Frosted (sand blasted) surface of temporarily seated cast restorations enables the patient to aid the identification of mediotrusive and laterotrusive potentially destructive contacts.

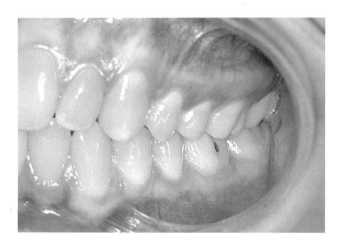

Fig. 3-14. C, Laterotrusive and mediotrusive movements require periodic clinical and radiographic review to verify an acceptable occlusion.

ing effect as constant pressure. When occlusal forces exceed the adaptive capacity of the periodontium, tissue injury results.[31-33]

Periodontal injury caused by occlusal forces is called trauma from occlusion. Occlusal traumatism does not affect the gingiva, nor does it cause bone formation. Inflammation causes horizontal bone loss.[34] However, inflammation in the presence of trauma from occlusion will alter the pathway of inflammation to allow it into the periodontal ligament space and lead to infraosseous pockets.[31] Thus trauma from occlusion does not affect the marginal gingiva, but affects the bone when inflammation is present. This is called the zone of codestruction: trauma from occlusion in the presence of inflammation[27] (Fig. 3-16). A classic example of trauma from occlusion leading to bone destruction is a poorly constructed RPD that causes gingival irritation with concomitant twisting force to the abutment tooth. When there is increased functional demand on the periodontium, this adaptive capacity varies. The principal fibers of the periodontal ligament best accommodate occlusal forces in the long axis of the tooth. With increased axial forces, there is a distortion of the periodontal ligament, compression of the periodontal fibers, and then resorption of the bone in the apical areas. Torque or rotational forces cause tension and pressure, which, under physiologic conditions, result in bone formation and resorption. Torque is the force most likely to injure the periodontium.[34]

Trauma from occlusion occurs in three stages: the first is injury, the second is repair, and the third is a change in the morphology of the periodontium. Tissue injury is produced by excessive occlusal forces. Natural repair of the injury and restoration of periodontal tissues occur if the force on the tooth diminishes or the tooth drifts away from the force. Moving away from the injurious force may result in mobility. If the force is chronic, the periodontal tissues are remolded to cushion the traumatic force: the periodontal ligament is widened at the expense of the bone, angular (vertical) bone defects occur without pockets, and the tooth becomes mobile.[33]

Occlusal Trauma in Gingivitis and Periodontal Disease

All periodontal tissues are affected by occlusion. Occlusion is a critical environmental factor in the life of the healthy periodontium and its influence expands in periodontal disease. Inflammation in the periodontal ligament cannot be separated from the influence of occlusion. Because occlusion is the constant monitor for the condition of the periodontium's health, it affects the response of the periodontium to inflammation and is a factor in periodontal disease. The role of trauma from occlusion in gingivitis and periodontitis is best understood if the periodontium is considered as having two zones, the zone of irritation and the

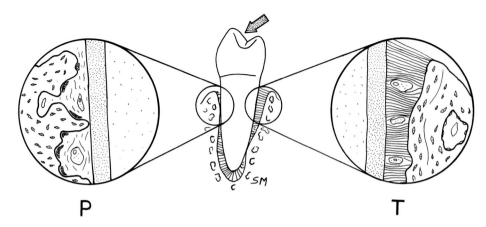

Fig. 3-15. Diagram showing center of rotation, x. P is pressure and T is tension.

zone of codestruction. The zone of irritation consists of the marginal and interdental gingiva, with its boundary formed by the gingival fibers. This is where gingivitis and periodontal pockets start.[35,36] They are caused by local irritation from plaque, bacteria, calculus, and by food impaction. With few exceptions, researchers agree that trauma from occlusion does not cause gingivitis or periodontal pockets.[37-39] In other words, such things as high restoration, orthodontic movement, or the poorly designed rest of any RPD causing tooth trauma can not lead to a periodontal pocket because the local irritants that start gingivitis and periodontal pockets affect the marginal gingiva, but trauma from occlusion affects only the supporting tissues. The marginal gingiva is not affected because its blood supply is sufficient to maintain it even when the vessels of the periodontal ligament are obliterated by excessive occlusal forces.[40] As long as the inflammation is confined to the gingiva, it is not affected by occlusal forces. When it extends from the gingiva to the supporting periodontal tissues, inflammation does enter into the zone of codestruction. The zone of codestruction begins with the transeptal fibers and consists of supporting periodontal tissues: the bone, periodontal ligament, and cementum. When inflammation reaches the supporting periodontal tissues, its pathway and the destruction it causes come under the influence of the occlusion[43] (Fig. 3-17).

In ordinary inflammation without trauma, the inflammation follows the path of least resistance. Its course is determined by the alignment of the transeptal fibers, and it goes into the crest of the bone by following a path along the circumvascular spaces[34] (Fig. 3-18, A to E). Trauma from occlusion changes the tissue environment around the inflammatory exudate in two ways: 1) it alters the alignment of the transeptal and alveolar crest fibers and thus changes the direction of the pathway of the inflammation so that it extends directly into the periodontal ligament, and 2) excessive occlusal forces produce periodontal

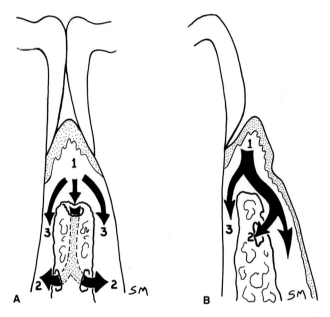

Fig. 3-16. Diagrams of pathways of inflammation. **A,** interproximal view. 1, inflammation, which passes to bone, 2, and then into periodontal ligament in inflammation, 3, pathway of inflammation with concomitant trauma from occlusion; inflammation goes directly into periodontal ligament space. **B,** Buccal view.

ligament damage and bone resorption which aggravate the tissue destruction caused by inflammation.[43] Combined with inflammation, trauma from occlusion leads to infraosseous pockets; angular (vertical), craterlike osseous defects; and excessive tooth mobility.

The response of the periodontium to the combination of inflammation and trauma from occlusion varies considerably. The inflammation may not be severe enough, or the anatomy of the tooth may not be conducive to pocket formation. In the absence of inflammation and local irritants, severe trauma from occlusion will cause excessive loosening of the teeth, widening of the periodontal ligament, and angular (vertical) defects in the alveolar bone *without pockets*.[41] Radiographic signs of trauma from occlusion are

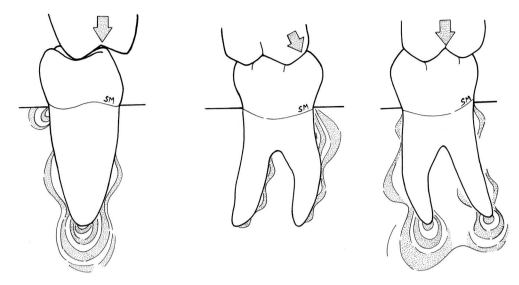

Fig. 3-17. A, A graphic depicting a photoelastic model of stress at apex when force is applied to cusp tip. **B,** A graphic depicting a photoelastic model of forces at mesial aspect of molar such as that found when mesial neighbor is removed. **C,** A graphic depicting a photoelastic model of forces at apex of root when force is in long axis of tooth.

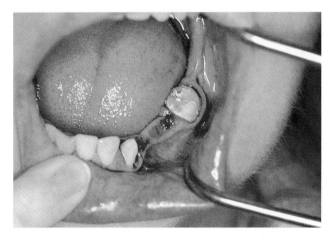

Fig. 3-18. A, Pretreatment condition of tissue after removal of a F.P.D. under traumatic occlusion. Determination of gingival margins depends upon healthy gingiva.

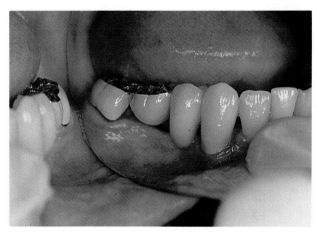

Fig. 3-18. C, Lateral view of four unit metal/ceramic F.P.D. illustrating tissue health postoperatively.

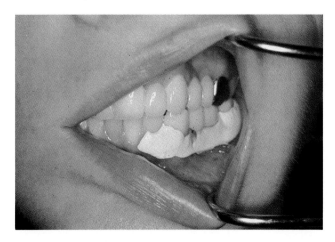

Fig. 3-18. B, Periodontal surgical pack.

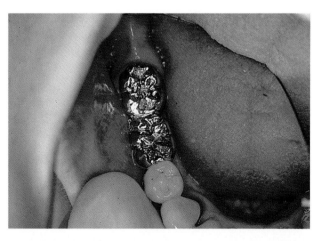

Fig. 3-18. D, Occlusal view of the four unit metal/ceramic F.P.D. (Courtesy Drs. Doug. Miley, St. Louis, Mo., Kevin Artime, Decatur, Ill. and W.F.P. Malone, Alton, Ill.)   *Continued*

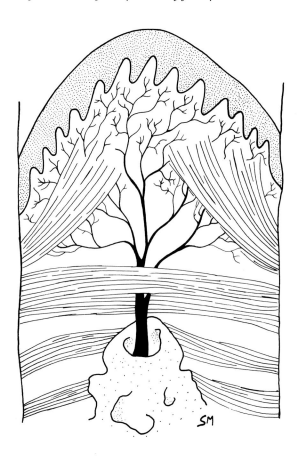

Fig. 3-18. E, Interdental area showing histologic features. Note the blood vessel passing through transseptial fibers into the crest of bone.

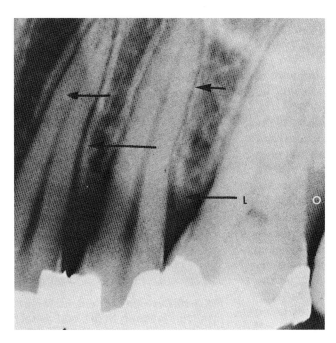

Fig. 3-19. Note widened lamina dura, arrows; trifurcation involvement, O; and loss of crestal lamina dura, L. These are classic signs of trauma from occlusion associated with inflammation.

seen in Fig. 3-19. Widening of the periodontal space, thickening of the lamina dura, and angular (vertical) bone loss can be observed rather than horizontal bone loss. The furcal area is the most sensitive to occlusal trauma.

Occlusal trauma may be caused by alterations in the occlusal forces, reduced capacity of the periodontium to withstand occlusal forces, or both. A malocclusion is not a prerequisite to trauma; it may be present when occlusion appears "normal."[42,43] Conversely, not all malocclusions are necessarily injurious to the periodontium.

Trauma from occlusion is primary or secondary. In primary occlusal trauma the forces are excessive and originate from compulsive habits such as clamping, clenching, or grinding the teeth. It is the parafunctional movements of bruxism that are significant in primary trauma from occlusion. Some other examples are "high" restorations, a prosthetic appliance that causes excessive forces on the abutment teeth or opposing teeth, orthodontic movement of teeth into functionally unacceptable positions, and the drifting of teeth into the spaces of unreplaced missing teeth.[40]

Secondary periodontal traumatism occurs from normal forces such as mastication, but the support of the tooth is weakened by the loss of a portion of its attachment apparatus and it cannot withstand normal forces. Pressure from mastication is short and light, and occurs infrequently during the day. Swallowing occurs frequently but is also only a light contact. Bruxism and other parafunctional habits appear to be the major cause of excessive traumatic forces in a twisting manner,[44,45] along with hastily constructed FPDs that violate prosthodontic guidelines and RPDs that exert excessive stress upon abutments.

Place of Margins of Restoration

Except for the risk of subgingival decay and esthetic considerations, it is best to terminate preparations above the gingival margin. If periodontal therapy has been performed and the gingiva has receded, the preparations should end at the cementoenamel junction. Even if the tissue does not recede, the margin of the tooth preparation should be away from the soft tissue.

Crown margins, when placed subgingivally, should be located at the base of the gingival sulcus,[46,47] which is the level reached when a thin blunt probe is positioned without pressure into the gingival sulcus. The gingival fibers can then brace the gingiva against the tooth and the margin of the completed restoration.

The margins of the preparation are not usually placed at the crest of the marginal gingiva, regardless of how precise the margins of the restoration (Fig. 3-20). Microscopically, the margin is rough and an excellent site to harbor bacteria. Since the margin of the gingiva rapidly collects plaque, this is the site of re-

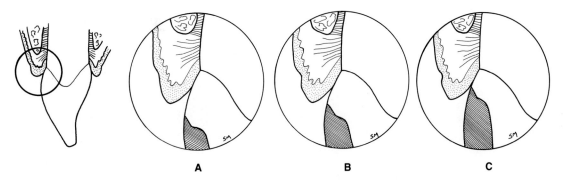

Fig. 3-20. The gingival termination of the tooth can be established: **A,** Above the gingival crest. **B,** At the gingival crest. **C,** Within the intracrevicular space.

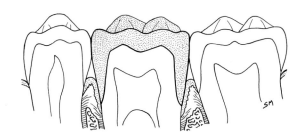

Fig. 3-21. Complete gold veneer crown within the epithelial attachment violating the biologic width.

current decay.[27] If decay does not result, the plaque causes periodontal disease at this most critical area which is not self-cleansing.

Conversely, restorations should not be forced subgingivally into the connective tissue, but placed in the intracrevicular space without violating biologic width. Tearing of the epithelial attachment causes it to migrate apically and the sulcus to deepen into a pocket (Fig. 3-21).

Biologic Width Embrasures

The teeth touch in an area called a proximal contact, the spaces below the contact are known as embrasures. In health, the embrasures are usually filled with tissue (Fig. 3-22). Embrasures protect the gingiva from food impaction and deflect the food to massage the gingival surface. They provide spillways for food during mastication and relieve occlusal forces when resistant food is chewed.

The proximal surfaces of dental restorations are important because they determine the embrasures essential for gingival health. In disease and periodontal therapy this tissue is reduced; the new restorations create another embrasure that will locate the restorations close to the new level of the gingiva. The proximal surfaces of crowns should taper away from the contact areas on all surfaces (Fig. 3-23, A and B). Excessively broad proximal contact areas and inadequate contour in the cervical areas surpress the gingival papillae. These prominent papillae trap food de-

bris, leading to gingival inflammation. Proximal contacts that are too narrow buccolingually create enlarged embrasures without sufficient protection against interdental food impaction.

Pontic Design in Fixed Prosthesis

Pontic design and construction is a controversial subject that is complicated by an array of confusing terms, an abundance of opinions, and lack of extensive research. A pontic is important to a FPD because it alters the functional and environmental demands directed onto the teeth and the ridge. Any factor acting on any part of the fixed restoration affects the entire prosthesis. The pontic mechanically unifies the abutment teeth, covers the residual ridge, assumes a dynamic role in the prosthesis, and is not considered to be a lifeless insert of material.[48-72] In this role the pontic restores the function of the missing tooth, ensures adequate sanitation, and is esthetically pleasing, comfortable, and biologically tolerable. Pontics are discussed in Chapter 18.

SPLINTING

Past explanations of splinting have been misleading and controversial. It has three purposes: 1) to protect loose teeth from injury during stabilization in a favorable occlusal relationship; 2) to distribute occlusal forces for teeth weakened by loss of periodontal support; and 3) to prevent a natural tooth from migrating. The number of teeth required to stabilize a loose tooth depends on the degree and direction of mobility, the remaining bone, the location of the mobile tooth, and designated function, i.e., whether it is to be used as an abutment tooth.

Reducing mesiodistal mobility is easier than reducing buccolingual mobility because of the approximating teeth that aid tooth support. In the reduction of buccolingual mobility, greater reliance is placed on nonmobile teeth in the splint. It is advisable to use more than one firm tooth to stabilize a mobile tooth. The more mobile the tooth, the greater the number of stable teeth required in the splint. The exact number required to splint the tooth varies with conditions.

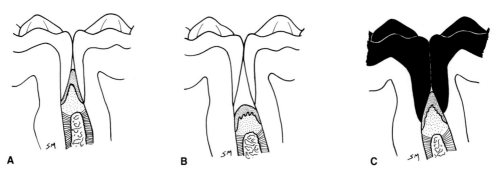

Fig. 3-22. A, Normal embrasure filled with tissue. **B,** Embrasure after periodontal surgery. **C,** Restructured crown shape restoring original embrasure.

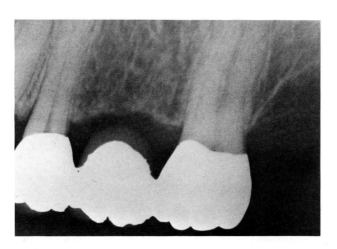

Fig. 3-23. A, Radiograph of a maxillary FPD with adequate margins, contour and embrasures. (Dr. W.F.P. Malone, Alton, Ill.)

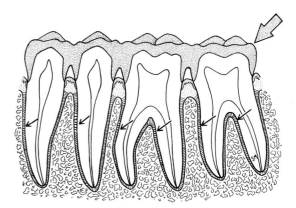

Fig. 3-24. Diagram showing how adverse force on splinted quadrant transmits force to all the teeth.

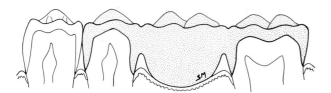

Fig. 3-23. B, Three-unit mandibular FPD with suitable embrasures and occlusal plane.

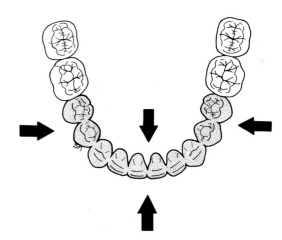

Fig. 3-25. Cross-arch splinting can withstand forces in all directions, but torquing of the mandible during opening must be considered.

If an FPD is used to replace missing teeth while stabilizing natural teeth, the following should be noted: When the distal abutment of an FPD is mobile, multiple firm anterior abutments are required because the splinting is only an added mechanical factor; it should be combined with redesign of the crown surfaces and in occlusal harmony with mandibular movements (Fig. 3-24).

Splinting refers to any joining together of two or more teeth for stabilization. Single or multiple mobile teeth with sufficient bone and evidence of parafunctional habits are rarely splinted. Occlusal correction and the construction of an appliance precede splinting. If the destructive forces are modified, the mobile teeth become firm. If the mobile teeth are splinted to ad-jacent teeth without correction of the occlusal traumatism or parafunctional habits, the entire splint can become unstable. Splinting is not recommended as the sole treatment for occlusal trauma mobility.

If splinting is required, it can redirect the offending forces. Splinting "around the corner" expands the base in two directions and redirects mesiodistal and buc-

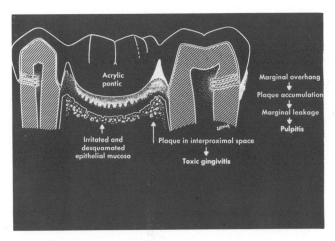

Fig. 3-26. A, Heat-cured acrylic treatment restorations are necessary for a favorable tissue response after F.P.D. preparation, but prolonged placement is undesirable. (Courtesy Dr. Maury Massler, Boston, Ma.)

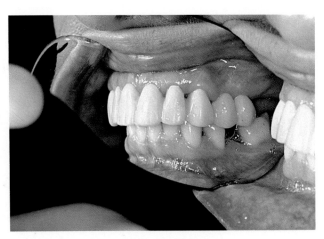

Fig. 3-26. B, Anterior long span treatment restoration with appropriate embrasures and occlusion (Courtesy Dr. Ted Sewitch, NY, NY)

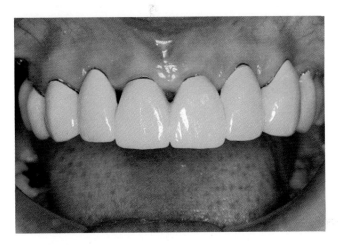

Fig. 3-26. C, Post surgical restoration of the anterior teeth with a F.P.D. splint creating exaggerated embrasures of the metal/ceramic abutment teeth (Dr. W.F.P. Malone, Alton, Ill.)

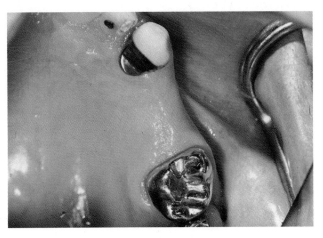

Fig. 3-26. D, Post-surgical insertion of complete crowns for R.P.D. The guide planes and rests are placed *within* the tooth preparations to minimize overcontouring while providing undercuts. This perceptive procedure avoids the labeling of RPDs as "chrome wonders" or "plaque traps". (Dr. W.F.P. Malone, Alton, Ill.)

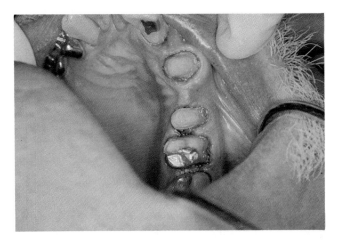

Fig. 3-26. E, Tissue management with "Ultra Cord" and improved astringents will afford predictable recovery of the tissue with smoother, more accurate margins. (Drs. Betsy Tedman and W.F.P. Malone, Alton, Ill.)

colingual forces (Fig. 3-25). Stress redirection permits effective treatment with minimal bone support. When teeth are joined together, any force on an individual tooth is redistributed to all of the splinted teeth. Root surfaces that resist stresses poorly in one direction may provide surprising resistance in another. Thus the combined effect of splinting weak teeth capitalizes on the strengths of individual teeth transferred to the group. Splinting also prevents teeth from migrating and supererupting.

If increased mobility is accelerating, this increasing mobility should be interrupted by joining teeth in a splint. The purpose of splinting is to completely eliminate mobility or at least to prevent its increase. Gradually increasing mobility (indicating the presence of extraction forces) can not be tolerated. Mobility that has increased but then stabilized can be tolerated,

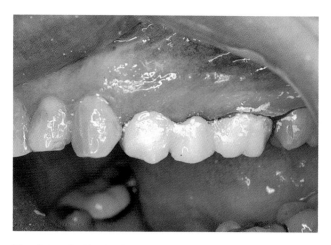

Fig. 3-27. A, Hastily fabricated "temporary" without adequate embrasures, etc.

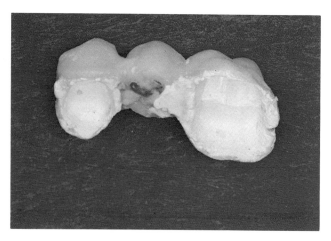

Fig. 3-27. B, "Temporary" in 3-27 A illustrating unfavorable tissue response.

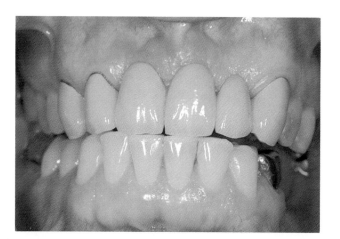

Fig. 3-27. C, Six unit, three abutment metal/ceramic F.P.D. with beveled shoulders and metal collars. Esthetic lip/smile lines were determined prior to preparation (Drs. Kevin Artime, Decatur, Ill. and W.F.P. Malone, Alton, Ill.)

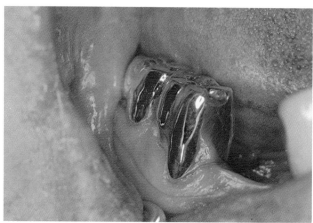

Fig. 3-27. D, Splinted, completed gold veneer crowns with guide planes, rests, facial flutes, .010 undercuts and monoplane occlusal anatomy that maintain the embrasures. (Drs. W.F.P. Malone, Alton, Ill. and Donald Lonergan, Jacksonville, Ill.)

provided that the periodontal tissues are healthy and the mobility only reflects a physiologic adaptation to the function.

Splinting Methods

Splinting may be classified as temporary or reversible, provisional, and permanent. Temporary splinting may or may not be followed with permanent splinting (Fig. 3-26, A to E). Some methods of reversible splinting are ligature wire, A-splint or circumferential wiring, removable appliances, and bonding.[73,75] The first two methods are rarely used and involve wrapping wire around the teeth, tying it in an intricate fashion, and then covering it with acrylic. Removable appliances include the Hawley retainer (after orthodontics) and a continuous clasp RPD. A swing-lock RPD is rare because it can be damaging and costly. It is used, however, for medically compromised patients.

Splinting by bonding

Newer materials have made splinting teeth easier. The composite resins have greater strength, and light-cured bonding permits better control of contours. Temporary splinting is accomplished with the composite material alone or in combination with extracoronal and intracoronal wires or screen meshes. Permanent splinting can also be performed with resin-bonded retainers (Maryland bridges) or bars and plates.

Provisional splinting with full-coverage acrylics.

This method is commonly used with periodontally compromised patients where there is a commitment to fixed splints after periodontal therapy. Before periodontal treatment, the teeth are prepared and heat processed acrylic treatment restorations are constructed and cemented with sedative cements (Fig. 3-27, A to D). These splints are then removed, peri-

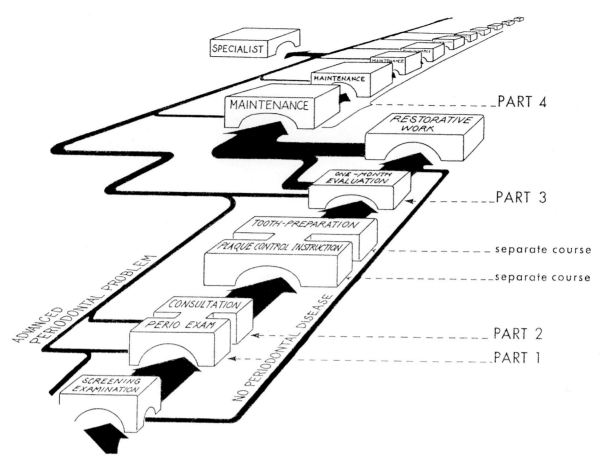

Table 3-2. Interspecialty Treatment Planning (courtesy Dr. Robert Parr)

odontal therapy performed, and the interim splints replaced. When tissue has healed and "matured" after surgery, cast splints are inserted.

Determination of abutments

Many factors are considered before abutment selection. The first is the crown-to-root ratio, because tooth stability is influenced by the leverage exerted upon the periodontium. The nature of this leverage depends on the amount of tooth retained in bone (clinical root). Increases in the length of the crown create unfavorable leverage upon the periodontium. The root can be short because of normal anatomy, orthodontic movement, bone loss, or a combination of these factors.

There are two methods of modifying the tooth form to change the unfavorable crown-to-root ratio. One is the construction of a complete crown; the other method is to change the occlusal surface of the tooth with an onlay. Lateral and tipping stresses arise during function when the cuspal inclines are steep or the occlusal topography is too broad.[76] Ideally, forces applied to the tooth fall within the periphery of the root structure in bone. In the mandible, this force is transmitted to the root by the buccal cusps. The location

of the cusp in relation to the root in the buccolingual direction influences the direction of the transmitted force upon the periodontium.[71] If the direction of the functional forces falls within the lateral borders of the clinical root, stress is directed vertically upon the periodontium.[77] Conversely, if the force is directed beyond the confines of the root, tipping stresses are induced. In most instances, the reduction in the length of the clinical crown changes the cuspal position, and modification of the cuspal inclines can be accomplished simultaneously with an artificial crown. Narrowing the buccolingual width of the occlusal surfaces of the reconstructed crowns encourages a more desirable location for the mandibular buccal and maxillary lingual (stamp) cusps in relation to the root.[78]

Teeth normally have a certain range of mobility, and one-rooted teeth are more mobile than multiple-rooted teeth. Mobility is usually in a horizontal direction, and it also occurs axially, but to a much lesser degree. Mobility beyond the physiologic range is termed "pathologic" and is attributable to: loss of alveolar bone or periodontal ligament support and severe trauma from occlusion. The mobility depends on the severity and distribution of the tissue lost on individual surfaces, the length and shape of the roots, and the root size compared with the crown. A tooth with short-tapered roots is more likely to be mobile than one with normal or bulbous roots with identical bone loss. The degree of mobility does <u>not</u> correspond to the amount of bone loss. Trauma caused by excessive occlusal forces and abnormal occlusal forces, aggravated by emotional stress, is a common cause of tooth mobility. Hypofunction, acute inflammation, pregnancy, and periodontal surgery increase mobility. Restoring tooth stability is inversely proportional to the extent of the alveolar bone loss.

Determining prognosis

Alveolar bone should be examined radiographically and three aspects should be considered: 1) the amount of remaining bone; 2) the distribution of the remaining bone; and 3) the pattern of bone loss. Obviously, the prognosis becomes less favorable as bone support diminishes. If bone loss extends to the apical third of the tooth, the prognosis is usually unfavorable. The prognosis varies as the distribution of the bone varies. If the bone is unevenly distributed around the tooth, but at least one third of the bone remains around the area of the greatest destruction, the prognosis is more favorable than if a similar amount of bone is distributed equally around the tooth.

The pattern of bone loss is also important. If the bony defect is surrounded by bone and a tooth surface, as in a three-walled infraosseous defect, there is greater chance for restoring bone than in a one-walled defect. Generally, the more bone that is around the defect, the better the prognosis. The dentist must observe the number of remaining teeth, their size, the shape of the crown and roots, and the crown-root ratio. It is also important to examine the roots to determine if they are within the bony housing; a tooth may appear radiographically to have bone on all sides, but a review of the arch position of the tooth might reveal that the tooth is in buccoversion without a bony housing on the buccal surface. Buccally, only gingiva soft tissue may cover the root. This is called a *dehiscence* and is common in teeth that are prominent in the arch: cuspids, maxillary and mandibular first premolars, mesiobuccal roots of the maxillary first molars, and also other teeth moved (after orthodontics) into a buccal position.

Maintenance

The primary goal of periodontal therapy is to establish optimal plaque control and prevent inflammation that promotes loss of periodontal attachment. This requires considerable effort from the patient in retaining a thorough program of home care. The dentist should scale and root plane at least every 3 months, continually monitor the patient's periodontal health, and motivate the patient to perform acceptable home care. This progressional assistance by the dentist and the hygienist is maintenance therapy (Table 3-2).

It has been suggested that the loss of periodontal support in population groups of the same age proceeds at almost the same rate in individuals who receive regular "traditional" dental care and in individuals who visit the dentist sporadically. The reason is that "traditional" dental care does not adequately emphasize plaque control with scaling and root planing.

The rate of periodontal breakdown and loss of the teeth has been estimated at between 0.001 and 0.04 mm per year. Available information indicates that loss of attachment over extended periods depends primarily upon the level of oral hygiene but also upon other measures taken to reduce the accumulation of plaque. In longitudinal studies on the effects of various modalities of periodontal therapy, Ramfjord recorded an annual loss of 0.04 mm per year even with professional tooth cleaning, polishing, and oral hygiene instruction *every 3 months!*

The success of fixed prosthodontics is measured by the longevity and durability of the prosthesis in healthy function. To achieve success, the fixed prosthesis should be biologically acceptable to the gingival tissues. The biologic principles involved are broad and all encompassing: 1) cleansability; 2) allowance for normal tissue shape and contour; 3) harmonious occlusion with the adaptive capacity of the periodontium; and 4) following the principles of occlusion in direction, duration, amount, and frequency of a force. It is also critical to diagnose subtle periodontal problems. Only in this manner can one proceed with confidence to construct a durable fixed prosthesis.

SELECTED REFERENCES

1. Gargiulo, A., Wentz, F.M., and Orban, B.J.: Dimensions and relations of the dento-gingival junction in humans, J. Periodontol. **32:**261, 1961.
2. Oliver, R.C., Holm-Pedersen, P., and Löe, H.: The correlation between clinical scoring, exudate measurements and microscopic evaluation of inflammation in the gingiva, J. Periodontol. **40:**201-209, April 1969.
3. Brill, N., and Krasse, B.: The passage of tissue fluid into the clinically healthy gingival pockets, Acta Odontol. Scand. **16:**233, 1958.
4. Grant, D., Stern, I., and Everett, P.: Orban's Periodontics, ed. 4, St. Louis, 1972, The C.V. Mosby Co., p. 206.
5. Ibid., p. 230.
6. Russell, A.L.: International nutrition surveys: a summary of preliminary dental findings, J. Dent. Res. **42:**233, 1963.
7. Löe, H., Theilade, E., and Jensen, S.P.: Experimental gingivitis in man, J. Periodontol. **36:**177, 1965.
8. Theilade, E., Wright, W.H., Jenson S.B., and Löe, H.: Experimental gingivitis in man. II. A longitudinal, clinical and bacteriological investigation, J. Periodont. Res. **1:**1, 1966.
9. Nisengard, R.: Immediate hypersensitivity and periodontal disease, J. Periodontol. **45:**344, 1974.
10. Ivanyi, L., Wilton, J.M.A., and Lehner, T.: Cell mediated immunity in periodontal disease; cytotoxicity, migration inhibition and lymphocyte transformation studies, Immunology **22:**141, 1972.

11. Brandtzaeg, P.: Local factors of resistance in the gingival area. J. Periodont. Res. **1**:19-42, 1966.
11a. Brandtzaeg, P.: Immunology of inflammatory periodontal lesions, Int. Dent. J. **23**:438, 1973.
12. MacKenzie, R.S., and Millard, H.D.: Interrelated effect of diabetes, arteriosclerosis and calculus on alveolar bone loss, J.A.D.A. **66**:191, 1963.
13. Wiener, R., Karshan, M., and Tenenbaum, B.: Ovarian function in periodontosis, J. Dent. Res. **35**:875, 1956.
14. Selye, H.: The general adaptation syndrome and the diseases of adaptation, J. Clin. Endo. 1950.
15. Chawla, T.N., and Glickman, I.: Protein deprivation and the periodontal structures of the albino rat, Oral Surg. **4**:578, 1951.
16. See reference 14.
17. Horton, L.: Requirement for macrophage-lymphocyte interaction, J. Dent. Res. **53**:337, 1974.
18. Macapanpan, L.C., and Weinmann, J.P.: The influence of injury to the periodontal membrane on the spread of gingival inflammation, J. Dent. Res. **33**:263, 1954.
19. Updegrave, W.J.: Simplifying and improving intraoral dental roentgenography, Oral Surg. **12**:704, 1959.
20. Goldman, H., and Cohen, D.W.: Periodontal therapy, ed. 5, St. Louis, 1973, The C.V. Mosby Co.
21. O'Leary, T.: Plaque control record, J. Periodontol. **43**:38, 1972.
22. Pritchard, J.: A technique for treating infrabony pockets based on alveolar process morphology. Dent. Clin North Am., p. 85, March 1960.
23. Ewen, S.J.: Bone swaging, J. Periodontol. **36**:57, 1956.
24. Robinson, R.E.: The osseous coagulum for bone induction technique, J. Calif. Dent. Assoc. **46**:18-27, Spring 1970.
25. Shellow, R.A., and Ratcliffe, P.A.: The problems of attaining new alveolar bone after periodontal surgery, J. West. Soc. Periodont. **15**:514, 1967.
26. Shallhorn, R.G.: Eradication of bifurcation defects utilizing frozen autogenous hip marrow implants, Periodontol Abstr. **15**:101, 1967.
27. Glickman, I.: Clinical periodontology, ed. 4, Philadelphia, 1972, W.B. Saunders Co., p. 329.
28. Glickman, I., Roeber, R.F., Brion, M., and Pameijers, J.: Photoclastic analysis of internal stresses in the periodontium created by occlusal forces, J. Periodontol. **41**:30-35, 1970.
29. Thurow, R.C.: The periodontal membrane in function, Angle Orthodont. **15**:18-29, 52-66, 1945.
30. Massoni, J., Gonzales, V., Haskel, E., and Sales, G.: Effect of traumatic forces applied on the molars of the rat, Odontológica Uruguaya **20**:5, 1964.
31. Glickman, I., and Weiss, L.: Role of trauma from occlusion in initiation of periodontal pocket formation in experimental animals, J. Periodontol. **26**:14, 1955.
32. Itoiz, M.E., Carranza, F.A., Jr., and Cabrini, R.L.: Histologic and histometric study of experimental occlusal trauma in rats, J. Periodontol. **34**:305, 1963.
33. See reference 18.
34. Orban, B.: Tissue changes in traumatic occlusion, J.A.D.A. **15**:2090, 1928.
35. Weinmann, J.P.: Progress of gingival inflammation into the supporting structures of the teeth, J. Periodontol, **12**:71, 1941.
36. Skillen, W.C., and Reitan, K.: Tissue changes following rotation of teeth in the dog, Angle Orthodont. **10**:149, 1940.
37. Bhaskar, S.N., and Orban, B.J.: Experimental occlusal trauma. J. Periodontol. **26**:270, 1955.
38. Stones, H.H.: An experimental investigation into the association of traumatic occlusion with periodontal disease, Proc. Roy Soc. Med. **31**:479, 1938.
39. Box, H.K.: Experimental traumatogenic occlusion in sheep. Oral Health **20**:642, 1930.
40. Glickman, I., Stein, R.S., and Smulow, J.B.: The effects of increased functional forces upon the periodontium of splinted and nonsplinted teeth, J. Periodontol. **32**:290, 1961.
41. Ramfjord, S.P., and Kohler, C.A.: Periodontal reaction to functional occlusal stress, J. Periodontol. **30**:95, 1959.
42. Goldman, H.: Gingival vascular supply in induced occlusal traumatism, Oral Surg. **9**:939, 1956.
43. Glickman, I., and Smulow, J.B.: Alterations in the pathway of gingival inflammation into the underlying tissues induced by excessive occlusal forces, J. Periodontol. **33**:7, 1962.
44. McCall, J.O.: Traumatic occlusion, J.A.D.A. **26**:519, 1939.
45. Robinson, J., Reding, G., Zepelin, H., Smith, V., and Zimmerman, S.: Nocturnal teeth-grinding: a reassessment for dentistry, J.A.D.A. **78**:1308, 1969.
46. Hirshberg, S.M.: Compatible temporary tooth health and gingival protection, J. Prosthet. Dent. **18**:151, 1967.
47. Waerhaug, J.: Tissue reactions around artificial crowns, J. Periodontol. **24**:172, 1953.
48. Boyd, J.R., Jr.: Pontics in fixed partial dentures, J. Prosthet. Dent. **5**:55, Jan. 1955.
49. Eissmann, H.F., Radke, R.A. and Noble, W.H.: Physiologic design criteria for fixed dental restorations, Dent. Clin. North Am. **15**:543, July 1971.
50. Harmon, C.B.: Pontic design, J. Prosthet. Dent. **8**:496, May 1958.
51. Hobo, S., and Shillingburg, H.T., Jr.: Porcelain fused to metal: tooth preparation and coping design. J. Prosthet. Dent. **30**:28, July 1973.
52. Allison, J.R., and Bliatia, H.L.: Tissue changes under acrylic and porcelain pontics, J. Dent. Res. Abstr. **37**:66, Feb. 1958.
53. Cavazos, E., Jr.: Tissue response to fixed partial denture pontics, J. Prosthet. Dent. **20**:143, Aug. 1968.
54. Coelho, D.H.: Pontic construction and assemblage, J. 2nd Dist. Dent. Soc. (N.Y.) **32**:162-168, April 1946.
55. Podshadley, A.G.: Gingival response to pontics, J. Prosthet. Dent. **19**:51-57, Jan. 1968.
56. Clayton, J.A., and Green, E.: Roughness of pontic materials and dental plaque, J. Prosthet. Dent. **23**:407, April 1970.
57. Adams, J.D.: Planning posterior bridges, J.A.D.A. **53**:647, Dec. 1956.
58. Gade, E.: Hygienic problems of fixed restorations, Int. Dent. J. **13**:318, June 1963.
59. Pine, B.: Pontics for gold-acrylic resin fixed partial dentures, J. Prosthet. Dent. **12**:347, 1962.
60. Stein, R.S.: Pontic residual ridge relationship: a research report, J. Prosthet. Dent. **16**:251, March-April 1966.
61. Wing, G.: Pontic design and construction in fixed bridgework, Dent. Pract. Dent. Rec. **12**:390, July 1962.
62. Masterson, J.B.: Recent trends in the design of pontics and retainers, Dent. Pract. Dent. Rec. **15**:131, Dec. 1964.
63. Swartz, M., and Philips, R.W.: Comparison of bacterial accumulations on rough and smooth enamel surfaces. J. Periodontol. **28**:304, Oct. 1957.
64. Waerhaug, J.: Effect of rough surfaces upon gingival tissues, J. Dent. Res. **35**:323, April 1956.
65. Kayser, A.F.: The gingival design of the pontic, Oral Res. Abstr. **5**:162, Feb. 1970.
66. Perel, M.L.: A modified sanitary pontic, J. Prosthet. Dent. **28**:589, Dec. 1972.
67. Meyers, G.E.: Textbook of crown and bridge prosthodontics, St. Louis, 1969, The C.V. Mosby Co.
68. Krajicek, D.D.: Periodontal consideration for prosthetic patients, J. Prosthet. Dent. **30**:15, July 1973.
69. Klaffenbach, A.O.: Biomechanical restoration and maintenance of the permanent first molar space, J.A.D.A. **45**:633, Dec. 1952.
70. Anderson, D.J., and Picton, D.C.: Masticatory stresses in normal and modified occlusion, J.Dent. Res. **37**:312, April 1958.

71. Ramfjord, S.P., and Ash, M.M.: Occlusion, ed. 2, Philadelphia, 1971, W.B. Saunders Co.

72. Morris, M.L.: Artificial crown contours and gingival health, J. Prosthet. Dent. **12**:1146, Nov.-Dec. 1962.

73. Hirschfeld, L.: The use of wire and silk ligatures, J.A.D.A. **41**:647, 1950.

74. Obin, J.N., and Arvens, A.N.: The use of self-curing resin splints for the temporary stabilization of mobile teeth due to periodontal involvement, J.A.D.A. **42**:320, 1951.

75. Block, P.: A wire band splint for immobilizing loose posterior teeth, J. Periodontol. **39**:17, 1968.

76. Pugh, C.E., and Smerke, J.W.: Rationale for fixed prosthesis in the management of advanced periodontal disease, Dent. Clin. North Am. **13**:243, 1969.

77. Glickman, I.: Role of occlusion in the etiology and treatment of periodontal disease, J. Dent. Res. **50**:199, 1971.

78. Burch, J.G.: Ten rules for developing crown contours in restorations, Dent. Clin North Am. **15**:611, 1971.

BIBLIOGRAPHY

Abrams, K., Canton, J., and Polson, A.: Histologic comparisons of interproximal gingival tissues related to the presence or absence of bleeding, J. Periodontol. 55-629-632, 1984.

Chambers, D., et al.: Aspartate aminotransferase increases in crevicular fluid during experimental periodontitis in beagle dogs, J. Periodontol. 55-526-530, 1984.

Davenport, R.H. Jr., Simpson, D.M., and Hassell, T.M.: Histometric comparison of active and inactive lesions of advanced periodontitis, J. Periodontol. **53**(5):285-295, 1982.

Goodson, J.M., Haffajee, A.D., and Socransky, S.S.: The relationship between attachment level loss and alveolar bone loss, J. Clin. Periodontol. **11**(5):348-359, 1984.

Greenstein, G.: The role of bleeding upon probing in the diagnosis of periodontal disease, J. Periodontol. **55**:684-688, 1984.

Greenstein, B., Caton, J., and Polson, A.M.: Histologic characteristics associated with bleeding after probing and visual signs of inflammation, J. Periodontol. **52**(8):420-425, 1981.

Haffajee, A.D., Socransky, S.S., and Goodson, J.M.: Comparison of different data analyses for detecting changes in attachment level, J. Clin. Periodontol. **10**(3):298-310, 1983.

Haffajee, A.D., Socransky, S.S., and Goodson, J.M.: Clinical parameters as predictors of destructive periodontal disease activity, J. Clin. Periodontol. **10**(3):257-265, 1983.

Hancock, E.B.: Determinations of periodontal disease activity, J. Periodontol. **52**(9):492-499, 1981.

Keyes, P., Wright, W., and Howard, S.: The use of phase-contrast microscopy and chemotherapy in the diagnosis and treatment of periodontal lesions—an initial report, Quintessence Int. **9**(1-2):51-76, 1978.

Kornman, K.: Microbiologic etiology of periodontal disease, Compend. Cont. Ed. (suppl. 7), 1986.

Loesche, W., et al: Treatment of periodontal infections due to anaerobic bacteria with short-term treatment with metronidazole, J. Clin. Periodontol. **8**:29-44, 1981.

Malone, W.F.P., Porter, Z.C., and Jameson, L.M.: Tooth preparation of periodontally comprised dentitions, Ill. State Dent. J. **53**:228, July/Aug, 1984.

Malone, W.F.P., Porter, Z.C.: Tissue management, Littleman, Mass., P.S.G. Publishers, Oct. 1982.

Morrison, E.C., et al: The significance of gingivitis during the maintenance phase of periodontal treatment, J. Periodontol. **53**(1):31-34, 1982.

Ortman, L.F., McHenry, K., and Hausmann, E.: Relationship between alveolar bone measured by R51 absorptiometry with analysis of standardized radiographs. In Bjorn technique, chap 2. J. Periodontol. **53**(5):3110-3145, 1982.

Peros W.J., et al: Rapid microbiologic tests as an adjunct to the diagnoses of periodontal disease, Compendium IX, 234-241 3/1988.

Reed, B., and Polson, A.: Relationship between bitewing and periapical radiographs in assessing crestal alveolar bone levels, J. Periodontol. **55**:22-27, 1984.

Slots, J., et al: The effects of scaling and root planing and of systemic tetracycline therapy on the subgingival microflora in patients with periodontal disease, J. Periodontol. Res. **14**:251-252, 1979.

Socransky, S.S.: Lecture—active destructive periodontal diseases, Atlanta, Am. Acad. of Periodontology, annual meeting, 1983.

Socransky, S.S., et al: New concepts of destructive periodontal disease, J. Clin. Periodontol. **11**:21-32, 1984.

Tanner, A., et al: A study of the bacteria associated with advancing periodontitis in man, J. Clin. Periodontol. **6**(5):278-307, 1979.

Wolf, L., Bakdash, B., and Bandt, C.: Microbial interpretation of plaque relative of the diagnosis and treatment of periodontal disease, J. Periodontol. **56**:281-284, 1985.

4

Donald H. Newell, Steven M. Morgano, and Robert F. Baima

FIXED PROSTHODONTICS WITH PERIODONTALLY COMPROMISED DENTITIONS

The dentist faces special problems in patients with a history of periodontitis requiring crowns or FPD's to restore carious or missing teeth. These problems include poor crown-to-root ratios, esthetic compromise, furcation invasions, progressive tooth mobility and migration, inadequate zones of attached gingiva, and prominent root concavities.[1]

If the patient is treated periodontally by one dentist and prosthodontically by another, it is critical to maintain a closely coordinated approach to treatment. This is accomplished by joint consultation; preferably after cause-related periodontal therapy,[2] when the patient's motivation, ability to remove the bacterial plaque, and the healing response to root planing can be assessed. Joint decisions are then made regarding questionable teeth, and a treatment sequence formulated that allows timely replacement of missing teeth or extractions.

PERIODONTAL SPLINTS
Contraindications

Early and moderate periodontitis. Most patients with moderate periodontitis, having only slight or no clinically detectable mobility after periodontal treatment, do not require fixed splints. This is because they still possess adequate hard and soft tissue attachment. Any pretreatment or residual posttreatment mobility in these cases is commonly attributable to periodontal inflammation, adaptation to excessive occlusal forces, or both.[3-6] Adaptive changes leading to increased mobility in the healthy tooth subjected to excessive functional forces are termed "primary occlusal traumatism."[7] In this situation bone resorption occurs along the periodontal ligament (PDL) and occasionally at the crest of the alveolar process, resulting in widening of the PDL.[8,9] Once the PDL widens to the point that the traumatic forces are nullified, no further resorption and widening occurs; detectable tooth mobility will stop increasing. Radiographs may exhibit angular osseous defects if the PDL widening is extensive. Probing attachment levels will not reveal loss of attachment in these situations, since the supra-alveolar connective tissue attachment has been unaffected, without apical downgrowth of the junctional epithelium.[8,9] The mobility is considered physiologic if it is *increased*, but not *increasing*, and does not impair function or cause patient discomfort.[10,11] As such, it is reversible once the source of the traumatic forces has been removed.[9] Lindhe described these conditions as follows:[12]

Situation I— increased mobility of a tooth with *increased width* of the periodontal ligament, but *normal height* of the alveolar bone.

Situation II—increased mobility of a tooth with *increased width* of the periodontal ligament and *reduced height* of the alveolar bone.

Splinting is contraindicated in patients with gingivitis and early or moderate periodontitis. Resolution of inflammation by root planing and reduction of occlusal prematurities will usually significantly reduce detectable mobility.[4,9,12] Even if mobility persists after completion of periodontal therapy, fixed splints are usually not indicated. The prosthodontist should determine by occlusal and periodontal evaluation if there are any persistent occlusal prematurities or residual inflammation. If the patient underwent periodontal surgery, residual mobility persists for approximately 6 months before returning to presurgical levels.[3]

Advanced periodontitis. Patients with advanced periodontitis have varying numbers of teeth that exhibit severe bone loss, advanced mobility, and edentulous areas.[13] Residual mobility after periodontal therapy is likely, but depends on factors other than advanced bone loss. Among these, the clinical crown to clinical root ratio and the root morphology are important determinants of mobility.[1,14] A tooth with a club-shaped root and 50 percent loss of circumferential bone height possesses a substantially greater area of remaining attachment than a tooth of equal length and bone height loss with a severely tapered, conical-shaped root (Fig. 4-1). When advanced bone loss has occurred on one or two surfaces of a tooth, but not on the others, the center of rotation of the tooth is nearer the crown.[14] This maintains more favorable leverage on the periodontium than the surfaces of advanced bone loss indicate, and mobility is surprisingly minimal.

Residual mobility of teeth or FPD may be present with advanced bone loss but not increasing. This would fit into Lindhe's classification as follows[12]:

Situation III—increased mobility of a tooth with reduced height of the alveolar bone and normal width of the periodontal ligament.

When this type of situation exists without increasing tooth or FPD mobility or migration and without discomfort during natural chewing, splinting is not indicated.

Indications for Splints

There is sparse literature regarding the indications for splints or the relative efficiency of different types. Well-documented studies have indicated that splinting teeth may *increase* mobility.[15,16] However, these studies tested removable splints and should not be quoted to condemn fixed splints. Usually, FPD's and splints are preferable to RPD's with advanced loss of periodontal support. They provide rigidity and a more favorable force distribution to the remaining periodontium.[17] Authors who disapproved of splints have singled out their frequent use to control mobility, but have not considered the causes of mobility or the presence of a diseased periodontium.[18] There is agreement that splinting of mobile teeth and FPD's, after periodontal and initial occlusal therapy, is indicated when mobility is increasing and interfering with chewing ability and comfort.[1,12,18-20] Lindhe candidates for splinting are[12]:

Situation IV—progressive (increasing) mobility of a tooth (teeth) as a result of gradually increasing width of the periodontal ligament in teeth with a reduced height of the alveolar bone.

Situation V—increased bridge mobility despite splinting.

Progressive mobility in Situation IV can often be controlled by unilateral splints, even though resistance to bucco or labiolingual mobility is less than to mesiodistal mobility (Fig. 4-2). Situation V mobility requires cross-arch splinting. The main objective of splinting is to produce an environment where the total mobility of the splint is normal or at least no longer increasing.[19] Nyman et al. have demonstrated long-term splint stability despite minimal periodontal support and hypermobility of isolated abutment teeth.[21-23] Mobility of a cross-arch splint can be accepted if the mobility does not cause patient discomfort or interfere with mastication and is not progressively increasing. If stability cannot be obtained, the prognosis is poor, and complete denture service is an eventuality.

Temporary and Provisional Splints

In patients with advanced periodontitis, it is difficult to predict in the early stages if an FPD or splint will exhibit increasing mobility after insertion. For these cases, provisional splints are made to gain greater insight into the prognosis. Provisional splints are also beneficial in guiding resistant patients into eventual acceptance of a complex treatment. Even intelligent, reasonably affluent patients are initially overwhelmed by the fear of extensive, painful dentistry with exhorbitant costs. Initial therapy, consisting of scaling and root planing, patient plaque control, occlusal therapy, and provisional splinting, is relatively nonthreatening. Once patients experience improved health, they are often more receptive to the long-term treatment plan.[24]

Types of treatment restorations. Stern[25] has described treatment restoration options as 1) external devices that are ligated or fixed to the intact tooth surface; 2) intracoronal internal devices that are bonded to cavity preparations within the tooth enamel and dentin; and 3) circumcoronal internal devices bonded to the surface of crown preparations.

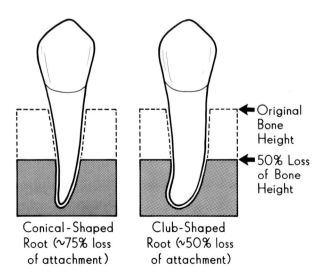

Conical-Shaped Root (~75% loss of attachment)

Club-Shaped Root (~50% loss of attachment)

← Original Bone Height

← 50% Loss of Bone Height

Fig. 4-1. Total attachment loss depends upon root configuration and the radiographic level of bone.

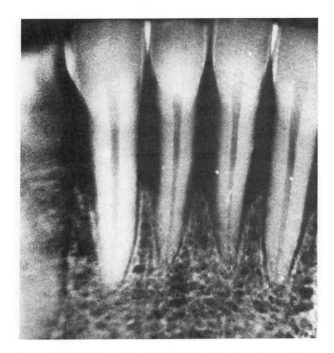

Fig. 4-2. A, Radiograph of Nos. 23 to 26 with advanced bone loss and widening of the PDL spaces.

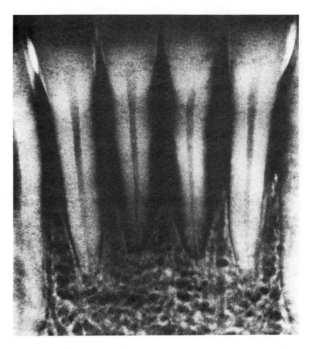

Fig. 4-2. B, Radiograph after 2 years with progressive attachment loss and widening of the PDL. Mobility was *increasing* despite resolution of inflammation with occlusal adjustment.

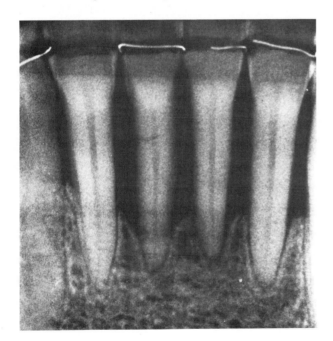

Fig. 4-2. C, Radiograph 2 years after periodontal therapy and provisional splinting from Nos. 22 to 27. Despite fractures in the splint, mobility of the teeth remained unchanged. Note narrower PDL spaces.

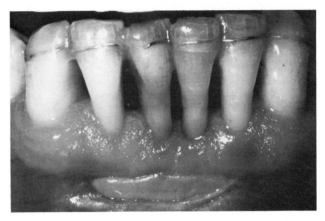

Fig. 4-2. D, Two years after therapy and immediately after repair of splint. Plaque control is good and the gingiva is not inflamed.

and to modify occlusal contacts that interfere with orthodontics.[26]

For information on treatment restorations, the reader is referred to publications listed in the Bibliography of this chapter by Amsterdam and Fox (1959), Grant et al. (1979), Pollack and Ponte (1981), Prichard (1979), and Schluger et al. (1977) and Chapter 11 in this text.

Permanent Splints

Permanent splints are commonly fabricated after completion of definitive periodontal therapy. Pretreatment dilemmas of questionable teeth will be solved, and a more predictable treatment plan can be formulated.

Modified Hawley bite planes are classified as removable splints and have limitations for use as provisional splints.[15,16] They are beneficial for the following reasons: to relieve the deleterious influences of bruxism, including the symptoms of myofascial pain dysfunction; as temporary stabilization in treating occlusal trauma associated with periodontal disease;

Removable Splints

Removable prostheses do not provide the rigidity or as favorable a force distribution as FPDs.[17] Removable splints have been shown to increase tooth mobility; this mobility can return to presplint levels within 2 to 3 years.[28] When splint design acknowledges the occlusal forces on periodontally compromised teeth, splints have proven to be compatible with periodontal health.[29,30] Detailed descriptions of RPDs for patients treated periodontally are presented by Carranza (1984), Goodkind (1984), Javid and Low (1984), Prichard (1979), Thayer and Kratochvil (1980), and Willarson (1969) in the Bibliography.

Rigid Connectors

Combined periodontal and prosthodontic treatment followed for over 10 years has shown gradual arrest of the progressive breakdown of periodontal disease.[22,23] In these studies, with a periodontal treatment and plaque control program, no teeth were lost from recurrent periodontal disease. Technical failures such as loss of retainer retention, fracture of metal components, and fracture of abutment teeth accounted for the nearly 8 percent failure rate.

Nonrigid Connectors

Nonrigid connectors are a precision dovetail lock design occupying more embrasure space buccolingually and occlusogingivally than cast rigid connectors. Broken stress connectors are indicated when tooth malalignment prevents a common path of insertion or to avoid an extensive single unit if cross-arch splinting is indicated.[31] They allow design flexibility in treating the multiple distributions of remaining teeth.[31]

The keyway should be on the distal surface of the abutment crown, with the key on the mesial surface of the adjacent pontic (Fig. 4-3). This arrangement encourages mesial drift to seat the key in the keyway of the connector. If the positioning of the component parts were reversed (keyway on the mesial, key on the distal), mesial drift would unseat the connection.[32]

Since nonrigid connectors restrict the interdental embrasure space more than rigid connectors due to greater bulk, they are used only with ample embrasure space. The gingival surfaces are convex buccolingually between the pontic and retainer, but concave mesiodistally, and well polished.[33,34] This allows plaque removal with floss or an interdental brush.

Telescope Crowns

Telescope crowns were first introduced as abutment retainers for RPD's by Peeso in 1916.[35] The technique consisted of covering the prepared teeth with thin gold copings, or thimbles, that incorporated shoulders at the gingival margin to which a superstructure was abutted with temporary luting agents.[36] The surfaces of the copings covered by the superstructure are left unpolished because cement will not adhere to a polished surface. The copings may be soldered or remain as individual units with the superstructure providing the splinting. Often these two approaches are integrated in a single case.[36] If complete arch splinting is necessary, cross-linkage of abutments across soldered copings allows a bilateral splint to be divided into manageable units (Fig. 4-4).[37]

The telescope principle has added great versatility to permanent splinting, but it has limitations.

Advantages:

1. Increased retention is achieved on single short clinical crowns or overtapered preparations. Overly tapered preparations have been shown to provide inadequate resistance to crown displacement.[38,39] It is difficult to prepare the axial walls of short teeth to a minimal taper for resistance form.[38] Copings are contoured with near-parallel axial walls to overcome this problem. Telescope crowns are not used on short abutment teeth for FPDs because of the space occupied by the additional casting.[1,40]

2. Paralleling of severely tipped abutment teeth without orthodontics is accomplished by adjusting the axial walls of the copings to a common withdrawal path. This often results in an increase in thickness of the copings of the malaligned teeth and creates overcontours. Paralleling of multiple splint abutments with minor alignment deviations can usually be achieved with minimal tooth reduction and only slight overcontouring of restorations.

3. Full-arch periodontal splinting is accomplished in multiple smaller segments. Accuracy is improved by reducing the number of solder joints if multiple superstructure units are cast. Dividing a bilateral splint also avoids removing the entire splint if one abutment crown requires repair.

4. Protection is provided to the abutment teeth by the permanently cemented copings if the superstructure is dislodged.

5. The superstructures, temporarily cemented, can be removed for treatment of recurrent periodontal disease. Teeth with a guarded prognosis, intentionally included in a splint, can also eventually be extracted with the abutment crown converted to a pontic.

6. Additional retention can be included on terminal abutments in long-span splints with tooth preparations for rods on the inside of the copings.

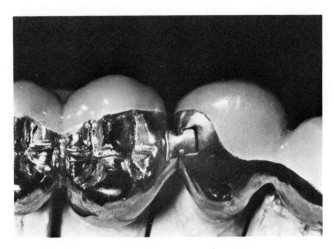

Fig. 4-3. Occlusal view of a nonrigid connector. Note keyway on the distal surface of the canine abutment and the key on the mesial surface of the premolar pontic. (Prosthesis by Dr. William Nagy, U.S. Army.)

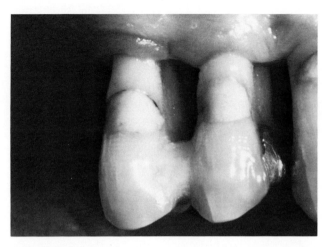

Fig. 4-4. A, Significant attachment loss and surgery have resulted in extensive exposure of root concavities. (Prosthesis by Dr. William Nagy, U.S. Army.)

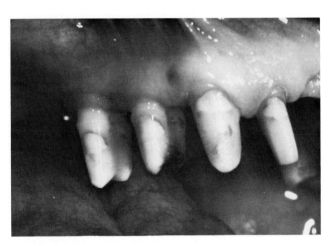

Fig. 4-4. B, After crown preparations for telescope copings with supragingival finish lines. Note fluted contours of the premolar preparation corresponding to root concavities.

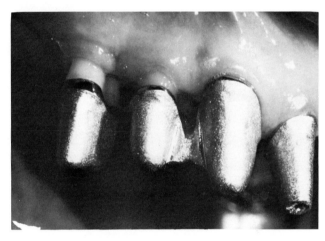

Fig. 4-4. C, Copings cemented as single copings except for soldered Nos. 5 and 6.

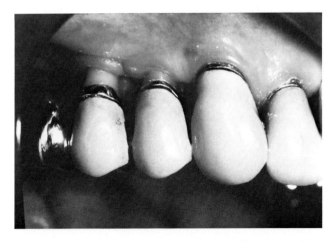

Fig. 4-4. D, Anterior superstructures temporarily cemented.

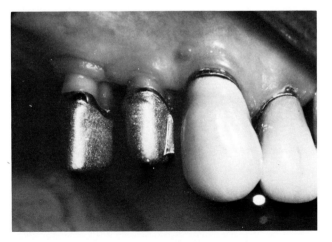

Fig. 4-4. E, Separate anterior and posterior superstructures temporarily cemented.

The outer surface of the copings can then incorporate internal grooves or external rods interlocking with opposing rods or grooves on the inner surface of the superstructure. This combination provides maximal resistance for the terminal abutments.

Disadvantages:

1. The retention between the coping and tooth must be greater than between the superstructure and the coping.
2. Fit is difficult between the superstructure margins and the coping finish lines. This is because it is difficult to apply wax accurately to gold for the wax pattern.
3. There are esthetic limitations in the anterior areas due to the bulk of the double castings with narrow embrasure spaces. Also, the supragingival margins where the superstructure meets the coping, plus the difficulty in achieving suitable fit (Disadvantages, Item 2) may be esthetically unacceptable (Fig. 4-4, E).
4. Telescoping is contraindicated with short abutment teeth or narrow embrasures. Strategic extraction of teeth jeopardizing neighboring teeth becomes critical with telescopic prostheses.[40,41]
5. Greater expense to the patients. Telescopes are nearly double the cost of a single restoration in some parts of the country,[40] while insignificant in others.[37]

Due to the complexities of telescopic prostheses, it is recommended that additional reading be pursued in the following publications listed in the Bibliography: Amsterdam and Abrams (1968), Gordon (1966), Prichard (1972), and Yuodelis (1977).

ORTHODONTIC THERAPY

Telescopic prostheses for malaligned abutment teeth are circumvented by orthodontics. Many patients demonstrate collapse of posterior occlusion,[1] which is characterized by mesial drift of the posterior teeth with tipping, extrusion, and loss of arch integrity.

Molar uprighting has been described as "minor tooth movement"[41,42] and is accomplished after initial periodontal therapy (not surgery) to reduce inflammation. Often after tooth realignment pocket depths are reduced, clinical crown length increased, and gingival contours improved, eliminating the need for surgery.[43] Conversely, soft tissue can become redundant on the advancing surface of a tooth and require surgery after orthodontics.[44]

Injuries to the teeth and periodontal tissues are possible during orthodontic movement. Usually the damage is reversible, unless the forces are uncontrolled. Significant root resorption and supportive tissue loss can occur in these situations.[45-47] The reader is directed to publications in the Bibliography of this chapter by Cooper (1979), Marks and Corn (1969), and Thilander (1983) for more detailed information on this subject.

OCCLUSAL CONSIDERATIONS

Occlusion in fixed prosthodontics is discussed in this textbook. The importance of occlusion in splint design cannot be overemphasized. A comfortable occlusal relationship with smooth movement during centric closure is necessary with advanced periodontal disease.[48] Permanent stability (no increasing mobility) of splints with minimal supporting tissues can be achieved by establishing a stable occlusion.[21]

Splinted teeth remain susceptible to the effects on the periodontium of trauma from occlusion caused by isolated premature contacts. When excessive occlusal forces are applied to one tooth in a splint, the attachment tissues of all splinted teeth suffer comparable injury. Nevertheless, splints dissipate forces so that no tooth is damaged as it would be if it received all the forces.[49]

Consideration of occlusion is paramount in treatment planning. Gross occlusal prematurities are corrected in the initial phases of periodontal treatment, but the prosthodontist is responsible for subsequent refinements.[1]

1. Splinting is not a substitute for periodontal therapy, and costly permanent splints are contraindicated without a cooperative patient in a long-term maintenance program (Fig. 4-5).
2. Provisional and permanent splinting have four basic indications: 1) to stabilize teeth with increasing mobility, that cause patient discomfort, or both in spite of adequate periodontal treatment, 2) to stabilize unstable teeth following orthodontics, 3) to replace missing teeth if the remaining teeth are suitable in distribution, and 4) to determine the success of therapy.
3. Splinting of periodontally treated, but compromised dentitions should be accomplished with minimal adverse effects and should not interfere with optimal plaque control procedures, ensuring that periodontal disease does not recur.[50]

ALTERATIONS IN THE PERIODONTAL ENVIRONMENT

Patients with a susceptibility to periodontal disease are a special challenge to the prosthodontist. Since they have had the disease, they are more susceptible to periodontal tissue insults from restorative procedures than healthy patients.[51]

After successful periodontal therapy there are morphologic alterations in the periodontal tissues. They exhibit a loss of hard and soft tissue attachment, with exposure of root anatomy and a greater crown-to-root ratio. As the severity of the periodontal disease in-

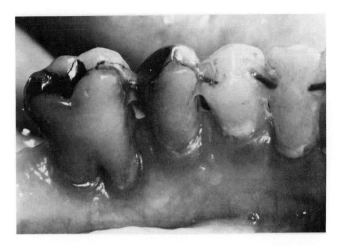

Fig. 4-5. Mandibular lingual gingiva of a nonconforming patient. Surgery was not performed and permanent splinting contraindicated. Provisional A-splints stabilized increasing mobility for patient comfort.

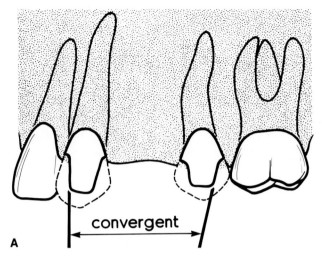

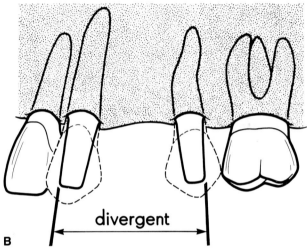

Fig. 4-6. A, Establishing withdrawal for FPDs is easier when preparations are on anatomic crowns. **B,** Divergent roots make withdrawal difficult if margins are on root surfaces of periodontally compromised teeth.

creases, these alterations become more complex,[1] particularly after pocket elimination.[52]

The exposed roots may have anatomic concavities and developmental grooves that complicate plaque removal and tooth preparation (Fig. 4-4, A).[53,54] The roots of adjacent abutment teeth with well-aligned crowns may also have root deviations that defy parallelism (Fig. 4-6).

The basic principles of fixed prosthodontics are identical for the periodontally compromised patient, but fewer abutment teeth and less support add complications.[17]

This chapter will not dwell on repetitious discussions for the periodontally sound patient. The emphasis is on problems encountered with an appreciably altered periodontium.

COMPLETE OR PARTIAL COVERAGE

The FPD includes the cementing agent, abutment teeth, PDL, and bone, in addition to metal and veneer. The PDL and bone are elastic tissues with the ability to resist permanent deformation.[17] Shortening pontic segments can control deformation of FPD's,[55] but is difficult to accomplish with periodontally compromised dentitions. Increased pontic stress is compensated for by increased height of the FPD in the direction of loading, including thicker solder joints.[19] This is usually not a problem with periodontal attachment loss with increased crown length.

Partial veneer crowns have less resistance to deformation than complete crowns,[55] and this increases cement fracture with loss of retention.[19] Silness also demonstrated that complete crowns accumulated more deposits, severe gingivitis, and increased pocket depths than abutments with partial veneer crowns.[56] This difference was not evident if the patients were instructed in methods to improve oral hygiene. Complete crowns are thus preferable as retainers in patients with long-span FPDs or splints with few abutment teeth.

MARGIN PLACEMENT
Supragingival Margin Placement

Whenever possible, margins are prepared supragingivally on the enamel of the anatomic crown (Fig. 4-6, A). In addition to the favorable reaction of the gingiva,[56-60] other advantages are gained: a common path of insertion[40]; wider shoulder tooth preparations can accommodate an adequate bulk of porcelain veneering material in the cervical area without pulpal injury (Fig. 4-7, A)[1]; and metal margin finishing techniques are easier.[61] Crown margins on exposed root surfaces, but still supragingival, are necessary for extensive FPD's to secure longer retainers while encouraging gingival health (Fig. 4-8).

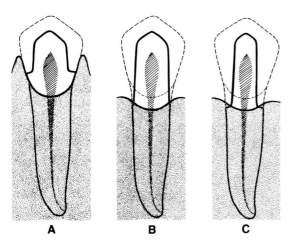

Fig. 4-7. A, Shoulder preparations on enamel with axial walls a safe distance from the pulp. **B,** Preparations on root surfaces require less tooth reduction to keep axial walls safely from the pulp. **C,** Shoulders placed on root surfaces may compromise the pulp, indicating intentional vital root canal therapy. (Modified from a drawing by Dr. David Kaiser, San Antonio, Tex.)

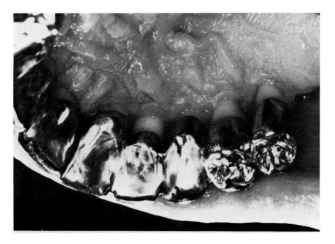

Fig. 4-8. An extensive, single-unit splint with supragingival margins on the roots near the CEJs and noninflamed gingiva.

Intracrevicular Margin Placement

The term *intracrevicular* for margin placement implies confinement within the gingival crevice.[62] It is preferable to the term *subgingival* margin because it is more specific; subgingival margins can extend into the junctional epithelium and connective tissue, which is a violation of the biologic width and results in localized gingivitis.[63]

Despite the advantages of supragingival margins, there are clinical situations requiring intracrevicular placement, even in periodontally treated dentitions.[61,64] They are: 1) esthetics[65]; 2) severe cervical erosion, restorations, or caries extending beyond the gingival crest; 3) adequate crown retention in short or broken-down clinical crowns; and 4) elimination of persistent root hypersensitivity. The comfort of the patient subjugates all guidelines.

Wound Healing Considerations

The time elapsed after completion of periodontal treatment is crucial when intracrevicular margins are anticipated. Healing of extensive periodontal surgery usually requires at least 3 months, and often more, to establish a new biologic width, crevice, and stable position of the gingival margin and papilla.[66] Even areas treated by scaling, root planing, and plaque control without surgery may take more than 1 or 2 months for their gingival margins to stabilize. Gingival margins after surgery commonly migrate coronally, whereas they tend to recede after scaling and root planing.[67] Margins prematurely placed intracrevicularly in the second situation often become exposed as healing progresses, and the result may be unesthetic.

Intracrevicular Depth

Accurate estimation of the true gingival crevice is important to ensure that margins do not impinge on the junctional epithelium or connective tissue attachment (biologic width). This requires accepted use of a periodontal probe. Position of the probe and probing force are critical for accuracy, as is the state of the gingival health.[68,69] In health, the probe is stopped by the junctional epithelium (JE), whereas gingivitis allows penetration of the JE and the connective tissue fibers.[70]

Authors have estimated the healthy crevice depth at 2 to 3 mm and recommend placing margins 1.5 to 2.0 mm beneath the gingival crest.[71,72] Others, reviewing histologic specimens, reported that the average sulcus depth in a healthy patient was 0.5 to 1 mm in depth and recommended margin placement not exceed this level.[73,74] The smaller measurements agree with those of Gargiulo et al., who discovered that the average crevice depth was between 0.5 to 1.0 mm whether adjacent to enamel or root surfaces (Fig. 4-9).[75] Therefore, the ideal intracrevicular position for margins is 0.5 mm beneath the gingival crest, especially when the crevice is adjacent to root surfaces. While the average crevicular depths are nearly identical for enamel or root surface, the average length of the junctional epithelium on the root is between 0.5 and 1.0 mm shorter than that on enamel.[75] Thus, overextension of margin placement beneath the gingiva on root surfaces impinges on the gingival connective tissue fibers and the junctional epithelium.

Pulpal Involvement

In posterior regions, intracrevicular margin placement after the gingival margins have receded is accomplished with minimal pulpal trauma if chamfer or knife-edge margins are prepared (Fig. 4-7, *B*). If a shoulder is prepared for a metal ceramic crown, the axial walls converge toward the pulp chamber with serious consequences (Fig. 4-7, *C*). This will be the

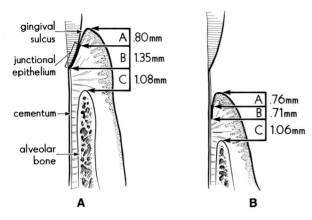

Fig. 4-9. A, Mean measurements of sulcus depth, junctional epithelium, and supracrestal fibers in a healthy periodontium. Zones B and C are the biologic width. **B,** Mean measurements of sulcus depth, junctional epithelium (JE), and supracrestal fibers if the attachment is on the root. Note differences in dimensions of JE. (From Gargiulo, A., et al., J. Periodontol., 32:261-267, 1961.)

case even if the axial walls are nearly parallel.

If there is divergent root anatomy without a clearly defined long axis, tooth preparation is impossible without exposing the pulp (Fig. 4-6, B). Intentional vital root canal therapy is indicated before crown completion[76,77] because endodontically treated teeth have a good prognosis in a periodontal prosthesis.[40] Belated pulpal necrosis develops approximately five times more frequently in abutment teeth than in nonabutment teeth.[78] At this time, damage to the prosthesis is unavoidable during endodontic therapy; therefore, intentional endodontics may solve technical problems in a periodontal prosthesis and prevent extraction.[76]

ATTACHED GINGIVA

The gingiva adjacent to intracrevicular crown margins is an important prepreparation consideration. The various steps in the fabrication of a crown are traumatic to the gingival sulcus,[79] and recession is common. Thin and friable mucosa is especially vulnerable during instrumentation.[80]

The width of keratinized and attached gingiva is often narrower in periodontal diseases, especially where surgery was performed.[81] Even gingival recession due to periodontal diseases and nonsurgical treatment narrows the zone of keratinized and attached gingiva, since the mucogingival junction does not change its position unless surgically moved.[82] Lang and Löe suggested that 2 mm of keratinized gingiva, including 1 mm of attached gingiva, is adequate to maintain gingival health,[83] but more recent studies question the need for keratinized gingiva.[84,85] Controlled studies have not been reported on the effect of restorative procedures on minimal keratinized or attached gingiva.

Empirical estimates have suggested 5 mm of keratinized tissue composed of 2 mm of free gingiva and 3 mm of attached gingiva for subgingival margins.[62] This may be excessive, since the authors recommended placing margins no further than 1.5 to 2.0 mm beneath the gingival crest,[72] whereas others concluded that beyond 0.5 to 1.0 mm is excessive.[73,74] Nevertheless, the avoidance of traumatic gingival recession usually depends on a zone of *thick* keratinized gingiva 4 to 5 mm in width, of which 2 to 3 mm is attached (Fig. 4-10).

The periodontal probe can be used to measure the clinical crevice depth, width of keratinized and attached gingiva, or estimate gingival thickness (Fig. 4-11). Despite tissue keratinization, if the probe is seen through the free gingival margin, the ability to resist trauma is doubtful. The surgical placement of a thicker, free autogenous gingival graft is indicated be-

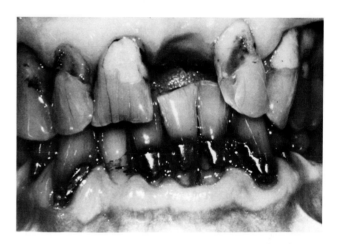

Fig. 4-10. A, Adequate marginal keratinized gingiva of 3 to 4 mm with 3 mm attached is present on the facial of No. 22 before tooth preparations. No keratinized or attached gingiva is evident, facial of No. 27. (Courtesy Dr. Roger Troendle, San Antonio, Tex.)

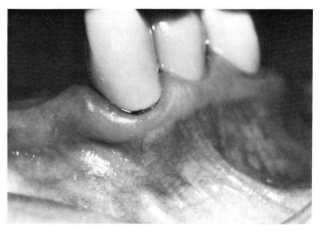

Fig. 4-10. B, A month post insertion shows the facial gingiva of No. 22 without recession. *continued*

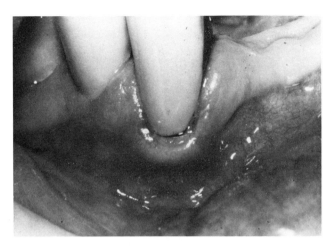

Fig. 4-10. C, One month after crown insertion the facial gingiva of No. 27 exhibits significant recession.

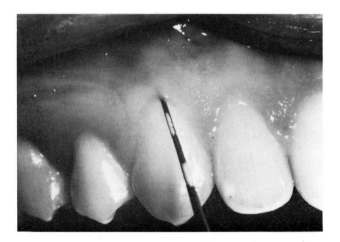

Fig. 4-11. The tip of a periodontal probe can just be seen through the free marginal gingiva of No. 6 indicating a thin gingiva. The crevice is approximately 1 mm, while the width of keratinized gingiva is approximately 3 mm, so the attached gingiva is about 2 mm wide.

fore the final tooth preparation of intracrevicular margins (Fig. 4-12).

ATRAUMATIC PREPARATION

The free and attached gingiva resists insults more effectively if the connective tissue fibers are intact and not inflamed. Dragoo and Williams have demonstrated that the placement of retraction cord into the sulcus before preparation protects the epithelium from damage.[86] Berman has described a technique of preparing a shoulder finish line to the gingival crest, then displacing the gingiva laterally and apically with retraction cord.[87] The shoulder is beveled with a supragingival finish line that is intracrevicular after cord removal. A modification of this technique using a conventional shoulder preparation without a bevel has been described by Kaiser and Newell (Fig. 4-13).[88]

Restoration of Endodontically Treated Teeth

Restoring teeth with endodontics is discussed elsewhere in this text; restoration of these teeth presents problems in periodontally compromised teeth not encountered with normal periodontal support. Posts are recommended to be extended to one-half the length of the root remaining in bone.[89] In the periodontal patient these posts often extend into the apical one-third of the root. This necessitates tapered posts instead of parallel posts to minimize thinning of dentin at the post apex, especially in teeth with cone-shaped roots. Tapered posts are also preferred because stresses are diminished surrounding the post apex compared to parallel posts.[90,91] Posts should not extend closer than 3 to 5 mm to the root apex to avoid disturbance of the seals of accessory canals more prevalent near the apex.[92]

Screw-type posts, while more retentive than cemented posts, produce greater stress on the root.[93] They are not used near the apex, since minute dentin fractures are likely to be present from the root canal instrumentation.[94,95]

Pin-retained amalgams alone or in combination with posts of modified lengths have been used if the attachment loss extends the posts too near to the root apices.[89,96] The use of composite resin cores has also been advocated with posts[89,97]; however, they were recently shown to be dimensionally unstable within an hour after exposure to moisture, adversely affecting the margins of the artificial crowns covering the composites.[98] Tooth preparation, impressions, and treatment restorations with composite cores at a separate appointment after placement—when moisture instability is less, may reduce marginal discrepancies. Until further research has clarified this possibility, it is prudent to use composite resins for core buildups judiciously.

GINGIVAL RETRACTION AND IMPRESSIONS

Supragingival finish lines with treated periodontal diseases are less traumatic to the gingival tissues if sufficient healing time has been allowed. Impressions of intracrevicular finish lines may be extremely injurious to the periodontium, depending to a great extent on the quality and quantity of the attached gingiva and the type of retraction. All retraction methods induce transient trauma to the junctional epithelium and connective tissue of the gingival sulcus.[99] If the retraction cord is placed against a clean tooth surface, healing is uneventful within a week.[100,101]

Retraction Cord

The retraction cord technique usually produces limited gingival recession[99] and can protect the sulcular tissues during preparation.[86-88] If used carelessly with

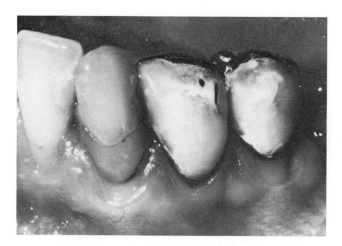

Fig. 4-12. A, The keratinized and attached gingiva on the facial of tooth No. 22 is minimal and nonexistent on No. 20. They appear healthy, but ceramic/metal crowns are planned with intracrevicular margins. These delicate gingival margins cannot withstand the trauma of prosthetic procedures, so gingival augmentation is indicated.

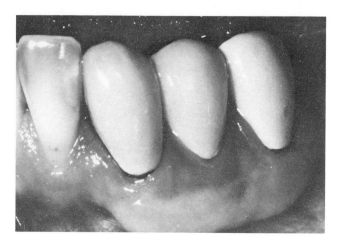

Fig. 4-12. B, Four months after a free gingival autograft and 1 month after cementation of metal/ceramic crowns. Note gingival health with minimal recession. (Prosthetics by Dr. Michael Conway, U.S. Army.)

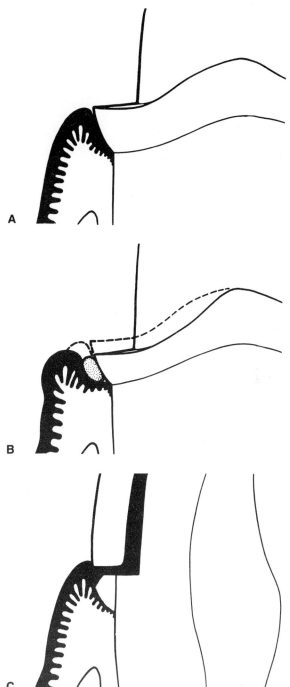

Fig. 4-13. A, Shoulder preparation to level of the gingival crest. **B,** Careful placement of a retraction cord into sulcus. This moves the gingival margin laterally and apically from its original position *(dotted line),* allowing the shoulder preparation to be slightly apical to its position before cord placement. **C,** Casting seated with the gingival margin at its original position before retraction cord. The margin is now ideally intracrevicular. (Courtesy Dr. Patrick Seeley, Santa Rosa, Calif.)

inadequate attached gingiva, injury to the gingival fibers occurs. This can allow impression material to be forced into the gingival connective tissue and bone, producing a foreign body reaction (Fig. 4-14, A-C).[102] This can manifest as a localized periodontal abcess or a diffuse cellulitis. Radiographs will reveal the radiopaque material and are a diagnostic aid when impression material is suspected as a cause of inflammation (Fig. 4-15).[67,103] Damage to the periodontium is more extensive and prolonged if the material is pressured into the marrow spaces of the alveolar process.[67,103] This requires multiple surgical procedures for debridement of the irritating material.

Electrosurgery

Various electrosurgical techniques are advocated to facilitate impressions.[104] Animal studies have demonstrated delayed healing and loss of periodontal attachment with electrosurgery.[105,106] These studies have been challenged for not using fully rectified, filtered

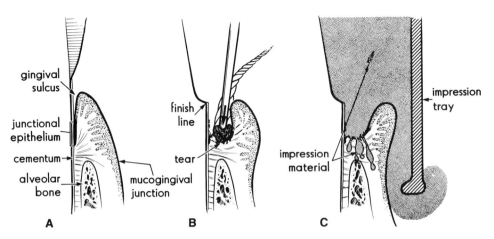

Fig. 4-14. A, Gingival margin completely on the root with thin gingiva and minimal attached gingiva. **B,** Forceful application of retraction cord into the delicate sulcus tearing the junctional epithelium and gingival fibers. **C,** Impression immediately after retraction. Impression material is forced through the epithelial and connective tissue into the mucosa, bone, and PDL.

electrosurgery units.[107] The use of modern units by dentists familiar with the limitations results in cellular healing comparable to a scalpel cut.[108] Controlled-depth cutting electrode tips avoid bone trauma but injure the gingival fibers if the tip is not angled properly in the sulcus.[86] These fibers heal if left undisturbed. Oringer's solution or a surgical pack may enhance healing. When followed immediately by the forceful insertion of impression material, the severed fibers allow deeper passage with potentially disastrous results.[67,103]

Rotary Gingival Curettage

Rotary gingival curettage combines subgingival crown preparation with removal of the soft tissue lining of the gingival sulcus with rotary stones. Clinically significant gingival recession has been noted compared to electrosurgery and plain cord.[99] Like electrosurgery, it effectively removes the sulcular epithelium, but the rationale for this technique is unclear. If hemorrhage is preventing a predictable impression of an intracrevicular finish line, electrosurgery will control this. Conversely, rotary curettage has resulted in increased bleeding and commonly requires a hemostatic cord. If the gingiva is healthy, normal coagulation occurs with gentle pressure from a nonmedicated retraction cord. With rotary curettage, the entire sulcular epithelium needs repair. This technique is illogical and without scientific justification.

TEMPORARY AND PROVISIONAL CROWNS

Temporary and provisional crowns are addressed in detail elsewhere in this text. Nevertheless, certain aspects regarding temporary and provisional crowns with intracrevicular margins in periodontally susceptible patients are considered here.

Temporary restorations with intracrevicular margins are usually associated with gingival recession.[109] The

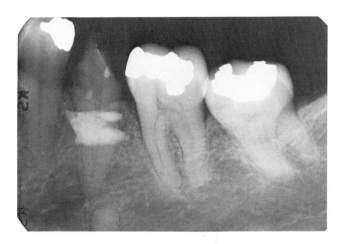

Fig. 4-15. Radiograph 1 week after impression of intracrevicular margins adjacent to minimal attached gingiva tooth No. 20 with a periodontal abscess. Radiopaque impression material embedded in alveolar mucosa was removed by surgical flap.

gingiva recovers its original position after the permanent crown is in place, but the possibility of permanent recession increases the longer the temporary restoration is in place. Some authors advise making temporary crowns slightly short and undercontoured so rough surfaces and poor margins are less irritating (Fig. 4-16).[67] Others advocate overcontouring to keep the gingiva away from the preparation during cementation.[110] Short, temporary margins do not restrict the gingiva and can allow migration over the finish line. This prevents seating of the final crown and results in a cement space with an eventual open margin as the cement dissolves (Fig. 4-16, B), gingival recession, or both.[111] Gingival recession is avoided around temporary crowns with careful preparations and by making contours of the treatment restoration resemble those of the natural tooth (Fig. 4-16, A and C).[112]

Treatment restorations for tooth preparations in periodontally susceptible patients require certain precautions. The microbial flora in the gingival sulcus is altered with artificial crowns if the margins are deficient, whether they are cast gold or acrylic resins.[113,114] Despite the characteristic of marginal shrinkage, suitable treatment restorations are possible.[115]

CROWN CONTOURS

The facial and lingual enamel bulge was formerly thought to protect the free gingival margin from the traumatic effects of mastication.[116] In 1962 this concept was challenged by Morris, who reported the response of gingival tissue around teeth prepared for complete artificial crowns but which had lost their temporary crowns.[117] He discovered healthy gingiva without plaque in the cervical regions compared with approximating, unprepared teeth. Since then the literature has been replete with descriptions of the adverse effects of overcontoured restorations, specifically, the effects of crown contours on gingiva whose margins were located on the coronal rather than on root surfaces. Periodontally compromised patients usually have the latter. This section addresses contours in the patients whose margins are placed intracrevicularly.

Esthetic Preprosthetic Surgery and Orthodontics

Patients treated for periodontal diseases are frequently left with unesthetic marginal gingival recession, open embrasures, and excessive edentulous ridge resorption. This presents an impossible cosmetic task with a patient who has a high lip line; these defects also cause speech problems. For these patients several reasonably successful corrective surgical and orthodontic procedures are available. Crown lengthening techniques[63,118] and/or forced eruption,[119,120] alone or in combination with root coverage[121,122] and ridge augmentation surgery,[65,123] are often indicated and produce excellent results.

Laboratory Soft Tissue Orientation

Conventional trimming of dies removes the gingival anatomy from the working casts and dies. Gingival morphology and position relative to finish lines and preparation contours, which are critical to establishing suitable artificial crown contours, are lost. The laboratory technician has no knowledge of the patient's gingival anatomy and commonly contours restorations to compensate for the enlarged spaces between the dies and adjacent teeth on the casts.[124]

A technique using Impregum was described by Martin[124] and applied by Ishii and Satoh.[125] It provides intact replication of the soft tissues, yet offers enough resiliency to allow seating of the restoration.

Facial and Lingual Sulcular Contours

In the patient whose gingival margins are apical to the cementoenamel junction (CEJ), the sulcular morphology differs from that of a healthy patient whose gingival margins are on enamel.[126,127]

Immediately after intracrevicular preparation, the sulcus is the widest when it was adjacent to enamel before preparation and in a healthy state. On the marginal or radicular surfaces, the enamel contours in the sulcular region flare from the vertical axis of the gingiva to support the gingiva (Fig. 4-17). This encourages a knifelike gingival margin. The intracrevicular contours of an artificial crown should be as close to the original enamel contour as possible. Wagman has estimated this angle of enamel flare from the CEJ to be approximately 22.5 degrees from the vertical axis of the gingival housing (Fig. 4-17).[128]

As the gingival margin progresses more apically, the sulcus narrows, and the intracrevicular contours of the tooth become the flat contours of the root rather than

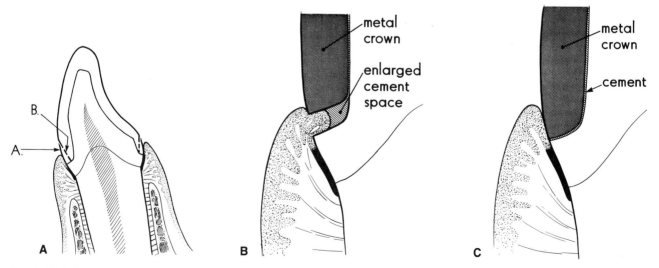

Fig. 4-16. A, Diagram of temporary crown with a margin completely to the finish line (A) and a short, but closed, margin *(dotted line at B).* **B,** With a short margin, the free gingiva migrates over the finish line, restricting complete seating of the permanent crown. **C,** With a well-contoured treatment restoration supporting the gingiva, the permanent crown seats completely, and the sulcus quickly adapts to the artificial crown.

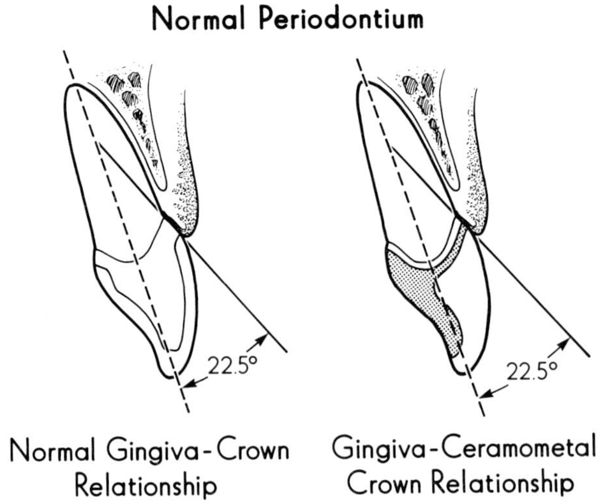

Normal Periodontium

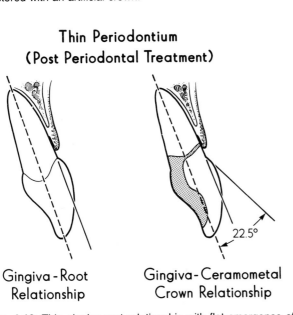

Normal Gingiva-Crown Relationship   Gingiva-Ceramometal Crown Relationship

Fig. 4-17. Normal gingiva-crown relationship with average enamel bulge of approximately 22.5 degrees and similar contour restored with an artificial crown.

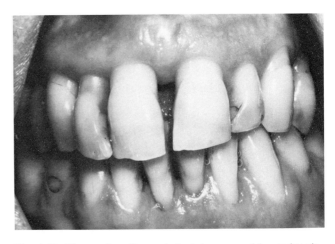

Fig. 4-19. Six months after periodontal surgery. All anterior gingival margins are radicular, but tissue on Nos. 6 to 8 is flat and thick, while that around Nos. 9 to 11 scalloped and thin. Note slight inflammation of the flat, thick margins, while the scalloped thin margins are healthy.

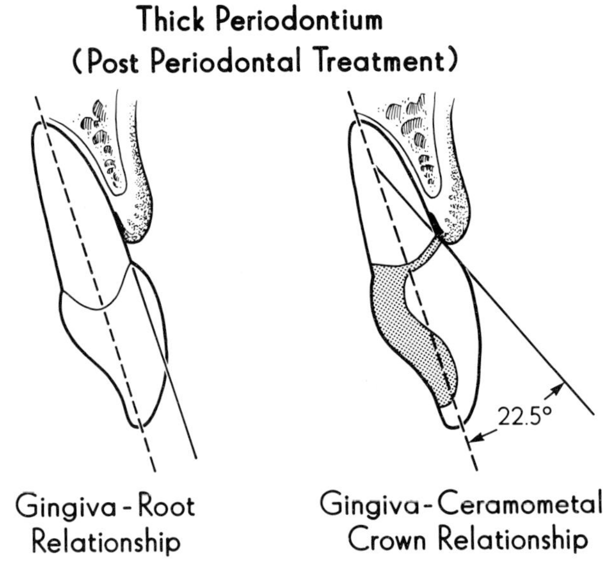

Thin Periodontium (Post Periodontal Treatment)

Gingiva-Root Relationship   Gingiva-Ceramometal Crown Relationship

Fig. 4-18. Thin gingiva-root relationship with flat emergence of the root from the gingiva; this same emergence angle reproduced in the artificial crown. The enamel bulge is added supragingivally for esthetics.

Thick Periodontium (Post Periodontal Treatment)

Gingiva-Root Relationship   Gingiva-Ceramometal Crown Relationship

Fig. 4-20. Thick gingiva-root relationship with a natural crown and the artificial crown incorporating the average enamel bulge angle to support the thick gingiva.

the convex surface of the anatomic crown (Fig. 4-18).[126,127] In this situation, the intracrevicular contours of the artificial crown do not mimic the root but depend on the adjacent gingival morphology.

Two general types of gingival forms have been described: scalloped-thin and flat-thick. Scalloped-thin gingiva usually accompanies ovoid or tapering teeth, whereas flat-thick gingiva is associated with square-shaped teeth. Scalloped-thin gingiva responds to irritation by receding; flat-thick gingiva enlarges, forms pockets, or both.[126] Depending upon factors other than crown shape, such as thickness of the alveolar process, root proximity, tooth position in the arch; the two

morphologic forms also manifest when the gingiva has migrated apically to the root surface (Fig. 4-19).

When intracrevicular margins are adjacent to thin gingiva on the root, the sulcular contours of the artificial crown should be flat, mimicking the shape of the root, to prevent overcontouring. In the anterior region, the normal facial contours are reestablished for esthetics, but this flare of the crown is far enough away from the gingival margin to avoid plaque accumulation (Fig. 4-18).

Often the gingiva adjacent to a flat root surface develops a thick free gingival margin when the underlying bone is thick.[117,126] This thick gingiva against a flat root often presents with a slight, chronic, marginal gingivitis despite minimal plaque accumulation (Fig. 4-19). In these situations it may be advisable to create a thicker intracrevicular crown contour similar to that of a natural crown (Fig. 4-20).[126] A clinical case incorporating these principles on two maxillary canines, one with thin marginal gingiva on the root and one with thicker gingiva, is shown in Fig. 4-21, A to G.

Supragingival Marginal Contours

When esthetics are not essential, contours emerging from thin gingiva on the root with a flat profile are designed to continue a flat surface, especially with concave surfaces that are frequently encountered in root anatomy.[53,54] The anatomy of the root emerging from the attachment dictates the finish line as it circumscribes the root.[1] Removal of undercuts coronal to the finish line results in a preparation where the occlusal outline mimics the outline at the most apical level.[129] The final restoration does not reproduce the original anatomic crown contours but instead continues the contours of the roots with flat axial walls.[130,131] When exceptional cosmetic measures are needed with flat intracrevicular crown contours, a cervical bulge is created far enough from the gingival margin for oral hygiene (Fig. 4-18).

Proximal Contours

The interdental embrasure is commonly the first site for gingivitis and the most frequently involved with periodontitis.[132,133]

Instead of a single interdental papilla, the interdental gingiva actually has separate facial and lingual peaks with a connecting valley under the contact area, which is referred to as a col.[134] The epithelial lining of the col is thin and nonkeratinized (similar to junctional epithelium) and permeable to bacterial toxins.[135] In the periodontally healthy patient, restoration of the proximal surfaces of artificial crowns without disrupting this gingival complex is a challenge.

With interdental gingival recession from periodontal diseases, the soft tissue is usually apical to the contact area. The interdental gingiva then is saddle-shaped, or a more pointed papilla, depending on the faciolingual width of the alveolar housing (Fig. 4-4B and 4-22). The epithelium covering this interdental gingiva is completely keratinized.[136]

The proximal contours of the crowns of natural teeth are usually flat, or concave, as are the transitional line angles.[116,126] In combination with crown length, the proximal contours establish the mesiodistal width of the healthy interdental embrasures. Usually, the more concave the proximal surfaces of teeth with long crowns, the wider the embrasure. Conversely, a flatter proximal surface on a short crown results in a narrow embrasure. Variation of flat or concave surfaces with

long and short crowns produces embrasures of varying intermediate widths.

A common error in normal periodontiums is over-contouring the proximal surfaces of artificial crowns by making them convex intracrevicularly and as they emerge from the sulcus.[126,136] This practice originates from imperceptive reduction, which leaves insufficient space for restorative materials. With narrow embrasures, the closely approximating teeth are prepared with more tooth reduction, especially at the line angle entrance to the embrasures.[126,136] However, with minimal embrasure space, it cannot be created by extensive tooth reduction without jeopardizing the pulp. In these situations, selective extraction, orthodontic realignment, or both are considered to gain embrasure space.[41,43] Crown lengthening alone or with forced eruption, can achieve this goal if there is sufficient diversion of the roots of the approximating teeth.

In maxillary anterior teeth, where esthetics and phonetics are a substantial concern, proximal root surfaces are usually flat, without distinct concavities (Fig. 4-4, B). Therefore, after emerging with flat contours from the receded interdental gingiva, anterior artificial crowns should have convex contours established more quickly as they progress incisally.[52] This restricts the embrasure space and improves esthetics and phonetics but limits the use of interdental cleaning devices to dental floss and tape.

Proximal root surface concavities on posterior teeth can be reduced in the contours of the final restoration if more tooth structure is reduced over the buccal and lingual prominences than over the concavities during preparation.[52]

The interdental brush was demonstrated as an effective proximal cleaning device in altered periodontal environments when root concavities were prevalent.[137,138] Dental floss is incapable of removing plaque from the concave surfaces (Fig. 4-23), so artificial crown contours and solder joints are created to accommodate the passage of this device (Fig. 4-24) or a floss threader; otherwise, gingivitis and possible recurrent periodontitis results from the patient's inability to clean this area (Fig. 4-25).

The larger interproximal spaces are not periodontal liabilities because of easy access to the proximal surfaces for hygiene[67]; however, the interdental brush is not effective in deplaquing the tooth surface at the gingival margin if it fits too loosely in a large embrasure (Fig. 4-26, A).[138] Proximal overcontouring is indicated to allow snug passage of the brush through the interdental embrasure (Fig. 4-26, B).

These problem areas are identified after periodontal therapy and before tooth preparation. The patient's success in deplaquing the proximal surfaces is evaluated during the treatment restoration phase, and per-

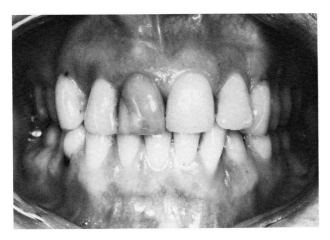

Fig. 4-21. A, Forty-two year old patient after periodontal therapy. Teeth Nos. 6 and 22 will receive ceramic/metal crowns. Note thin gingival margin No. 11 and slightly thicker gingiva No. 6.

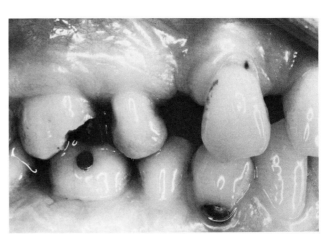

Fig. 4-21. B, Facial view of No. 6 and No. 4 prior to preparation for three-unit FPD. Note thick gingiva, facial No. 4 and thick gingiva on the root surface of No. 6.

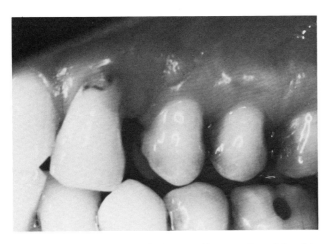

Fig. 4-21. C, Facial view of No. 11 with recession of the thin marginal gingiva prior to crown preparation.

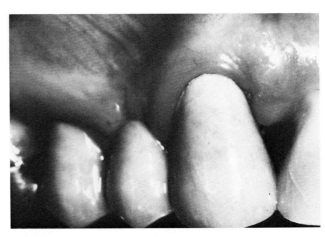

Fig. 4-21. D, Facial view of FPD No. 6 three months post insertion. Note convex facial intracrevicular and supragingival contours to support the moderately thick gingiva.

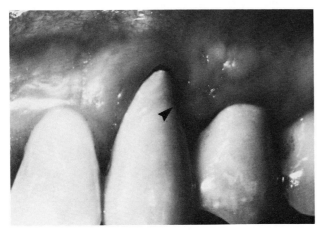

Fig. 4-21. E, Mesial profile of crown No. 6 three years post cementation. Note convex contours for thicker gingival support.

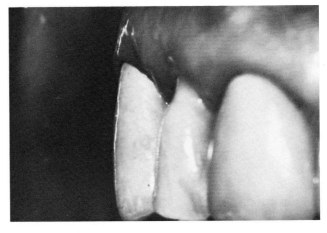

Fig. 4-21. F, Facial view of No. 11 three months postinsertion. Note flat emergence profile with enamel bulge (arrow) approximately 3 mm supragingivally for esthetics.

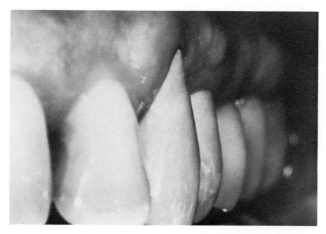

Fig. 4-21. G, Mesial profile of crown No. 11 three years post cementation. Note flat emergence profile with thin gingiva. (Periodontal therapy by Dr. Carol Brownstein; prosthodontics by Dr. David Kaiser, San Antonio, Tex.)

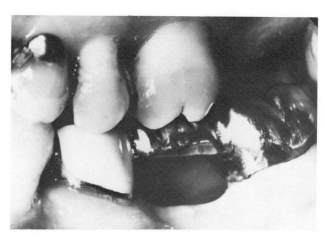

Fig. 4-22. Buccal view of undercontoured sanitary pontic. The patient is acutely aware of the space and lack of musculature support.

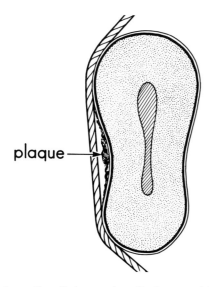

Fig. 4-23. A maxillary first premolar with deep mesial and distal concavities; dental floss is totally ineffective.

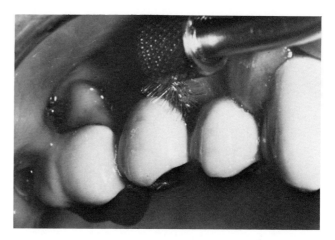

Fig. 4-24. An interdental brush entering the buccal embrasure between abutment No. 4 and pontic No. 5. The embrasure is adequate to accept the brush easily, but snugly, for thorough deplaquing. (Prosthetics by Dr. Thomas Smith, Tacoma, Wash.)

manent crown contours are designed accordingly. This is a situation where reproduction of gingival position and contours on the master cast will be extremely helpful to the technician in achieving the ideal artificial crown contours.[124] In addition to food impaction and phonetic problems, collapse of the tongue and buccal musculature into large edentulous areas is bothersome to many patients. Teeth support the oral musculature and enhance normal facial contours (Fig. 4-22 and 4-27) and patient comfort.[71]

Cementation

Cast restorations are intended to be cemented indefinitely. All intracrevicular margins are checked carefully after cementation for excess cement.[67] The cement material is tolerated by the gingiva,[139-141] but retains plaque as an overhanging margin regardless of the margins. These cement excesses are often subgingival, so the material is unnoticed and slowly dissolves. The pathogenic flora of the plaque associated with the cement overhang causes gingival irritation, violates the periodontal attachment, and causes bone loss (Fig. 4-28).[109,112,114]

RESTORATION OF MOLAR TEETH WITH FURCATION INVASIONS

In long-term studies of tooth longevity, molars are the teeth that are most often lost.[142,143] This is due to the complex root anatomy and furcations that make periodontal therapy and plaque control difficult for the patient. In addition, their posterior location is close to the condyle, which is the fulcrum for the mandible

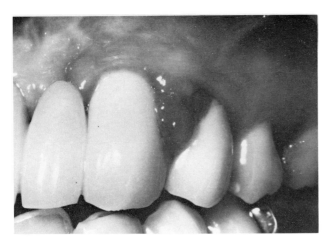

Fig. 4-25. A, A splint with double abutments Nos. 11 and 12 exhibits gingival inflammation and enlargement between the soldered abutments. The solder joint was so thick occlusogingivally that the patient could not insert a floss threader through the embrasure.

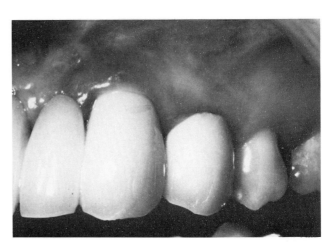

Fig. 4-25. B, The No. 11 and No. 12 area three months after crown lengthening to create an embrasure without compromising esthetics.

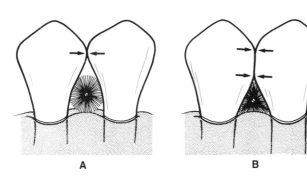

Fig. 4-26. A, Mesiodistal diagram of an interdental brush in a wide embrasure both mesiodistally and occlusogingivally. Note the narrow contact area and the lack of bristle contact in the critical dentogingival junction regions. **B,** Mesiodistal diagram of the embrasure space after alteration of the adjacent proximal contours of artificial crowns. The interdental brush enters the embrasure snugly and the bristles now contact the dentogingival regions.

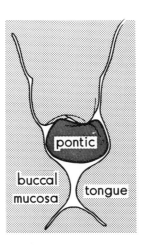
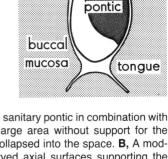

Fig. 4-27. A, Undercontoured sanitary pontic in combination with a resorbed ridge. Note the large area without support for the tongue and buccal mucosa collapsed into the space. **B,** A modified sanitary pontic with curved axial surfaces supporting the musculature while the apex is sufficiently short of ridge contact to avoid entrapping food particles.

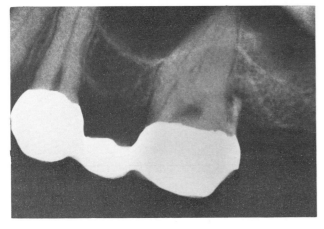

Fig. 4-28. A, Radiograph of a three-unit FPD No. 12 to No. 14 with a cement overhang distal No. 14 with bone resorption.

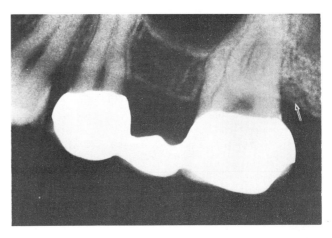

Fig. 4-28. B, No. 14 immediately after removal of excess cement. The area of bone resorption is now more easily visible (arrow).

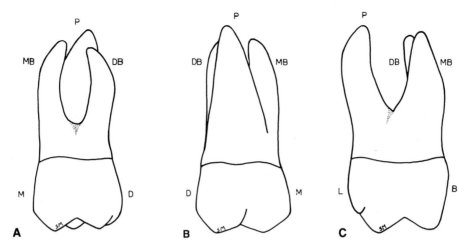

Fig. 4-29. A, Buccal view of a typical maxillary first molar. **B,** Palatal view. **C,** Mesial view. Note wide buccolingual width of the mesibuccal root.

and is a class III lever.[144] This produces moments of force on the molar teeth that exceed those on premolars.[145] These inordinate forces may exceed the adaptation of the attachment apparatus, and attachment loss is accelerated more than in periodontitis.[146,147]

It is important to retain molar teeth if possible[40] because their presence means the difference between needing an FPD and an RPD. Also, early loss of molars and inclusion of anterior teeth in a prosthesis shortens the life of the dentition.

The restoration of molar teeth with exposed supragingival furcations, or that had root resection, is similar to conventional restorations. However, such teeth have anatomic characteristics that present difficulties and lead to unpredictable results. Knowledge of molar furcation and root anatomy is necessary for an accurate prognosis and a practical treatment plan for these compromised molars.

Anatomy

Maxillary molars. Maxillary molars have three roots: mesiobuccal, distobuccal, and palatal (Fig. 4-29). As molar teeth progress distally in the arch there are variations of root anatomy, and root fusion is more common.[148] The morphology of the crown and root trunk coronal to the furcations causes changes in tooth preparation (Fig. 4-30).

The distobuccal and palatal roots are often located in the same plane on their distal surfaces. This distal position of the palatal root creates more mesial space to accommodate the increased buccolingual width of the mesiobuccal root (Fig. 4-31). The distal furcation is usually more apical on the tooth than the mesial furcation. It is less frequently involved with periodontal attachment loss than the mesial and buccal furcations.[149] The furcal surfaces of the distobuccal and palatal roots are less frequently concave (31 percent and 17 percent respectively) than the mesiobuccal root, which is concave approximately 94 percent of

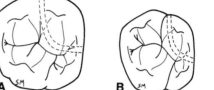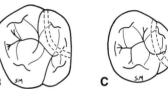

Fig. 4-30. Change to occlusal outline of maxillary molars from (A) first molar to (C) third molar. Note increasingly ovoid shape of occlusal outline after resection of the distobuccal root of the second and third molar compared to "L" shape of the first molar.

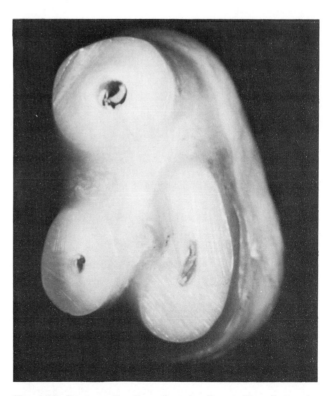

Fig. 4-31. Cross-section through roots of a maxillary first molar 2 mm apical to furca entrances. Note wide mesiobuccal root with deep distal concavity and ribbonlike pulp canal. Note more nearly circular palatal and distobuccal roots whose distal surfaces are in nearly the same plane.

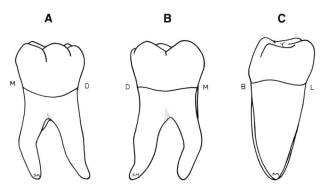

Fig. 4-32. A, Buccal view of a typical mandibular first molar. **B,** Lingual view. **C,** Distal view with a narrower buccolingual width of distal root compared to mesial root.

the time (Fig. 4-31).[150] The concavities and root alignments result in a furcation chamber that is wider than the entrances. In addition, the roofs of furcations are coronal to the root separations in approximately 50 percent of the teeth.[151]

The mesiobuccal root has a root surface area comparable to the palatal root.[151] This is due to its club-shaped morphology, furcal surface concavity, and buccolingual width that is greater than that of the palatal root.

Mandibular molars. Mandibular molars normally have two roots: mesial and distal (Fig. 4-32). As with the maxillary molars, there are slight anatomic variations in the shapes of the crowns and root trunks with distal progression in the arch, which causes the configuration of the tooth preparations to vary.

The root surfaces facing the furcation both have a high prevalence of concavities. The mesial root is concave 100 percent of the time, and the distal root 99 percent, with the mesial root concavity being substantially deeper (Fig. 4-33, A).[150] This also results in the furcation chamber being wider than the buccal and lingual entrances. The mesial root is normally wider buccolingually than the distal root but narrower mesiodistally, with a greater surface area of attachment.[152,153]

The roof of the furcation exhibits a structure known as the intermediate bifurcation ridge approximately 73 to 77 percent of the time.[154,155] It consists of varying thicknesses of cementum and transends the bifurcation connecting the mesial and distal roots. This further complicates the treatment of the mandibular furca when it is periodontally involved. Both maxillary and mandibular molars have a change in furcal position as the teeth are positioned distally in the arch. The trunks of the second molars are longer than the first molars, and the furcations farther apically from the CEJ's (Fig. 4-33, B).[156] Root proximity is also greater in second molars with narrower furcations.[156]

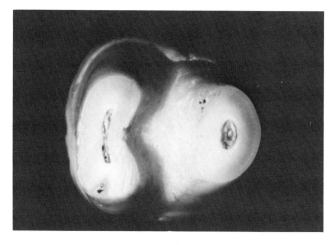

Fig. 4-33. A, Cross-section of a mandibular first molar 2 or 3 mm apical to furcal entrances. Note buccolingual width of mesial root is greater than that of distal root and also the deep distal concavity of mesial root, ribbonlike pulp canal, and mesiodistal width less than distal root. The mesial root is a poor candidate for a post.

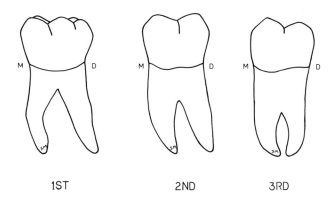

1ST   2ND   3RD

Fig. 4-33. B, Buccal view of mandibular first, second, and third molars. Note more apically positioned furcas and closer root proximity with second and third molars.

Classification of Furcation Invasions

The classifications of furcation invasions are numerous. Many are simply slight modifications of Glickman's classification, which was one of the first described and still commonly used.[157] This classification will be compared with the normal furcation.

Normal furcation (Fig. 4-34). There is no bone or attachment loss involving the furcation per se or the flute leading into the furcation. There may be early attachment loss and pocket formation coronally, but the flute cannot be detected with clinical probing.

Grade I involvement (Fig. 4-35). This is an incipient lesion. The pocket is suprabony, involving the soft tissue, and the flute concavity can be detected with the probe. There may be slight bone loss in the furcation area, but a curved probe cannot enter the furca. Radiographic change is unusual.

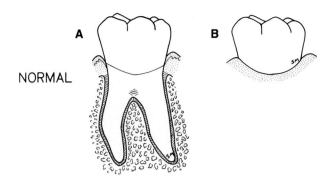

Fig. 4-34. A normal, healthy furcation of a mandibular first molar. **A,** Mesiodistal cross-section showing intact intrafurcal bone and PDL. **B,** Clinical appearance.

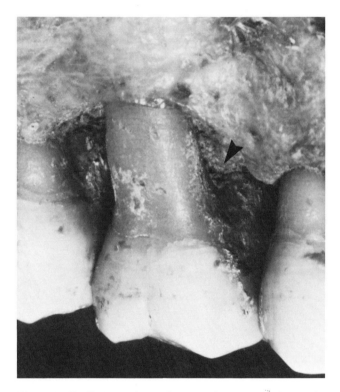

Fig. 4-35. D, Skull specimen illustrates bone loss apical to the furcation entrance but not within.

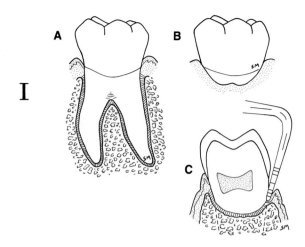

Fig. 4-35. Grade I furcation invasion (FI). **A,** Intrafurcal bone and PDL are intact. **B,** Clinical view may show some gingival recession. **C,** Buccolingual section exhibits pocket depth into the flute of the furcation, but no horizontal component into the furca proper.

Grade II involvement (Fig. 4-36). This lesion is a cul-de-sac. Bone is destroyed on one or more aspects of the furcation (mesial, distal, buccal, or buccal and lingual), but a portion of the alveolar bone and PDL remains intact, permitting only partial penetration of the probe into the furca. Radiographs may reveal changes within the furca due to variables, i.e., thickness of remaining bone, root proximity, angle of the x-ray beam, or presence of the palatal root. The Grade II involvement may be shallow, with most of the furcal bone intact (Fig. 4-36, D) or deep, if most of the furcal bone has been lost (Fig. 4-36, E and F).

Grade III involvement (Fig. 4-37). Interradicular bone is completely absent horizontally, but the entrances to the furcation are occluded by gingival tissue. It is possible to pass a probe completely through the furcation (Fig. 4-37, C and D). Radiographic radiolucency is usually visible between the roots if the roots are divergent and the x-ray beam angle is optimal (Fig. 4-37, E).

Grade IV involvement (Fig. 4-38). The interradicular bone is completely destroyed in a horizontal direction, and the gingival tissue has receded apically so that the furcation is visible (Fig. 4-38, D and E). This is usually seen after therapeutic "tunneling" procedures rather than in the disease process.

In addition to the horizontal bone loss, vertical bone loss also occurs surrounding the furcations. This vertical loss is more critical in the prognosis for the tooth than the horizontal loss.[157] Tarnow and Fletcher have devised a subclassification for vertical attachment loss in the furcations that is combined with Glickman's horizontal classification.[158] Their subclassification is as follows:

Subclass A: 0 to 3 mm probable depth from the roof of the furca

Subclass B: 4 to 6 mm probable depth from the roof of the furca

Subclass C: 7 mm or greater probable depth from the roof of the furca

Furcations would thus be classified as IA, IB, IC, IIA, IIB, IIC, IIIA, IIIB, IIIC, and IVA, IVB, IVC. This joint classification is an aid in prognosis and treatment planning, especially if root resection is considered.

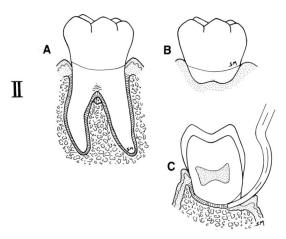

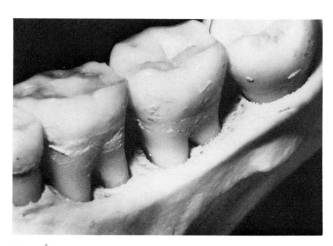

Fig. 4-36. Grade II FI. **A,** Intrafurcal bone and PDL were lost within the furca but not completely through to the other entrance. **B,** Clinically there may be gingival recession, but the furcation entrance is invisible. **C,** A curved probe can penetrate into the furca indicating the approximate attachment loss.

Fig. 4-36. D, Skull specimen shows two shallow Grade II FI on lingual of teeth Nos. 30 and 31. There is so little bone loss within furca No. 31 that clinically, the biologic width restricts probing to a Grade I.

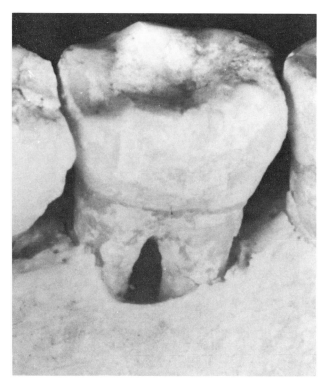

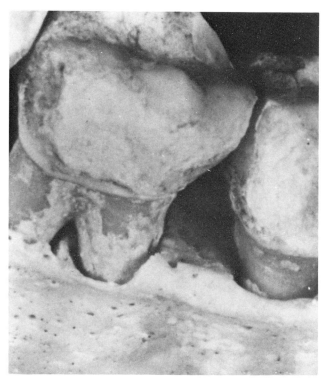

Fig. 4-36. E, Skull specimen demonstrates lingual view of deep bone loss within furca of tooth No. 19.

Fig. 4-36. F, Buccal view of No. 19 shows intact buccal bone within furca. The inverted V shaped space was occupied by the PDL.

Diagnosis of Furcation Invasion

Since radiographic evidence of furcal invasion is inconsistent, the extent of furcal invasion is determined by probing. Straight periodontal probes are used for detecting the extent of vertical bone and attachment loss, whereas curved probes are necessary to probe the horizontal pockets if the furcas are subgingival

(Fig. 4-39). Bone sounding may also be indicated to determine the exact morphology of the bony defects.[68,159,160] The information gained from thorough examination before therapy will expedite a more accurate prognosis and sound treatment plan, but these procedures are often uncomfortable to the patient and are best performed under local infiltration anesthesia.[161]

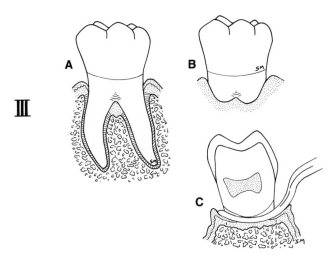

Ⅲ

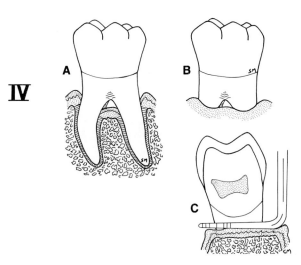

Ⅳ

Fig. 4-37. Grade III FI. **A,** Intrafurcal bone and PDL were destroyed to the other entrance. **B,** Clinically there may be gingival recession, but the furca entrances are not visible. **C,** A curved probe can penetrate the furca from one entrance to the other in a horizontal direction.

Fig. 4-38. Grade IV FI. **A,** There is loss of attachment within the furca through one entrance to the other, with apical gingival recession. **B,** Clinically, gingival recession allows visualization of the furca. **C,** A straight probe is now able to traverse the furca from one entrance to the other due to a patent furca.

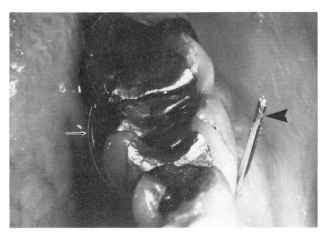

Fig. 4-37. D, Clinical view of tooth No. 19 showing a bent silver cone passing through the furca (white and black arrows).

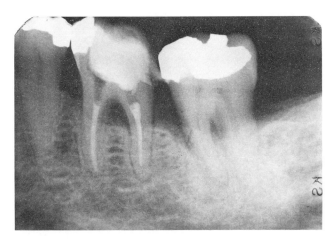

Fig. 4-37. E, X-ray of No. 19 shows distinct furca radiolucency. A root canal filling and interim restoration were placed prior to bisection.

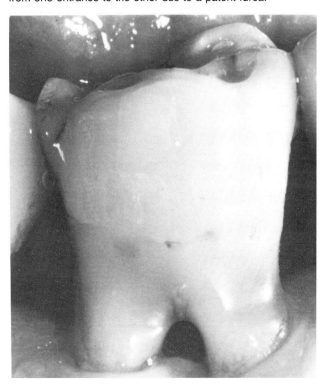

Fig. 4-38. D, Buccal view of open FI, tooth No. 30 (note narrow mesiodistal width of mesial root compared to distal root.

Probing of mandibular molar furcations is easier because there are only two entrances, one on the buccal and one on the lingual surface, located midway mesiodistally (Fig. 4-33). The distal and buccal furcations of maxillary molars are also accessible, as they are located midway buccolingually and mesiodistally (Fig. 4-31). The mesial furcation, however, is not situated midway buccolingually but toward the palate due to the wide buccolingual width of the mesiobuccal root

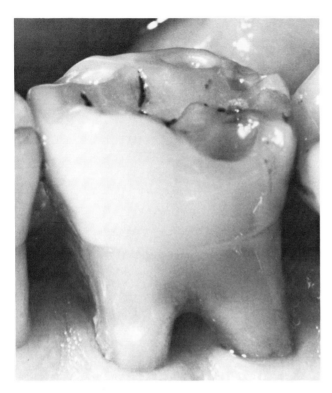

Fig. 4-38. E, Lingual view of open FI No. 30.

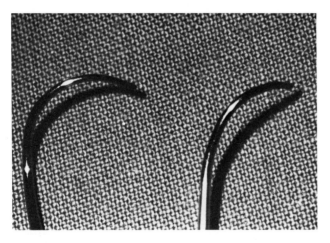

Fig. 4-39. Nabers No. 2 curved probe *(left)* and No. 1 curved probe *(right)*. The No. 1 probe is shorter and has a narrower arc. It was designed to probe the proximal furcas of maxillary molars, but the narrow arc makes probing beneath the gingival margin difficult.

(Fig. 4-31). This furca must be probed from the palatal aspect with the curved probe entering the pocket near the mesiopalatal line angle and curving apically, buccally, and distally into the palatally oriented furca (Fig. 4-40). If the mesial furca is probed at the midpoint buccolingually, the examiner will feel only the mesial surface of the mesiobuccal root and be led to the possibly erroneous conclusion that there is no furcal invasion.

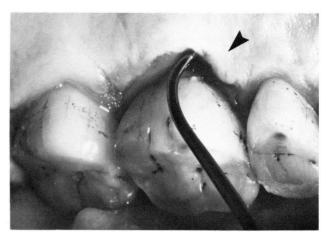

Fig. 4-40. A No. 2 Nabers shown probing the palatally inclined mesial furca of a maxillary first molar.

Prognosis and Treatment Planning

A comprehensive flow chart designed by Morgano efficiently organizes the extensive number of facts gained from examination and diagnosis and indicates treatment consideration regarding root resective and nonresective procedures (Fig. 4-41).

Treatment

This chapter does not discuss specific periodontal and endodontic aspects of root resections but reviews procedures that bear directly on restoring molar teeth treated with root resection. For more detailed information about the management of furcal invasions, the reader is referred to Basaraba (1969, 1977), Hamp and Nyman (1983), Newell (1981), Saadoun (1985), Staffileno (1969) (see Bibliography) and Chapter 3.

Molars with Grade I and shallow Grade II furcation invasions are prepared following the accepted guidelines.

After osseous surgery and pocket elimination, the teeth have increased crown length and exaggerated contours in furcations and areas apical to the CEJ. The gingival finish line of the preparation ideally remains coronal to the soft tissue whenever possible. However, if there are indications for placing margins intracrevicularly or on the root surfaces, the preparation needs to be fluted or barreled into the anatomic depressions for emphasis.[162]

Knowledge of pulp anatomy is critical, especially when working with the maxillary molars. The pulp chamber in maxillary first molars is within the root trunk and follows the external contours of the trunk.[129] At the level of the furcal plane, formed by the levels of the separation points of the three roots, the average thickness of dentin is only 2.0 mm, which is the thickness required for desirable pulpal protection from injury during preparation.[163] Dentin is thickest in a maxillary molar on the distal surface, followed by the lin-

INDICATIONS AND CONTRAINDICATIONS

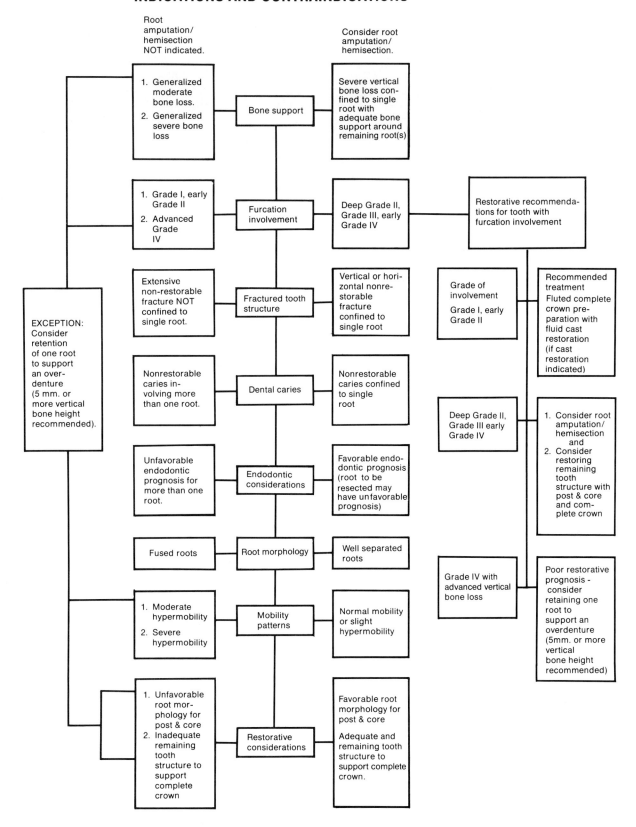

Fig. 4-41. Diagnosis and treatment planning flow chart for root treatment.

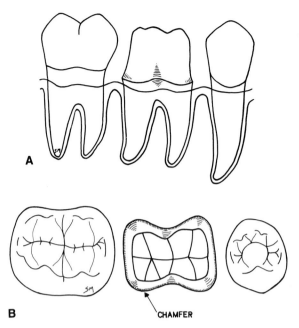

Fig. 4-42. Preparation of a mandibular molar with furca invasion treated by osteoplasty/odontoplasty without root resection. **A,** Ideal taper and reduction obtained with fluting. **B,** Occlusal preparation that mirrors gingival finish line profile.

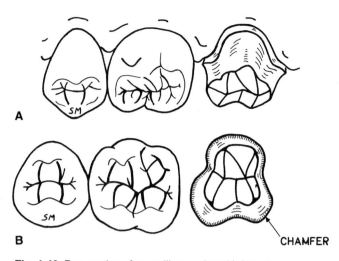

Fig. 4-43. Preparation of a maxillary molar with furcation invasion treated by osteoplasty/odontoplasty without root resection. **A,** Preparation is fluted to prevent overcontouring. **B,** Note Y shaped outline assumed by both occlusal outline and gingival finish line outline.

gual, buccal, and mesial surfaces, respectively. The lingual pulp horn often approaches the mesial tooth surface near the furcation; the dentist should take extra care when barreling into this furcation.

In mandibular first molars, the average thickness of dentin is 3.0 mm on the buccal surface, 2.7 mm on the distal surface, 2.5 mm on the mesial surface, and 2.4 mm on the lingual surface.[164] Therefore, barreling a preparation into a lingual furcation is more likely to result in pulp exposure than is barreling into a buccal furcation.

The final preparation can exhibit gingival seats that have figure eight configurations on mandibular molars (Fig. 4-42) and Y-shaped configurations on maxillary molars (Fig. 4-43). Whatever the shape of the gingival finish line, the gingival margins of the casting are a mirror image of the outline of the finish line of the preparation (Fig. 4-44).

The proximal artificial crown surfaces emerge from the gingival crevice with a flat profile that flares to establish contact with the adjacent tooth. On the facial and lingual surfaces, flat emergence angles are undercontoured from the gingival margin to the cusp tips.[130] If the technician restores normal crown contours coronal to the flat gingival emergence of the flute of the casting, a difficult-to-clean supragingival cul-de-sac is created for plaque retention and subsequent gingival inflammation (Fig. 4-45, A). Conversely, when the fluted margin from the crevice is continued occlusally without a cervical bulge, access for plaque control is effective (Fig. 4-45, B).

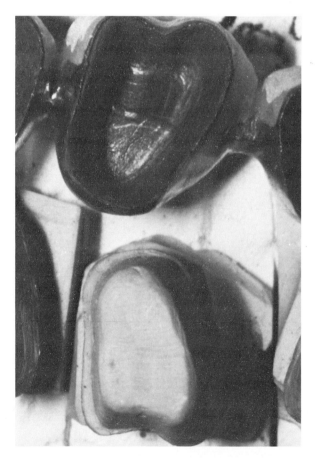

Fig. 4-44. Die and casting of a maxillary molar with a buccal Grade II FI treated by osteoplasty/odontoplasty without resection. Note that the gingival margin outline of the casting mirrors the finish line. Proximal surfaces of casting are flat in the apical third of the crown and then flare with concave surfaces. (Courtesy Dr. David Kaiser, San Antonio, Tex.)

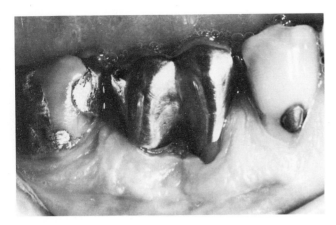

Fig. 4-45. A, Tooth No. 30 with buccal Grade II FI treated by osteoplasty/odontoplasty. Gold crown has been overcontoured without a flat emergence to the occlusal plane. Note plaque and gingivitis.

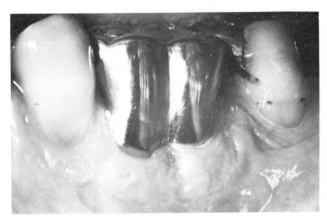

Fig. 4-45. B, Tooth No. 19 in same patient. The extent of the FI was comparable to No. 30 with identical surgical treatment. The gold crown was contoured with flat emergence profiles extending to the occlusal surface. Note lack of plaque and health of gingiva.

RESTORATION OF ROOT-RESECTED MOLARS

The earliest evidence of root amputation is that performed by Farrar in 1884.[165] In 1886, G. V. Black termed resection of one or more roots "radectomy."[166] The concept of retaining portions of a tooth or root along with its periodontal ligament (PDL) after elimination of disease has been refined in subsequent years.[167,168]

Terminology

The terminology for the various approaches in resecting the different roots of molar teeth is far from uniform and very confusing. Hiatt used the term hemisection for the removal of a palatal root of a maxillary molar,[169] while Augsberger limited the term to the buccolingual sectioning of a mandibular molar.[170] Polson described the removal of two maxillary roots and the accompanying crown as trisection,[171] while Greenstein et al. used the term for any combination of root

and crown removal in a maxillary molar.[172] Eastman and Backmeyer have attempted a logical terminology,[173] but in the interest of approved acceptability, the terms published by the American Academy of Periodontology will be used here[174]:

Root amputation: The removal of a root from a multirooted tooth.

Root resection: Surgical removal of all or a portion of the root before or after endodontic treatment.

Hemisection: Surgical separation of a multirooted tooth through the furcation area in such a way that a root, or roots, may be surgically removed along with the associated portion of the crown. The procedure is most frequently performed on the lower molars but may be performed on any multirooted tooth.

Since the *Glossary of Periodontic Terms* does not have a term for splitting and retaining the roots and accompanying crowns of a mandibular molar, or any two roots of a maxillary molar, the term *bisection* will be used. On the rarely indicated occasions when three roots and crown portions of a maxillary molar are retained, the term *trisection* is applicable.

Success of Molar Root Resection

There is agreement concerning short-term success of root resections, hemisections, and bisections. Klavan,[175] Erpenstein,[176] and Hamp et al.[177] have reported high retention rates of 88 to 100 percent, but the average follow-up periods ranged from 3 to 5 years. The long-term results are more questionable. Langer et al. identified increasing failure rates that started low but increased to 38 percent 8 to 10 years after treatment.[178] Nearly 75 percent of the failures resulted from nonperiodontal problems, i.e., root fracture, endodontic failure, or cement washouts; 82 percent of the failures occurred after the first 5 years. Based on their evaluation of these failures the authors discussed factors regarding case selection and treatment precautions that improve the long-term success. These factors are discussed in the following sections.

Prognosis

The prognosis for teeth with resected roots depends upon the supporting bone, the treatment plan, patient motivation, and oral hygiene. The prognosis can be improved by following criteria for patient and tooth selection.

Teeth with large roots and clinical crowns are easier to treat, and pocket elimination ensures a predictable result. Complete instrumentation of the root canals without weakening the root structure is essential, and the remaining root should have adequate bulk for a

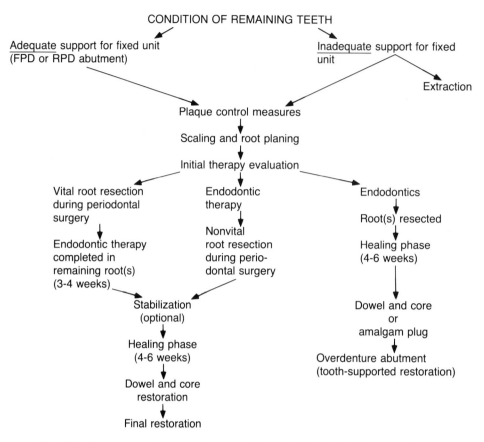

Fig. 4-46. Diagnosis and treatment planning flow chart for teeth with resected roots.

dowel and core. In addition, fabrication of the cast restoration and a biologic occlusion play a fundamental role in the prognosis.

The patient must also assume responsibility for maintaining a healthy environment. If carefully considered, the following indications should encourage a favorable prognosis for molar root resections.

Indications

1. Vertical bone loss around one root but not others
2. Furcation invasions with limited vertical bone loss around roots to be retained
3. Fracture into the middle or apical one third of one root
4. Unfavorable root proximity
5. Caries or unrestorable tooth structure into the furcation or into the middle one third of a root
6. A root with an untreatable apical lesion or endodontic perforation
7. Inability to obturate root canals
8. Severe dehiscence and root sensitivity
9. Impaired prognosis of an adjacent root

Individual Root Considerations for Retention

1. Extent of periodontal furcation invasion
2. Anatomy and topography of supporting bone
3. External root morphology and root canal anatomy
4. Periapical and periodontal health of remaining roots

Contraindications

1. Systemic conditions prohibiting extensive dental procedures
2. Inadequate bone support or unfavorable crown-root ratio of retained roots
3. Adjacent teeth could support an FPD
4. Periodontal therapy that cannot produce an acceptable gingival architecture without removing supportive bone from adjacent teeth
5. Patient unwilling or unable to control plaque
6. Retained roots cannot be endodontically treated
7. Fused roots
8. Economics

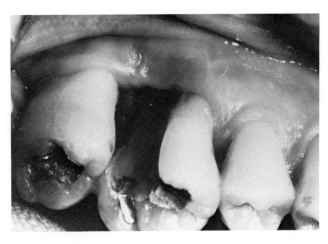

Fig. 4-47. A, Tooth No. 3 after distobuccal hemisection to treat a Grade III distal to buccal FI. A flap was not raised, and the root and its crown portion were removed occlusally. Note soft tissue ledge and crater interdentally over the resected root with deep pockets.

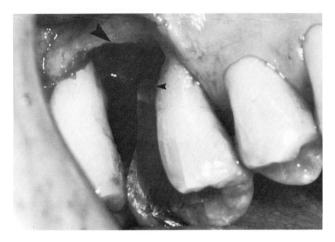

Fig. 4-47. B, Flap raised to treat residual periodontal defects. Large arrow shows ridge of bone beneath soft tissue ridge. Small arrow shows residual distobuccal root left because of lack of visibility.

Diagnosis and Treatment Planning

Ideally, the dentist is consulted in the original treatment plan before the root resection. If a patient has already had a molar root resection, it is prudent to evaluate the situation. Fig. 4-46 shows some of the basic considerations in treatment planning for the restoration of root-resected molars.

Postsurgical Healing

Postsurgical healing is critical with intracrevicular margins. A minimum of 4 to 6 weeks of healing after surgery is required before the soft tissues can resist the trauma of tooth preparation. Three months or more are required for the biologic width and crevice to develop with a stable gingival margin.[66] A 3 to 6-month period between resection and cast restoration is suggested for evaluation of residual

soft or hard tissue defects.[173] Revisional surgery is then performed before the restorative phase of treatment. This would include mucogingival procedures to establish a zone of keratinized and attached gingiva adequate to resist traumatic prosthodontic procedures.[62]

HIDDEN RESIDUAL FURCATION LIPS, ROOTS, AND LEDGES

When root resective procedures are indicated to treat periodontal lesions, they are combined with root and soft tissue debridement and osseous recontouring to establish a healthy dentogingival junction.[179] This requires a surgical flap procedure. Some advocate a technique to elevate the root and its portion of the crown from the socket without raising a flap, especially for a root with a severe periodontal lesion.[180] This frequently leads to residual bony defects and roots without eliminating the furcal invasion (Fig. 4-47).

A surgical flap allows root resection after thorough debridement for improved visibility has occurred. Any residual furcation lip that remains after the initial cut is then removed before soft tissue readaptation (Fig. 4-48). Even with flap surgery, visibility is compromised by excessive bleeding and accessibility in the posterior regions. To avoid cutting too far into the crown and root to be retained, the surgeon may cut short of the furcation, leaving a lip (Fig. 4-49, A). This is not serious if the lip is supragingival after healing, because the dentist can remove it during preparation (Fig. 4-49, B). If hidden subgingivally, it may be undetected and retained.

Backman reported four cases of incomplete root resection with substantial portions of the resected root remaining.[181] Other authors have commented on this problem, but they have not reported on its prevalence.[182] An unpublished retrospective study of over 100 root-resected molars has revealed an inordinate number of residual roots, furcation lips, and cul-de-sac ledges "hidden" subgingivally (Fig. 4-50).[183] Residual roots were more routinely found with mesiobuccal root amputations in maxillary molars (nearly 40 percent of the time) and often initially observed radiographically (Fig. 4-51). This root is incompletely removed because its exceptional buccolingual width is not perceived (Fig. 4-31). Ledges that acted as cul-de-sac furcation invasions were usually associated with distobuccal and palatal root amputations (Fig. 4-50, B and C). Teeth with subgingival residual root furcation lips or ledges were observed approximately 30 percent of the time.

Most faulty root resections were asymptomatic, but the sites were often associated with bleeding when probed, and several presented with periodontal abcesses (Fig. 4-52, A). When a root is resected with a horizontal cut that creates a ledge rather than with a long beveled section, visibility of the furcation is se-

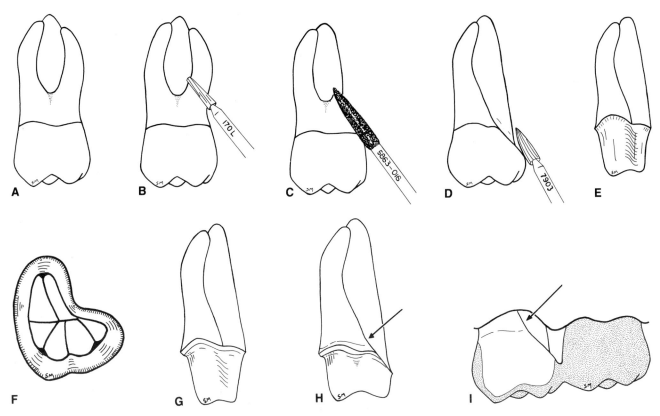

Fig. 4-48. Root amputation for maxillary first molar. **A,** Intact maxillary molar. **B,** Initial bur position for amputation of distobuccal root. **C,** After root is delivered, lip of furcation is contoured to remove area of furcation. **D,** Final shape of tooth after lip of furcation is removed. **E,** Buccal view of preparation for a complete crown. **F,** Occlusal view of preparation; Note L shape. **G,** A modification of the preparation in Figs. 14-48.E, and 14-48.F, for an esthetic veneer complete crown. A facial beveled shoulder blends with the lingual chamfer. **H,** A more conservative preparation design that maintains much of the distobuccal portion of the crown. The lip of the furcation should be eliminated and the opening to the root canal sealed with amalgam (arrow). **I,** Splinting of the resected tooth to a continuous tooth is recommended if mobility is increasing or causing the patient discomfort. The tooth can be prepared for an onlay or ¾ crown that is soldered to an adjacent artificial crown. The opening to the root canal is sealed with amalgam (arrow).

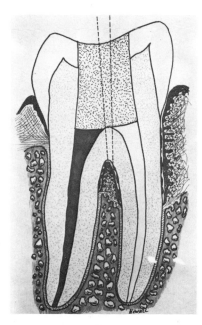

Fig. 4-49.A, Diagram of mandibular molar requiring a mesial hemisection. Dotted lines show planes of bur cuts positioned toward the root to be removed without notching the remaining root.

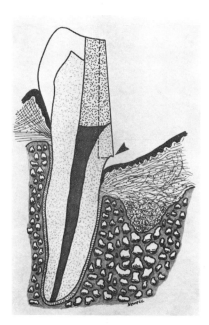

Fig. 4-49. B, This approach often leaves a furcation lip *(arrow)* to be removed by the surgeon or the dentist during preparation. If located supragingivally, it is easy to see; if subgingivally, the dentist probes to confirm the presence.

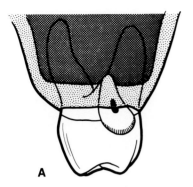 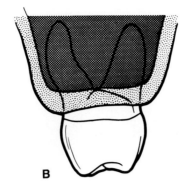 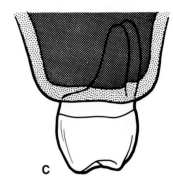

Fig. 4-50. A, The residual subgingival mesiobuccal root is difficult to locate without probing. **B,** The distobuccal root has been removed except for a lip, but the cut has left a subgingival ledge and cul-de-sac. **C,** The palatal root is often removed with a flat cut to preserve palatal crown structure, leaving an uncleansable ledge. This also creates a cantilever to the palatal aspect without support from adjacent teeth.

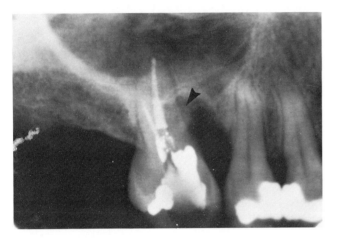

Fig. 4-51. A, X-ray of a maxillary first molar 2 years after a mesiobuccal root amputation. Note the radiopaque shadow of a residual mesiobuccal root and bone resorption.

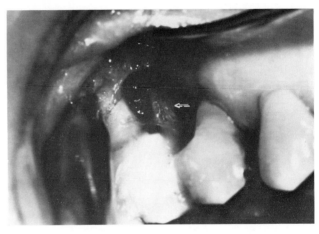

Fig. 4-51. B, Surgical flap shows a large residual section of the incompletely amputated mesiobuccal root seen in the radiograph.

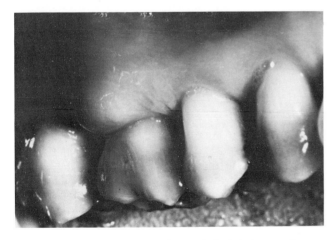

Fig. 4-52. A, A buccal view of a periodontal abscess from a Grade III FI between the buccal roots of No. 3 after faulty palatal root amputation.

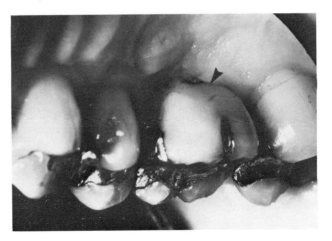

Fig. 4-52. B, Palatal view shows a residual ledge partially subgingival with an internal furcation between the buccal roots *(arrow)*.

verely limited (Fig. 4-52, B). It is difficult in maxillary molars to detect internal furcation invasions between the remaining two roots that progress to Grade III invasions.[182] The frequency of faulty root resections requires the dentist to probe thoroughly around root-resected teeth to detect any residual structures.

VITAL OR NONVITAL ROOT RESECTION

Endodontic treatment is usually completed before root resection when it is definitely indicated. After the canals of the retained roots are filled with gutta-percha, the pulp chamber can be filled with amalgam and the canal of the root to be amputated can be filled to half its length.[184] This acts as a retrofill seal after amputation and facilitates tooth restoration. Root resection may not be confirmed until after surgical exposure of the defect, however. Gerstein concluded that vital root amputation can be performed at that time with endodontics completed when practical.[185] Pulps were asymptomatic two weeks after vital root resection, allowing time for surgical healing before endodontics.[186] If vital root resection was performed, however, prosthetic treatment should not begin until after root canal therapy to determine the need for a crown buildup.

POST AND CORES

Brittleness of the pulpless root-resected tooth is a primary reason for root fractures over time[187]; however, the intact, arch-shaped roof of the pulp chamber is extremely resistant to pressure and stress. Removal of the roof for endodontic access weakens the tooth, which requires strong interior and exterior support.[188] For these reasons, complete protective coverage of root-resected teeth is recommended,[189,190] especially over the area of resection.[191]

When roots have been removed from vital teeth, final tooth preparations are deferred until endodontic procedures are completed.

Endodontically treated teeth usually have a post inserted before cast restorations.[89] There is no evidence that this is beneficial in resected teeth, and it could be detrimental (Fig. 4-53). Cast post and core restorations are usually applicable only to maxillary palatal roots and mandibular distal roots. The maxillary mesiobuccal root and mandibular mesial root are narrower mesiodistally than the palatal root and mandibular distal root. Their pulp canals are elongated or ribbon shaped when compared to the other root canals, and are located nearer to the furcal surfaces (Figs. 4-31 and 4-33). Abou-Rass et al. discovered that in preparation of spaces for posting in mandibular molars, the distal wall of the mesial root was often perforated, whereas in maxillary molars it was the distal wall of the mesiobuccal root.[192] Depending on the roots retained, post and cores without perforation or fracture are difficult.

CROWN PREPARATION

Whenever possible, crown margins should be placed supragingivally for ease of impressions, margin finishing, and overall periodontal health.[172]

Intracrevicular margin placement may be required to cover portions of the root-resected area.[191] Koth demonstrated no significant difference in gingival fluid as an indicator of inflammation in patients with healthy gingiva who were motivated in plaque control, regardless of the location of gingival crown margins.[193]

The crown margin should be apical to the pulp chamber floor or root canal that was exposed by resection,[172] especially if these structures have not been

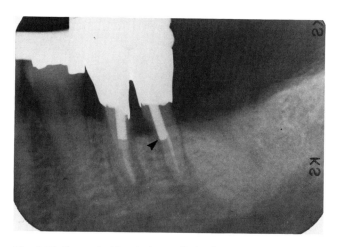

Fig. 4-53. X-ray of a bisected mandibular first molar with soldered permanent crowns cemented over post and cores. Note mesial perforation of the distal root due to a large malaligned post *(arrow)*. Note diffuse radiolucency surrounding the apical half of the distal root due to fracture from the perforation. The mesial post is too large for this narrow root mesidistally.

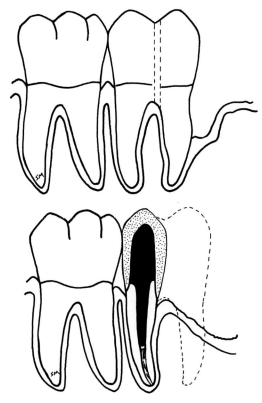

Fig. 4-54. Diagram of a hemisection of the mesial root of a mandibular second molar restored as a single crown.

sealed with amalgam. To prevent impingement on the biologic width; intracrevicular margins to cover the pulpal canal structures should be no closer than *3 mm* to the alveolar crest.[172] This may necessitate additional lengthening.

To preserve remaining tooth structure and encourage a better-fitting restoration, a less complicated

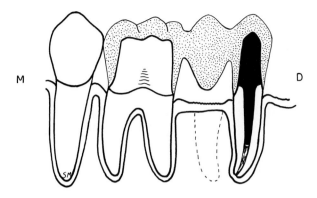

Fig. 4-55. Diagram of a single root of a mandibular molar retained after hemisection and restored as an abutment for a short-span three unit FPD.

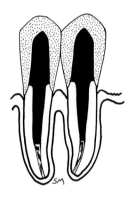

Fig. 4-56. Diagram of a bisected mandibular molar and restoration of each root. The units may be independent or soldered together, depending on the mobility.

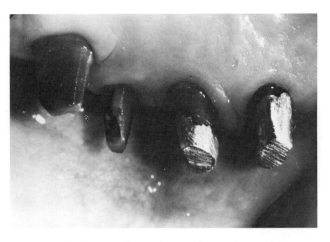

Fig. 4-57. A, Maxillary first and second premolars and the separated mesiobuccal and palatal roots of the first molar prepared for complete crowns.

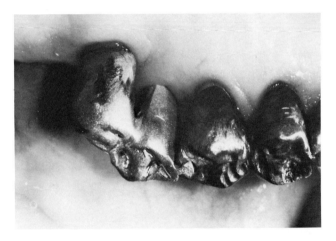

Fig. 4-57. B, Unpolished castings seated but uncemented. A nonrigid connector was used to improve withdrawal planes without sacrificing tooth structure.

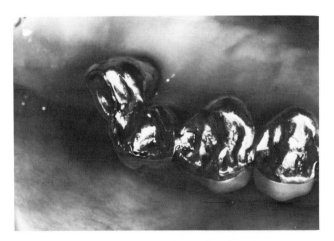

Fig. 4-57. C, Occlusal view of polished and cemented crowns. Note lack of excessive occlusal contours of resected molar. There is adequate function without unsupported forces on this tooth. (Courtesy Dr. David Kaiser, San Antonio, Tex.)

preparation utilizing a knife edge finish line[194] or a chamfer is recommended.[191]

This preparation eliminates residual ledges, roots, furcation lips, or horizontal components of the furcation.[194] In maxillary molars this includes eliminating remaining *internal furcation invasions* (IFI). This may present problems if an IFI is deeper than estimated. Barreling this preparation to eliminate the IFI may reduce tooth structure to a critically narrow isthmus. The tooth may then be too weak in the preparation to support a prosthesis, or the remaining intrafurcal attachment may soon be lost, resulting in a Grade III furca invasion. This may require hemisection of one of the remaining roots and retention of only one root (Fig. 4-54). This root can serve as an abutment, especially if the retained root is the distal root of a mandibular molar (Fig. 4-55). The remaining roots with a narrow connecting isthmus can also be bisected and restored as a Grade IV "tunnel" with metal axial walls to resist recurrent caries. These separated roots may be restored with individual crowns (Fig. 4-56) or with a solder joint (Fig. 4-57). If the separated roots are too close to permit adequate cleansing by the patient, orthodontic separation may be necessary.

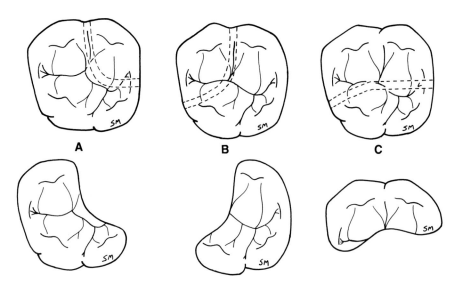

Fig. 4-58. Hemisections for the maxillary first molar. **A,** Distobuccal hemisection and crown contour before preparation. **B,** Mesiobuccal hemisection and prepreparation crown form. **C,** Palatal hemisection and prepreparation crown form. Note that the mesial cuts and posthemisection contours deviate slightly toward the palate to accommodate the wide mesiobuccal root.

Stabilization

Splinting sectioned teeth is not always necessary. Even slight, increased mobility is acceptable as long as it is not increasing and the patient is comfortable. If there is uncertainty as to how a resected molar will function, a treatment restoration can be fabricated and the mobility observed for several months before a cast restoration is inserted.[172]

Crown contours

The health of the periodontium is the objective in restoring a tooth with resected roots. The gingival third of the restoration is fabricated with a flat emergence profile from the gingiva to facilitate oral hygiene. Open embrasures between individual crowns and apical to rigid connectors allow proximal cleaning with an interdental brush.

The various root resections and the resultant contours should be reviewed by the dentist. With maxillary molars, the distobuccal root is the most frequently removed root (Fig. 4-58, A).[183] The mesiobuccal root is also commonly removed (Fig. 4-58, B), and occasionally, the palatal root is removed (Fig. 4-58, C). The palatal root can be retained alone, but deviates severely toward the midline from the vertical axis of the crown and buccal roots, and is less tolerant of occlusal forces (Fig. 4-50, A, B). Two remaining maxillary roots can be bisected and retained as a soldered unit consisting of the two buccal roots, the distobuccal and palatal root, or the mesiobuccal and palatal root (Fig. 4-57).[171]

Mandibular molars have only three combinations of remaining roots, since they have only two roots. The mesial root can be hemisected, leaving the distal root and a portion of the crown (Fig. 4-59, A). This is the

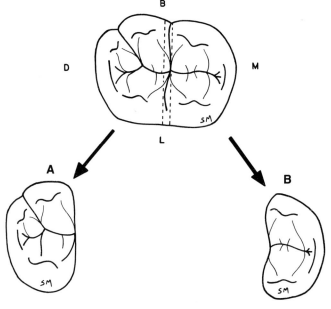

Fig. 4-59. Hemisection of the mandibular first molar and forms of the remaining crowns. **A,** Hemisection of the mesial root with a relatively flat mesial surface of the distal root and crown. **B,** Hemisection of the distal root with a concavity on the distal surface of the mesial crown portion that is an extension of the pronounced root concavity.

preferrable arrangement, as the root is more symmetrical when it has shallower concavities and a more circular pulp canal to accommodate a post or dowel (Fig. 4-33, A). When necessary, the distal root and crown portion is hemisected, leaving the mesial root and its crown (Fig. 4-59, B). This root is not as desirable to retain because of a deep distal surface concavity, its narrow mesiodistal width, and its ribbonlike pulp canal system, which makes placing a post difficult (Fig. 4-33, A).

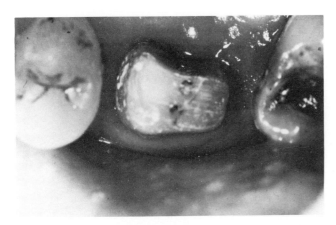

Fig. 4-60. A, Occlusal view of prepared buccal portion of a maxillary first molar with a hemisected palatal root. The mesial portion is wider due to the wider mesiobuccal root.

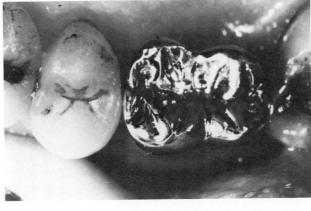

Fig. 4-60. B, Occlusal view of permanent crown. Note contact areas with adjacent teeth and palatal extention of occlusal surface only far enough to establish centric stops with lower molar.

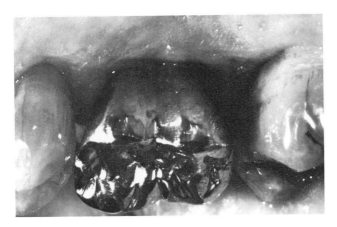

Fig. 4-60. C, Lingual view of permanent crown showing flat emergence profile with slight lingual flare towards the occlusal surface for centric stops.

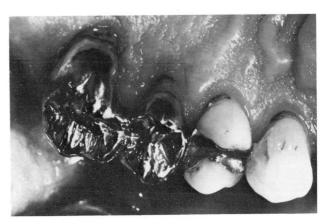

Fig. 4-61. A, Occlusolingual view of soldered castings on teeth Nos. 13 and 14. The mesiobuccal root of No. 14 has been hemisected, and there was a diastema between No. 13 and 14. Extensive restoration of No. 13 was required, so splinting was performed for mesiodistal stability to No. 14. Note extremely steep cuspal inclines that generated lateral forces.

Occlusion

The restored axial surface adjacent to the resected root has a flat profile, and the occlusal outline mirrors the gingival margin outline. The occlusal table may require extension over the area of the missing root in the following instances: establishing the contact with an adjacent tooth; when the bulk of metal is required for a solder joint; and establishing centric stops, such as the lingual cusps of a maxillary molar (Fig. 4-60, A to C).

Lateral forces are controlled by minimizing cuspal inclines on the resected molar and the teeth stabilizing it.[49] Should inflammatory periodontal diseases recur around a resected tooth with excessive lateral forces from steep cuspal inclines, rapid attachment loss is common (Fig. 4-61, A and B). With controlled occlusal forces and inflammatory periodontal diseases, even resected teeth with severely compromised support can function for extended periods (Fig. 4-61, C to E).

Maintenance

Silness reported a study of 73 FPDs in 73 patients,

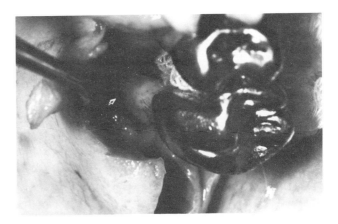

Fig. 4-61. B, One year after root resection the patient returned with a palatal abscess No. 14. Surgical exploration revealed loss of bone support around the palatal root (arrow).　*continued*

only a few of whom had received oral hygiene instruction.[56] He discovered that there was more soft deposit

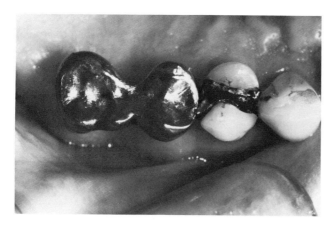

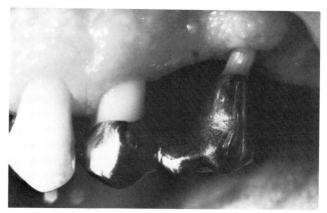

Fig. 4-61. C, Occlusal view of splint No. 13-14 five years after palatal root amputation and occlusal equilibration to reduce the cuspal inclines for light centric stops.

Fig. 4-61. D, Buccal view of splint No. 13-14 with distobuccal root providing terminal support five years post palatal root amputation. Buccolingual mobility of the splint is only Class I and stable. The patient can chew without limitations, has acceptable gingival health; shallowed cuspal inclines and crevices around the abutments do not exceed 2 mm.

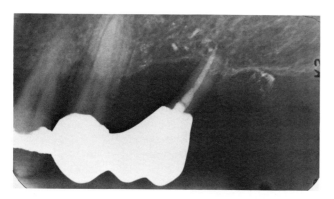

Fig. 4-61. E, X-ray of No. 13 and distobuccal root No. 14 five years postoperatively. The PDL spaces are slightly widened, but mobility is slight and not increasing.

accummulation, more severe gingivitis, and increased pocket depth around complete crowns than in contralateral natural teeth. The periodontal conditions were better in patients who had received oral hygiene instruction. Axelsson and Lindhe reported a 6-year study of 375 treated patients who received instruction and practice in oral hygiene techniques and meticulous prophylaxis every 2 to 3 months compared to 180 treated patients who were examined annually and received only symptomatic treatment.[195] In the maintained group, the progress of gingivitis, periodontitis, and caries was effectively prevented. Long-term success with periodontic or prosthodontic patients requires a coordinated maintenance program.

SELECTED REFERENCES

1. Keough, B.E., Kay, H.B., Rosenberg, M.M., and Holt, R.L.: Periodontal prosthetics: management of the patient with advanced periodontal disease. In Clark, J.: Clinical dentistry **4:** Chap. 41, 1-106, 1982.
2. Nassif, J., and Blumenfeld, W.L.: Joint consultation services by the periodontist and prosthodontist, J. Prosthet. Dent. **29:**55-60, 1973.
3. Selipsky, H.: Osseous surgery: how much need we compromise? Dent. Clin. North Am. **20**(1):79-106, 1976.
4. Kegel, W., Selipsky, H., and Phillips, C.: The effect of splinting on tooth mobility. I. During initial therapy, J. Clin. Periodontol. **6:**45-58, 1979.
5. Perlitsh, M.: A systematic approach to the interpretation of tooth mobility and its clinical implications, Dent. Clin. North Am. **24**(2):177-193, 1980.
6. Wank, G.S., and Kroll, Y.J.: Occlusal trauma: an evaluation of its relationship to periodontal prosthesis, Dent. Clin. North Am. **25**(3):511-532, 1981.
7. Goldman, H.M., and Cohen, D.W.: Periodontal therapy, ed. 4, St. Louis, 1968, The C.V. Mosby Co., p. 241.
8. Wentz, F., Jarabak, J., and Orban, B.: Experimental occlusal trauma imitating cuspal interferences, J. Periodontol. **29:**117-127, 1958.
9. Polson, A.M., Meitner, S.W., and Zander, H.A.: Trauma and progression of marginal periodontitis in squirrel monkeys. IV. Reversibility of bone loss due to trauma alone and trauma superimposed upon periodontitis, J. Periodont. Res. **11:**290, 1976.
10. Vogel, R., and Deasy, M.: Tooth mobility: etiology and rationale of therapy, N.Y. Dent. J. **43:**159, 1977.
11. Zander, H., and Polson, A.M.: Present status of occlusal therapy in periodontics, J. Periodontol. **48:**540-544, 1977.
12. Lindhe, J.: Textbook of clinical periodontology, Copenhagen, 1983, Munksgaard, pp. 451-465.
13. Grant, D.A., Stern, I.B., and Everett, F.G.: Periodontics: In the Tradition of Orban and Gottlieb, ed. 5, St. Louis, 1979, The C.V. Mosby Co., p. 444.
14. Carranza, F.A.: Glickman's Clinical Periodontology, ed. 6, Philadelphia, 1984, W.B. Saunders Co., p. 537.
15. Mühlemann, H.R., Herzog, H., and Vogel, A.: Occlusal trauma and tooth mobility, Schweiz. Mschr. Zahnhk. **66:**527-544, 1956.
16. Mühlemann, H.R., Savdir, S., and Rateitschak, K.H.: Tooth mobility—its causes and significance, J. Periodontol. **36:**148-153, 1965.
17. Lindhe, J.: Textbook of Clinical Periodontology, Copenhagen, 1983, Munksgaard, pp. 466-479.
18. Waerhaug, J.: Justification for splinting in periodontal therapy, J. Prosthet. Dent. **22:**201-208, 1969.
19. Lindhe, J., and Nyman, S.: The role of occlusion in periodontal disease and the biological rationale for splinting in treatment of periodontitis, Oral Sci. Rev. **10:**11-43, 1977.
20. Polson, A.M., and Haijl, L.C.: Occlusion and periodontal disease, Dent. Clin. North Am. **24**(4):783-795, 1980.

21. Nyman, S., Lindhe, J., and Lundgren, D.: The role of occlusion for the stability of fixed bridges in patients with reduced periodontal support, J. Clin. Periodontol. **50:**163-169, 1979.

22. Nyman, S., and Lindhe, J.: A longitudinal study of combined periodontal and prosthetic treatment of patients with advanced periodontal disease, J. Periodontol. **50:**163-169, 1979.

23. Nyman, S., and Ericsson, I.: The capacity of reduced periodontal tissues to support fixed bridgework, J. Clin. Periodontol. **9:**409-414, 1982.

24. Stein, S.D., and Moloff, R.L.: Realities in addressing the emotional, economic and sequential aspects of certain advanced periodontal prosthetic cases, Int. J. Periodont. Restor. Dent. **3(2):**59-73, 1983.

25. Stern, I.B.: The status of temporary fixed splinting procedures in the treatment of periodontally involved teeth, J. Periodontol. **31:**217-223, 1960.

26. Caffessee, R.G.: Management of periodontal disease in patients with occlusal abnormalities, Dent. Clin. North Am. **24(2):**215-230, 1980.

27. Amsterdam, M.: Periodontal prosthesis: twenty-five years in retrospect. IV. Modified Hawley bite plane, Compend. Contin. Ed. **5(6):**500-506, 1984.

28. Rateitschak, K.H.: The therapeutic effect of local treatment on periodontal disease assessed upon evaluation of different diagnostic criteria. I. Changes in tooth mobility, J. Periodontol. **34:**540-544, 1963.

29. Rudd, K.D., and O'Leary, T.J.: Stabilizing periodontally weakened teeth by using guide plane removable partial dentures: a preliminary report, J. Prosthet. Dent. **16:**721-730, 1966.

30. Stewart, K.L., and Rudd, K.D.: Stabilizing periodontally weakened teeth with removable partial dentures, J. Prosthet. Dent. **19:**475-482, 1968.

31. Thayer, K.E.: Fixed Prosthodontics, Chicago, 1984, Year Book Medical Publishers, Inc., p. 223.

32. Shillingberg, H.T., and Fisher, D.W.: Nonrigid connectors for fixed partial dentures, J.A.D.A. **87:**1195-1199, 1973.

33. Crispin, B.J.: Tissue response to posterior denture base-type pontics, J. Prosthet. Dent. **42:**257-262, 1979.

34. Becker, C.M., and Kaldahl, W.B.: Current theories of crown contour, margin placement, and pontic design, J. Prosthet. Dent. **45:**268-277, 1981.

35. Peeso, F.A.: Crown and Bridge Work for Students and Practitioners, Philadelphia, 1916, Lea and Febiger.

36. Prichard, J.F., and Feder, M.: A modern adaptation of the telescopic principle in periodontal prosthesis, J. Periodontol. **33:**360-364, 1962.

37. Pugh, C.E., and Smerke, J.W.: Rationale for fixed prosthesis in the management of advanced periodontal disease, Dent. Clin. North Am. **13(1):**243-262, 1969.

38. Woolsey, G.D., and Matich, J.A.: The effect of axial grooves on the resistance form of cast restorations, J.A.D.A. **97:**978-980, 1978.

39. Weed, R.M., and Baez, R.J.: A method for determining adequate resistance form of complete cast crown preparations, J. Prosthet. Dent. **52:**330-334, 1984.

40. Amsterdam, M.: Periodontal prosthesis: twenty-five years in retrospect. V. Final treatment plan, Compend. Cont. Ed. **5:**577-591, July/August 1984.

41. Yulzari, J.C.: Strategic extraction in periodontal prosthesis, Int. J. Periodont. Restor. Dent. **2(6):**51-63, 1982.

42. Lubow, R.M., Cooley, R.L., and Kaiser, D.: Periodontal and restorative aspects of molar uprighting, J. Prosthet. Dent. **47:**373-376, 1982.

43. Brown, J.S.: The effect of orthodontic therapy on certain types of periodontal defects. I. Clinical findings, J. Periodontol. **44:**742-756, 1973.

44. Rönnerman, A., Thilander, B., and Heyden, G.: Gingival tissue reactions to orthodontic closure of extraction sites. Histologic and histochemical studies, Am. J. Orthodont. **77:**620-625, 1980.

45. Morse, P.H.: Resorption of upper incisors following orthodontic treatment, Dent. Practitioner **22:**21-35, 1971.

46. Zachrisson, B., and Alnaes, L.: Periodontal condition in orthodontically treated and untreated individuals. I. Loss of attachment, gingival pocket depth and clinical crown height, Angle Orthodontists **43:**402-411, 1973.

47. Zachrisson, B., and Alnaes, L.: Periodontal condition in orthodontically treated and untreated individuals. II. Alveolar bone loss: radiographic findings, Angle Orthodontist **44:**48-55, 1974.

48. Kaleta, A., and Malone, W.F.P.: A preview for the rationale of centric closure position, Ill. Dent. J. **43:**83-86, 1974.

49. Glickman, J., Stein, R.S., and Smulow, J.B.: The effect of increased functional forces upon the periodontium of splinted and non-splinted teeth, J. Periodontol. **32:**290-300, 1961.

50. Silness, J.: Fixed prosthodontics and periodontal health, Dent. Clin. North Am. **24(2):**317-329, April 1980.

51. Levinson, E.: Periodontal postulates for the prosthodontist, Int. J. Periodont. Restor. Dent. **1(1):**45-49, 1981.

52. Kay, H.B.: Criteria for restorative contours in the altered periodontal environment, Int. J. Periodont. Restor. Dent. **5(3):**43-63, 1985.

53. Gher, M.E., and Vernino, A.R.: Root morphology—clinical significance in pathogenesis and treatment of periodontal disease, J.A.D.A. **101:**627-633, 1980.

54. Gher, M.E., and Vernino, A.R.: Root anatomy: a local factor in inflammatory periodontal disease, Int. J. Periodont. Restor. Dent. **1(5):**53-63, 1981.

55. Timoshenko, S.P., Goodier, J.N.: Theory of Elasticity, ed. 3, New York, 1970, McGraw-Hill Book Co.

56. Silness, J.: Periodontal conditions in patients treated with dental bridges. II. The influence of full and partial crowns on plaque accummulation, development of gingivitis and pocket formation, J. Periodont. Res. **5:**219-224, 1970.

57. Waerhaug, J.: Histologic considerations which govern where the margins of restorations should be located in relation to the gingiva, Dent. Clin. North Am. **4(2):**161-176, 1960.

58. Silness, J.: Periodontal conditions in patients treated with dental bridges. III. The relationship between the location of the crown and margin and the periodontal condition, J. Periodont. Res. **5:**225-229, 1970.

59. Newcomb, G.M.: The relationship between the location of subgingival crown margins and gingival inflammation, J. Periodontol. **45:**151-154, 1974.

60. Jameson, L.M.: Comparison of the volume of crevicular fluid from restored and nonrestored teeth, J. Prosthet. Dent. **41:**209-214, 1979.

61. Kishimoto, M., Hobo, S., Duncanson, M.G., and Shillingburg, H.T.: Effectiveness of margin finishing techniques on cast gold restorations, Int. J. Periodont. Restor. Dent. **1(5):**21-29, 1981.

62. Wilson, R.D., and Maynard, J.G.: The relationship of restorative dentistry to periodontics. In Prichard, J.F., editor: The Diagnosis and Treatment of Periodontal Disease, Philadelphia, 1979, W.B. Saunders Co., pp. 538-576.

63. Ingber, J.S., Rose, L.F., and Coslet, J.G.: The "Biologic Width"—a concept in periodontics and restorative dentistry, Alpha Omegan **70:**62-65, 1977.

64. Nevins, M., Skurow, H.M.: The intracrevicular restorative margin, the biologic width, and the maintenance of the gingival margin, Int. J. Periodont. Restor. Dent. **4(3):**31-49, 1984.

65. Kay, H.B.: Esthetic considerations in the definitive periodontal prosthetic management of the maxillary anterior seg-

ment, Int. J. Periodont. Restor. Dent. **2**(3):45-59, 1982.

66. Rosen, H., and Gitnick, P.J.: Integrating restorative procedures into the treatment of periodontal disease, J. Prosthet. Dent. **14**:343-354, 1964.

67. Ramfjord, S.P., and Ash, M.M.: Periodontology and Periodontics, Philadelphia, 1979, W.B. Saunders Co., pp. 675-693.

68. Tibbetts, L.S.: Use of diagnostic probes for detection of periodontal disease, J.A.D.A. **78**:549-555, 1969.

69. Listgarten, M.A.: Periodontal probing: what does it mean? J. Clin. Periodontol. **7**:165-176, 1980.

70. Armitage, G.C., Svanberg, G.K., and Löe, H.: Microscopic evaluation of clinical measurements of connective tissue attachment levels, J. Clin. Periodontol. **4**:173-190, 1977.

71. Eismann, H.F., Radke, R.A., and Noble, W.H.: Physiologic design criteria for fixed dental restorations, Dent. Clin. North Am. **15**(3):543-568, 1971.

72. Wilson, R.D., and Maynard, I.G.: Intracrevicular restorative dentistry, Int. J. Periodont. Restor. Dent. **1**(4):35-49, 1981.

73. Mount, G.J.: Crowns and the gingival tissues, Austral. Dent. J. **15**:253-258, 1970.

74. Dragoo, M.R., and Williams, G.B.: Periodontal tissue reactions to restorative procedures, Int. J. Periodont. Restor. Dent. **1**(1):9-23, 1981.

75. Gargiulo, A.W., Wentz, F.M., and Orban, B.J.: Dimensions and relations of the dentogingival junction in humans, J. Periodontol. **32**:261-267, 1961.

76. Bohannan, H.M., and Abrams, L.: Intentional vital pulp extirpation in periodontal prosthesis, J. Prosthet. Dent. **11**:781-789, 1961.

77. Mullaney, T.P., and Laswell, H.R.: Iatrogenic blushing of dentin following full crown preparation, J. Prosthet. Dent. **22**:354-359, 1969.

78. Bergenholtz, G., and Nyman, S.: Endodontic complications following periodontal and prosthetic treatment of patients with advanced periodontal disease, J. Periodontol. **55**:63-68, 1984.

79. Löe, H.: Reactions of marginal periodontal tissues to restorative procedures, Int. Dent. J. **18**:759, 1968.

80. Hall, W.B.: Periodontal preparation of the mouth for restoration, Dent. Clin. North Am. **24**(2):195-213, 1980.

81. Takei, H.H., and Carranza, F.A.: The periodontal flap. In Carranza, F.A., editor: Glickman's Clinical Periodontology, ed. 6, Philadelphia, 1984, W.B. Saunders Co., pp. 797-802.

82. Ainamo, A.: Influence of age on the location of the maxillary mucogingival junction, J. Periodont. Res. **13**:189-193, 1978.

83. Lang, N.P., and Löe, H.: The relationship between the width of keratinized gingiva and gingival health, J. Periodontol. **43**:623-627, 1972.

84. Wennström, J., and Lindhe, J., and Nyman, S.: The role of keratinized gingiva in plaque-associated gingivitis in dogs, J. Clin. Periodontol. **9**:75-85, 1982.

85. Wennström, J., and Lindhe, J.: Role of attached gingiva for maintenance of periodontal health, J. Clin. Periodontol. **10**:206-221, 1983.

86. Dragoo, M.R., and Williams, G.B.: Periodontal tissue reaction to restorative procedures, Int. J. Periodont. Restor. Dent. **1**(1):9-23, 1981.

87. Berman, M.H.: The complete-coverage restoration and the gingival sulcus, J. Prosthet. Dent. **29**:301-309, 1973.

88. Kaiser, D., and Newell, D.H.: Technique to diminish the display of metal margin of ceramic/metal crowns. Submitted for publication.

89. Fagin, M.D.: Restoration of endodontically treated teeth, Int. J. Periodont. Restor. Dent. **1**(2):9-29, 1981.

90. Rheinhardt, R.A., Krejci, R.F., Pao, Y.C., and Stannard, J.G.: Dentin stresses in post-constructed teeth with dimin-

ishing bone support, J. Dent. Res. **62**:1002-1007, 1983.

91. Pao, Y.C., Rheinhardt, R.A., and Krejci, R.F.: Root stresses with tapered-end post design in periodontally compromised teeth, J. Prosthet. Dent. In press.

92. Bender, I.B., Seltzer, S., and Saltanoff, W.: Endodontic success—a reappraisal of criteria, Oral Surg. **22**:780-789, 1966.

93. Standlee, J.P., Caputo, A.A., Holcomb, J., and Trabert, K.: The retentive and stress distributing properties of a threaded endodontic dowel, J. Prosthet. Dent. **44**:398, 1980.

94. Pitts, D.L., Matheny, H.H., and Nicholls, J.I.: An in-vitro study of spreader loads required to cause vertical root fracture during lateral condensation, J. Endodont. **9**:544-550, 1983.

95. Gher, M.E., Dunlap, R.M., Maxwell, H.A., and Kuhl, L.V.: Clinical survey of fractured teeth, J.A.D.A. **114**:174-177, 1987.

96. Halpern, B.G.: Restoration of endodontically treated teeth, Dent. Clin. North Am. **29**(2):293-303, 1985.

97. Appleton, I.E.: Restoration of root-resected teeth, J. Prosthet. Dent. **44**:150-153, 1980.

98. Oliva, R.A., and Lowe, J.A.: Dimensional stability of composite used as a core material, J. Prosthet. Dent. **56**:554-559, 1986.

99. Azzi, R., Tsao, T.F., Carranza, F.A., and Kenney, E.B.: Comparative study of gingival retraction methods, J. Prosthet. Dent. **50**:561-565, 1983.

100. Löe, H., and Silness, J.: Tissue reactions to string packs used in fixed restorations, J. Prosthet. Dent. **13**:318-323, 1963.

101. Taylor, A.C., and Campbell, M.M.: Reattachment of gingival epithelium to the tooth, J. Periodontol. Dent. **43**:281-293, 1972.

102. Price, C., and Whitehead, F.I.: Impression materials as foreign bodies, Br. Dent. J. **133**:9-14, 1972.

103. O'Leary, T.J., Standish, S.M., and Bloomer, R.S.: Severe periodontal destruction following impression procedures, J. Periodontol. **44**:43-48, 1973.

104. Malone, W.F.P., and Manning, J.L.: Electrosurgery in restorative dentistry, J. Prosthet. Dent. **20**:417-425, 1968.

105. Pope, J.W., Gargiulo, A.V., Staffileno, H., and Levy, S.: Effects of electrosurgery on wound healing in dogs, Periodontics **6**:30-37, 1968.

106. Wilhelmsen, N.R., Ramfjord, S.P., and Blankenship, J.R.: Effects of electrosurgery on the gingival attachment in Rhesus monkeys, J. Periodontol. **47**:160-170, 1976.

107. Oringer, M.J.: Electrosurgery for definitive, conservative, modern periodontal therapy, Dent. Clin. North Am. **13**(1):53-73, 1969.

108. Malone, W.F.P., Eisenmann, D., and Kusek, J.: Interceptive periodontics with electrosurgery, J. Prosthet. Dent. **22**:555-564, 1969.

109. Donaldson, D.: Gingival recession associated with temporary crowns, J. Periodontol. **44**:691-696, 1973.

110. Waerhaug, J.: Temporary restorations: advantages and disadvantages, Dent. Clin. North Am. **24**(2):305-316, 1980.

111. Dragoo, M.R., and Williams, G.B.: Periodontal tissue reactions to restorative procedures. II. Int. J. Periodont. Restor. Dent. **2**(2):35-45, 1982.

112. Donaldson, D.: The etiology of gingival recession associated with temporary crowns, J. Periodontol. **45**:468-471, 1974.

113. Waerhaug, J.: Tissue reactions around temporary crowns, J. Periodontol. **24**:172-185, 1953.

114. Lang, N.P., Kiel, R.A., and Anderhalden, K.: Clinical and microbiological effects of subgingival restorations with overhanging or clinically perfect margins, J. Clin. Periodontol. **10**:563-578, 1983.

115. Kaiser, D.A., and Cavazos, E.: Temporization techniques in fixed prosthodontics, Dent. Clin. North Am. **29**(2):403-412, 1985.

116. Wheeler, R.C.: Complete crown form and the periodontium, J. Prosthet. Dent. **11**:722-734, 1961.

117. Morris, M.L.: Artificial crown contours and gingival health, J. Prosthet. Dent. **12**:1146-1156, 1962.

118. Baima, R.F.: Extension of clinical crown length, J. Prosthet. Dent. **55**:547-557, 1986.

119. Ingber, J.S.: Forced eruption. I. A method of treating isolated one and two wall infrabony osseous defects-rationale and case report, J. Periodontol. **45**:199-206, 1974.

120. Inger, J.S.: Forced eruption. II. A method of treating nonrestorable teeth-periodontal and restorative considerations, J. Periodontol. **47**:203-216, 1976.

121. Miller, P.D.: Root coverage using a free soft tissue autograft following citric acid application. I. Technique, Int. J. Periodont. Restor. Dent. **2**(1):65-70, 1982.

122. Holbrook, T., and Ochsenbein, C.: Complete coverage of denuded root surface with a one stage graft, Int. J. Periodont. Restor. Dent. **3**(3):8-27, 1983.

123. Allen, E.P., Gainza, C.F., Farthing, G.G., and Newbold, D.A.: Approved technique for localized ridge augmentation: a report of 21 cases, J. Periodontol. **56**:195-199, 1985.

124. Martin, D.: Soft tissue master cast, Int. J. Periodont. Restor. Dent. **2**(4):35-43, 1982.

125. Ishii, M., and Satoh, N.: Fabrication of collarless porcelain fused to metal restorations without using a platinum matrix, Int. J. Periodont. Restor. Dent. **6**(3):65-73, 1986.

126. Weisgold, A.S.: Contours of the full crown restoration, Alpha Omegan **70**:77-89, 1977.

127. Sachs, R.I.: Restorative dentistry and the periodontium, Dent. Clin. North Am. **29**(2):261-279, 1985.

128. Wagman, S.S.: Tissue orientation of the crown in the laboratory, J. Prosthet. Dent. **43**:357-358, 1980.

129. Waller, M.J.: The anatomy of the maxillary molar furcal plane crown preparation, J.A.D.A. **99**:978-982, 1979.

130. Perel, M.L.: Axial crown contours, J. Prosthet. Dent. **25**:642-649, 1971.

131. Yuodelis, R.A., Weaver, J.D., and Sapkos, S.: Facial and lingual contours of artificial complete crown restorations and their effects on the periodontium, J. Prosthet. Dent. **29**:61-66, 1973.

132. Schour, I., and Massler, M.: Prevalence of gingivitis in young adults, J. Dent. Res. **27**:733-734, 1948.

133. Nevins, M.: Interproximal periodontal disease—the embrasure as an etiologic factor, Int. J. Periodont. Restor. Dent. **2**(6):9-27, 1982.

134. Cohen, D.W.: Morphological factors in the pathogenesis of periodontal disease. Br. Dent. J. **107**:31-39, 1959.

135. Caffesse, R.C., and Nasjilet, C.E.: Enzyme penetration through intact sulcular epithelium, J. Periodontol. **47**:391-397, 1976.

136. Boner, C., and Boner, N.: Restoration of the interdental space, Int. J. Periodont. Restor. Dent. **3**(2):31-45, 1983.

137. Gjermo, P., and Flötra, L.: The effect of different methods of interdental cleaning, J. Periodont. Res. **5**:230-236, 1970.

138. Waerhaug, J.: The interdental brush and its place in operative and crown and bridge dentistry, J. Oral Rehabil. **3**:107-113, 1976.

139. Waerhaug, J.: Effect of zinc-phosphate cement fillings on gingival tissues, J. Periodontol. **27**:284-290, 1956.

140. Newell, D.H.: Gingival reactions to restorative materials in rat molars, M.S. thesis, Chicago, University of Illinois at the Medical Center, 1964.

141. Newell, D.H.: Gingival reactions to restorative materials: a review, J. Israeli Dent. Med. **19**:9-12, 1970.

142. Hirschfeld, L., and Wasserman, B.: A long-term survey of tooth loss in 600 treated periodontal patients, J. Periodontol. **49**:225-237, 1978.

143. McFall, W.T.: Tooth loss in 100 treated patients with periodontal disease: a long-term study, J. Periodontol. **53**:539-549, 1982.

144. Gabel, A.B.: The American Textbook of Operative Dentistry, ed. 9, Philadelphia, 1961, Lea and Febiger Book Co., pp. 163-167.

145. Mansour, R.M., and Reynik, R.J.: In vivo occlusal forces and moments. I. Forces measured in terminal hinge position and associated moments, J. Dent. Res. **54**:114-120, 1975.

146. Lindhe, J., and Svanberg, G.: Influence of trauma from occlusion on progression of experimental periodontitis in the beagle dog, J. Clin. Periodontol. **1**:3-13, 1974.

147. Ericsson, I., and Lindhe, J.: The effect of longstanding jiggling on experimental marginal periodontitis in the beagle dog, J. Clin. Periodontol. **9**:497-503, 1982.

148. Ross, J.F., and Evanchik, P.A.: Root fusion in molars: incidence and sex linkage, J. Periodontol. **52**:663-667, 1981.

149. Larato, D.C.: Furcation involvements: incidence and distribution, J. Periodontol. **41**:499-501, 1970.

150. Bower, R.C.: Furcation morphology relative to periodontal treatment. Furcation root surface anatomy, J. Periodontol. **50**:366-374, 1979.

151. Gher, M.W., and Dunlap, R.W.: Linear variation of the root surface areas of the maxillary first molar, J. Periodontol. **56**:39-43, 1985.

152. Dunlap, R.M., and Gher, M.E.,:Root surface measurements of the mandibular first molar, J. Periodontol. **56**:234-238, 1985.

153. Anderson, R.W., McGarrah, H.E., Lamb, R.D., and Eick, J.D.: Root surface measurements of mandibular molars using stereophotogrammetry, J.A.D.A. **107**:613-615, 1983.

154. Everett, F.B., Jump, E.B., Holder, T.D., and Williams, G.C.: The intermediate bifurcation ridge: a study of the morphology of the bifurcation of the lower first molar, J. Dent. Res. **37**:162-169, 1958.

155. Burch, J.G., and Hulen, S.: A study of the presence of accessory foramina and the topography of molar furcations, Oral Surg. **38**:451-455, 1974.

156. Wheeler, R.C.: Dental anatomy, physiology and occlusion, ed. 4, Philadelphia, 1974, W.B. Saunders Co., pp. 238-259;267-290.

157. Glickman, I.: Clinical Periodontology, ed. 2, Philadelphia, 1958, W.B. Saunders Co., pp. 694-696.

158. Tarnow, D., and Fletcher, P.: Classification of the vertical component of furcation involvement, J. Periodontol. **55**:283-284, 1984.

159. Easley, J.: Methods of determining alveolar osseous form. J. Periodontol. **38**:112-118, 1967.

160. Greenberg, J., Laster, L., and Listgarten, M.A.: Transgingival probing as a potential estimator of alveolar bone level, J. Periodontol. **47**:514-517, 1976.

161. Baima, F.R.: Considerations for furcation treatment. I. Diagnosis and treatment planning, J. Prosthet. Dent. **56**:138-142, 1986.

162. Eskow, R.N., and Kapin, S.H.: Furcation invasions: correlating a classification system with therapeutic consideration. II. Periodontal and restorative considerations in furcation management, Compend. Cont. Dent. Ed. **5**:527-532, 1984.

163. Stanley, H.R.: Changing concepts of the dental pulp based on recent investigation, J. D.C. Dental Soc. **37**:6-9, 1962.

164. Stambaugh, R.V., and Wittrock, J.W.: The relationship of the pulp chamber to the external surface of the tooth, J. Prosthet. Dent. **37**:537-546, 1977.

165. Farrar, J.N.: Radical heroic treatment of alveolar abscess by amputation of roots of teeth, Dent. Cosmos **26**:79-81, 1884.

166. Black, G.V.: In Litch, W., editor: American System of Dentistry, Philadelphia, 1886, Lea Brothers, p. 990.

167. Messinger, T.F., and Orban, B.: Elimination of periodontal pockets by root amputation, J. Periodontol. **25:**213-215, 1954.

168. Amen, C.R.: Hemisection and root amputation, Periodontics **4:**197-204, 1966.

169. Hiatt, W.H.: Periodontal pocket elimination by combined endodontic-periodontic therapy, Periodontics **1:**152-158, 1963.

170. Augsberger, R.A.: Root amputations and hemisections, Gen. Dent. **24:**35-38, 1976.

171. Polson, A.M.: Periodontal considerations for functional utilization of a retained root after furcation management, J. Clin. Periodontol. **4:**223-230, 1977.

172. Greenstein, G., Caton, J., and Polson, A.: Trisection of maxillary molars, Compend. Cont. Dent. Ed. **5:**624-628, 1984.

173. Eastman, J.R., and Backmeyer, J.: A review of the periodontal, endodontic, and prosthodontic considerations in odontogenous resection procedures, Int. J. Periodontol. Restor. Dent. **6**(2):35-51, 1986.

174. Glossary of periodontic terms, J. Peridontol. vol. 57 (suppl.), November, 1986.

175. Klavan, B.: Clinical observations following root amputation in maxillary molar teeth, J. Periodontol. **46:**1-5, 1975.

176. Erpenstein, H.: A 3-year study of hemisectioned molars, J. Clin. Periodontol. **10:**1-10, 1983.

177. Hamp, S.E., Nyman, S., and Lindhe, J.: Periodontal treatment of multirooted teeth. Results after 5 years, J. Clin. Periodontol. **2:**126-135, 1975.

178. Langer, B., Stein, S.D., and Wagenberg, B.: An evaluation of root resections: a ten-year study, J. Periodontol. **52:**719-722, 1981.

179. Staffileno, H.J.: Surgical management of the furca invasion, Dent. Clin. North Am. **13**(1):103-119, 1969.

180. Weine, F.S.: Endodontic Therapy, ed. 2, St. Louis, 1976, The C.V. Mosby Co., pp. 358-366.

181. Backman, K.J.: The incomplete root resection—case presentations, Int. J. Periodont. Restor. Dent. **2**(3):61-71, 1982.

182. Rosenberg, M.M.: Management of osseous defects, furcation involvement and periodontal-pulpal lesions. In Clark, J.W., editor: Clinical Dentistry, vol. 3, Philadelphia, 1979, Lippencott-Harper, Chap. 10.

183. Newell, D.H., and Brunsvold, M.B.: Prevalence of faulty root resections. Submitted for publication.

184. Krichoff, D.A., and Gerstein, H.: Pre-surgical crown contouring for root amputation procedures, Oral Surg. **27:**379-384, 1969.

185. Gerstein, K.A.: The role of vital root resection in periodontics, J. Periodontol. **48:**478-483, 1977.

186. Tagger, M., and Smukler, H.: Microscopic study of the pulps of human teeth following vital root resection, Oral Surg. **44:**96-105, 1977.

187. Helfer, A.R., Melnick, S., and Schilder, H.: Determination of the moisture content of vital and pulpless teeth, Oral Surg. **34:**661-670, 1972.

188. Weine, F.S.: Endodontic Therapy, ed. 2, St. Louis, 1976, The C.V. Mosby Co., pp. 4-44.

189. Healey, H.J.: Coronal restoration of the treated pulpless tooth, Dent. Clin. North Am. **1**(3):885-896, November 1957.

190. Frank, A.L.: Protective coronal coverage of the pulpless tooth, J.A.D.A. **59:**895-900, 1959.

191. Ward, H.E.: Preparation of furcally involved teeth, J. Prosthet. Dent. **48:**261-263, 1982.

192. Abou-Rass, M., Jann, J.M., Jobe, D., and Tsutsui, F.: Preparation of space for posting: effect on thickness of canal walls and incidence of perforation in molars, J.A.D.A. **104:**834-837, 1982.

193. Koth, D.L.: Full crown restoration and gingival inflammation

in a controlled population, J. Prosthet. Dent. **48:**681-685, 1982.

194. Kastenbaum, F. The restoration of the sectioned molar, Int. J. Periodont. Restor. Dent. **6**(6):9-23, 1986.

195. Axelsson, P., and Lindhe, J.: Effect of controlled oral hygiene procedures on caries and periodontal disease in adults: results after 6 years, J. Clin. Periodontol. **8:**239-248, 1981.

BIBLIOGRAPHY

Amsterdam, M., and Fox, L.: Provisional splinting-principles and technics, Dent. Clin. North Am. **3**(1):73-99, 1959.

Amsterdam, M., and Abrams, L.: Periodontal prosthesis. In Goldman, H.M., and Cohen, D.W., editors: Periodontal Therapy, ed. 4, St. Louis, 1968, The C.V. Mosby Co., pp. 962-971.

Basaraba, N.: Root amputation and tooth hemisection, Dent. Clin. North Am. **13**(1):121-132, 1969.

Basaraba, N.: Furcation invasions. In Schluger, S., Yuodelis, R.A., and Page, R.C., editors: Periodontal Disease, Philadelphia, 1977, Lea & Febiger, pp. 540-558.

Carranza, F.A.: Glickman's Clinical Periodontology, ed. 6, Philadelphia, 1984, W.B. Saunders Co., pp. 934-945.

Cooper, M.B.: Minor tooth movement in the management of the periodontal patient. In Prichard, J.F., editor: The Diagnosis and Treatment of Periodontal Disease, Philadelphia, 1979, W.B. Saunders Co., pp. 462-504.

Flocken, J.: Electrosurgical management of soft tissues and restorative dentistry, Dent. Clin. North Am. **24**(2):247-269, 1980.

Goodkind, R.J.: Precision attachment removable partial dentures for the periodontally compromised patient, Dent. Clin. North Am. **28**(2):327-336, 1984.

Gordon, T.: Telescope reconstruction: an approach to oral rehabilitation. J.A.D.A. **72:**97-105, 1966.

Grant, D.A., Stern, I.B., and Everett, F.G.: Periodontics: in The Tradition of Orban and Gottlieb, ed. 5, St. Louis, 1979, The C.V. Mosby Co., pp. 898-905.

Hamp, S.E., and Nyman, S.: Treatment of furcation involved teeth. In Lindhe, J., editor: Textbook of Clinical Periodontology, Copenhagen, 1983, Munksgaard, pp. 433-450.

Javid, N.S., and Low, S.B.: The removable partial denture as a periodontal prothesis, Dent. Clin. North Am. **28**(2):337-348, 1984.

Kornfeld, M.: Mouth Rehabilitation: Clinical and Laboratory Procedures, ed. 2, vols. 1 and 2, St. Louis, 1974, The C.V. Mosby Co.

Malone, W.F.P., Porter, Z.C., and Jameson, M.L.: Tooth preparation of periodontally compromised teeth. Ill. State Dent. J. **53:**228-231, July/August 1984.

Marks, M.H., and Corn, H.: The role of tooth movement in periodontal therapy, Dent. Clin. North Am. **13**(1):229-241, 1969.

Newell, D.H.: Current status of the management of teeth with furcation invasions, J. Periodontol. **52:**559-568, 1981.

Pollack, R.P., and Ponte, P.M.: Treatment of type III and IV periodontal cases without crown and bridge splinting, Int. J. Periodont. Restor. Dent. **1**(2):27-49, 1981.

Prichard, J.F.: Advanced Periodontal Disease: Surgical and Prosthetic Management, ed. 2, Philadelphia, 1972, W.B. Saunders Co., pp. 905-909.

Prichard, J.F.: The Diagnosis and Treatment of Periodontal Disease, Philadelphia, 1979, W.B. Saunders Co., pp. 608-633.

Prichard, J.F.: The Diagnosis and Treatment of Periodontal Disease, Philadelphia, 1979, W.B. Saunders Co., pp. 505-524.

Saadoun, A.P.: Management of furcation involvement, Perio. Abstracts, J. West. Soc. Periodont. **33:**91-125, 1985.

Schluger, S., Yuodelis, R.A., and Page, R.C.: Periodontal Disease: Basic Phenomina, Clinical Management, and Occlusal and Restorative Interrelationships, Philadelphia, 1977, Lea & Febiger, pp. 638-656.

Staffileno, H.J.: Surgical management of the furca invasion, Dent. Clin. North Am. **13**(1):103-119, 1969.

Thayer, H.H., and Kratochvil, F.J.: Periodontal considerations with removable partial dentures, Dent. Clin. North Am. **24**(2):357-368, 1980.

Thilander, B.: Orthodontic tooth movement in periodontal therapy. In Lindhe, J., editor: Textbook of Clinical Periodontology, Copenhagen, 1983, Munksgaard, pp. 480-500.

Willarson, K.S.: Removable partial denture prosthesis for the periodontal patient, Dent. Clin. North Am. **13**(1):263-279, 1969.

Wise, R.J., and Kramer, G.M.: Predetermination of osseous changes associated with uprighting tipped molars by probing, Int. J. Periodont. Restor. Dent. **3**(1):69-81, 1983.

Yuodelis, R.A.: Long-term stabilization. In Schluger, S., Yuodelis, R.A., and Page, R.C., editors: Periodontal Disease, Philadelphia, 1977, Lea & Febiger, pp. 658-699.

Yuodelis, R.A., and Faucher, R.: Provisional restorations: an integrated approach to periodontics and restorative dentistry, Dent. Clin. North Am. **24**(2):285-303, 1980.

5

W.F.P. Malone, Edmund Cavazos, Jr., and Gerald J. Re

BIOMECHANICS OF TOOTH PREPARATION

TOOTH PREPARATION

Tooth preparation is defined as the mechanical treatment of dental disease or injury to hard tissues that restores a tooth to original form. Perceptive diagnosis and disciplined tooth preparation can determine the success of a fixed prosthodontic denture (FPD) because abutment teeth have the additional responsibility of supporting a fixed prosthesis over an edentulous space. Reduction of tooth structure is preceded by a mental image of the design of the artificial crown and the anticipated occlusion (Fig. 5-1, A and B).

Sound preparation design enhances longevity for the majority of cast restorations. The current focus is

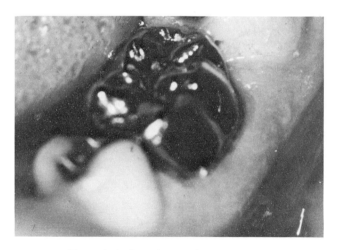

Fig. 5-1. A, Complete gold veneer crown.

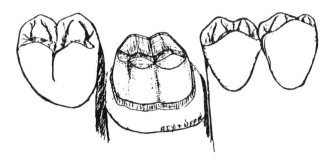

Fig. 5-1. B, Die of a prepared mandibular first molar with two plane reduction on stamp cusps.

on conservative tooth preparation that is noninvasive and that minimally involves dentin (Fig. 5-2, A to D). This trend is rational in light of the reduction of the caries rate by fluorides, nutritional counseling, and oral hygiene programs. Black's[1] principles of cavity preparation and Tylman's[2] principles of tooth preparation are both presently being modified to accommodate imaginative approaches, i.e., acid etching with minimum reduction. Dentistry is changing from macrotooth preparation to an environment of molecular chemistry, i.e., esthetic bonding (Fig. 5-3, A to D). These techniques are not presently supported by longitudinal studies, but are exciting and promising.[3]

A premise that should be communicated to the patient and understood by the technician and dentist is that crowns are usually placed on compromised teeth. Despite these advances, traditional crowns are still indicated for the majority of patients. The classic design for the preparation must be visualized so modifications can be instituted (Fig. 5-4). Diagnosis and disciplined tooth preparation are essential to successful fixed prosthodontics.[4]

Objectives of Tooth Preparation

The objectives of preparation remain clearly defined, but the methods of securing these goals are constantly being revised:

1. Reduction of the tooth in miniature to provide retainer support
2. Preservation of healthy tooth structure to secure resistance form
3. Provision for acceptable finish lines
4. Performing pragmatic axial tooth reduction to encourage favorable tissue responses from artificial crown contours, i.e., fluting of molars

Caries Control Program

Comprehensive patient care is commonly initiated with a caries control program and concomitant periodontal evaluation so that the disease can be eliminated before restorative treatment begins. Caries control also allows a programmed sequence of treatment so that fixed prosthodontics can be accomplished over

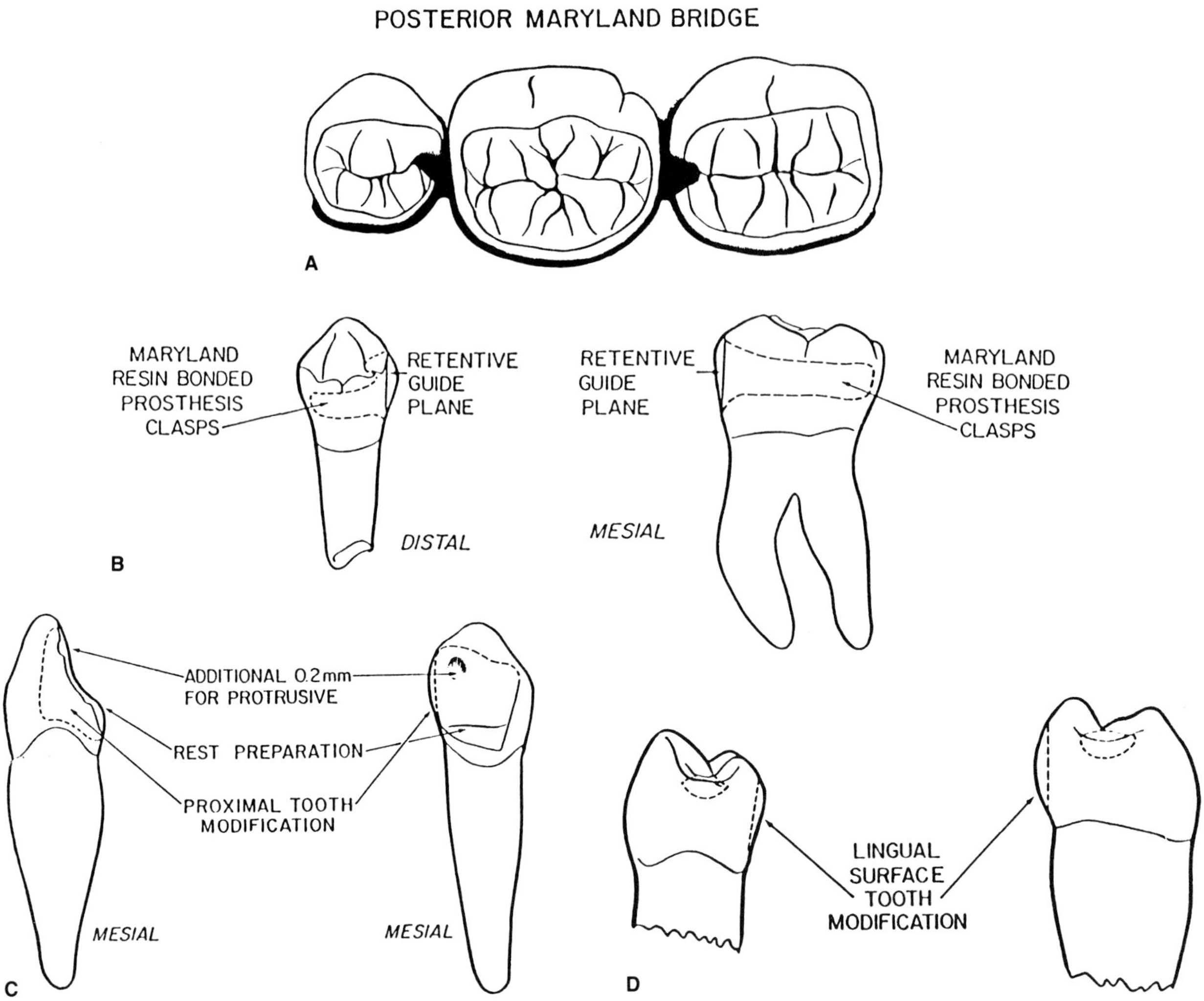

POSTERIOR MARYLAND BRIDGE

Fig. 5-2. A, Posterior resin-bonded prosthesis with lingual clasp extension. **B,** Proximal retentive guide planes should be at least 2 mm vertically. **C,** Anterior tooth reparation emphasizing the rest preparation, protrusive accommodation, and proximal guide plane. **D,** Rest preparations and lingual modification for a mandibular posterior.

a period of time within the patient's priorities, comfort, esthetics, and/or functional needs. Further benefits include:

1. Patient accommodation to biologic restorations
2. Time for financial planning by patient
3. Evaluation of the patient's oral hygiene

The caries control program can then be followed by more complex treatment within a mutually agreeable time period.

REMOVAL OF CARIES

The removal of caries during tooth preparation is only possible when there is limited involvement. In these cases, carious tooth structure and existing restorations are removed while accomplishing the traditional preparation. This procedure allows the dentist to preserve tooth structure and vitality of the teeth. Removal of caries or existing restorations without a preconceived concept of the final tooth preparation commonly renders the tooth inoperable. Conversely,

the most common error associated with caries removal is incomplete excavation of active caries in the dentinoenamel junction under the cusps.

A common practice is to remove caries or existing restorations during preparation and to "base out" defects on the working dies. One liability of this practice is the effect of severe undercuts, which compromises the elastic memory of the impression materials. Extensive caries involvement or the presence of large restorations requires a caries control program. These procedures are initiated as quadrant cavity preparations using a rubber dam and placement of amalgam restorations or glass ionomer cements.[5] There are three classic steps involved in caries control programs:

1. Preparation of traditional outline form with removal of the infected carious tooth structure and existing restoration (Fig. 5-5, A to D)
2. Protection of tooth vitality or initiation of endodontic therapy
3. Restoration of tooth structure with amalgam res-

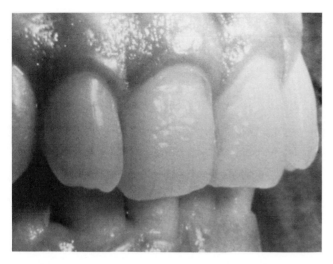

Fig. 5-3. A, Lemon and salt sucking habit showing pretreatment facial erosion of maxillary central incisors.

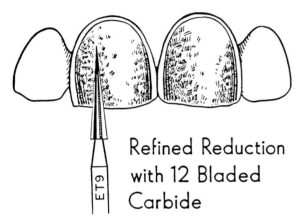

Refined Reduction with 12 Bladed Carbide

Fig. 5-3. B, Refinement of facial surface and proximal extension.

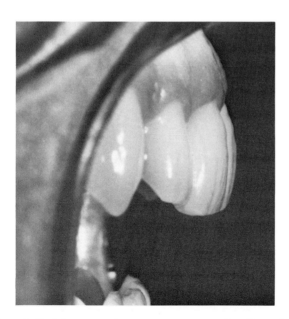

Fig. 5-3. C, Adjustment of protrusive movement is critical. Final product illustrating facial surface without overcontour.

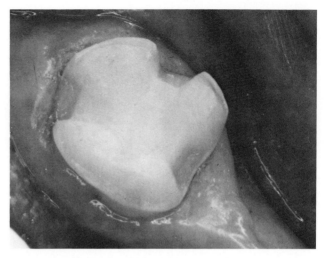

Fig. 5-4. Onlay RPD abutment with supragingival margins and boxing to allow rest preparation and paralleling guide plane.

torations or glass ionomer cements before preparing cast restorations (Fig. 5-5, E and F)

Carious tooth structure is removed by a slowly revolving No. 6 or No. 8 round bur without pressure (Fig. 5-5 G). Spoon excavators are avoided in deep caries removal because carious dentin is in layers, and the pulp's incomplete response to the caries can be easily dislodged (Fig. 5-5 H). Glass ionomer cements are indicated when less than 30 percent of the tooth is missing (Fig. 5-5, I to O). They have the additional advantage of gradual fluoride release.[6]

Sequence of Caries Control

Canines and terminal molars are given priority after the dentist has addressed patient discomfort, emergency esthetics, or pain relief. The first molars would be treated after the canines and terminal molars because of critical arch position.[7] In summary:

1. A control program removes dental caries as an infectious disease.
2. Caries control makes possible a logical sequence for complex treatments.
3. A programmed excavation of caries and replacement with liners, amalgams, or glass ionomer cements effectively completes the initial caries control program.
4. Whenever complex treatment is anticipated, a caries control program is recommended to restore the critical teeth with concomitant periodontal and endodontic therapy.

Uniform tooth reduction

When preparing teeth with ultra speed, the removal of tooth structure is swift and irreversible. Previously, preparations were performed by a combination of cleavage, planing, and abrasion, with increments of tooth structure tediously removed. A conservative tooth preparation design has become popular due to

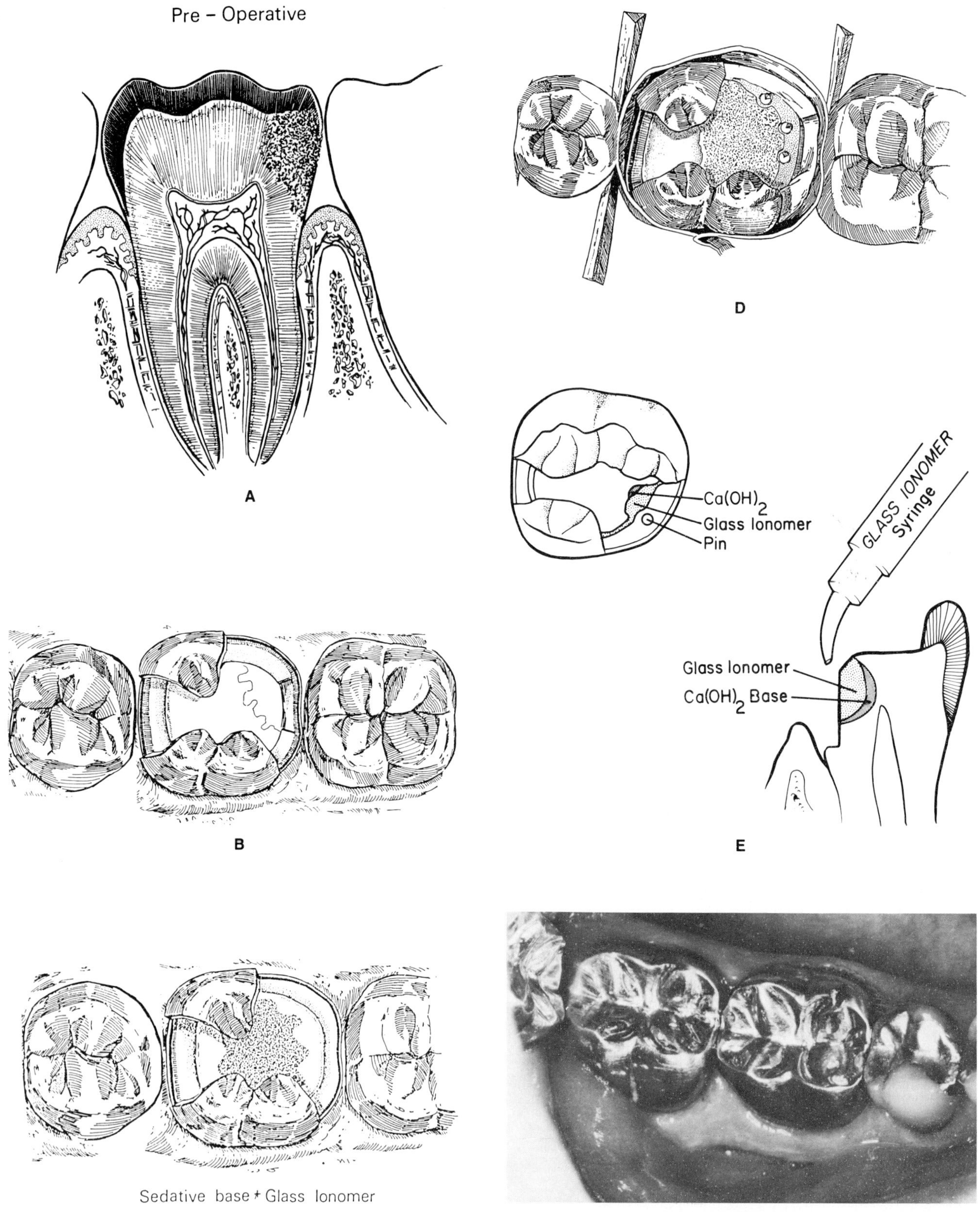

Pre – Operative

A

B

Ca(OH)$_2$
Glass Ionomer
Pin

GLASS IONOMER Syringe

Glass Ionomer
Ca(OH)$_2$ Base

E

D

Sedative base + Glass Ionomer

C

F

Fig. 5-5. A, Carious lesion undermining distal lingual cusp of mandibular first molar. **B,** Establishing the outline form for tooth reconstruction. **C,** Sedative base or liner placed prior to glass ionomer cement. **D,** Glass ionomer over sedative base with pin placement. **E,** Glass ionomer placement with syringe glass ionomer base. **F,** Complete gold veneer crowns after pin reconstruction. (A to D, courtesy L. Paul Lustig, Boston, Mass., and W.F.P. Malone, Alton, Ill.; E, Garcia Godoy et al.: Texas Dent. J. 103:4, October 1986; F, courtesy James N. Ciesco, Park Ridge, Ill.) *Continued*

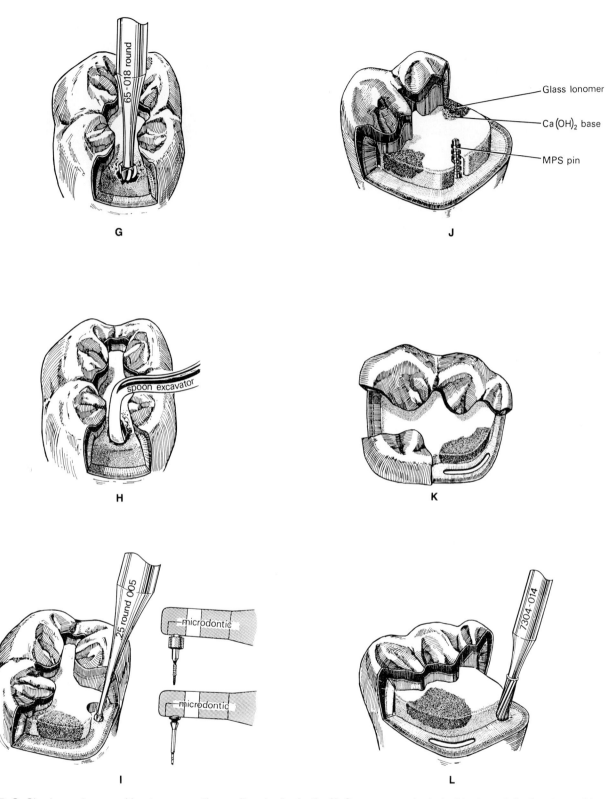

Fig. 5-5. G, Slowly moving round bur to remove "layered" caries in dentin. **H,** Spoon excavator to test texture of dentin; ¼ round bur is suggested for removing caries in DE junction (see Chapter 2). **I,** MPS pin placement and glass ionomer base for mandibular second molar prior to amalgam restoration followed by cast restoration. Bur for pin placement has a corresponding pin diameter for frictional retention. **J,** Glass ionomer base, Ca(OH)₂ liner and MPS for compromised molar prior to tooth preparation for a cast restoration. Placement of more than three pins is discouraged. **K,** Chamber or slot formations have been encouraged as an alternate method. Distal lingual cusp of mandibular first molar is a common fracture site. **L,** Lingual slot, proximal retentive grooves, glass ionomer base with "well preparation" for a single pin is considered adequate support for compromised tooth prior to amalgam restoration. (G to L, courtesy L. Paul Lustig, Boston, Mass., and W.F.P. Malone, Alton, Ill.)

Continued

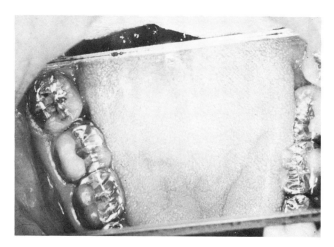

Fig. 5-5. M, Amalgam reconstruction prior to tooth preparation for cast restorations. Amalgams remain undisturbed after reconstruction to assess occlusion and patient comfort. Third molars remain as vertical stops until cast restorations "feel natural."

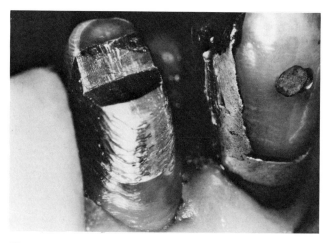

Fig. 5-5. O, Amalgam reconstruction with central groove development and two-plan reduction on buccal cusps. (Courtesy W.F.P. Malone and Z.C. Porter: Tissue Management, Littleton, Mass., 1982, PSC Publishing.)

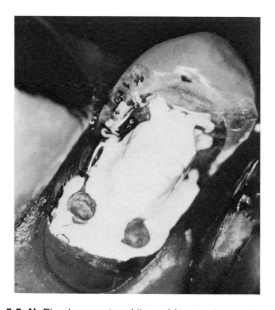

Fig. 5-5. N, Pin placement and liner of fractured premolar.

the reduction of caries by fluoride programs. Conservative tooth preparation is not to be confused with underpreparation of traditional preparations, which result in overcontoured cast restorations.

Uniform tooth reduction is desirable but not possible when teeth are in poor arch position. These teeth warrant a more perceptive diagnosis and treatment plan sequence, including diagnostic waxups to develop a suitable occlusion (Fig. 5-6, A to I). The dentist can then program the reduction of tooth surfaces to provide parallelism and improve arch position with selective tooth reduction. Deviations from uniform reduction become more apparent in gross disparities of the maxillomandibular relationship, i.e., class III malocclusions and cross-bites.

Sequence of uniform tooth reduction Diagnostic casts are helpful in avoiding insufficient or excessive reduction during tooth preparation (Fig. 5-7, A and B) and are a necessity when preparations are planned. *Steps in tooth preparation are:*

1. Occlusal or incisal reduction for sufficient clearance
2. Axial reduction and proximal, facial, and lingual reduction to establish optimal contours and embrasures
3. Resistance and retention form for predictable results
4. Refinement and smoothing to reduce stress during function
5. Establishment of finish lines to control microleakage

INCISAL/OCCLUSAL REDUCTION

Occlusal or incisal reduction is performed to provide adequate clearance between the prepared surface and the opposing teeth. Two millimeters is considered adequate, but variations occur depending upon the occlusion, type of restoration, and patient's age (Fig. 5-8, A to H). The dentist should examine border movements and stamp cusp positions so that adequate clearance is secured in the areas of occlusal load. Surfaces of minimal load can be conservatively prepared to provide resistance and retention.[8]

Additional forms of retention may be required when shorter axial walls fail to supply sufficient retention and resistance form (Fig. 5-8, I and J). A template designed from diagnostic casts can aid in establishing a satisfactory occlusal reduction. A registration gauge in centric and eccentric positions during preparation helps in determining interocclusal clearance. The final occlusal reduction should be uniform to permit an even thickness of metal, and resemble the original

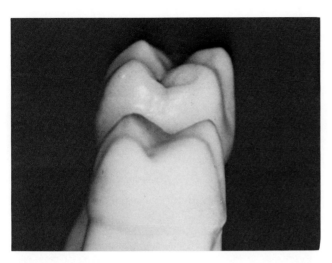

Fig. 5-6. A, Uniform reduction of maxillary first molar for complete gold veneer crown.

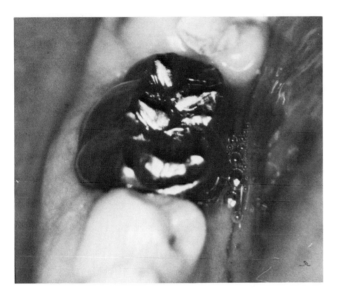

Fig. 5-6. B, Complete gold veneer crown on mandibular first molar with gingival margins at the crest.

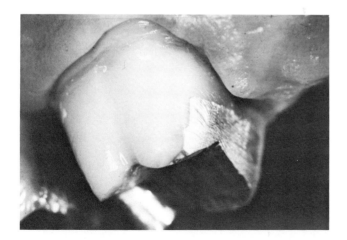

Fig. 5-6. C, Exaggerated facial chamfer on reconstructed maxillary first molar with a buccal flute. (Courtesy Dr. Thomas E. Yuhas, Palos Heights, Ill.)

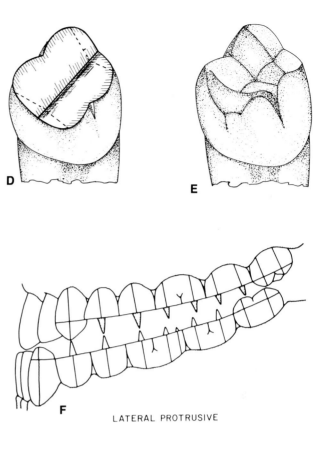

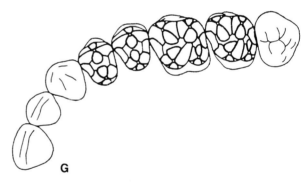

LATERAL PROTRUSIVE

Fig. 5-6. D, Uniform reduction is started with central groove preparation for suitable arch position and sufficient occlusal clearance in eccentric movements. **E,** Occlusal topography serves as a prescription during laboratory fabrication. **F,** Programmed placement of cusps to develop a smooth protrusive movement. **G,** Waxing of maxillary arch, occlusal view. Note triangular cuspal formation and programmed placement of marginal ridges.

anatomy of the tooth. Placement of treatment restorations can reaffirm the validity of tooth reduction and clearance. If the interim restoration is extremely thin, tooth preparation should be reevaluated before impressions (Fig. 5-8 K).

The "corrugated" occlusal reduction aids in cusp placement and in avoiding the pulp. Flat plane reduction may be acceptable on older patients when interocclusal relationships are worn.

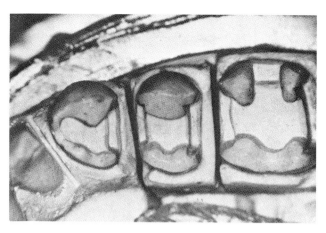

Fig. 5-6. H, Quadrant of onlay preparations showing multicolored wax addition technique. Former restorations usually dictate buccolingual extensions.

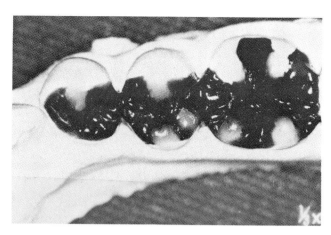

Fig. 5-6. I, Quadrant of onlay preparations showing multicolored wax addition technique. Former restorations usually dictate buccolingual extensions.

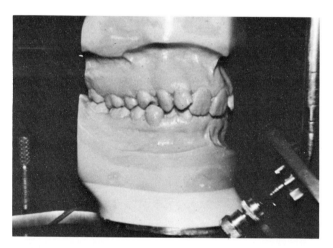

Fig. 5-7. A, Diagnostic casts identifying the need for an orthodontic consultation.

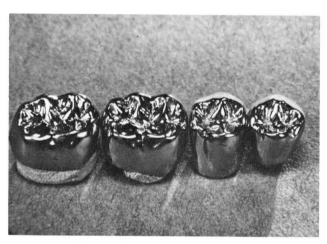

Fig. 5-7. B, Programmed cast interim nonprecious restorations for occlusal treatment.

Narrowed Occlusal Table

Narrowing the occlusal table of a restoration is possible only if the buccolingual width is reduced in the preparation. When indicated, the occlusal table should be reduced to direct the occlusal stresses toward the long axis of the tooth or to reduce the incidences of prematurities during lateral excursions of the mandible (Fig. 5-9, A and B).

Axial Reduction

Axial reduction commonly encompasses the entire circumference of the tooth. Preparation of the proximal axial walls should display a 5 to 10 degree taper occlusogingivally from the long axis of the preparation. The distal surface of mandibular molars may be an exception because some patients cannot accommodate the combined height of the bur and handpiece.

Insufficient preparation of the proximal axial walls

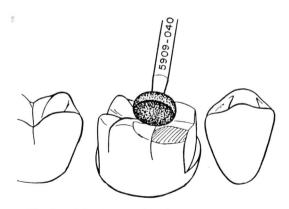

Occlusal Reduction for Complete Crown

Fig. 5-8. A, Tooth preparation of mandibular first molar illustrating occlusal reduction of rotated tooth with diamond stone. Occlusal reduction usually precedes proximal preparation. *Continued*

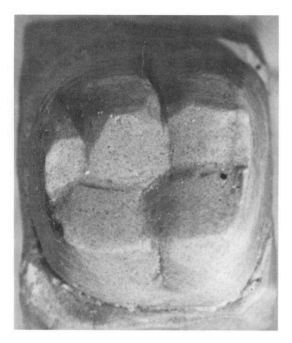

Fig. 5-8. B, Die of completed preparation for CGVC of mandibular first molar with two-plane reduction of the buccal cusps while preserving the occlusal anatomy of the original tooth. The distal surface has an increased convergence angle because patient cannot accommodate bur and handpiece in full vertical position.

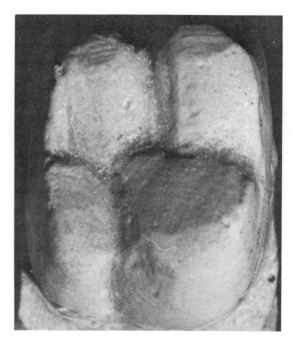

Fig. 5-8. C, Occlusal view of prepared maxillary first molar with two-plane reduction lingually and buccally. Bur striations are reason for die spacers.

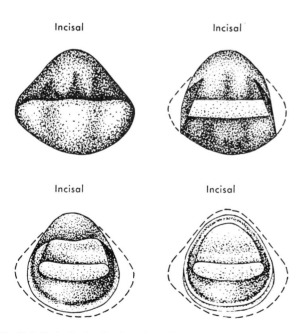

Incisal   Incisal

Incisal   Incisal

Fig. 5-8. D, Incisal reduction should be at least 2 mm to secure clearance in various occlusal positions. Note the proximal reduction to ensure adequate embrasure.

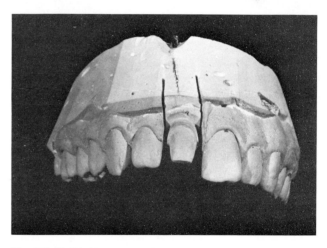

Fig. 5-8. E, Working cast with removable die to facilitate developing the gingival margin. Note the incisal reduction of over 2 mm to accomodate protrusive movements of the mandible. *Continued*

results in inadequate embrasures with predictable periodontal implications (Fig. 5-10, A and B). Conversely, excessive reduction in the proximal axial walls reduces the resistance and retention form, which resists functional forces. Splinted multiple restorations compensate for the need of traditional tapers mesiodistally, but splinting of additional teeth should be defensible (Fig. 5-10, C and D). (See Chapter 1.) The preparation of the axial surfaces of both anterior and posterior teeth requires support of the proximal tissue (Fig. 5-10 E).

Contour

Contours on the artificial crown enhance accessibility for cleaning. Acceptable buccal and lingual contours of the retainer begin with axial tooth preparation.

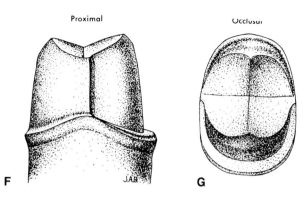

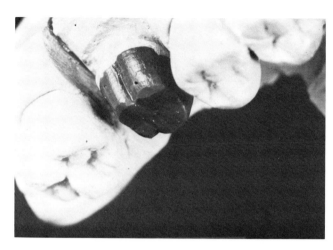

Fig. 5-8. F, PFM preparation for a maxillary premolar with occlusal reduction of central grooves on the height of proximal tissue support. **G,** PFM preparation for a maxillary premolar with occlusal reduction of central grooves on the height of proximal tissue support.

Fig. 5-8. H, Occlusal clearance of a maxillary first molar with two-plane buccal reduction and die spacer to accommodate cement.

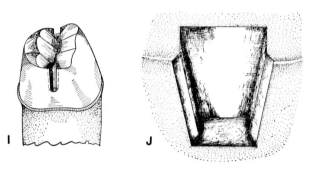

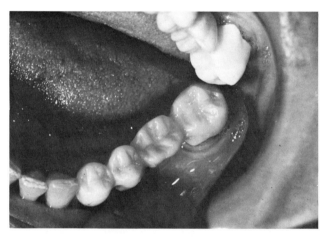

Fig. 5-8. I, Proximal groove for additional resistance to displacement. **J,** Proximal box added for stability, but combined extracoronal intracoronal retention makes seating of the casting arduous.

Fig. 5-8. K, Heat cured treatment restoration fabricated from diagnostic casts. (K, courtesy Dr. Hanna Sweetnam, Joliet, Ill.)

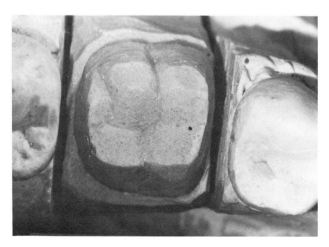

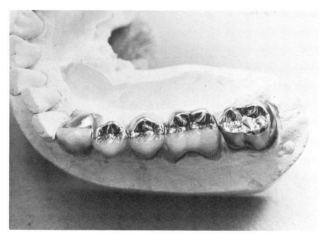

Fig. 5-9. A, Tooth preparation of the mandibular first molar with a reduced buccolingual width.

Fig. 5-9. B, Narrowed buccolingual width of four-unit FPD and a complete gold crown on a remounting cast. (Courtesy Dr. F.W. Summers, Westchester, Ill.)

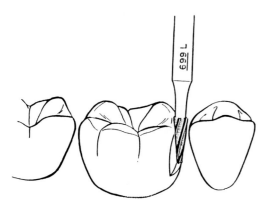

Proximal Tooth Reduction

Fig. 5-10. A, Proximal reduction for mandibular first molar. Occlusal reduction is usually performed prior to this step, but open contacts and rotation present a more pressing concern.

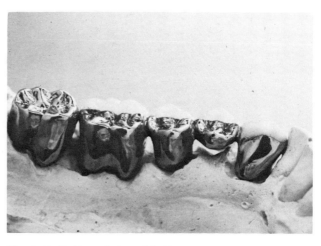

Fig. 5-10. D, Lingual view of C; Note pontic-tissue relationship. (Courtesy Dr. F.W. Summers, Westchester, Ill.)

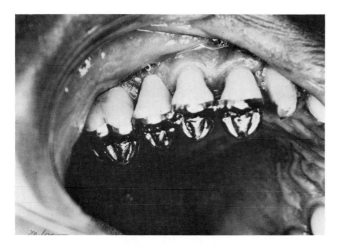

Fig. 5-10. B, Four-unit FPD with wide embrasures using three-quarter crowns to replace first maxillary despite drift of second molar.

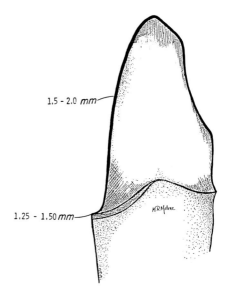

1.5 - 2.0 *mm*

1.25 - 1.50 *mm*

Fig. 5-10. E, Tooth preparation for PFM anterior restoration demonstrating the proximal support required for tissue support. (Courtesy Ms. M.R. Malone-Pleak, San Antonio, Tex.)

According to Yuodelis et al.,[9] the restoration should not mimic the original anatomic crown but recreate the contour of the root portion (Fig. 5-11 A). Tooth preparations for periodontally compromised patients are fluted short of the furca, avoiding the triangular region formed by the crevicular emergence and the roots. The flattened, undercontoured restoration creates a more cleanable area for home care (Fig. 5-11, B to G). Supervised technical construction is necessary to ensure that "flat not fat" contours result (Fig. 5-11, H to L). The slopes and contour of the restorations should reflect the fluted preparation, which enhances gingival health. Sections of Chapter 6 provide a more detailed discussion of crown contouring.

1. Retention is influenced by occlusogingival length of the axial walls.

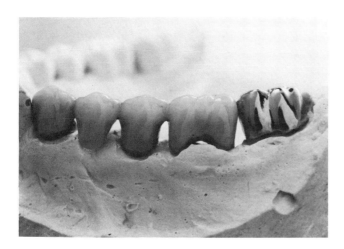

Fig. 5-10. C, Buccal view of four-unit FPD and CGVC on second molar. Note cleansible interproximal embrasure despite splinted second premolar and first mandibular molar. Gold lingual surfaces permit accommodation of lingual maxillary stamp cusps. (Courtesy Dr. F.W. Summers, Westchester, Ill.)

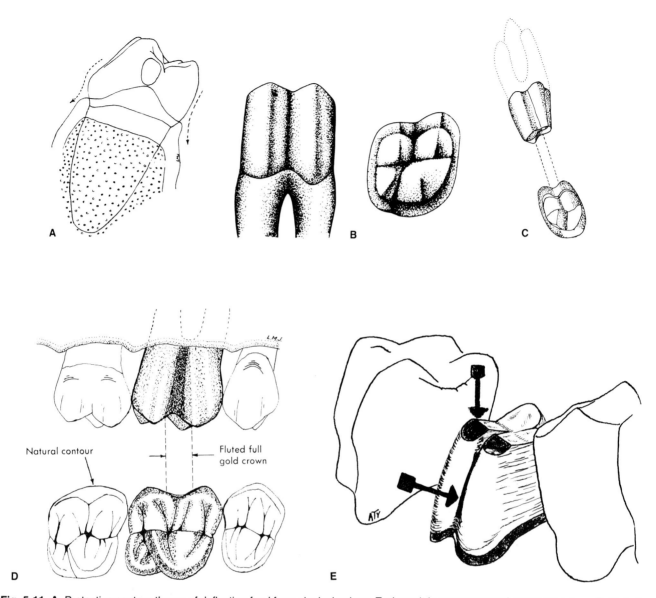

Fig. 5-11. A, Protective contour theory of deflecting food from gingival sulcus. End result is overcontoured complete crown. **B,** Fluted maxillary first molar. **C,** Fluted maxillary first molar with preservation of flute in cast restoration. (Courtesy L.M. Jameson and W.F.P. Malone: J. Prosth. Dent. 47:620, 1982.) **D,** Cast restoration should reflect flute the entire length of the buccal surface. **E,** Supragingival margins in periodontally involved teeth illustrating fluted facial surface and two-plane reduction of stamp cusps. *Continued*

2. Proximal walls should be nearly equal in vertical length because the retention of the retainer is only as effective as the shortest wall.
3. Proximal walls ideally possess a 5 to 8-degree taper, except distal surfaces of molars.
4. Facial and lingual walls are more convergent from the occlusal one-third to provide a narrowed occlusal table.
5. Short axial walls require accessory methods of retention: boxing, groove, and pins.

APPLIED PHYSICAL FORCES

Basic principles of resistance and retention form are commonly compromised in preparations for fixed prostheses because of the condition of the abutment teeth. Modifications to satisfy the needs of individual and multiple tooth preparations, esthetics, and occlusion cannot be oversimplified. Forces develop on teeth from a myriad of angles. A force placed on a retainer can result from mastication, bruxism, dietary intake, and a host of intangible, unpredictable stresses (Fig. 5-12, A to C).

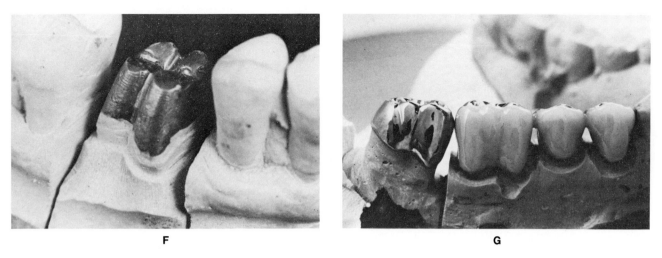

Fig. 5-11. F, Trimmed die of clinical preparation with die spacer due to vertical length of axial surfaces. **G,** Three-unit ceramic/metal FPD replacing No. 29 with a complete gold crown as a single unit. Note the buccal flutes and broad embrasures. (E and F from W.F.P. Malone, et al.: Ill. State Dent. J. July-August 1984; G, courtesy F.W. Summers, Westchester, Ill.)

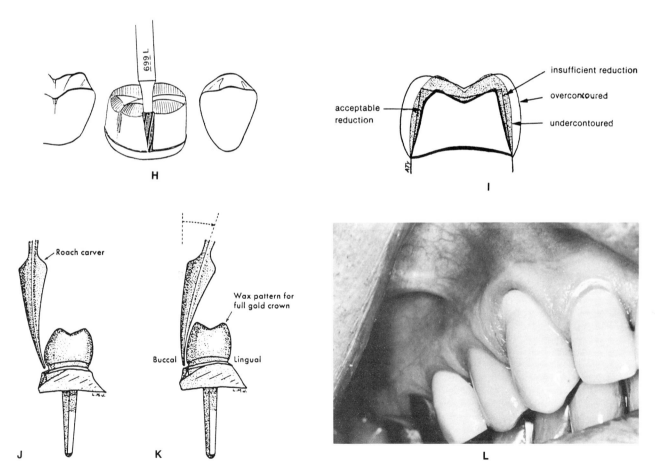

Fig. 5-11. H, Preparation of buccal flute while maintaining a supragingival margin. **I,** Crown contours are directly affected by perceptive tooth preparation. **J,** Developing physiologic contours in wax. **K,** "Protective-deflective bulges" are avoided and eliminated by changing the angulation of carving instrument. **L,** Dual deflective profiles were devised to avoid over-contouring the gingival third of teeth that had periodontal surgery. Note maxillary right canine with a metal collar plus the recessed area immediately incisally. (I, from W.F.P. Malone and Z.C. Porter, Tissue management, Littleton, Mass., 1982, P.S.F. Publishing.)

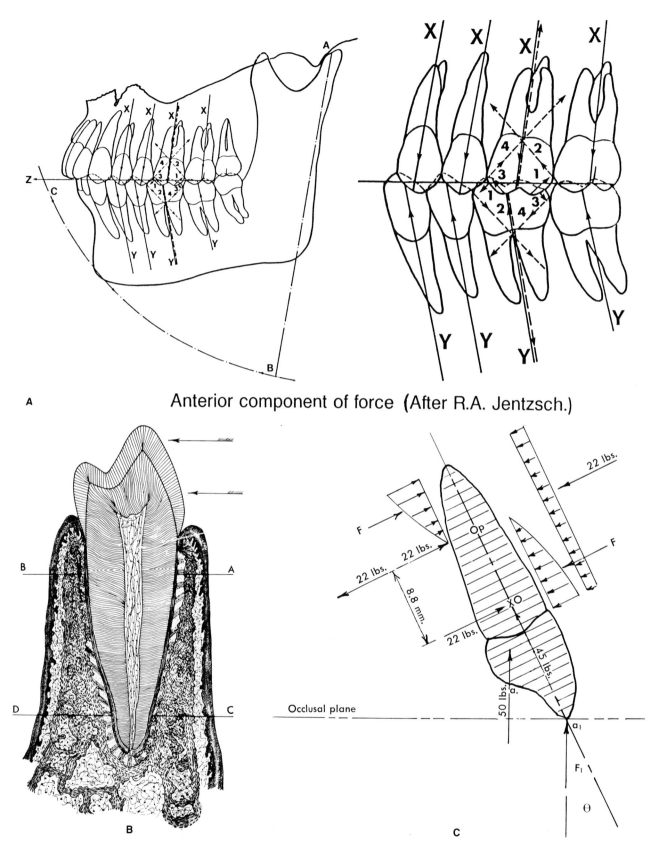

Anterior component of force **(After R.A. Jentzsch.)**

Fig. 5-12. A, Graphic illustration of how teeth can move: X = the maxillary vector; Y = the mandibular vector with resultant vector 2. Diverse secondary vectors are represented on the maxillary and mandibular first molars. **B,** Areas of tension (A and D) and compression (B and C) in periodontal membrane; center of rotation lies between apical one-third and occlusal two-thirds of root. **C,** Analysis of effects of incisal force on maxillary central incisor.

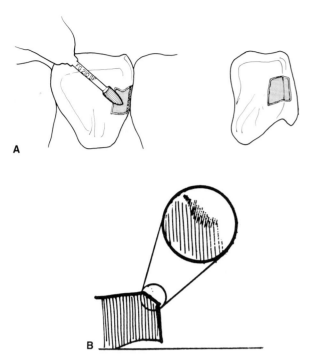

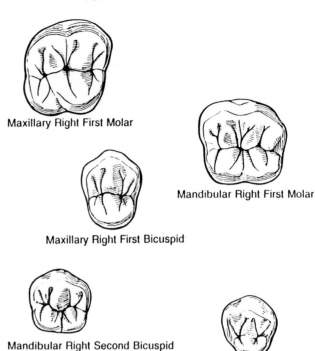

Maxillary Right First Molar

Mandibular Right First Molar

Maxillary Right First Bicuspid

Mandibular Right Second Bicuspid

Mandibular Right First Bicuspid

Fig. 5-13. A, Beveled cavosurfaces for increased retention are also indicated if intracoronal designs are used for FPDs. **B,** Beveled cavosurface angle for increased microretention represents a new surface chemistry environment. (From F. Godoy and W.F.P. Malone, Quintessence, Int. 17:621 1987.)

Fig. 5-14. A, Commonly restored teeth with triangular cuspal inclines. *Continued*

Intracoronal Designs

Intracoronal retainers for FPDs have increased in popularity since reduction and microretentive techniques became available (Fig. 5-13, A and B). An advantage of intracoronal preparations is that gingival tissues are undisturbed, while occlusal relationships are maintained. A disadvantage is the wedgelike effect, although onlays have minimized this problem. Deleterious pulpal responses are not uncommon with intracoronal preparations. The ideal marginal seal with intracoronal retainers has also been an elusive aim for even the most fastidious dentists. In addition, intracoronal tooth preparations are contraindicated for patients with a high DMF rate and malpositioned or supererupted teeth.

Traditional boxes are also placed with resin-bonded prostheses to increase retention, but this removes the advantage of reversibility for the Maryland bridge. Grooves and boxes for R.B.P. are common modifications in teeth of the indigent, elderly, and medically compromised patients.

Extracoronal Designs

Complete crowns have the distinct advantage of allowing cusps to warp during wax formation to a desired arch position (Fig. 5-14 A). Complete crowns provide added strength to teeth that are incapable of withstanding the forces of mastication. Improved esthetics,

retention, and laboratory implementation have made complete veneer crowns the standard-bearer for fixed prosthodontics (Fig. 5-14, B and C).

One liability of complete veneer crowns is the replacement of occlusal topography so that it is not in harmony with its approximating and opposing teeth (Fig. 5-14 D). Subgingival placement of margins does not promote favorable tissue response. In addition, anterior esthetics with various finish lines has been and continues to be a problem (Fig. 5-14 E).

Additional Retention

One method of increasing resistance and retention without lengthening axial surfaces is with grooves or boxes. A seven-eighth or three-quarter crown preparation is an example of effective use of retentive grooves (Fig. 5-15, A to D). Pins are also used to increase retention. Theoretically, pins improve retention by increasing surface area (Fig. 5-15, E to G). Two types of pins are commonly used. The tapered pin provides a strong form of additional retention; parallel-walled pins have failed to demonstrate stability when tested experimentally. Guyer has detailed a review of pin and box configuration for retention and resistance.[10] Five ways to resist displacing forces are:

1. Maintaining 4 to 10 degrees axial taper (Fig. 5-16 A)

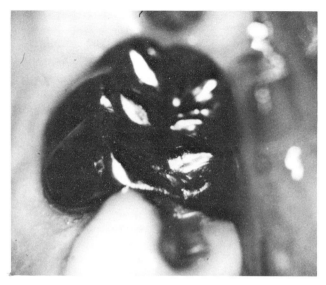

Fig. 5-14. B, Complete gold veneer crown with acceptable gingival tissue response.

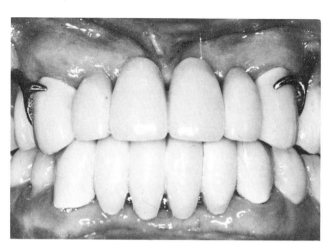

Fig. 5-14. E, Periodontal prostheses FPD anteriorly with metal gingival collars and broad embrasures; posterior is restored with a RPD. (From W.F.P. Malone and Z.C. Porter: Tissue Management, Littleton, Mass., 1982, P.S.D. Publishing.)

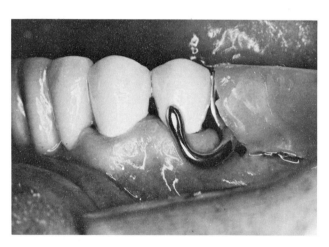

Fig. 5-14. C, Anterior porcelain fused-to-metal FPD with mesial rests and distal surface guide planes with splinted abutments for RPI clasps. Esthetics have encouraged increased use of complete veneer crowns.

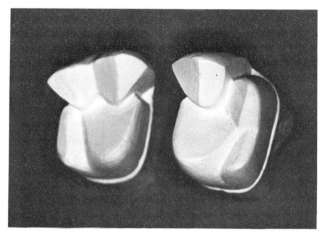

Fig. 5-15. A, Three-quarter crown on left with Tinker's proximal grooves and a seven-eight crown on the right with facial and mesial grooves.

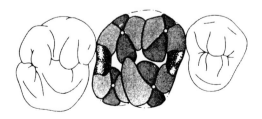

Fig. 5-14. D, Programmed appositional wax technique for a complete crown. Note triangular formation of cuspal inclines.

posterior three-quarter crown molar

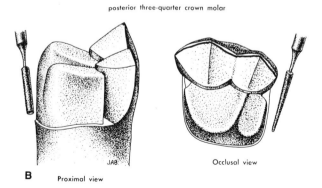

B Proximal view   Occlusal view

Fig. 5-15. B, Traditional three-quarter crown preparation with deep central groove to accommodate the buccal stamp cusp of the mandibular molar. Diamond stones are replaced with 12 fluted carbide burs to smooth the preparation. *Continued*

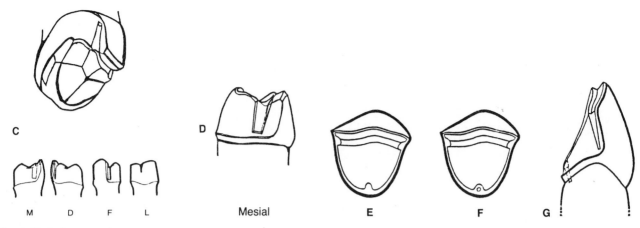

Fig. 5-15. C, Seven-eight crown with facial groove, proximal box, and gingival chamfer M = mesial, D = distal, F = facial, L = lingual surfaces. **D,** Mesial box on a seven-eight crown; depth of the 170L and width twice of diameter. **E,** Lingual surface of three-quarter preparation with well preparation for cingulum pin. **F,** Pin hole after well preparation. **G,** Proximal view to parallel direction of lingual pin to proximal grooves. (C and D, courtesy D.A. Kaiser, San Antonio, Tex.; E and F, courtesy E. Schelb, San Antonio, Tex.; drawings by E. Schelb.)

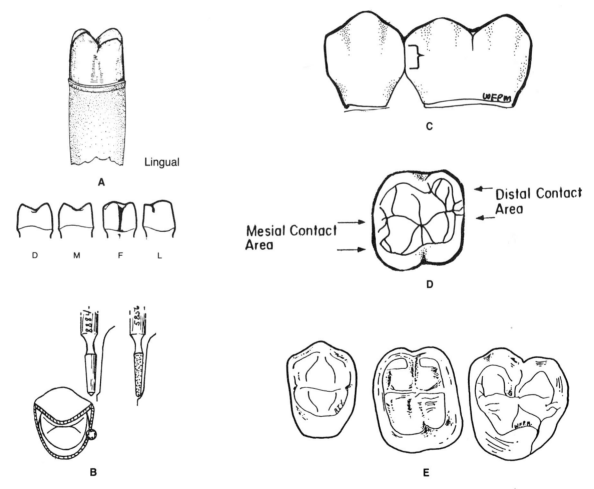

Fig. 5-16. A, Rigid parallelism is usually possible for patients with a large mouth, but the convergence angle is commonly increased due to vertical height of handpiece and bur. D = distal, M = mesial, F = facial, L = lingual. **B,** Instrumentation for preparation of the gingival margin can vary, but chamfer is preferable. **C,** Facial view of maxillary first molar and second premolar illustrating contact area and embrasure space. **D,** Mesial contact of maxillary first molar is farther buccal; distal contact is usually more lingual. **E,** Prepared tooth for CGVC emphasizing sufficient proximal reduction to create suitable contact areas. (C-E from drawings by W.F.P. Malone, Alton, Ill, and A.T. Young, Westchester, Ill.)

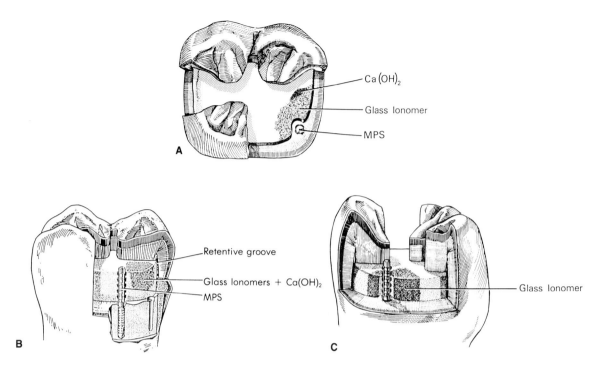

Fig. 5-17. A, Fractured distal lingual cusp of a mandibular first molar with Ca(OH)$_2$ liner, glass ionomer base, and single MPS pin. MPS pins remain vertical. **B,** Sagittal view of a gingival margin at the CEJ. **C,** Gingival margin on cementum may require finishing the cast restoration on amalgam to avoid violating the biologic width. (Courtesy L. Paul Lustig, Boston, Mass., and W.F.P. Malone, Alton, Ill.)

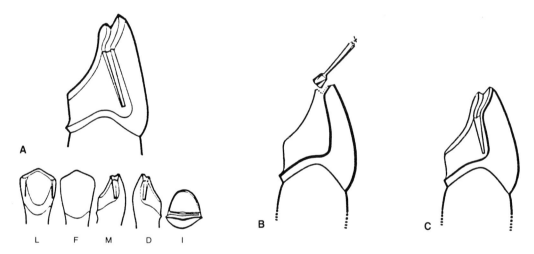

Fig. 5-18. A, Three-quarter crown preparation on maxillary canine. L = lingual, F = facial, M = mesial, D = distal, I = incisal surface. **B,** Preparation of incisal groove for additional retention. **C,** Note that the remaining tooth structure is considerable. (Courtesy E. Schelb, San Antonio, Tex.)

2. Preparing suitable gingival finish line (Fig. 5-16 B)
3. Contouring and placing suitable contact areas (Fig. 5-16, C to E)
4. Incorporating occlusal locks, i.e., dovetail, boxes, and grooves
5. Adding tapered or parallel pins

Individual tooth preparations with an accompanying bibliography are available in Chapter 6.

Conservation of Tooth Structure

One objective of tooth preparation is to preserve healthy tooth structure. The preparation design also enhances the resistance and retention of the classic preparations. Parallelism provides opposition to displacement and is synonymous with conservatism in most cases. The taper of the proximal walls of a preparation could exceed 8 degrees if the axial length of the tooth is excessive or inaccessible. Additional retention is required to compensate for excessive taper or diminished tooth surface. Pin-supported amalgam restorations are an alternate method for reconstructing compromised teeth (Fig. 5-17, A and B). Extension of the gingival margin of the cast restoration beyond the amalgam acts as a collar for protection of the abutment. Termination of the gingival margin of the cast restoration on the amalgam is necessary in some patients (Fig. 5-17 C). Periodontal crown lengthening is indicated for these patients to avoid violating the biologic width.

The three-quarter crown is one of the most conservative preparations, because it requires less tooth reduction (Fig. 5-18 A). This preparation was the standard-bearer until the advent of high-speed tooth reduction. It has limited application in patients with high DMF rates, esthetic priorities, or both (Fig. 5-18, B and C).

Intracoronal preparations are the antithesis of three-quarter crowns. They are not conservative if the number of dentinal tubules involved is considered; they are conservative if evaluated for undisturbed enamel and minimal soft tissue involvement. Stress caused by an intracoronal retainer may eventually split the tooth. Consequently, inlays appear more conservative but are considered inappropriate as retainers because of stress concentration and microleakage. Onlays are preferable because of cuspal protection and retention of favorable gingival tissue response. The introduction of resin-bonded prostheses with different stresses encourages increased use of intracoronal designs, while fluoride programs protect the patient from caries. The verdict on this treatment must be verified in longitudinal studies.

Gingival Termination of Tooth Preparation

Tooth preparations terminate in a finish line. Some terminate on the occlusal and axial surfaces and are referred to as cavosurface angles. The most controversial, however, are the gingival finish lines. Increased use of complete coverage restorations, research, and emphasis on periodontal support are responsible for repudiating the traditional extension of crown margins into the gingival crevice. The previous recommendation was to extend crown margins into the intracrevicular space because the gingival crevice was purported to be immune to caries. Deviation from this norm was viewed as irresponsible, despite the fact that strong evidence supported supragingival margins. Conversely, subgingival margins are considered necessary for the following reasons:
1. Esthetics
2. Presence of existing restorations extending into the intracrevicular space
3. Insufficient vertical length for retention
4. Inordinately high DMF rate of younger patients

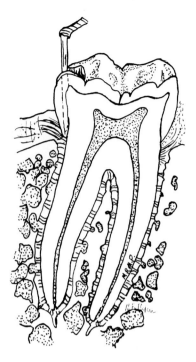

Fig. 5-19. Interproximal redundant tissue is removed prior to preparation to allow unobserved, unobscured vision of the gingival finish line. (Drawing by Mary Ruth Malone-Pleak, San Antonio, Tex.)

One commonly omitted precept is that the soft tissue approximating the tooth is usually unhealthy before preparation.[12] The original contours supporting the soft tissue have been altered by caries or modified by existing restorations. Therefore, the removal of tissue with questionable architecture and regrowth of healthier tissue is a rational direction of treatment (Fig. 5-19). Interceptive periodontics resulting from the early recognition of tissue symptoms is recommended.[14,15]

Generalities about where finish lines should be placed for an optimal contour require astute analysis.[16-24] The subgingival area is <u>not</u> an immune area. Additionally, if there is any validity to the theory of passive eruption, the subgingival margin could become supragingival in a surprisingly short time. Therefore, the dentist's evaluation should include inquiry into the longevity of the restoration.

Supragingival Versus Subgingival Margins

Ideally, the most innocuous position of the margin for soft tissue health is above the gingival crest (Fig. 5-20, A to E). An esthetic position for anterior restorations would be midpoint subgingivally between the epithelial attachment and the crest of the gingiva (Fig. 5-20, F and G). Gentle air pressure from a syringe would reveal the condition of the margin. The area immediately above the gingival crest is desirable, but considered offensive by some patients. Serious thought should precede a supragingival approach for

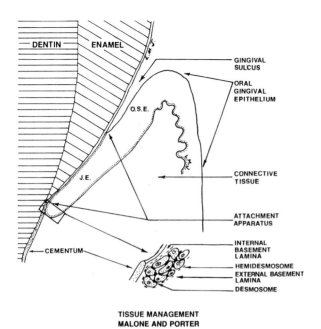

TISSUE MANAGEMENT
MALONE AND PORTER

Fig. 5-20. A, Intracrevicular space is the Bermuda Triangle of dentistry, and its response is magnified by rough, irregular margins of restorations. (Drawing by Dr. L.M. Jameson, Chicago, Ill.)

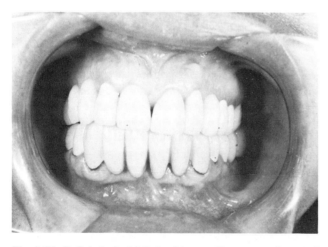

Fig. 5-20. C, Subgingival full shoulder maxillary restorations and supragingival mandibular margins with a metal collar at the crest.

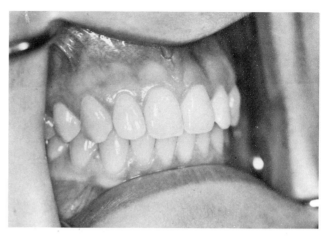

Fig. 5-20. B, Naturally occurring neutroocclusion reflecting desirable soft tissue health.

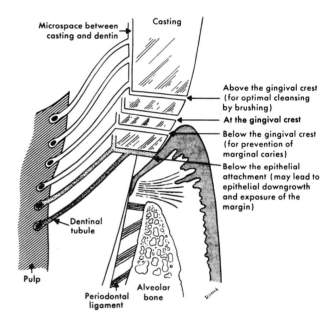

Fig. 5-20. D, Cervical margin of crown at various levels. Most dentists favor placement of cervical margin just below gingival crest, especially on proximal surfaces, for maximal protection against plaque accumulation and penetration of bacteria in the margins of restoration. Care must be exercised to place the margin of the crown at least 2 mm from the crest of the alveolar bone to preserve the biologic width. *Continued*

a younger patient with a high DMF rate or an older patient who exhibits decalcification in the gingival third of a potential abutment. Reduced caries rates have rendered the supragingival margins more feasible despite the age of the patient.

Overcontoured restorations in the gingival third, regardless of types of gingival termination, are objectionable. Supragingival margins are usually advocated for restorations placed subsequent to periodontal surgery and for elderly patients who exhibit a normal recession (Fig. 5-20, H to J). The exceptions to these guidelines are usually esthetic demands by the pa-

tients, increased vertical length for retention, and gingival extension of previous restorations.

Types of Finish Lines

There are four basic types of finish lines (Fig. 5-21 A): shoulder, bevel shoulder, chamfer, and knife edge. Four fundamental criteria for successful margins are:

1. Acceptable marginal adaptation
2. Tissue-tolerant surfaces
3. Adequate contour
4. Sufficient strength

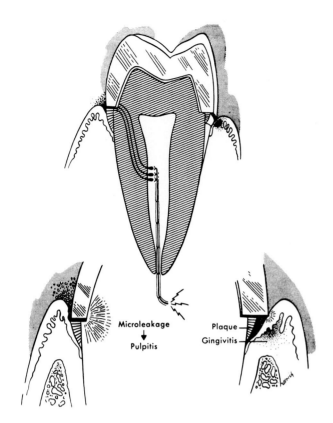

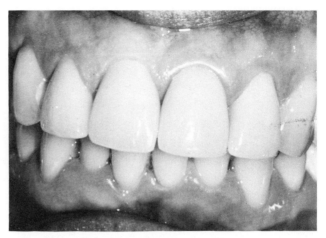

Fig. 5-20. G, Porcelain jacket crowns placed subgingivally on four incisors; canines are retained in their natural state, encouraging a mutually protected occlusion.

Fig. 5-20. E, All castings leave a microspace, which is filled by cement. The smaller the micromargin, the less likely that the cement will wash out.

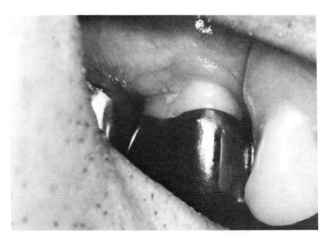

Fig. 5-20. H, Supragingival margins for complete gold crown with a precision attachment and RPD abutment. The increased axial surfaces of the abutment resulted from periodontal surgery.

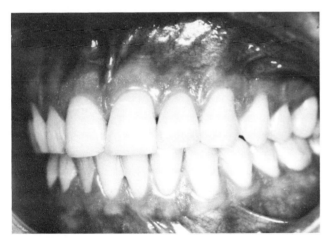

Fig. 5-20. F, Patient desiring esthetic appearance that eliminates black spaces between teeth with PJC on lateral.

Shoulders

The shoulder finish line is usually associated with complete porcelain crowns or at times with porcelain-fused-to-metal crowns and presently, injectable porcelains. If the external line angle of the preparation is perpendicular to the long axis of the tooth, a shoulder results (Fig. 5-22 A). It is arduous to prepare, difficult to obtain an accurate margin, and more likely to pro-

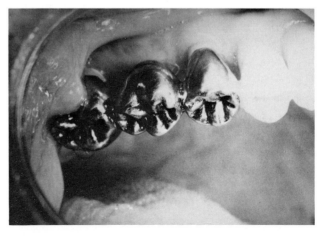

Fig. 5-20. I, Three-unit FPD after crown lengthening with supragingival finish lines. Patient oral hygiene is facilitated. *Continued*

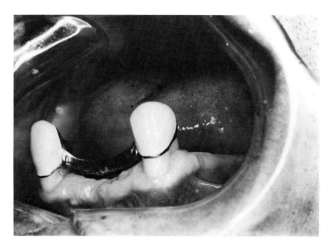

Fig. 5-20. J, Supragingival margins of mandibular splint bar. Programmed professional prophylaxis and fluoride treatments are necessary.

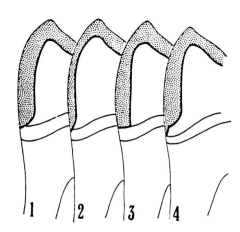

Fig. 5-21. Types of finish lines. 1, Chamfer provides bulk at the finish line. 2, Knife-edge provides minimal reduction. 3, Shoulder used for porcelain jacket crowns. 4, Chamfer or shoulder with bevel used for porcelain fused-to-metal crown. (Courtesy D.A. Kaiser, San Antonio, Tex.)

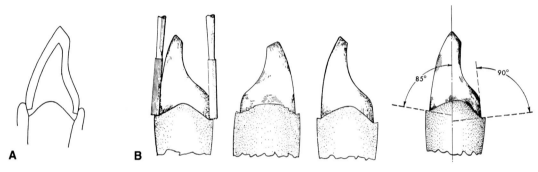

Fig. 5-22. A, Full shoulders have been traditionally associated with complete ceramic crowns, i.e., aluminous porcelain, PJCs and currently injectable porcelain crowns namely Dicor and Cerestore. **B,** Use of plain fissure, left, and end-cutting burs (right) for shoulder. Sharp-line angles are rounded and polished with discs. Plane of shoulder at right angle to axial surface of tooth.

mote adverse pulpal involvement. Controlled removal and pulpal avoidance are paramount during preparation. Caries or existing restorations make it difficult to prepare a shoulder with a uniform width around the circumference of the tooth (Fig. 5-22 B). The gingival crest should be followed to provide adequate tissue support. Shoulders for posterior teeth also are extremely difficult because of belated microleakage and accessibility on distal surfaces of molars. Conversely, the increased tooth reduction performed during shoulder preparation permits more latitude for the gingival contour of the cast restoration. Full shoulder usage has increased after the introduction of "injectable ceramic" crowns such as Dicor and Cerestore.

Beveled shoulders

Modification of the full shoulder with a bevel is considered a more judicious course of treatment. The angle of this bevel approaches the path of insertion of the restoration and improves marginal adaptation. The bevel with a rounded axial angle is indicated for porcelain-fused-to-metal preparations (Fig. 5-23). This preparation has a smooth, evenly distributed bevel from proximal to proximal on the lingual surface. A rounded axial angle allows the metal bulk to resist functional distortion.

Chamfer

A chamfer is an obtuse-angled gingival termination. It is a concave extracoronal finish line that possesses greater angulation than a knife-edge with less width than a shoulder (Fig. 5-24). According to El-Ebrashi et al.,[25] margins with chamfers provide a gingival area with an acceptable stress distribution and an adequate seal and required minimal uniform tooth reduction.[26] The chamfer also enhances accurate die trimming for technical fabrication of the cast restorations.

Knife-edge finish line

The knife-edge finish line is more expedient during preparation but arduous to fabricate because of the difficulty in determining the finish line during laboratory procedures. Waxing and polishing features of construction become critical, and casting the knife-edge restoration is challenging. There are situations

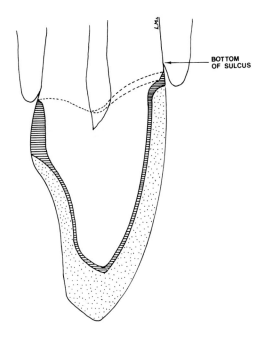

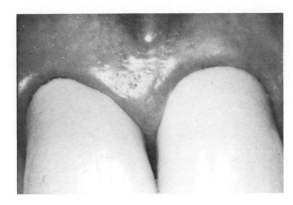

Higher margin of metal collar on two P.F.M. crowns after treatment.

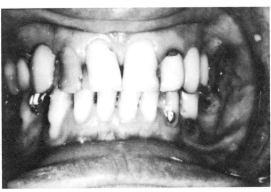

Pretreatment

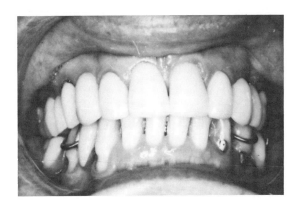

Posttreatment

Fig. 5-23. Porcelain-fused to metal crowns with metal collars placed subgingivally. The tissue rarely fully recovers without incidence. Despite obvious improvement in the patient's appearance in the inset, the gingival tissue sustains a "rolled appearance," with metal in the intracrevicular space. (Drawing courtesy L.M. Jameson, Chicago, Ill.)

when knife-edge margins are a distinct advantage, i.e., in younger patients, inaccessible areas of the oral cavity, and in cementum. Knife-edge finish lines are also employed in areas other than gingival termination, i.e., pinledge preparations and the outline of partial veneer crowns (Fig. 5-25, A and B).

Summary

1. Complete shoulders are the classic finish lines for completed porcelain crowns and injectable ceramic restorations.
2. Beveled shoulders are used in preparations for veneers and selected posterior teeth.
3. The chamfer possesses internal bulk and satisfactory marginal adaptation extracoronally; it is the traditional gingival termination for posterior crowns and the lingual surface of anterior ceramic/metal crowns.

4. Knife-edge finish lines are used for younger patients, pinledge three-quarter crowns, inaccessible areas of the oral cavity, and finish lines on the cementum.

Common Errors of Tooth Preparation

1. Insufficient occlusal or incisal reduction.
2. Lack of uniform reduction of labial or buccal surface compromising esthetics (Fig. 5-26 A).
3. Minimal axial reduction on the buccal and lingual surfaces of posterior teeth, which increases the incidence of working prematurities. The distinction between reduction and clearance is crucial.
4. Inappropriate proximal reduction, which prevents having a cleanable embrasure space (Fig. 5-26 B).
5. Overreduction of teeth and/or violation of the

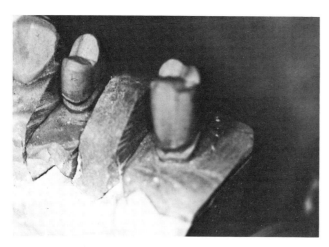

Fig. 5-24. Lingual chamfer on the PFM preparation of a premolar for a FPD and knife edge on the proximals.

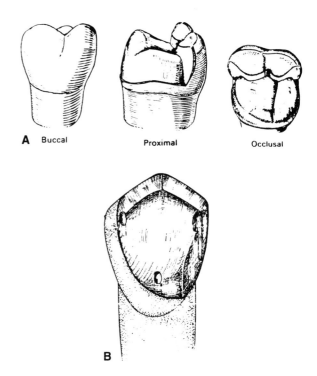

Fig. 5-25. A, Proximal knife-edge slice on posterior three-quarter crown with a chamfer. **B,** Pin and groove placement for retention of a partial veneer. Similarity of preparation for resin bonded prostheses (without pins). (From H.H. Kabnick, Dental Items Interest 53:376, 1931.)

biologic width (Fig. 5-26 C).

6. Insufficient gingival reduction to accommodate a definite finish line.
7. Undercuts on the distolingual surface of the preparation and/or lack of parallelism of an FPD abutment (Fig. 5-26, D and E).
8. Failure to contour proximal surfaces of adjacent teeth to allow seating of a restoration (Fig. 5-26, F and G).

SELECTION OF RETAINERS

The retainers are the coronal extension of the preparation on the abutment teeth for a fixed prosthesis. Any omission during tooth preparation is magnified during the construction of the retainer.[27-31] All facts concerning the patient are weighed in a regimented differential diagnosis. The patient's oral hygiene, occlusion, or both may preclude intracoronal retainers, while complete crowns are not always ideal. There is a considerable latitude in the selection of retainers when the patient has a low DMF rate and a healthy periodontium.

Although the periodontal ligament of the abutment teeth determines the limit of force that an FPD endures, the span and type of FPD also determines the retainers. Retainer selection for terminal abutments is critical and is dictated by the following:

1. Age
2. DMF rate
3. Edentulous space
4. Periodontal support
5. Arch position of the teeth
6. Skeletal relationships
7. Interocclusal and intraocclusal conditions, such as crown length
8. Oral hygiene of the patient
9. Vitality of the abutment

Step-by-step procedures of the most frequently used preparations are in Chapter 6.

COMMON SENSE OCCLUSION FOR RESTORATIVE DENTISTRY

Common occlusal problems must be recognized to enable the dentist to deliver complex treatment uneventfully.

1. *Evaluate occlusal planes opposing edentulous areas in the oral cavity.* Discrepancies in the plane of occlusion may occur because of supraeruption or gravitation of a tooth without an antagonist. The tooth in poor arch position must then be removed or be treated through endodontics, crown lengthening, and a cast restoration to modify the occlusal plane. These procedures must be performed before restoring the opposing edentulous area (Fig. 5-27 A). Diagnostic waxups are essential for these patients (Fig. 5-27 B).
2. *Record the occlusal contact of the stamp cusps.* Stamp cusps may be elongated because of undercarved multiple opposing restorations. This omission of enamelplasty on the opposing arch can foster unfavorable intercuspal relationships.

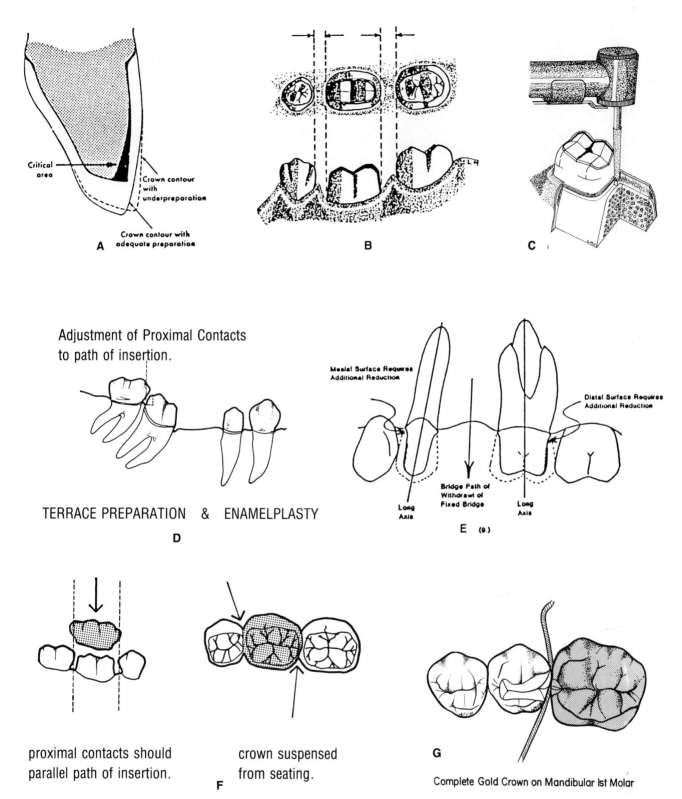

Fig. 5-26. A, Insufficient labial reduction is common on the incisal one-third of the tooth. Two-plane reduction to accommodate an adequate facing is required. **B,** Stagnation of interdental papillae and col area are avoided with perceptive tooth reduction. **C,** The biologic width must not be violated with subgingival margin placement. **D,** The proximal surfaces of adjacent teeth commonly require enamelplasty to permit insertion and appropriate embrasure areas. **E,** Parallelism can be disconcerting for the neophyte. Study of casts procured during preparation aids selective reduction to secure retention and enamelplasty of adjacent tooth while establishing a path of insertion. **F,** Proximal contacts should be parallel to path of insertion to allow crowns to seat. **G,** Dental floss can be used to test and measure the magnitude of contact areas. (D and G drawn by W.F.P. Malone, Alton, Ill.; E drawn by Richard Wells, Chicago, Ill.)

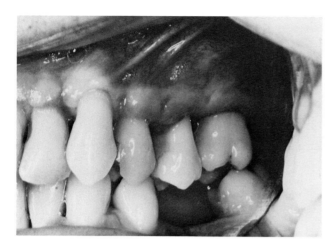

Fig. 5-27. A, Postsurgical "periodontal ramping." Note the supraeruption of second premolar opposing edentulous area, tilting of second molar, and root proximity of anterior teeth. Orthodontics should be entertained prior to restorative dentistry.

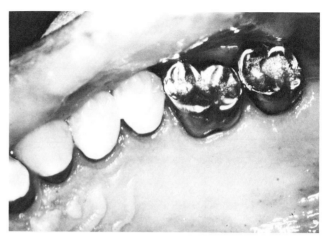

Fig. 5-27. C, Terminal molars in gold while premolar maintain the same marginal ridge level for smooth movement from CRO to CO. Ideally the lingual cusps of premolar would have metal occluding against mandibular natural dentition. Patient preference prevails.

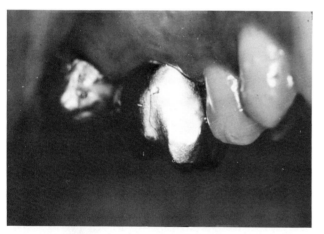

Fig. 5-27. B, Overcontoured restoration placed without evaluation of occlusal plane. Crown lengthening is also necessary to attain a suitable occlusal plane and endodontics.

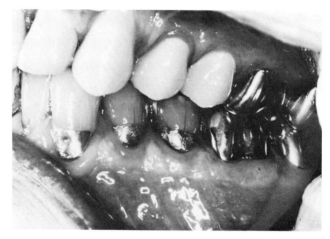

Fig. 5-27. D, Interdigitation of **C.**

3. *Keep the marginal ridges of proximal teeth congruent.* The marginal ridges of the anticipated restorations are kept at the same level as the existing dentition if the plane of occlusion is to be acceptable. If there is a discrepancy between CRO and CO, the slide should be smooth (Fig. 5-27, C and D).
4. *Remove malpositioned third molars.* Third molars may be poor abutments with inconsistent root configuration and bone support. Poor hygiene is common because of their arch position.
5. *Maintain the vertical dimension of occlusion.* Alteration of vertical dimension (opening the bite) is a common cause of failure of restorative dentistry. Posterior occlusal stops should be preserved in one of four ways:
   a. Restore the second molars first, frost (sandblast) occlusal surfaces of cast restorations, ce-

ment provisionally, and wait an appropriate time to ensure patient comfort. Conversely, leave the terminal molar untouched and use it as a reference during extensive restorative dentistry.
   b. Place cast restorations in alternate quadrants and postpone further treatment until the patient functions naturally. The posterior quadrants are completed before the anterior quadrants, hopefully preserving the sanctity of the canines. Every alternative should be explored to maintain the integrity of the anterior mandibular arch.
   c. Formulate the anterior incisal guidance after establishing and/or recording the vertical dimension. Ideally, one canine should remain untouched to provide a morphologic template for the prepared side.

d. If the vertical dimension is reestablished, it is accomplished progressively with removable appliances and/or prolonged evaluation of cemented heat cured treatment restorations. The final restorations are seated with interim cements and frosted occlusal surfaces to monitor patient tolerance.

6. *Judicious selection of materials to be used.* Porcelain-to-porcelain occlusal surfaces do not afford the latitude for periodic adjustment or the wear resulting from eccentric movements. Conversely, gold occlusal surfaces allow an attrition rate similar to that of enamel. Therefore, complete gold veneer crowns are recommended for terminal molars and bizarre occlusal relationships (Fig. 5-28).

Porcelain-to-porcelain occlusals are usually a patient dictate, and the dentist is obliged to comply after informing the patient of biologic incompatibilities. Gifted ceramists are capable of compensating for the noted disadvantages, but porcelain-to-porcelain surfaces are unyielding and unforgiving. A canine disengagement of the posterior teeth may permit the use of porcelain on opposing surfaces.

Longitudinal studies are necessary to provide further guidelines for the dentist to monitor supporting structures with different occlusions and materials while maintaining chewing efficiency.

Organized Occlusal Treatment

Because of the introduction of high-velocity instrumentation and the speed of tooth reduction, a mythical Armageddon looms within each dentist. Specific courses of study should be attended before performing complex restorative dentistry. The high-speed handpiece has an insatiable desire for tooth structure and requires a disciplined approach to conservative tooth preparation.

In the early 1950s the arduous task of tooth preparation for a maxillary canine with a 6,000 to 11,000 rpm handpiece prevented the creation of many occlusal disharmonies by limiting the reduction of tooth structure (Figs. 5-29). Today there are many excellent texts, postgraduate courses in occlusion, and curricular revisions aimed at improving the pedogogic ability of faculty in dental schools. Dawson's text presents an in-depth comprehensive approach to the subject; Payne's systematic addition of colored wax emphasized principles of articulation based on Angle's neutro-occlusion with group function. P.K. Thomas then introduced a similar method that stresses a modified cusp-fossa relationship to direct articular forces along the long axes of teeth.

In the 1980's, the beneficial results of two decades of fluoride have reduced the need for extensive rehabilitation[32] and have dramatically increased the

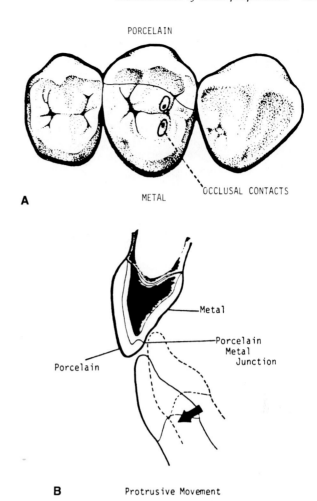

Fig. 5-28. A, Occlusal contact. It is preferable to locate centric contacts on metal. Abrasion is likely on the opposing dentition when centric contacts are in porcelain. **B,** Excursive and protrusive contacts on maxillary anteriors could initially be located on metal and, if possible, at least 1 mm away from porcelain-metal junction. (**B,** courtesy David A. Kaiser, San Antonio, Tex.)

need for interaction of dental specialities for total care. This level of health care delivery requires more correlation and knowledge of allied specialities. Above all, it suggests that health care providers realize the limitations of each other's treatments.

Difficult Restorative Treatment

Oral rehabilitation is time consuming and costly. It also depends upon the recognition of complex problems if success is to be realized. The following conditions require an inordinate amount of supervision and extensive preoperative preparation.[33-36]

1. Occlusion at different levels
2. Occlusion with excessive vertical overlap (Fig. 5-30 A)
3. Occlusion with excessive horizontal overlap (overjet)
4. Occlusion with a prognathic mandible
5. Occlusion with mobile teeth

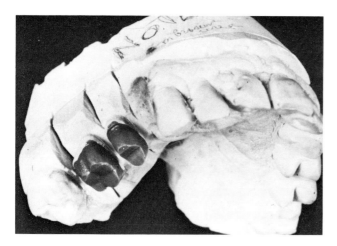

Fig. 5-29. A, Splinted first molar and second premolar with cantilever first promolar pontic to preserve "the sanctity" of the canine.

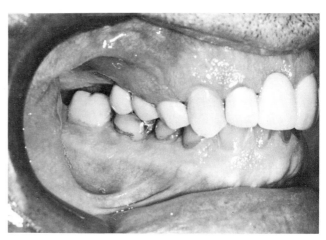

Fig. 5-30. A, Vertical overlap severe with supraeruption of mandibular second molar. Occlusal plane modification is necessary.

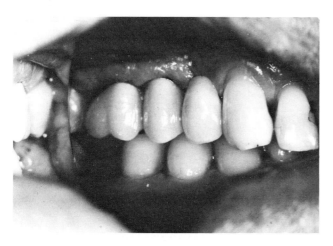

Fig. 5-29. B, Facial views of A with broad embrasures. (From W.F.P. Malone et al.: Ill. State Dent. J. July/Aug. 1984.)

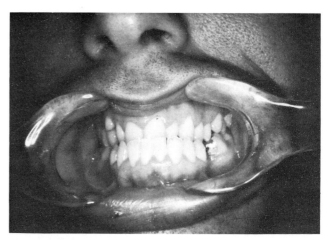

Fig. 5-30. B, Although patient possesses a pleasant smile, the forces of occlusion will precipitate bone loss. Skeletal Class III suggest interspecialty treatment before loss of tooth from insurmountable occlusal forces.

6. Occlusion influenced by wear from bruxism
7. Occlusion with an anterior or posterior cross bite (Fig. 5-30 B)
8. Occlusion with abnormal tongue and swallowing habits
9. Occlusion treated previously
10. Abnormal but functional occlusion of convenience

Additional problems are:

11. Temporomandibular joint disturbances
12. Patients with congenital anomalies, i.e., amelogenesis imperfecta[37] (Fig. 5-30 C)
13. Patients with a history of mental disturbance or conversion hysteria

Success rates in restorative dentistry are adversely effected by capricious vertical dimension alteration, identical occlusal schemes for all patients, and limitations of dental materials. Recognition of difficult cases and timely institution of prerestorative measures ensures success in the majority of patients. However,

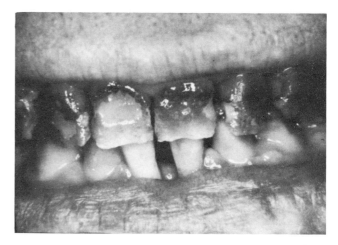

Fig. 5-30. C, Amelogenesis imperfecta presents formidable restorative problem.

the combination of two or three of the difficult clinical conditions in one patient jeopardizes the outcome of treatment in spite of technical advances or the dentist's ability. The patient should be informed of these limitations in explicit terms.[39,40]

SELECTED REFERENCES

1. Black, G.V.: Operative Dentistry, ed. 7, Vol. 2, Chicago, 1956, Medico-Dental Publishing Co.
2. Tylman, S.D., and Malone, W.F.P.: Theory and Practice of Crown and Fixed Partial Prosthodontics, ed. 7, St. Louis, 1978, The C.V. Mosby Co.
3. Godoy-Garcia, F., and Malone, W.F.P.: The effect of acid etching on two glass ionomer lining cements, Quint. Int. **17**:621, October 1986.
4. Douglass, D.: Principles of preparation design in fixed prosthodontics, J. Acad. Gen. Dent. **21**:25-29, March-April 1973.
5. Malone, W.F.P., and Balaty, J.: The rubber dam dilemma, Ill. State Dent. J. **37**:138-143, March 1968.
6. Muzynski, B.L., Greene, E., Jameson, L.M., and Malone, W.F.P.: Fluoride release from glass ionomer used as luting agents, J. Prosth. Dent. (in press).
7. Malone, W.F.P., and Manning, L.: Caries control, Ill. State Dent. J. **36**:724-729, November 1967.
8. Gilbar, D.B., and Teteruck, W.R.: Fundamentals of extracoronal tooth preparation. I. Retention and resistance form, J. Prosth. Dent. **32**:651-656, 1974.
9. Yuodelis, A., Weaver, J.D., and Sapkos, S.: Facial and lingual contours of artificial complete crown restorations and their effects on the periodontium, J. Prosth. Dent. **27**:61-65, 1973.
10. Guyer, S.E.: Multiple preparations for fixed prosthodontics, J. Prosth. Dent. **23**:529-553, 1970.
11. Loe, H.: Reactions to marginal periodontal tissues to restorative procedures, Int. Dent. **18**:4, 759-778, December 1968.
12. McElroy, D.L., and Malone, W.F.P.: Handbook of Oral Diagnosis and Treatment Planning, Springfield, Ill., 1969, Charles C Thomas, Publisher.
13. Stein, R.S.: Residual pontic ridge relationships, J. Prosth. Dent. **26**:251, March-April 1969.
14. Eisenmann, D., Malone, W.F.P., and Kusek, J.: Interceptive periodontics with electrosurgery, J. Prosth. Dent. **22**:502, November 1969.
15. Mahajan, M.: Tissue responses to dental rehabilitative procedures, postdoctoral master's, Chicago, Loyola Medical Center, Loyola University, 1976.
16. Gavelis, J.R., Morency, J.D., Riley, E.D., and Sozio, R.B.: The effect of various finish line preparations on the marginal seal and occlusal seat of full crown preparations, J. Prosth. Dent. **45**:138, 1981.
17. Glickman, I., Stein, R.S., and Smulow, J.B.: The effect of increased function forces upon the periodontium of splinted and non-splinted teeth, J. Periodont. **32**:290, 1961.
18. Jameson, L.M., and Malone, W.F.P.: Crown contours and gingival response, J. Prosth. Dent. **47**:620, June 1982.
19. Perel, M.L.: Artificial crown contours and gingival health, J. Prosth. Dent. **12**:1146-1156, 1962.
20. Marcum, J.S.: The effect of crown marginal depth upon gingival tissues, J. Prosth. Dent. **17**:479-487, 1967.
21. Waerhaug, J.: Histological considerations which govern where the margins of restorations should be located in relation to the gingiva, Dent. Clin. North Am. **8**:161-176, March 1960.
22. Volchansky, A., Cleton, J.P., and Retief, D.H.: Study of surface characteristics of natural teeth and restoration adjacent to gingiva, J. Prosth. Dent. **31**:411-421, April 1974.
23. Heilando, R.E., Lucca, J.J., and Morris, J.L.: Forms, contours and extension of full coverage restorations in occlusal reconstruction, Dent. Clin. North Am. **6**:147-162, 1958.
24. Larato, D.: Effect of cervical margins on gingiva, J. Calif. Dentists' Assoc. **45**:19-22, 1969.
25. El-Elbrashi, M.K., Craig, R.C., and Peyton, F.A.: Experimental stress analysis of dental restorations, J. Prosth. Dent. Parts II to IX, 1967 to 1970.
26. Farah, J.W., and Craig, R.G.: Stress analysis of three marginal configurations of full posterior crons by three dimensional photoelasticity, J. Dent. Res. **53**(5):1219, 1974.
27. Hood, J.A., Farah, J.W., and Craig, R.G.: Modifications of stresses in alveolar bone induced by tilted molar, J. Prosth. Dent. **345**(4):415, 1975.
28. Behrend, D.A.: Posterior tilted molar, J. Prosth. Dent. **37**:622, June 1977.
29. Gordon, T.: Where to avoid pitfalls in periodontal prosthetics, Bull. Acad. Gen. Dent., Issue 11, p. 24, June 1965.
30. Brewer, A.A., and Morrow, R.M.: Overdentures, St. Louis, 1975, The C.V. Mosby Co.
31. Dawson, P.E.: Evaluation, Diagnosis and Treatment of Occlusal Problems, St. Louis, 1974, The C.V. Mosby Co.
32. Murakami, I., and Barrack, G.M.: Relationship of surface area and design to the bond strength of etched cast restorations: an in vitro study, J. Prosth. Dent. **56**:539, November 1986.
33. Brecker, S.C.: Conservative occlusal rehabilitation, J. Prosth. Dent. **9**(6):1001-1016, 1959.
34. Miller, L.: Tooth preparation and the design of metal substructures for metal ceramic restorations. In McLean, J.W., ed.: Dental ceramics: Proceedings of the First International Symposium on Ceramics, Chicago, 1983, Quintessence Publishing Co., pp. 699-716.
35. Hobo, S.: Accuracy of porcelain occlusals. In McLean Dental ceramics: Proceedings of First International Symposium on Ceramics, Chicago, 1983, Quintessence Publishing Co., pp. 699-716.
36. Ingber, J.S., Rose, L.F., and Coslet, J.G.: The "biologic width": a concept in periodontics and restorative dentistry, Alpha Omega, December 1980.
37. Malone, W.F.P., and Bazola, F.N.: Amelogenesis imperfecta, J. Prosth. Dent. **16**:540, May 1964.
38. Carlyle, L.W., Duncan, J.M., Richardson, J.T., and Garcia, Lily: Magnetically retained implant denture, J. Prosth. Dent. **56**:583, November 1986.
39. Moretti, R.J., et al.: Controlling anxiety in the dental office—emphasis, J.A.D.A. **113**:728, November 1986.
40. Sawyer, H.F.: Presentation, Madigan Army Hospital, Tacoma, Wash., April, 1956.

BIBLIOGRAPHY

Aiach, D., Malone, W.F.P., and Sandrik, J.L.: Dimensional accuracy of epoxy resins and their compatibility with impression materials, J. Prosth. Dent. **52**:500, October 1984.

Barghi, N., King, C.J., and Draughn, R.A.: A study of porcelain surfaces as utilized in fixed prosthodontics, J. Prosth. Dent. **34**:314-319, 1975.

Barghi, N., Alexander, L., and Draughn, R.A.: When to glaze—an electron microscope study, J. Prosth. Dent. **35**:648-653, 1976.

Berman, H., and Lustig, L.P.: Primary substructures and removable telescopic superstructures in dental reconstruction, J. Prosth. Dent. **10**:724-732, 1960.

Brill, N.: Adaptation and the hybrid protheses, J. Prosth. Dent. **5**:811, 1955.

Brukl, C.E., and Reisbick, M.H.: Accuracy of singly and quadruply cast gold and nonnoble crowns, J.A.D.A. **105**:1002, December 1982.

Brukl, C.E., and Philip, G.K.: The fit of Cerestore, twin foil and conventional ceramic crowns, IADR Program and Abstracts No. 1989, 1985.

Campbell, S.D., Riley, E.J., and Sozio, R.B.: Evaluation of a new epoxy resin die material, J. Prosth. Dent. **54**:136-140, 1985.

Ciesco, J.N., Malone, W.F.P., Sandrik, J.L., and Mazur, B.: Comparison of elastomeric impression materials used in fixed prosthodontics, J. Prosth. Dent. **45**:89, January 1981.

Contino, R.M., and Stallard, H.: Instruments essential for obtaining data needed in making a functional diagnosis of the human mouth, J. Prosth. Dent. **7**:66, 1957.

Cronin, R.J., Wardle, W.L.: Prosthodontic management of vertical root extrusion, J. Prosth. Dent. **46**:5, 1986.

Dodge, W.W., Weed, R.M., Baez, R.J., and Buchanan, R.N.: The effect of convergence angle on retention and resistance form, Quint. Int. **3**:191, 1985.

Dolder, E.J.: The bar joint mandibular denture, J. Prosth. Dent. **11**:689, 1961.

Douglas, H.B., Jr., Moon, P.C., Eshleman, J.R., and Lutins, N.D.: The occlusal dimensional change upon glazing porcelain, J. Dent. Res. **60**:828-829, 1981.

Eames, W.B., O'Neal, S.J., Monteiro, J., et al.: Techniques to improve the seating of castings, J.A.D.A. **96**:432, 1978.

Eglitis, I.I., Malone, W.F.P., Toto, P.D., and Gerhard, R.J.: The presence of immunoglobulin IgG and complement factor C_3 in inflammatory papillary hyperplasia associated with maxillary dentures, J. Prosth. Dent. **46**:201, August 1981.

Fusayama, T., Ide, K., and Hosoda, H.: Relief of resistance of cement of full cast crowns, J. Prosth. Dent. **14**:95, 1964.

Gardner, F.M.: Margins of complete crowns—literature review, J. Prosth. Dent. **48**:396, 1982.

Garguilo, A.W., Wentz, F.M., and Orban, B.: Dimensions of the dentinogingival junction in humans, J. Periodontol. **32**:261, July 1961.

Gordon, T.: Telescope reconstruction: an approach to oral rehabilitation, J.A.D.A. **72**:97-105, 1966.

Grajower, R., and Lewinstein, I.: A mathematical treatise on the fit of crown castings, J. Prosth. Dent. **49**:663, 1983.

Hollenback, G.M.: A plea for a more conservative approach in certain dental procedures, J. Alabama Dent. Assoc. **46**:16, 1962.

Hudgins, J.L., Moon, P.C., and Knap, F.J.: The particle-roughened resin-bonded retainers, J. Prosth. Dent. **53**:471, April 1985.

Ishikiriama, A., Oliveira, D.F., and Mondelli, J.: Influence of some factors on the fit of cemented crowns, J. Prosth. Dent. **45**:400, 1981.

Jameson, L.M.: Comparison of the volume of crevicular fluid from restored and non-restored teeth, J. Prosth. Dent. **41**:2, 1979.

Jorgensen, K.D., and Petersen, G.F.: The grain size of zinc phosphate cements, Acta Odont. Scandinav. **21**:255-270, 1963.

Josephson, B.A., Schulman, A., Dunn, Z.A., and Hurwitz, W.A.: A compressive strength study of an all-ceramic crown, J. Prosth. Dent. **53**:301-303, 1985.

Kaiser, D.A., Brukl, C.E., and Kiser, G.C.: Film thickness of disclosing wax, J. Prosth. Dent. **50**:510, October 1983.

Kornfeld, M., ed.: Mouth Rehabilitation, St. Louis, 1967, The C.V. Mosby Co., Vol. 1, pp. 118-120.

Koyano, E., Iwaku, M., and Fusayama, T.: Pressuring techniques and cement thickness for cast restoration, J. Prosth. Dent. **40**:544, 1978.

Kuwata, M.: Theory and Practice for Ceramo Metal Restorations, Chicago, 1980, Quintessence Publishing Co.

Levin, E.I.: Dental esthetics and the golden proportion, J. Prosth. Dent. **40**:244, September 1978.

Lutz, F., Phillips, R.W., Roulet, J.F., and Setcos, J.C.: In vivo and in vitro wear of potential posterior composites, J. Dent. Res. **63**:914, 1984.

Malone, W.F.P., Geehard, R.J., Ensing, H., and Morganelli, J.: Imaginative prosthodontics, J. Acad. Gen. Dent. **18**:21-24, June 1970.

Malone, W.F.P., and Porter, Z.C.: Tissue Management and Restorative Dentistry, Littleton, Mass., 1982, P.S.G. Publ.

Maruyama, T., Simoosa, T., and Ojima, H.: Morphology of gingival capillaries adjacent to complete crowns, J. Prosth. Dent. **35**:179-184, 1976.

McAllister, H.H.: The tilted molar abutment, Dent. Clin. North Am. **10**:25-32, March 1965.

McDermott, T., Lutz, F., Lufi, A., et al.: Quantitative evaluation of in vivo occlusal wear of acrylic resin bridges and wear resistance of three different materials—results after 6 months, Helv. Odont. Acta **25**:1001, 1981.

McKinney, J.E., and Wu, W.: Relationship between subsurface damage and wear of dental restorative composites, J. Dent. Res. **61**:1083, 1982.

Miller, P.A.: Complete dentures supported by natural teeth, J. Prosth. Dent. **8**:924-928, 1958.

Morrow, R.M., Feldmann, E.E., Rudd, K.D., and Trovillion, H.M.: Tooth supported complete dentures: an approach to preventive prosthodontics, J. Prosth. Dent. **21**:513-521, 1969.

Morrow, R.M., Brown, C.E., Larkin, J.P., et al.: Evaluation of methods for polishing denture teeth, J. Prosth. Dent. **30**:222-226, 1973.

Munoz, C.A., Goodacre, C.J., Moore, B.K., and Dykema, R.W.: A comparative study of the strength of aluminous porcelain jacket crowns constructed with the conventional and twin-foil techniques, J. Prosth. Dent. **48**:271-281, 1982.

Muttall, E.B.: Abutment preparations using high speed instruments, J. Kentucky Dent. Assoc. **13**:161, 1961.

Pardo, G.: A full cast restoration design offering superior marginal characteristics, J. Prosth. Dent. **48**:539, 1982.

Pascoe, D.F.: An evaluation of the marginal adaptation of extracoronal restoration during cementation, J. Prosth. Dent. **49**:657, 1983.

Philip, G.K., and Brukl, C.E.: Compressive strengths of conventional, twin foil and all-ceramic crowns, J. Prosth. Dent. **2**:215-220, 1981.

Philips, R.W.: Skinner's Science of Dental Materials, ed. 8, Philadelphia, 1982, W.B. Saunders Co., pp. 502-529.

Potts, R.G., Schillingburg, H.T., and Duncanson, M.G.: Retention and resistance of preparations for cast restorations, J. Prosth. Dent. **43**:303, March 1980.

Prichard, J.F., and Feder, M.: Modern adaptation of the telescopic principle in periodontal prosthesis, J. Periodontol. **33**:360-364, 1962.

Oliva, R.A., and Lowe, J.A.: Dimensional stability of composite resin used as a core material, J. Prosth. Dent. **56**:554, 1986.

Ramfjord, S.P., and Ash, M.M.: Occlusion, Philadelphia, 1984, W.B. Saunders Co.

Ricketts, R.M.: The biologic significance of the divine proportion and Fibonacci series, Am. J. Ortho. **81**:351, May 1982.

Riley, E., Sozio, R., Shklar, G., and Krech, K.: Shrink-free ceramic crown versus ceramometal: a comparative study in dogs, J. Prosth. Dent. **49**:766-771, 1983.

Schlissel, E.R., Newitter, D.A., Renner, R.R., and Gwinnett, A.J.: An evaluation of postadjustment polishing techniques for porcelain denture teeth, J. Prosth. Dent. **43**:258-265, 1980.

Seltzer, S., and Bender, I.B.: The Dental Pulp: Biological Considerations in Dental Procedures, Philadelphia, 1965, J.P. Lippincott.

Smith, D.E.: Fixed bridge with tilted mandibular second or third molar as an abutment, J. South. Calif. Dent. Assoc. **6**:131, 1939.

Sozio, R.B., and Riley, E.J.: The shrink free ceramic crown, J. Prosth. Dent. **49**(2):182-187, February 1983.

Stein, R.S., and Glickman, I.: Prosthodontic considerations essential for gingival health, Dent. Clin. North Am., March 1962.

Stewart, G.P., Bagley, R.L., and Froemling, R.A.: Evaluation of reversible hydrocolloid impression material in a wet field, J. Prosth. Dent. **51**:797, June 1984.

Schweitzer, J.M., Schweitzer, R.D., and Schweitzer, J.: The telescoped complete denture: a research report at the clinical level, J. Prosth. Dent. **10**:724-732, 1960.

Suthers, M.D., and Wise, M.D.: Influence of the cementing medium on the accuracy of the remount procedure, J. Prosth. Dent. **47**:377, 1982.

Tjan, A.H.L., Sarkissian, R., and Miller, G.D.: Effect of multiple axial grooves on the marginal adaptation of full cast-gold crowns, J. Prosth. Dent. **46**:399, 1981.

Van Nortwick, W.T., and Gettleman, L.: Effect of internal relief, vibration, and venting on the vertical seating of cemented crowns, J. Prosth. Dent. **45**:395, 1981.

Vryonis, P.: A simplified approach to the complete porcelain margin, J. Prosth. Dent. **42**:592, November 1979.

Waller, M.I.: The anatomy of the maxillary molar furcal plane crown prep, J.A.D.A. **99**(6):978-982, 1979.

Ward, Herbert E.: Preparation of furcally involved teeth, J. Prosth. Dent. **48**:261, September 1982.

Webb, E.L., Murray, H.V., Holland, G.A., and Taylor, D.F.: Effects of preparation relief and flow channels on seating full coverage castings during cementation, J. Prosth. Dent. **49**:777, 1983.

Waerhaug, J.: Histological considerations which govern where the margins should be located in relation to the gingiva, Dent. Clin. North Am. **8**:161-176, March 1960.

Wiley, M.G., Huff, T.L., Trebilcock, Charles, and Girvan, T.B.: Esthetic porcelain margins: modified porcelain wax technique, J. Prosth. Dent. **56**:527, November 1986.

6

INDIVIDUAL TOOTH
PREPARATION

**William F.P. Malone, D.J. Maroso,
D.A. Kaiser, Karen B. Troendle,
G. Roger Troendle, Gaylord J. James, Jr.,
Antony T. Young, James R. Schmidt,
Maria Lopez-Howell, Steven M. Morgano,
and Boleslaw Mazur**

INTRODUCTION TO TOOTH PREPARATION: ROTARY INSTRUMENTS WITH PRIMARY SHAPES AND USES

The primary rotary instruments used to prepare teeth for cast metals, dental porcelains, acrylic resins, or their combinations, are cutting or abrading instruments. Burs are classified as cutting instruments; diamond points are abrading instruments. The shapes of each are designed to perform a specific task.

Generally, diamond rotary instruments are preferred for preparing teeth for fixed prosthodontics. However, for certain preparations a combination of diamonds and burs is needed to incorporate all the retentive and resistance features required for that restoration. An example would be a preparation requiring pins and, occasionally, grooves.

The friction grip burs and diamonds are available in short or regular length shanks. The latter are used for most procedures, but limited access requires a shorter shank. If a short shank is not readily available, a regular shank can be modified.

There are quality differences in manufacturing of burs and diamonds. In some instances irreparable damage to tooth structures results from the lower quality instrument. Carefully examine (preferably with magnification) burs for irregularities of cutting edges, shape, and concentricity. After limited use, examine them again for dullness of cutting edges. Diamonds should be examined for excessive projection of diamond particles and concentricity. Dressing stones are available for correcting projecting particles, but particles are also removed by this process. After limited use, inspect the diamonds to determine if the bond of diamond to the instrument is satisfactory. Low quality diamonds lose particles rapidly due to a poor bond.

Concentricity is determined by viewing the rotary instrument in profile while it is being rotated at the maximum speed recommended for that instrument.

A nonconcentric instrument produces a "whipping" action seen as a blurred image at the tip of the instrument. This not only causes major preparation irregularities, but may cause pulpal damage.

Diamond rotary instruments are manufactured to produce three abrasive qualities: coarse, medium, and fine. The instrument with the largest diameter and the coarsest surface is intended to reduce the tooth most efficiently. A fine-particle diamond point is designed for finishing prepared surfaces. The medium particle surface produces a prepared surface texture somewhere between the coarse and fine particle.

Cutting Instruments

The primary rotary cutting instruments are carbide burs, which reduce tooth structure, or diamond points, which reduce a tooth surface. Diamonds are intended for restorative dentistry and prosthodontics. They are easier to control than burs because of increased tactile sense.

The dentist should be familiar with the dimensions of diamonds and burs. Reduction of tooth structure is in proportion to the size of the cutting instrument, so an efficient instrument should be used to save effort and energy during tooth preparation.

Generally, efficient bulk cutting is performed with the largest, coarsest diamond instrument that can be accommodated. Finer diamonds are less efficient but give the preparation a fine matte finish. Cutting instruments are kept in motion to control the instrument and produce smoother reductions. Development of the tactile sense and a light touch at high speed also provides greater control. Eccentric rotating and worn diamonds and burs are worthless. The following pages list the commonly used instruments:

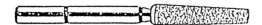

Fig. A. Flat-ended, tapered diamond cylinder

A flat-end, tapered cylinder is used for bulk axial and occlusal reduction and shoulder preparation on PJC and PFM tooth preparations. End cutting burs are also used to develop and lower shoulder preparation. They are kept perpendicular to the plane being reduced (Fig. A).

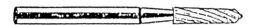

Fig. C. Twelve-fluted carbide bur

Twelve-fluted carbide burs are specifically matched with the different-sized Tinker diamonds and give a highly finished surface to a preparation. The greater the number of blades on a bur, the smoother the cut. Also, blades in a spiral or diagonal to the shaft produce a smoother surface than blades parallel to the instrument shaft. The slightly spiral, multibladed 12-fluted carbide is a smooth-cutting instrument (Fig. C).

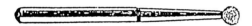

Fig. E. Round diamonds

Round diamonds facilitate establishing depth grooves before reduction. They vary in size and are measured to determine the cut depth. Round diamonds and burs are true and do not tend toward apical migration. It is possible to delineate margins on preparations precisely and accurately using this technique. Round diamonds are also used to establish rest seats and reduce lingual surfaces of anterior teeth (Fig. E).

Fig. G. Oblong diamonds (football)

Variously shaped football diamonds are available for lingual reduction of anterior teeth. They are available in sizes that uniformly reduce the fossae (Fig. G).

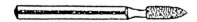

Fig. I. Tapered oblong diamond (flame)

Small flame-shaped diamonds are used in bevel placement. There are many multifluted flame-shaped carbides that have identical functions (Fig. I).

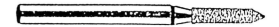

Fig. B. Straight cylinder diamond with a tapered point

A suitable instrument for chamfer placement is a Tinker diamond; a straight cylinder with a tapered point. This tapered point creates a chamfer with greater control than the round-end tapered diamond. It is usually indicated for molars, not premolars and incisors (Fig. B).

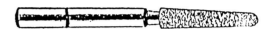

Fig. D. Round-ended tapered diamond cylinders

Round-end, tapered cylinders are available in various sizes. They are used for axial and occlusal reduction and developing chamfer margins. Less than half the diameter of the tip is used for chamfer margins. Cutting to a depth greater than one-half the diameter of the tip produces a shoulder. Tapered cylindrical diamonds also have a tendency to creep apically; this proclivity must be recognized and avoided (Fig. D).

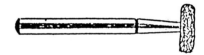

Fig. F. Round diamond wheels (donut)

Round wheels are gross reduction instruments and also used in anterior teeth lingual reductions (Fig. F).

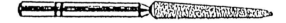

Fig. H. Thin tapered diamond cones (needle)

Thin tapered cones are used for proximal slices to isolate teeth from adjacent teeth. They tend to lose their sharpness sooner than coarse diamonds and are replaced frequently (Fig. H).

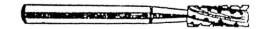

Fig. J. Cross cut fissure burs

Cross-cut fissure burs come in varying sizes, both tapered and cylindrical. The tapered burs are used for groove placement in three-quarter crowns, flutes, and for seating grooves in complete gold crowns. They work efficiently in sectioning gold restorations removed clinically (Fig. J).

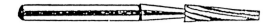

Fig. K. Plain fissure burs

Plain fissure burs cut smoothly and come in a variety of sizes, both tapered and cylindrical. They may also be used for groove placement and finishing of preparations. The long tapered variety, such as the 169L, can be used in lieu of the narrow-tapered diamonds in proximal slices on teeth (Fig. K).

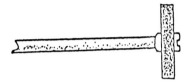

Fig. M. Heatless stone (laboratory)

Large heatless stones will remove the remnant of the sprue attached to the casting (Fig. M).

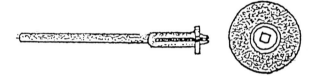

Fig. O. Sand paper discs

Sandpaper discs of various grits are excellent in finishing marginal areas of castings while maintaining contours. They may also be used in finishing tooth preparations (Fig. O).

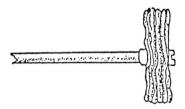

Fig. Q. Chamois wheels (laboratory)

Chamois wheels are used only with dental rouge and give a lustre to the casting (Fig. Q).

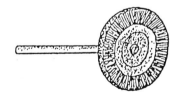

Fig. S. Robinson brushes (laboratory)

Robinson brushes (stiff, medium, soft) are used with pumice or tripoli. Slow speed with pressure produces greater cutting potential; high speed with light pressure produces a high-lustre finish (Fig. S).

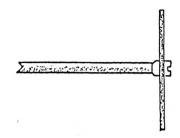

Fig. L. Large Carborundum disc (laboratory)

Mounted stones, discs, and wheels are all used in finishing cast gold, procelain, acrylics, and tooth structure. Large, thin carborundum discs quickly section a sprue from a casting. Similar diamond discs can be used to shape bulk procelain (Fig. L).

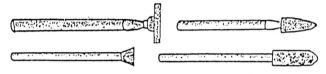

Fig. N. Mounted green and white stones (low speed)

Various mounted green and white stones exist for straight and contraangle handpieces. They are not for high speeds. They can be altered by grinding against a coarse/heatless stone. White stones have a finer texture than green stones and are preferable (Fig. N).

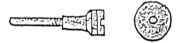

Fig. P. Small pin discs

Small-pin sandpaper discs are fine for accessible margins in the mouth and finishing axial walls in inlay preparations (Fig. P).

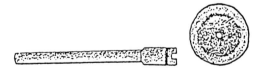

Fig. R. Rubber burlew discs (laboratory)

Rubber burlew discs used after the fine sandpaper stage of finishing provide a smooth surface to the casting. Smaller sulci discs exist for smaller ridge and groove areas but are rarely used intraorally (Fig. R).

SECTION A

Complete Metal Veneer Crown: Maxillary Molar

William F.P. Malone, Steven M. Morgano, Anthony T. Young, and James R. Schmidt

---

DEFINITIONS

Anatomic Crown. Portion of a natural tooth that extends from its cementoenamel junction to the occlusal surface or incisal edge.

Clinical Crown. Portion of a natural tooth that extends from the bottom of the sulcus (epithelial attachment) to the occlusal surface or incisal edge.

Artificial Crown. Fixed restoration of the major surfaces or the entire coronal part of a natural tooth that restores anatomy, function, and esthetics; usually of metal, porcelain, synthetic resin, or combinations.

Advantages

1. Strength imparted to tooth.
2. Contact areas can be conveniently developed.
3. Embrasure areas can be enhanced for periodontally compromised dentitions.
4. Buccal flutes can be developed for preferred contours.
5. Occlusal plane modifications facilitated.
6. Complete metal crowns are the posterior retainers for the majority of FPD's and provide desirable guide planes for RPD's.
7. Indicated for endodontically treated teeth.
8. Ideal for restoring patients with craniofacial anomalies.[1]

Disadvantages

1. Unesthetic.
2. Restricted to posterior teeth.
3. Tooth preparation is more arduous than believed at outset.
4. Belated supportive tissue responses.
5. Hastily underreduced teeth commonly result in overcontouring of axial surfaces without fluting.
6. Occlusion can be capricious without provisional seating; i.e., frosted (sand-blasted) occlusal surfaces.
7. Uniform gingival finish lines are challenging due to accommodation of the patient to vertical height (distal of molars) from the combined height of the handpiece and diamonds.
8. Time-consuming treatment restorations are critical for favorable soft tissue responses.
9. Postcementation gingival caries is difficult to detect.
10. Laboratory implementation requires supervision.

General Indications

1. Any posterior tooth in the nonesthetic zone with existing restorations unable to withstand normal occlusion.
2. An FPD or RPP retainer requiring maximum retention.
3. Short clinical crowns dictating complete coverage for artificial crowns. The complete artificial metal crown is indicated for a single-restoration RPD and/or an FPD retainer (Fig. 6-1). The complete metal crown is usually the last resort when reclaiming a carious or fractured tooth. Some are so undermined that the insertion of a complete crown prevents fracture of the remaining tooth structure.[2]

Complete veneer crowns possess fewer margins than intracoronal restorations. Therefore, for a patient with a history of active caries and poor hygiene, a complete veneer crown is indicated rather than an intracoronal restoration with multiple cavosurface margins. However, all cast restorations are deferred until a caries control program has eliminated caries and preventive measures are instituted (Fig. 6-2).

A complete gold veneer crown may be constructed on both vital and pulpless, anterior or posterior teeth (Fig. 6-3). The esthetic requirements are met by a porcelain or acrylic resin veneer on facial surfaces of the crown. The complete metal veneer artificial crown is rarely used for anterior teeth.

Requirements

Every precaution is exercised during tooth preparation and after the crown has been cemented not to

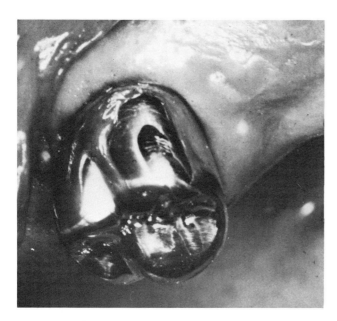

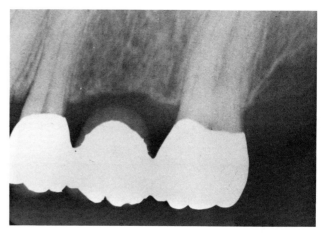

Fig. 6-1. B, Complete crowns as retainers for maxillary three tooth FPD.

Fig. 6-1. A, Complete gold veneer crown for maxillary second molar with healthy tissue. Guideplane and rest are required before cementation.

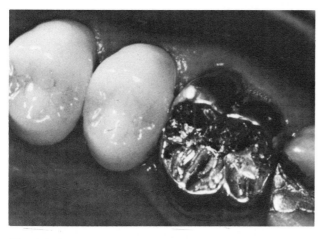

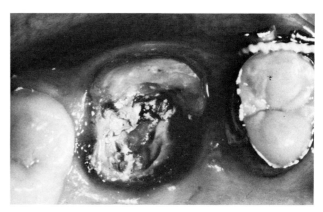

Fig. 6-3. A, Maxillary first molar after endodontic treatment. Note preliminary preparation before cast posts and core.

Fig. 6-2. A complete cast gold crown on a maxillary right first molar. Note buccal flute.

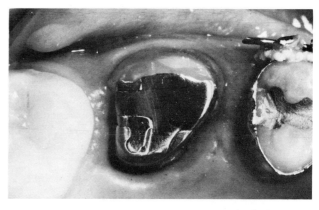

jeopardize the vitality of the pulp. Hasty preparation of a tooth can result in belated degeneration or death of the pulp.[3] Uniform reduction in a regimented sequence after amalgam core reconstruction for missing tooth structure provides orientation and reduces inadvertent pulpal involvement during tooth preparation (Fig. 6-4).

Restoring Function and Anatomy

Establishment of suitable contours with a harmonious occlusion is the intent of treatment. Crowns are commonly placed on compromised teeth, so carefully designed preparations are needed for the tooth to return to function.[4-6] Because the initial carious or traumatic insult often exceeds the recovery capacity of the

Fig. 6-3. B, Cast, "interlock" coronal radicular stabilization before crown lenghtening, treatment restoration, and orthodontic extrusion.

tooth, belated endodontics is not uncommon after crown insertion. Establishing prescribed contours and physiologic occlusion ensures uneventful treatment in most patients.

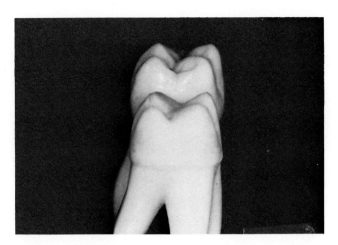

Fig. 6-4. A, Tooth preparation on a maxillary right first molar. The gingival finish line is a chamfer while reduction is uniform. Deviations from the geometric form are common due to lost tooth structure.

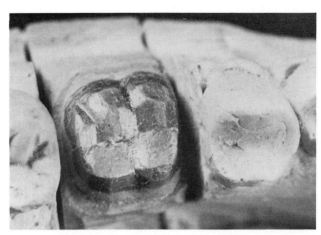

Fig. 6-4. B, Tooth preparation for a complete gold crown of a mandibular left first molar on a dissected stone die with spacer applied.

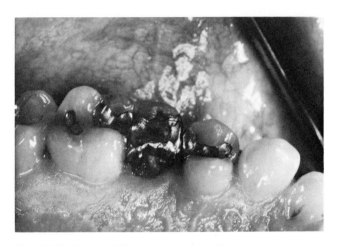

Fig. 6-5. A, Fractured lingual cusp of maxillary second premolar. (Courtesy Dr. Alan Schneider, Los Angeles, Calif.)

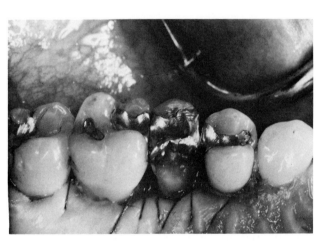

Fig. 6-5. B, Tooth in A after crown lengthening to avoid violating the biologic width. (Courtesy Dr. Alan Schneider, Los Angeles, Calif.)

Gingival Finish Lines and Supportive Tissue

A successful cast or porcelain restoration usually implies a smooth gingival margin with a supportive relationship to the gingival margin.[8,9] The gingival finish lines are not overextended gingivally to violate the biologic width (Fig. 6-5). Crown lengthening, orthodontic extrusion, or both may be necessary for teeth with margins that encroach upon the biologic width. Another preparation problem is root proximity, which presents an almost insurmountable dilemma without orthodontic movement of the offending teeth. Increased proximal reduction to enlarge the embrasure area is a short-term, palliative measure. Chapter 5 also addresses tooth preparation of questionable abutments.

Uniformity of Tooth Reduction

The original occlusal anatomy is sustained during both preparations so that reduction occurs in miniature. Cusps and grooves remain in the same relative position, but at a lower level; however, normal occlusal anatomy of prepared teeth is reduced to a configuration (cuspal warpage) to favor strength, stability, and retention of the artificial crown (Fig. 6-6). Axial surfaces are prepared to remove undercuts, provide sufficient reduction for cleansible embrasures, encourage narrowed occlusal tables with fluted buccal surfaces, and accommodate a veneer (Fig. 6-7).[10,11] Note: the subtle object of all tooth preparation for cast restorations of compromised teeth is to provide a geometric form that encourages greater compression of the cement.

Alloys

An acceptable metal crown has intrinsic strength with resistance to wear. Although the proliferation of metal with reduced noble alloy content has made mon-

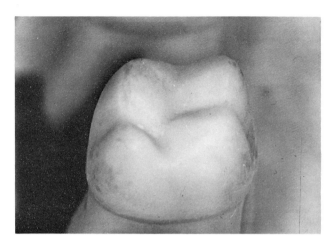

Fig. 6-6. Tooth preparation of a complete gold veneer crown on a maxillary first molar. The occlusal surface should be a prescription to the laboratory for cusp placement.

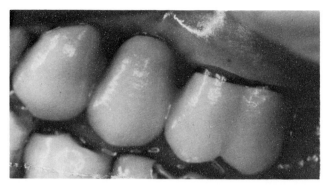

Fig. 6-7. Three-unit maxillary FPD with adequate embrasures, fluted buccal surface on molar, and supragingival margins.

itoring of alloy content difficult, alloy should respond favorably to an oral environment. Metal selection is based upon open communication between dentist and technician. The role of tarnish and corrosion of metals and general biocompatibility are the focus of concentrated research; preliminary results indicate that corrosion can intimately effect cementation.[12-15]

Most teeth requiring a complete crown are reconstructed with amalgam before tooth preparation (see Chapter 2). The step-by-step preparation for complete gold veneer crowns is as follows:[16,17]

1. *Uniformly finish* the gingival margin 1 mm coronal to the CEJ, but variations are commonly instituted by the dentist.
    a. Determine a suitable finish line before tooth preparation. The DMF rate, height of gingival tissue, and oral hygiene directly influence the decision (Fig. 6-8).
    b. Make maxillary and mandibular impressions and mount diagnostic casts.
    c. Reproduce the cast of the intended preparation; prepare the tooth on the second cast; wax to achieve desired occlusion and esthetic results.
    d. Prepare a template from a vacuum-formed shell (metal or resin crown form) for a treatment restoration (temporary) before tooth preparation.
2. *Rotary instruments* for complete gold veneer crowns.
    a. Conventional and ultraspeed handpieces
        (1) Conventional for finishing procedures, minor modifications, and groove refinement.
        (2) Ultraspeed for major tooth reductions.
    b. No. 2 round bur for occlusal depth guides
        (1) Cutting head approximates a 1.0 mm.

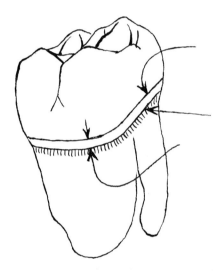

Fig. 6-8. The gingival finish line requires careful review before preparation, and the tissue response can reflect the validity of the determination.

diameter dimension.
    c. Diamond instruments
        (1) No. 870-012 tapered tip cylinder and/or No. 857-014 (safe-end); axial and occlusal surface reduction.
        (2) No. 30006-060-012 (thin tapering shape), proximal slices and initial groove formation; refinement of prepared axial surfaces and margins (conventional speed).
    d. Burs (conventional speed)
        (1) No. 700; groove refinement
        (2) No. H375-014; groove refinement
        (3) No. H282-010; margin and axial wall refinement
    e. Mounted stones
        (1) Flame shaped (green); smooth occlusal surfaces and round line angles.
    f. Mandrel and 5/8 inch felt wheel; polish modified gingival base.

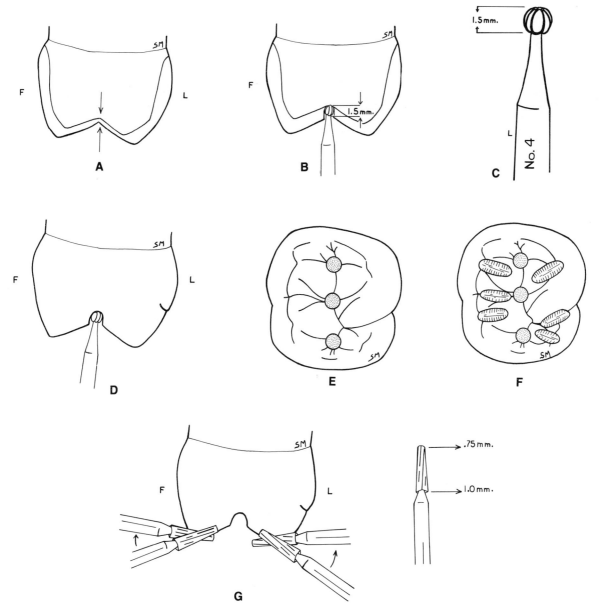

Fig. 6-9. A, Inadequate occlusal reduction causes: lack of occlusal morphology, perforation of occlusal metal, and supraocclusal relationship. **B,** Uniform reduction allows more latitude. **C,** A No. 2 round bur is placed slightly less than the long axis diameter for depth in the mesial central and distal fossa. **D,** Depth wells are placed at the three major occlusal pits with a No. 2 round bur. **E,** The three major occlusal pits to receive depth wells. **F,** The shaded areas are for cusp depth guides and dotted areas to continue the central groove. **G,** A No. 700 fissure bur can also be used to develop depth penetration grooves by placing the bur at the tips of the cusps and gradually increasing the angulation.

3. In *occlusal reduction*, depth guides are helpful for teeth in critical arch position with a reduced interocclusal clearance (Fig. 6-9).
   a. No. 2 round bur slightly less than the long-axis diameter is used for depth in mesial (M), central and distal (d) fossae (Fig. 6-9).
   b. The three main occlusal pits are located to place the depth wells.
   c. Secure depth wells while observing any caries. This is one method of ensuring uniform occlusal reduction.

d. Cusp depth penetration indices are placed in shadowed areas and then addressed with a No. 700 fissure bur (Fig. 6-9, F and G). A second method uses the No. 2 round bur and the No. 700 fissure bur.
   e. Optional depth guide placement, cuspal tips: A third, method equally effective is using a diamond instrument to reduce the occlusal surface.
4. *Depth Guide Grooves*
   a. The full diameter of the No. 877-012 or 878-

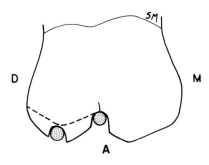

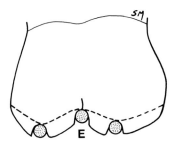

Fig.6-10. E, Orientation of the bur or diamond if a complete crown is confirmed for a CGVC.

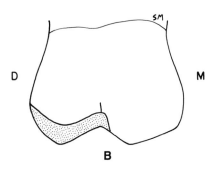

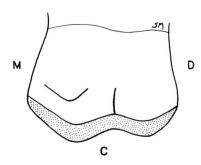

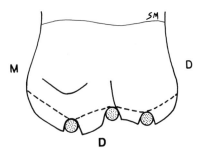

Fig. 6-10. **A,** Depth penetration grooves are usually started on the distal buccal cusps. **B,** The distal buccal cusp is reduced at approximately 45 degree angle, mimicking the inclination of the cusp. If there is sufficient mesial buccal cusp, use of a seven-eighth crown can be considered. **C,** The mesial and distal lingual cusps are then notched and gauged for full occlusal reduction. **D,** The lingual cusps are selectively reduced using the depth penetration guides.

012 diamond (approximately 1.0 mm diameter) or the No. 2 round bur may be used. The advantage of the diamond is that the remaining occlusal reduction can then be accomplished without a bur change (Fig. 6-10, A to D).

b. Occlusal reduction is the first step in tooth preparation, and underreduction is the commonest omission in fixed prosthodontics. This is particularly true when the occlusal surfaces are restored in full porcelain. Uniform reduction aided by predetermined depth grooves ensures adequate clearance (Fig. 6-10 E).

5. Following proper technique for *tooth preparation,* the occlusal surface is a reduced uniformly by 2.0 mm so that the occlusal surface is a replica of the original tooth.

a. Establish a depth groove starting from the central fossa with depth pits extending through the groove between the mesial and distal buccal cusps to a depth of 1.5 mm using a cross-cut tapered fissure, Nos. 1157 or 700 (Fig. 6-11, A and B).

b. Make a similar depth cut along the developmental groove between the mesial and distal palatal cusps (Fig. 6-11 B).

c. Develop a depth cut through the cusp tips and the triangular ridges of the buccal cusps and the mesiopalatal cusp but <u>not</u> the distal lingual cusp unless the tooth is rotated.

d. Reduce the inclined planes between the depth guides in the developmental grooves and those along the triangular ridges.

e. Reduce the marginal ridge by 1.5 mm (Fig. 6-11 C).

f. Smooth the occlusal surface so that it duplicates the unprepared tooth in miniature at a level 2.0 mm pulpally. This requires an additional 0.5 mm reduction for a total of 2.0 for static reduction. Further tooth preparation may be necessary to establish clearance during excursions of the mandible, par-

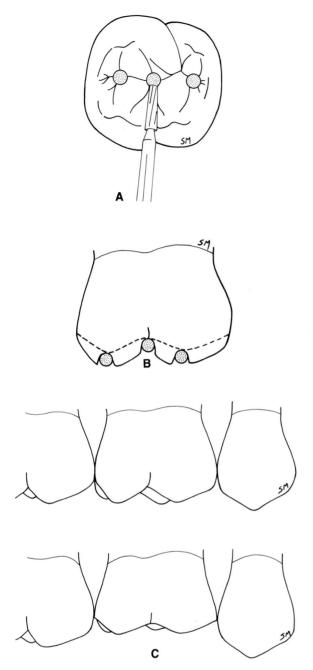

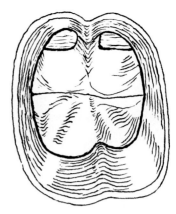

Fig. 6-12. The occlusal surface should appear as a prescription for cusp placement to the technician.

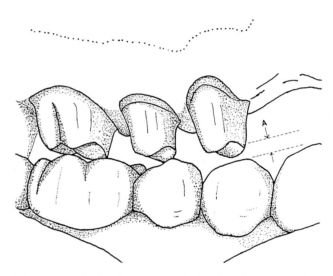

Fig. 6-13. Patient with open bite in left lateral excursion but insufficient clearance during movement. Static reduction of 2 mm can appear adequate, but when evaluated for clearance, it may be insufficient.

Fig. 6-11. A, Occlusal view of No. 700 bur placement to central pit. **B,** The occlusal is reduced in miniature to the dotted line. **C,** Uniform reduction should be checked in excursions of the mandible.

ticularly with ceramic/metal or injectible ceramic restorations (Fig. 6-12).

g. Modify the preparation to accommodate excursive movements of the mandible. Reduction indicates static centric occlusion that is usually adequate, while occlusal clearance infers sufficient tooth preparation without occlusal contact during excursive movements of the mandible (Fig. 6-13).

6. The initial *proximal surface reduction* is performed to break contact with the adjacent tooth only, so as <u>not</u> to establish a proximal finish line (Fig. 6-14 A).

a. The tooth adjacent to the tooth being prepared is to be protected during preparation (Fig. 6-14, B and C), however, excessive proximal contours are routinely modified with enameloplasty to permit seating of the casting.

b. Position the No. 669L carbide bur or thin tapered diamond with the long axis of the preparation to provide 2 to 5 degrees convergence on the mesial surface of the tooth. (Note that the tip of the bur is not used in preparation.)

c. Prepare the mesial surface (Fig. 6-14 D).

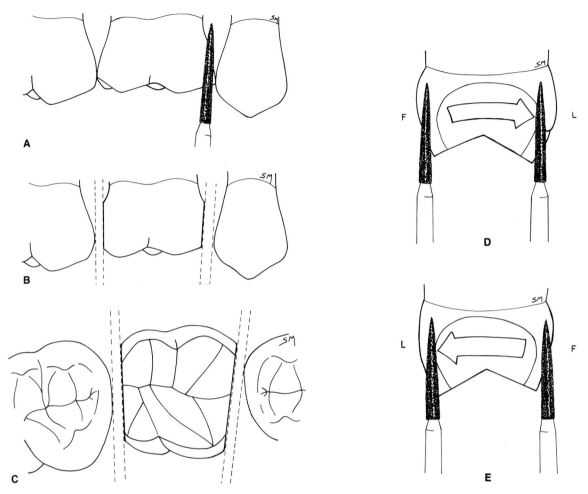

Fig. 6-14. A, The contacts between adjacent teeth are broken with a thin diamond. **B,** A tofflemire matrix or a "T" band can be inserted before proximal preparations; however, many teeth require enameloplasty to provide adequate embrasures. **C,** A long thin diamond is directed through the contact to establish 2 to 5 degree convergence. Angulation exceeding 10 degrees are not uncommon because the diamond and the vertical length of the handpiece is not easily accommodated by most patients. **D,** The mesial slice reduction should be a flat plane forming a knife edge at the juncture of the prepared and unprepared tooth structure. **E,** The distal surface is prepared similarly, but the contacts on the mesial are more buccal and the distal contacts more lingual than the mesial surface.

   d. Do <u>not</u> create the gingival finish line at this time. (Fig. 6-14 E).

   e. Repeat Steps 1 to 3 for the distal surface.

 7. *Facial* and *lingual reduction.* During the facial and lingual reduction, an appropriate taper is established on the axial walls. The anatomy of the tooth converges occlusally-naturally more than the ideal 2 to 5 degrees. Therefore, the walls of the preparation are developed in relation to the path of insertion rather than the existing anatomy (Fig. 6-15, A and B).

   a. Place the diamond next to the buccal surface of the tooth at an angle parallel to the long axis of the tooth <u>not</u> parallel to the axis of the buccal surface (Fig. 6-15 C).

   b. Maintaining the desired angulation of the bur, position the tip of the bur immediately above the finish line.

   c. Reduce the tooth in miniature using a brushing motion.

   d. Control the tip of the bur so it does <u>not</u> pass beyond the finish line or does not exceed the depth of one-half the diameter of the bur.

   e. Reexamine the buccal surface and determine the areas that are <u>not</u> uniformly reduced.

   f. Position the bur parallel with the surface of the uncut tooth and reduce it uniformly (Fig. 6-15 C <u>not</u> Fig. 6-15 D).

   g. Repeat Steps 1 to 4 for the lingual surface without changing the angulation of the bur that undercuts the preparation (Fig. 6-15 B).

h. Recall that the lingual cusps on maxillary molars are "stamp cusps" and require a "two-plane" reduction (Fig. 6-15 E).

i. Using a diamond bur, provide a two-plane reduction by modifying the occlusal one-third of lingual wall of the preparation at a 45-degree angle to the long axis of the tooth (Fig. 6-15 F). A two-plane reduction is also not uncommon on the facial surface of the maxillary molar for esthetics or for stamp cusp modification in patients with a cross-bite (Fig. 6-15 G). Boxes improve retention but reduce the vertical seat of the artificial crown.

8. *Axial angle reduction.* It is necessary to smooth the sharp line angles created after the proximal, facial, and lingual surfaces have been reduced. The axial reductions are directly related to the physiologic contours of fluting (Fig. 6-16 A) and cleansible embrasures.

a. Position the 30006-012 diamond parallel to the long axis of the tooth at the four line angles (Fig. 6-16 B).

b. Blend the buccal and lingual reduction into the interproximals, rounding the sharp line angle (Fig. 6-16, C and D).

9. *Margins.* The proximal finish lines are now established, and margins are reviewed for smoothness and continuity.

a. Prepare the mesial and distal knife edge finish lines with the diamond to a level approximately 1 mm above the CEJ (Fig. 6-17 A).

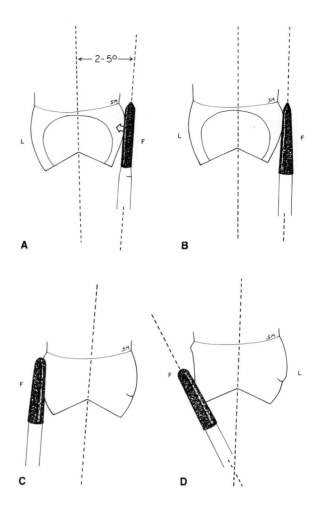

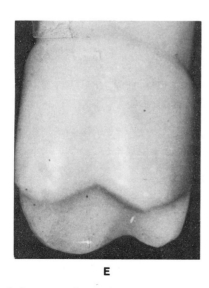

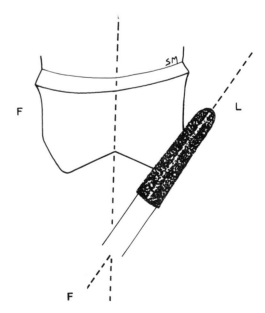

Fig. 6-15. A, A coarser diamond is used for gross reduction along the path of insertion, *not* existing anatomy. **B,** A coarse diamond is then used to develop the lingual wall along the path of insertion *not* as in A or D. **C,** The coarse diamond is placed parallel to the long axis of the tooth, *not* the angle demonstrated in D. **D,** Inappropriate angulation for axial surface reduction. Use the path of insertion as a guideline. **E,** The lingual surface requires a two-plane reduction for the stamp cusps. **F,** Angulation of reduction to ensure sufficient bulk metal or metal/ceramic crowns.

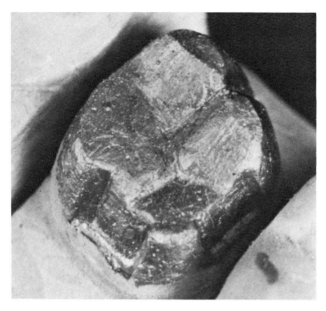

Fig. 6-15. G, Two-plane reduction on buccal surface for posterior cross bite. Boxes are for additional retention.

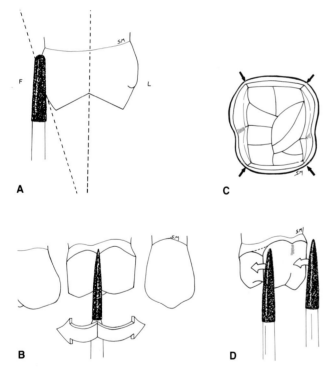

Fig. 6-16. A, Preliminary barreling of the mesial and distal cusps but short of the furca cove is an embryonic flute. **B,** Mesiodistal planning of the long axis at the four line angles is the initial step of finishing the preparation surface. **C,** Smooth strokes will accomplish the line angle smoothing. **D,** The lingual mesial and distal line angles are rounded. Caution must be observed to avoid excessive angulation of the hand piece and produce excessive occlusal convergence or divergence. A lingual groove is placed to separate distal and mesial lingual cusps that terminate in knife edge margins at this stage.

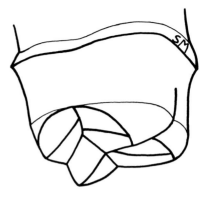

Fig. 6-17. A, A smooth and continuous gingival finish line is placed supporting the gingival tissue.

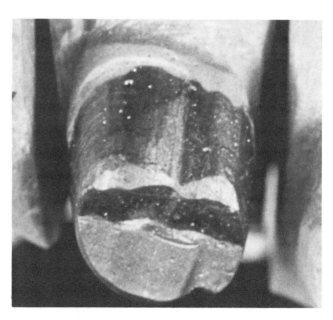

Fig. 6-17. B, Dissected die using spacer with a slight buccal flute and exaggerated bevel on the mesial buccal gingival finish line. The occlusal morphology is maintained in miniature and the distal surface convergence angle is exceptionally rigid.

    b. The traditional 2 to 5 degree convergence on the interproximal surface is preserved if possible (Fig. 6-17 B).

10. Finish the preparation by refining the line angles and point angles.

    a. Smooth sharp angles or surface irregularities with the diamond or a matching "duet" carbide bur and, lastly, with a cuttle fish disc.

    b. Occlusal anatomy is placed in a wax pattern to provide harmonious contact (Fig. 6-18 A). Narrowed occlusal tables are encouraged, but are related to opposing teeth (Fig. 6-18, B and C).

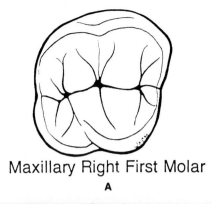

Maxillary Right First Molar

A

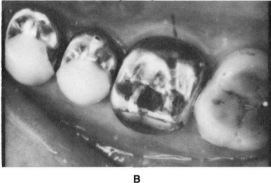

B

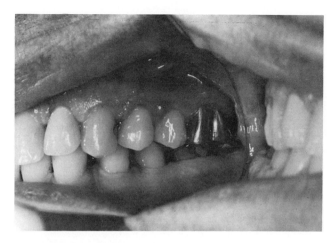

Fig. 6-18. C, Fluted buccal surface of a maxillary first molar complete gold crown. A metal crown was indicated with the reduced interocclusal clearance.

Fig. 6-18. A, Basic occlusal anatomy for a maxillary first molar. **B,** Complete gold veneer crown on the maxillary molar. Note the reduced buccolingual width to diminish the frequence of balancing side prematurities.

SELECTED REFERENCES

1. Tylman, S.D. and Malone, W.F.P.: Tylman's Theory and Practice of Fixed Prosthodontics, St. Louis, 1978, The C.V. Mosby Co.
2. Guyer, S.E.: Multiple preparations for fixed prosthodontics, J. Prosthet. Dent. **23:**529, 1970.
3. Walton, J.N., Gardner, F.M., and Agar, J.R.: A survey of crown and fixed partial denture failures: length of service and reasons for replacement, J. Prosthet. Dent. **56:**416, 1986.
4. Owens, C.P.: Factors influencing the retention and resistance of preparation for cast intracoronal restorations, J. Prosthet. Dent. **55:**674, 1986.
5. Owens, C.P.: Retention and resistance in preparation for extracoronal restorations, II, Practical and clinical studies, J. Prosthet. Dent. **56:**148, 1986.
6. Cavazos, E. and Acosta, J.: Tooth preparation taper of extracoronal retainers, J. Prosthet. Dent., in press.
7. Jameson, L.M. and Malone, W.F.P.: Crown contour in fixed prosthodontics, J. Prosthet. Dent. **41:**620, 1982.
8. Wiley, M.C., Huff, T.L., Trebilcock, C., and Girvan, T.B.: Esthetic porcelain margins: a modified porcelain-wax technique, J. Prosthet. Dent. **56:**527, 1986.
9. Lofstron, L.H. and Asgar, K.: Scanning electromicroscope evaluation of techniques to extend deficient cast gold margins, J. Prosthet. Dent. **56:**416, 1986.
10. Malone, W.F., Porter, S.C., and Jameson, L.M.: Tooth preparation for periodontally compromised dentitions, IL State Dent. J. **53:**228, 1984.
11. Neuhas, R.K.: Crown preparation (II), Quint. Int. **5:**429, 1984.
12. Broze, B.: The Cerestore crown—is this the future of dental restorative veneering materials? Trends Tech. Contemp. Dent. Lab. **1:**15, 1984.
13. Johnson, L.N.: The physical properties of some alternate alloys, Int. Dent. J. **33:**41, 1983.
14. Christensen, Gordon J.: The use of porcelain fused to metal restorations in current dental practice: a survey, J. Prosthet. Dent. **56:**1, 1986.
15. Brukl, Charles E., and Reisbeck, M.H.: Accuracy of singly and quadruply cast gold and non-noble crowns, J.A.D.A. **105:**1002, 1982.
16. Troendle, Karen: The University of Texas San Antonio Freshman Fixed Prosthodontic Technique Manual, 1988.
17. Schmidt, J.R.: Southern Illinois University School of Dental Medicine Fixed Prosthodontic Manual, 1979.
18. Maroso, D.J.: Southern Illinois University School of Dental Medicine DRMO 711 Operative Dentistry Lab. Manual, 1987.

BIBLIOGRAPHY

Crim, G.A., Tobias, R.S., and Browne, R.M.: Pulpal response to an experimental adhesion promotor, J. Oral Pathol. **15:**196, 1986.

Dodge, W.W., Weed, R.M., and Baez, R.J.: the effect of die space on casting fit, J. Dent. Res. 61 (special issue), 1982 (Abst. No. 1300).

Douglass, Gordon D.: Principles of preparation design in fixed prosthodontics, J. Am. Acad. Gen. Dent., April 1973.

Eams, W.B., O'Neal, S.J., Monterior, J., et al.: Techniques to improve the seating of castings, J.A.D.A. **96:**432, 1978.

Eissmann, H., Radke, R., and Noble, W.: Physiologic design criteria for fixed dental restorations, Dent. Clin North Am. **15:**543, 1971.

El-Ebraski, M.K., Craig, R.C., and Peyton, F.A.: Experimental stress analysis of dental restorations, J. Prosthet. Dent. 1967, 1970, Parts I-IX.

Farah, J.W., and Craig, R.G.: Stress analysis of three marginal configurations of full posterior crowns by three dimensional photoelasticity, 53, No. 5, Part 2, September-October, 1975, P. 1219.

Farer, J., and Isaacson, D.: Biologic contours, J. Prev. Dent. **1:**4, August 1974.

Fusayama, T., Ide, K., and Hosoda, H.: Relief of resistance of cement of full cast crowns, J. Prosthet. Dent. **14:**95, 1964.

Gardner, F.M.: Margins of complete crowns—literature reviews, J. Prosthet. Dent. **48:**396, 1982.

Gavelis, J.R., Morency, J.D., Riley, E.D., and Sozio, R.B.: The effect of various finish line preparations on the marginal seal and occlusal seat of full crown preparations, J. Prosthet. Dent. **45**:138, 1981.

Gilbar, Dennis B., and Tetruch, Walter R.: Fundamental of extracoronal tooth preparation I. Retention and resistance form, J. Prosthet. Dent. **32**:651-656, 1974.

Glickman, I., Stein, R., and Smulson, M.: Function forces upon the periodontium of splinted and non splinted teeth, J. Perioton. **32**:290, 1961.

Grajower, R., and Lewinstein, I.: A mathematical treatise on the fit of crown castings, J. Prosthet. Dent. **49**:663, 1983.

Guyer, S.E.: Multiple preparations for fixed prosthodontics, J. Prosthet. Dent. **23**:529-553, 1970.

Harrison, J.D.: Crown and bridge preparation, design and use, Dent. Clin. North Am. pp. 105-191, March 1966.

Herlands, R.E., Lucca, J.J., and Morris, M.L.: Forms, contours, and extensions of full coverage restorations in occlusal reconstruction, Dent. Clin. North Am. **6**:147, 1962.

Horn, H.R.: A new lamination: porcelain bonded to enamel, N.Y. State Dent. J. **49**:401, 1983.

Ibsen, R.L., and Strassler, H.E.: An innovative method for fixed anterior tooth replacement utilizing porcelain veneers, Quint. Int. **17**:455, 1986.

Ishikiriama, A., Olivira, J.F., Vieira, D.F., and Mondelli, J.: Influence of some factors on the fit of cemented crowns, J. Prosthet. Dent. **45**:400, 1981.

Ishu, M., and Satoh, N.: Fabrication of collarless porcelain fused to metal restorations without using a plaintum matrix, Int. J. Periodont. Restor. Dent. **6**:64, 1986.

Jameson, L.M.: Comparison of the volume of crevicular fluid from restored and non restored teeth, J. Prosthet. Dent. **41**:2, 1979.

Jendresen, M.D., Hamilton, A.E., McLean, J.W., Phillips, R.W., and Ramfjord, S.P.: Report of the Committee on Scientific Investigation of the Amer. Acad. of Restor. Dent., J. Prosthet. Dent. **51**:823, 1984.

Kelly, J.R., and Rose, T.C.: Nonprecious alloys for use in fixed prosthodontics: a literature review, J. Prosthet. Dent. **49**:363, 1983.

Kemper, W.W., et al.: Periodontal tissue changes in response to high artificial crowns, J. Prosthet. Dent. **10**:160, 1968.

Klecinic, E.P.: Periodontal preparation for fixed prosthodontics, J. Prosthet. Dent. **20**:511, 1968.

Koyano, E., Iwaku, M., and Fusayama, T.: Pressuring techniques and cement thickness for cast restorations, J. Prosthet. Dent. **40**:544, 1978.

Larato, Dominick C.: Effect of cervical margins on gingiva, J. Calif. Dent. Assoc. **45**:19-22, 1969.

Machert, J.R., Jr., Parry, E.E., Hashinser, T., II, and Fairhurst, C.W.: Measurement of oxide adherence to PFM alloys, J. Dent. Res. **63**:1335, 1984.

Malone, W.F.P.: Electrosurgery in Dentistry, Springfield, Ill., 1975, Charles C Thomas Publishing Co., chapter 6.

Malone, W.F.P., Mazur, B., Tylman, S.D., et al.: Biomechanical considerations of tooth preparation for fixed prosthodontics. In Tylman, S.D., and Malone, W.F.P.: Tylman's Theory and Practice of Fixed Prosthodontics, Ed. 7, St. Louis, 1978, The C.V. Mosby Co., pp. 96-127.

McCune, R.J., Phillips, R.W., and Swartx, M.L.: The effect of occlusal venting and film thickness on the cementation of full cast crowns, J.S. Calif. Dent. Assoc. **39**:361, 1971.

McLean, J.W., and Wilson, A.D.: Butt joint versus bevelled gold margin in metal/ceramic crowns, Dent. Clin. North Am. **24**:242, April 1980.

Newman, G.V.: Bonding to porcelain, J. Clin. Orthodon. **17**:53, 1983.

Ohno, H., and Kanzowa, Y.: Structural changes in the oxidation zones of gold alloys for porcelain bonding containing small amounts of Fe and Sn, J. Dent. Res. **64**:67, 1985.

Owen, C.P.: Factors influencing the retention and resistance of preparations for cast intracoronal restorations, J. Prosthet. Dent. **55**:674, 1986.

Pardo, G.: A full cast restoration design offering superior marginal characteristics, J. Prosthet. Dent. **48**:539, 1982.

Pascoe, D.F.: An evaluation of the marginal adaptation of extracoronal restoration during cementation, J. Prosthet. Dent. **49**:657, 1983.

Pascoe, D.F.: Analysis of the geometry of finishing lines for full crown restorations, J. Prosthet. Dent. **40**:157, 1978.

Perel, M.: Axial crown contours, J. Prosthet. Dent. **25**:642, 1971.

Preston, J.D.: The metal-cermac restorations: the problem remains, Int. J. Periodont. Restor. Dent. **4**:8, 1984.

Romanelli, J.H.: Considerations in tooth preparation for crown and bridges, Dent. Clin. North Am. **24**:271, April 1980.

Shillingburg, H.T., Jr., Hobo, S., and Whitsett, L.D.: Fundamentos de Prostodoncia fija. Berlin, Buch-und Zeitschriften-Verlag "Die Quintessenz," pp. 67-83, 1978.

Shoher, I.: Reinforced porcelain system: concepts and techniques, Dent. Clin North Am. **29**:805, 1985.

Stein, R.S.: J. Prosthet. Dent. March-April 1966, P. 251.

Stein, R.S., and Glickman, I.: Prosthodontic consideration essential for gingival health, Dent. Clin. North Am. March 1962.

Tjan, A.H.L.: Sarkissian, R., and Miller, G.D.: Effect of multiple axial grooves on the marginal adaptation of full cast-gold crowns, J. Prosthet. Dent. **46**:399, 1981.

Tylman, S.D., and Malone, W.F.P.: Tylman's Theory and Practice of Fixed Prosthodontics, ed. 7, St. Louis, 1978, The C.V. Mosby Co., pp. 99-217.

Van Northwick, W.T., and Gettleman, L.: Effect of internal relief vibration and venting on the vertical seating of cemented crowns, J. Prosthet. Dent. **45**:395, 1981.

Watson, Philip: Cast Restorations in Operative Dentistry, Current Treatment in Dental Practice, Philadelphia & London, 1986, W.B. Saunders Co., pp. 108-110.

Watson, Philip: Preparation design, current treatment in dental practice, Philadelphia and London, 1986, W.B. Saunders Co., pp. 110-115.

Webb, E.L., Murray, H.V., Holland, G.A., and Taylor, D.F.: Effects of preparation relief and flow channels on seating full coverage castings during cementation, J. Prosthet. Dent. **49**:777, 1983.

Yuodelis, R.A., and Faucher, R.: Provisional restorations, Dent. Clin. North Am. **24**:285, April 1980.

Yuodelis, Ralph A., Weater, James D., and Sapkos, Stanley: Facial and lingual contours of artificial complete crown restorations and their effects on the periodontium, J. Prosthet. Dent. **27**:61-65, 1973.

Zarb, G.A., Bergman, B., Clayton, J.A., et al: Placement of margins. In Zarb, G.A., et al: Prosthodontic Treatment for Partially Edentulous Patients, St. Louis, 1978, The C.V. Mosby Co., pp. 333-344.

SECTION B

Complete Metal Veneer Crown: Mandibular Molar

William F.P. Malone, Delmo J. Maroso,
Gaylord J. James, Jr., and James R. Schmidt

MANDIBULAR MOLARS
General Indications

1. A posterior tooth in a nonesthetic zone containing extensive restorations that can not withstand occlusal forces (Fig. 6-19, A and B).
2. A retainer requiring maximum retention for an FPD and/or an RPD (Fig. 6-19 C).
3. Short clinical crowns requiring a complete restoration (Fig. 6-19 D).

General Contraindications

1. Extensively restored or cariously involved teeth within an esthetic zone, both physically and psychologically.

Advantages

1. Protects the coronal integrity of a natural tooth compromised by extensive carious involvement or restorations (Fig. 6-19 E).
2. Provides the maximum retention, favorable contours, and guide planes for retainers.

Disadvantages

1. Marginal adaptation is time consuming and arduous.
2. Difficult to develop axial contours in wax patterns.
3. Caries detection is elusive after fabrication.
4. Vitality tests are unreliable.
5. Belated untoward tissue responses.

SEQUENTIAL PREPARATION PROCEDURES
Diagnosis

1. Isolate the tooth, identify the CEJ, and estimate the clearance necessary for occlusion of patient.
2. Identify the gingival crest contours extending beyond the 1.0 mm above the CEJ.
   a. Evaluate the condition of the supporting structures with a PDL explorer and radiographs.
   b. Make the impressions for diagnostic casts to shape the vacuum celluloid form for a treatment restoration following preparation.

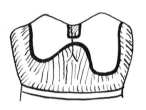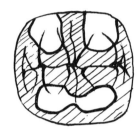

Fig. 6-19. A, Second molar with extensive restorations indicating the need for a complete crown.

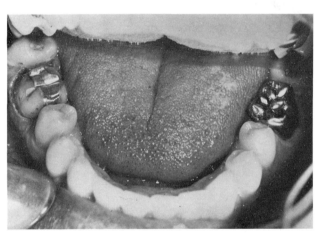

Fig. 6-19. B, Complete gold veneer crown *(left)* with preparation and tissue dilation of an endodontically treated mandibular first molar *(right)*. A chamfer is placed on the facial and lingual surfaces; a knife edge finish line was placed on the proximal surfaces below the amalgam reconstruction.

3. Mentally scribe a line corresponding to the long axis of the tooth on the mesial surface.
4. Observe the tooth from the sagittal and note that a horizontal plane touching cuspal tips is not perpendicular to the long axis.
5. Acknowledge that the long axis is inclined lingually; the lingual cusp tips appear on the same plane as the buccal cusp tips (Fig. 6-20).
6. The extent of lingual inclination will vary among individuals. Its significance is minimal for single unit preparations but may be a major factor for retainers of FPD's.

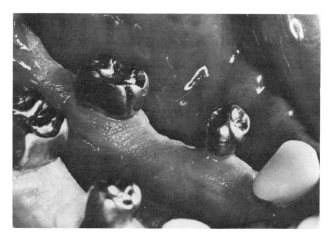

Fig. 6-19. C, Complete crowns as abutments for RPD. Note the rests and guideplanes that were prepared in the tooth prior to the wax patterns to incorporate the .010 undercut without over-contouring.

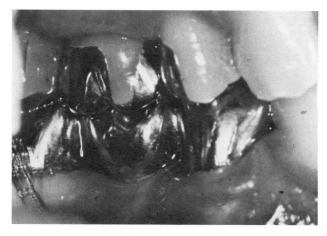

Fig. 6-19. D, Complete metal crowns allow magnified embrasures for short clinical crowns.

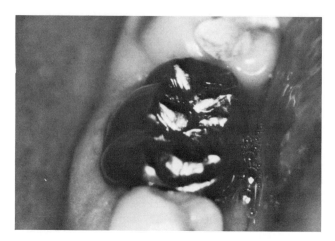

Fig. 6-19. E, Complete crown on the mandibular first molar with a smooth buccal surface and a narrow buccolingual width.

Armamentarium and Uses

1. *Diamonds*
   a. 3000006-060-012 coarse tapering; the tip diameter is approximately 0.25 mm, and the base is approximately 1.0 mm.
      i. Uses include axial reductions, but not as efficient as larger-diameter diamonds.
      ii. General use is for proximal reductions when there are adjoining teeth.
      iii. Taper is approximately 2 or 3 degrees.
      iv. The tip is a good gauge for approximating the depth of a chamfer finish line for cast metals.
      v. The base is a good gauge for approximating the depth of cusp tip reduction on nonfunctional cusps.
   b. 877-012 coarse/round tip cylinder; the diameter of the cylinder is approximately 1.0 mm. Not recommended for preclinical preparations.
      i. Uses include axial and occlusal reduction (the long axis of the shank must be inclined 2 or 3 degrees in relation to the path of insertion to attain the proper axial wall inclinations.
      ii. One-half the diameter is acceptable for the depth of a chamfer finish line for cast metals. The full diameter is acceptable for a porcelain-bonded-to-metal preparation on the facial surface if a large chamfer is desired for the preparation.
      iii. Its efficiency is probably twice that of the 3000006-060-012 diamond.
2. *Burs*
   a. No. 2 round carbide; depth guide wells and/or grooves (conventional or ultraspeed handpiece)
   b. No. 7801 tapered/round tip (optional); chamfer finish line and adjacent axial wall surface (conventional speed only).

Occlusal Reduction

1. *Depth guide wells* (optional)
   a. Place at center of each of the three major occlusal pits (1, 2, and 3), marginal ridge grooves (4 & 5), and the buccal and lingual developmental grooves at the cuspal ridge emminences (6 & 7).
   b. Use the full diameter of the bur for each well (Fig. 6-21, A and B).
   c. Conventional speed is recommended for ivorine teeth.
2. *Depth guide grooves* (optional), No. 2 round bur.
   a. Join each well centering on and following the major developmental grooves.
   b. The groove vertical contour will rise and fall

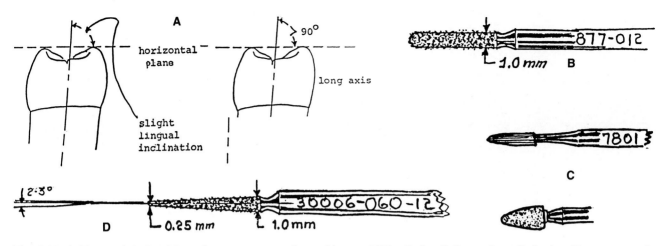

Fig. 6-20. A, The teeth inclined lingually present more of a problem on FPDs. **B,** Small diamond needle for breaking contacts. **C,** Round tipped cylinder for axial surfaces. **D,** Tapered finishing bur (7801) and mounted white stone for smoothing.

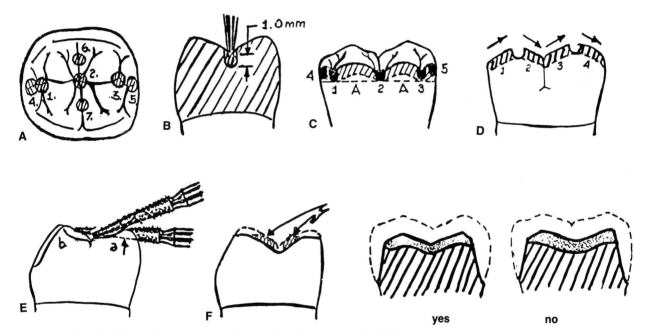

Fig. 6-21. A, Depth guide wells are placed at three major pits, two marginal ridge grooves, and two cuspal ridges. **B,** A No. 2 round bur is used to place depth wells. **C,** The depth guide wells vary with the cuspal contours. **D,** Functional cusp reduction ensures clearance in lateral movements. **E,** Tooth reduction is accomplished at a 45 degree angle to the long axis. **F,** The inner inclines are formed but not completed. **G,** Occlusal topography is not obliterated but preserved.

in conjunction with the rise and fall of cuspal contours <u>not</u> at a constant level mesiodistally (A) (Fig. 6-21 C).

3. Cusp height reduction guides (Fig. 6-21, D and E)

   a. Functional cusp reduction provides clearance in lateral movements. The tooth reduction is accomplished at a 45 degree angle to the long axis of the tooth.

4. *Gross occlusal reduction*

   a. With the diamond stone at a horizontal position, follow the cuspal contours and remove an equal amount of cuspal ridge structure. <u>Do</u> <u>not</u> strive for final occlusal height reduction at this time. Allow for preparation finishing procedures.

   b. Reduce cuspal inner inclines, maintaining rounded cuspal contours (Fig. 6-21, F and G).

   c. A two-plane reduction is performed on the occlusobuccal surface to provide sufficient bulk of metal to accommodate the stamp cusps.

   d. This strategic reduction can be performed after proximal and axial reduction or during

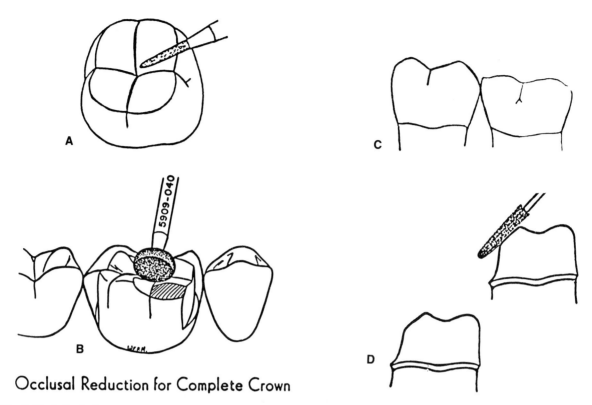

Occlusal Reduction for Complete Crown

Fig. 6-22. A, Preliminary anatomy is established. **B,** Some dentists prefer a "donut" diamond for two-plane reduction. **C,** Approximately 1.5 mm is adequate at this stage. **D,** A two-plane reduction on the buccal stamp cusps for strength.

occlusal reduction. The occlusal reduction is approximately 2 mm, but the reduction may be inadequate for clearance during mandibular movements (Fig. 6-22, A to D).

Buccal and Lingual Reduction

1. *Buccal surface*. The buccal surface reduction can be accomplished with a coarse, round-ended, high-speed diamond, i.e., 770-8p. The reduction is performed parallel to the long axis of the tooth and extended gingivally to the gingival crest with as much mesial and distal extension as possible. Although inadvertent contact with adjacent teeth is strongly discouraged, the convexity of the proximal teeth must be stressed. An open embrasure for cleansing is fundamental (Fig. 6-23, A and B).
2. *Lingual surface*. The lingual surface does not require extensive reduction in the cervical area because of the lingual inclination of the tooth. More tooth structure is removed from the occlusal third than from the gingival extension, which is directed to the gingival crest with the No. 770-8p.
3. *Proximal reduction*
   a. Protect the proximal surface of the adjacent

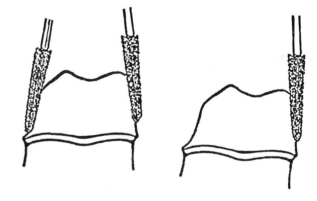

Fig. 6-23. A, The buccal surface reduction is accomplished with a coarse rounded diamond. The buccal and lingual reduction is performed prior to breaking the proximal contacts. **B,** The lingual surface requires minimal reduction due to its inclination (See Fig. 6-20).

tooth with matrix material (Tofflemire or T-Band) (Fig. 6-24 A).
   b. If the facial and lingual surfaces are prepared before the proximal surfaces, the contact can be broken more easily. A thin "needle" diamond is commonly used. The contact areas of the adjacent teeth should be evaluated for extreme convexity (Fig. 6-24 B).

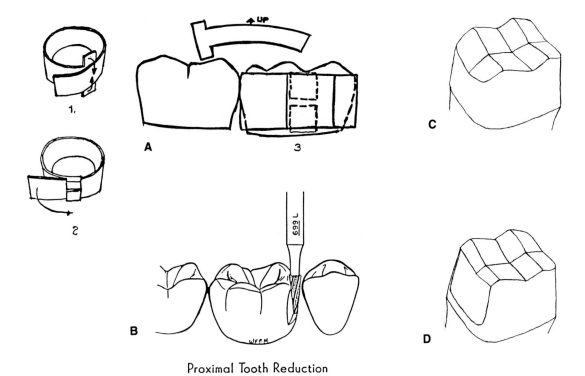

Proximal Tooth Reduction

Fig. 6-24. A, Proximal reduction after facial and lingual preparation does not require protection. **B,** Fissure burs are indicated for teeth reconstructed with amalgam. **C,** Occlusal clearance proceeds proximal or facial reduction. **D,** When the tooth is an abutment for an FPD, the proximal reduction is completed after occlusal clearance to ensure parallelism. A long, medium-coarse diamond is used to address the surfaces *first* that would deviate from the path of insertion.

c. When a tooth is malposed or extensively restored, a fissure 699L is the recommended bur.

d. On proximal surfaces, after the occlusal, buccal, and lingual surfaces are prepared, the mesial and distal surfaces are more accessible with a long, thin taper diamond and a thin carbide bur. The distal surfaces are notoriously difficult to prepare because of prolonged vertical opening by the patient to accommodate the high-speed handpiece with diamond. Lack of visibility tests the perseverance of the most skilled, experienced dentists. This delicate procedure is completed with a cuttle disc (Fig. 6-24, C and D).

e. When the tooth is designated as an abutment for an FPD, the proximal surface that would deviate from the path of insertion is prepared first; i.e., the distal surface of the distal abutment and the mesial surface of the proximal abutment. Over-reduction is common when the more accessible surfaces are prepared before the arduous areas; i.e., mesial surface of the distal abutment and the distal surface of the proximal abutment.

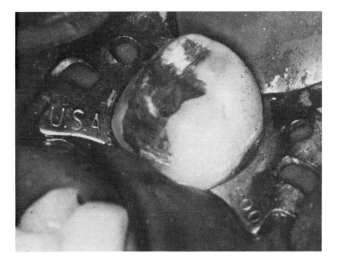

Fig. 6-24. E, The distal surface of the distal abutment is always difficult because of arch position, particularly with a three quarter crown as an anterior abutment.

Axial Refinement

The axial lines are blended to complete the gross reduction and develop smooth surfaces. The mesio-buccal angle has easy access and is commonly overre-

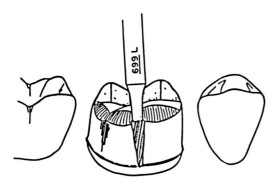

Preparation of Buccal Flute and Gingival Termination

Fig. 6-25. A, A No. 699L is used to create initial flute of molar.

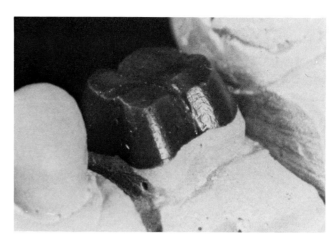

Fig. 6-25. B, Mandibular first molar with exaggerated two-plane reduction and normal flute.

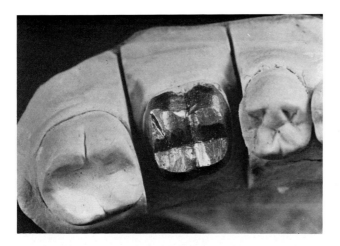

Fig. 6-25. C, Mounted casts of preparation for complete crowns with die spacers. Note the occlusal topography, fluted facial surface and functional two-plane reduction.

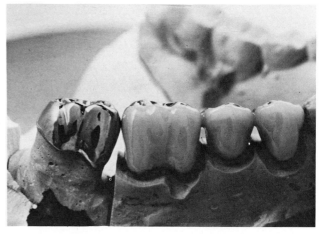

Fig. 6-25. D, Fluted buccal surfaces in porcelain and metal. Open communication with the laboratory is necessary or the flute is routinely obliterated.

duced, while the distolingual is underprepared due to poor visibility and obstruction by the tongue and cheek (Fig. 6-25).

Patient fatigue also accounts for considerable difficulty in developing a smooth surface in the later stages of the tooth preparation. The buccal surface is fluted, so the facial surface is not overcontoured and is continuous with the root surface. A smooth "flat not fat" surface is desired, but the tooth preparation dictates final form. The flute also aids cementation but does <u>not</u> contribute appreciably to retention.

Finish

The functional bevel and the axiocclusal angles are refined to finish the preparation (Fig. 6-26, A and B).

1. A chamfer is the common gingival finish line when the gingiva is at a normal level, accessible, and does not hamper cleansing. However, a chamfer prepared on the same tooth with the gingiva more apically can endanger the pulp and violate the biologic width, so a knife-edge finish may be more appropriate. Gingival margins should be characterized by continuity, uniformity, and definition. With clinical experience, each dentist can decide the most beneficial approach for the patient's specific needs (Fig. 6-26, C and D).

2. The fundamental factors of margin development are definition, uniformity, and continuity. These three desirable characteristics of tooth preparation are used to describe the measures necessary to create geometric forms that allow greater compression of cement with compromised teeth (Fig. 6-26 B).

3. After prudent tooth removal, the hasty formulation of a wax pattern can jeopardize the health

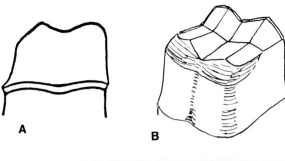

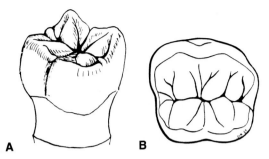

Fig. 6-27. A, Wax form of a mandibular second molar. **B,** Occlusal morphology of a mandibular first molar.

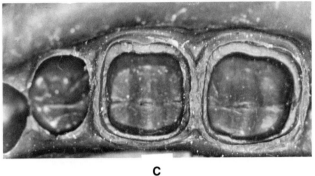

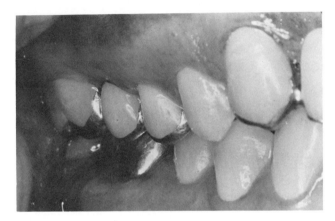

Fig. 6-27. C, Mandibular first molar inserted opposing a three-unit FPD. The reduced space necessitated complete metal coverage heavy boxes and provisional cementation with frosted occlusal surfaces for a determined period.

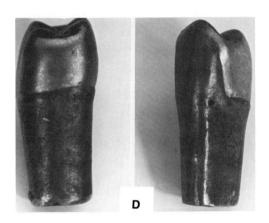

Fig. 6-26. A, Proximal view of mandibular molar with a bevel on the facial and lingual and a knife edge on the proximal surfaces. **B,** Finish preparation emphasizing the geometric configurations. **C,** Polyether impression of full shoulder finish lines for complete crowns. This gingiva configuration is becoming more popular with expanded usage of metal/ceramic and injectible porcelain crowns. **D,** Clinically acceptable crowns. (From Bruhl, C.E., and Reesbick, M.H.: J.A.D.A. **105:**1002, 1982).

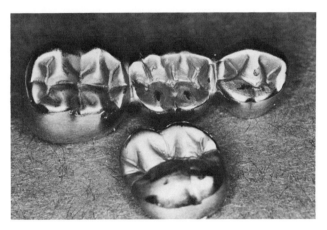

Fig. 6-27. D, Frosted (sand blasted) occlusal surfaces after interim placement to identify occlusal disharmony.

of the gingival tissue with overcontouring or encourage microleakage without focusing on the gingival finish. Complete gold veneer crowns remain the standard bearer of conventional fixed prosthodontics, despite metal display. The complete crown is well suited for a patient with a reduced interocclusal space (Fig. 6-27, A to D).

4. Finishing of restorations is necessary to avoid debris and plaque accumulation that would sponsor gingival inflammation and recurrent caries. Consideration should be given to the fact that the process is initiated at the wax pattern stage.

Pits and voids in wax mean a prolonged and sometimes impossible task at the finishing stage of fabrication. The dentist must understand the difference between finishing and polishing. Finishing is a step by step procedure using abrasive agents from a coarse to fine texture that are slightly finer than the roughness of the surface to be finished. When the surface is reduced to the finer stage, the process is continued with polishing abrasives until the surface is free of scratches and has a smooth surface.

5. If the tooth preparation required an inordinate amount of time, the smoothing of the tooth surface should be postponed and a suitable treatment restoration placed. Hasty fabrication of the interim coverage jeopardizes predictable results, while prolonged opening by the patient sponsors discomfort. Studies are now being conducted to determine the untoward results of repeated long appointments.

Table 6-1. CGVC retainer preparation for mandibular second molar.

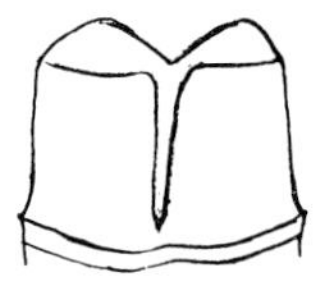

FACIAL

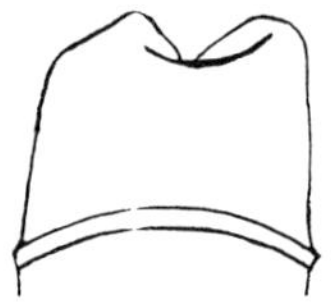

DISTAL

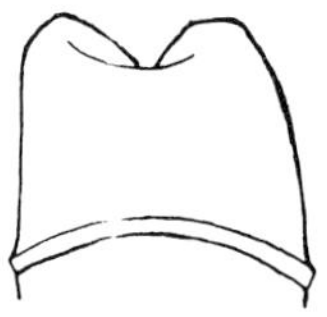

MESIAL

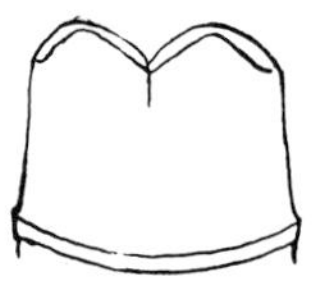

LINGUAL

Occlusal
Reduction _____

Proximal
Reduction _____

Facial
Reduction _____

Lingual
Reduction _____

Lingual
Reduction _____

Surface
Finish _____

Finish
Margin _____

Preparation
Characteristics _____

Courtesy Dr. J.R. Schmidt, Fixed Prosthodontics Manual, 1979, Southern Illinois University School of Dental Medicine

Table 6-2. Evaluation form for cast CGVC on mandibular second molar

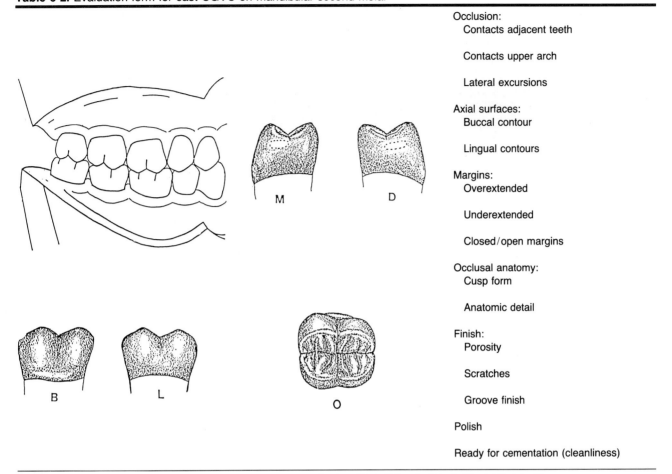

Occlusion:
  Contacts adjacent teeth

  Contacts upper arch

  Lateral excursions

Axial surfaces:
  Buccal contour

  Lingual contours

Margins:
  Overextended

  Underextended

  Closed/open margins

Occlusal anatomy:
  Cusp form

  Anatomic detail

Finish:
  Porosity

  Scratches

  Groove finish

Polish

Ready for cementation (cleanliness)

Courtesy Dr. D. J. Maroso, Operative Dentistry Laboratory Manual, 1987, Southern Illinois University School of Dental Medicine.[18]

SECTION C

Partial Veneer Crowns

Karen B. Troendle and G. Roger Troendle

A partial veneer crown is a restoration covering two or more surfaces of a tooth. The surfaces usually covered are the lingual, proximal, occlusal, or incisal. The rationale for preserving part of the tooth is to enhance the esthetics of the restoration and to conserve tooth structure (see flow sheet No. 1). There are three types of partial veneer crowns: three-quarter crown, seven-eighth crown, and mesial half crown. Other types of partial veneer crowns are considered variations of the three fundamental types.

The three-quarter crown covers three fourths of the gingival circumference of the tooth, leaving one surface intact (Fig. 6-28). The facial surface commonly remains untouched. To conserve tooth structure, however, the lingual surface of a mandibular posterior tooth is occasionally preserved and is referred to as a reverse three-quarter crown. Reverse three-quarter crowns are indicated on mandibular molars with severe lingual inclination used as FPD abutments.

Because they are esthetically pleasing, three-quarter crowns can be used in the anterior or posterior and can serve as a single unit or as an FPD retainer.

The seven-eighths partial veneer crown encompasses seven eighths of the gingival circumference of the tooth. It is generally indicated for maxillary molars and premolars that are sound mesially but have extensive carious involvement or a previous restoration on the distal surface. Occasionally, a seven-eighths veneer crown is used on a mandibular premolar that is to serve as an abutment for an FPD. The seven-eighths crown preparation extends the distal finish line to the midfacial surface, avoiding an unnecessary display of metal on the mesial surface (Fig. 6-29).

The mesial half crown is actually a three-quarter crown rotated 90 degrees, preserving the distal surface of the tooth while veneering the remaining surfaces. This preparation design is primarily indicated for the distal retainer of a mandibular FPD with tilted molar abutment (Fig. 6-30). The restoration is also used as a single retainer where there has been drifting and tipping of a mandibular molar. Mesial half crowns are contraindicated if there are blemishes on the distal surface of the tooth.

Variations of the three fundamental types of partial veneer crown preparations have been described in the literature. These modifications are often used to further enhance esthetics and minimize metal display.

Indications

Partial veneer crowns are a conservative measure and are preferable to the complete veneer restoration. Indications include:
1. Intact or minimally restored teeth.
2. Teeth with crown length that is average or that exceeds the average.
3. Teeth with normal anatomic crown form, i.e., without excessive cervical constriction.
4. Anterior teeth with adequate labiolingual thickness.

Contraindications

The contraindications for partial veneers are:
1. High caries rate. Cast restorations in general are not indicated with a high caries rate. This consideration is critical with a partial veneer restoration where both the unveneered surface and the increased margin to finish line interface are susceptible to decay.
2. Teeth with extensive core restorations. Before a partial veneer restoration can be placed, the unveneered tooth surface must be sound. When the intact tooth surface is undermined, or if a core restoration extends onto the surface, a complete veneer crown is indicated.
3. Deep cervical abrasion. If the unveneered surface has deep cervical abrasion, it is difficult to establish a finish line. If the abraded area is sensitive, it is preferable to cover that surface with a complete veneer crown.
4. Short teeth. Teeth with short clinical crowns are usually not suitable for partial veneer crowns. The difficulty is in establishing adequate retention and resistance form. Also, the esthetics of a partial veneer crown are compromised on a short tooth. Complete veneer restorations are more suitable for teeth with short clinical crowns.
5. Bell-shaped teeth. Teeth severely constricted at the cervical require more axial reduction to provide adequate groove length. The additional

Flow Sheet 1

DIAGNOSIS AND TREATMENT PLANNING
FOR PARTIAL VENEER CROWNS

Oral hygiene and periodontal
support adequate?   No ◆   Casting contraindicated
                    Yes
                     ◆

More conservative treatment is   Yes ◆   Casting contraindicated
possible?   No
                                            ◆

| Complete veneer crown vs Partial veneer crown |

Consider complete veneer crown   Consider partial veneer crown

Tooth length average too long?
◆ No   Yes
         ◆

Large amounts of sound tooth
structure remain?
◆ No   Yes
         ◆

Patient has low DMF rate?
◆ No   Yes
         ◆

Retainer is for single unit or
small to medium span FFD?
◆ No   Yes
         ◆

Tooth alignment normal?
No   Yes ◆
 ◆

Can malalignment be overcome
with a modified partial veneer
crown preparation?
◆ No   Yes ◆

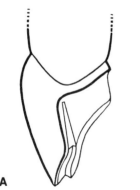 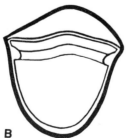

Fig. 6-28. A, A proximal view of a three-quarter crown preparation on a maxillary cuspid. **B,** Incisal view.

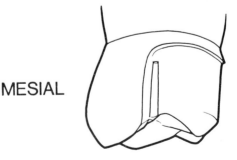

Fig. 6-29. A seven-eighths crown preparation on a maxillary molar.

depth required to place proximal grooves or boxes can jeopardize pulpal health.

6. Thin teeth. It is difficult to prepare grooves of suitable length in teeth with insufficient buccolingual width without undermining the facial enamel.

Advantages

Partial veneer crowns have several advantages over complete crowns:

1. The tooth reduction is conservative.
2. The esthetics surpass the complete veneer cast crown and the three-quarter crown can be used on anterior teeth.
3. Having fewer margins in the intracrevicular space increases biocompatability with supportive tissues.
4. Margin accessibility for finishing and cleaning is improved.
5. Complete seating of the casting is more easily verified with at least one margin visible.
6. Complete seating of the casting during cementation is enhanced by diminished hydraulic pressure.
7. Electric pulp testing can be conveniently accomplished on the intact enamel surface.

Disadvantages

Partial veneer crowns have the following disadvantages:

1. The partial veneer crown is <u>not</u> as retentive as a complete veneer crown.
2. There is a limited display of metal with the partial veneer crown.

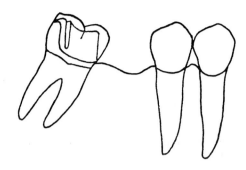

Fig. 6-30. A mesial half crown preparation on a tilted mandibular molar.

3. Skillful preparation is critical to avoid metal display.
4. The partial veneer crown preparation is limited to fairly intact teeth with normally shaped, average length clinical crowns.

Preparation

The seven steps for preparation of partial veneer crowns are:

1. Occlusal or incisal reduction
2. Lingual reduction
3. Interproximal reduction
4. Proximal box or groove placement
5. Occlusal or incisal offset placement
6. Facial bevel
7. Finishing the preparation

The technique for each step may vary, depending upon whether the tooth is in the maxillary or mandibular arch, or anterior or posterior.

ANTERIOR MAXILLARY PARTIAL VENEER CROWNS

The following subsection describes a three-quarter crown preparation on a maxillary cuspid.

Technique: Maxillary Cuspid

Three-quarter crown preparation:

1. *Incisal reduction.* Using a tapered, round-ended diamond, reduce the incisal edge 1 mm at a 45 degree angle to the long axis of the tooth. Follow the facial contour of the tooth, uniformly removing 1.0 to 1.5 mm (Fig. 6-31).

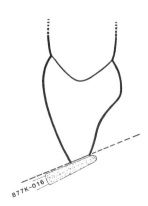

Fig. 6-31. Incisal reduction: 877K-106 diamond.

2. *Lingual reduction*. The lingual surface reduction is accomplished in two steps.
   a. Lingual surface reduction. Using a football-shaped diamond, reduce the lingual surface in two planes, leaving a slight ridge running incisogingivally along the center of the lingual surface. Clearance with the opposing tooth is at least 0.7 mm to 1 mm (Fig. 6-32). (Caution: Do <u>not</u> overreduce the height of the cingulum shortening the lingual gingival wall.)

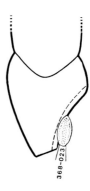

Fig. 6-32. Lingual surface reduction: 368-023 diamond.

   b. Lingual gingival reduction. Using a tapered, round-ended diamond, make a chamfer 0.5 mm deep at the cervical finish line. The reduction parallels the long axis of the preparation. On anterior teeth, this is usually the incisal two thirds of the labial surface. Extend the chamfer to include the lingual line angles (Fig. 6-33).

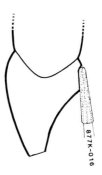

Fig. 6-33. Lingual gingival reduction: 877K-016 diamond.

3. *Interproximal reduction* involves three steps.
   a. Using a 169L carbide bur, reduce the proximal surface by moving the bur from the lingual to the facial surface. Position the bur so that the tip of the bur is farther facial than the shank. Do <u>not</u> break contact with the adjacent teeth at this time (Fig. 6-34). The facial line angles must remain intact to produce esthetically acceptable results.

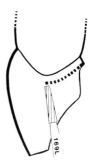

Fig. 6-34. Interproximal reduction: 169L bur.

   b. Using a narrow chamfer diamond, establish a light chamfer finish line on the proximal surface, blending it with the lingual chamfer.
   c. Using a hatchet instrument from the facial surface, the contact with the adjacent teeth is broken to establish the labial proximal extensions. A flame-shaped diamond is used to finish the flare (Fig. 6-35).

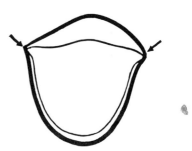

Fig. 6-35. Contact broken with adjacent teeth from the facial with hand instrument.

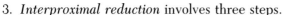

4. *Proximal grooves.* The grooves are initiated with a 167 carbide bur to determine if alignment is appropriate. Using a 169L carbide bur, place the proximal grooves parallel to the incisal two thirds of the facial surface. The groove can be expanded with a 701 bur if sufficient tooth structure is present. The lingual wall of the proximal grooves has a 2- to 5-degree incisal convergence with the lingual gingival wall of the preparation (Fig. 6-36). The grooves are designed to create a definite lingual wall that resists lingual displacement (Fig. 6-37). The facial wall of the groove should be continuous with the proximal flare to contribute bulk to the facial margin. The grooves are a minimum of 3 mm long and terminate within 0.5 mm of the gingival finish line. The facial and lingual walls of the grooves have a 2 to 5 degree incisal divergence.

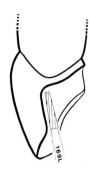

Fig. 6-36. Proximal groove placement: 169L bur.

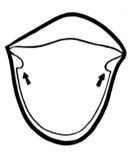

Fig. 6-37. Grooves have a definite lingual wall.

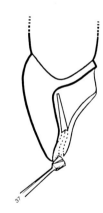

Fig. 6-38. Incisal groove: 37 inverted cone.

5. *Incisal groove.* Using a 37 inverted cone carbide bur, develop a 0.5 to 1 mm groove connecting the proximal grooves (Fig. 6-38). The groove should be in dentin and parallel to the DEJ. The groove is not placed at the expense of the incisal edge (Fig. 6-39).

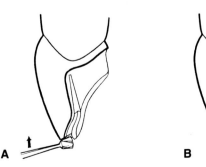

Fig. 6-39. A, Incorrect placement of inverted cone. **B,** Incisal groove placed at expense of incisal edge.

6. *Facial bevel.* Using a fine, flame-shaped diamond bur, develop a narrow bevel <0.5 mm on the labioincisal finish line at right angles to the incisal two thirds of the facial surface (Fig. 6-40).

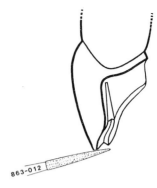

Fig. 6-40. Facial bevel: 863-012 diamond.

7. *Finishing the preparation.* Using a carbide finishing bur, round the line angles to ensure continuity of all finish lines (Fig. 6-41).

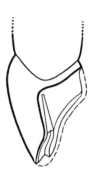

Fig. 6-41. Finish of preparation: carbide finishing bur.

8. *Cingulum modification.* This variation is used for additional retention:
   a. Parallel a 170 bur to the long axis on the proximal grooves and prepare a ledge into the cingulum (Fig. 6-42).

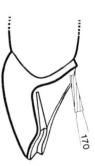

Fig. 6-42. Ledge for cingulum modification: 170 carbide bur.

   b. Cut a pilot hole in the ledge with a No. 1/2 round bur (Fig. 6-43).

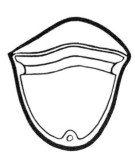

Fig. 6-43. Pilot hole: No. ½ round bur.

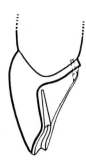

c. Prepare a pinhole 1.5 to 2 mm deep with a No. 027 twist drill (Fig. 6-44). The drill must parallel the path of insertion.

Fig. 6-44. Pinhole prepared 1.5 mm to 2.0 mm deep with a No. .027 twist drill.

POSTERIOR PARTIAL VENEER CROWNS

Posterior partial veneer crowns differ from anterior partial veneers because the path of insertion is usually parallel with the long axis of the tooth. In addition, mandibular partial veneers are prepared differently because the buccal cusp is the stamp/working cusp. The steps in preparation are described for a three-quarter crown on a maxillary premolar and mandibular premolar, and for a seven-eighth crown on a maxillary molar.

Technique: Maxillary Premolar

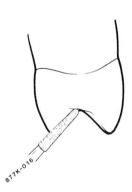

Three-quarter crown preparation on a maxillary premolar.
1. *Occlusal reduction* has two steps.
   a. Using a tapered, round-ended diamond, reduce the inner and outer inclines of the lingual cusp to obtain 1.5 to 2 mm clearance for the range of mandibular motion (Fig. 6-45).

Fig. 6-45. Reduce lingual cusp 1.5 mm to 2.0 mm using 877K-016 diamond.

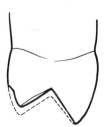

b. Using the same bur, reduce the inner incline of the buccal cusp to obtain 1.5 mm occlusal clearance at the depth of the central groove and 1 mm of clearance at the cusp tip (Fig. 6-46).

Fig. 6-46. Reduce buccal cusp 1 mm at tip 1.5 mm in central groove using 877K-016 diamond.

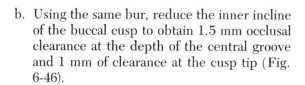

2. *Lingual reduction*. Using the same bur, reduce the lingual surface to create a 0.5 mm chamfer at the cervical finish line. Carry the chamfer into the line angles (Fig. 6-47).

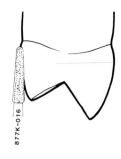

Fig. 6-47. Lingual reduction: 877K-106 diamond.

3. *Interproximal reduction* involves three steps.
   a. Using a 169L carbide bur, reduce the proximal surface by moving the bur from the lingual to the facial surface. Do not break contact with the facial surface of the adjacent tooth at this time (Fig. 6-48).

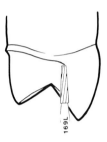

Fig. 6-48. Proximal reduction: 169L carbide bur.

   b. Using a narrow-diameter, round-edged diamond, establish a light chamfer finish line on the interproximal surface (Fig. 6-49).

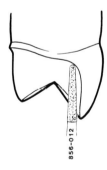

Fig. 6-49. Proximal chamfer: 856-012 diamond.

   c. Using a hatchet instrument from a facial direction, break contact with the adjacent teeth (Fig. 6-50). Use a narrow, round-ended carbide bur to finish the flare.

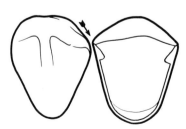

Fig. 6-50. Proximal contact broken with adjacent teeth from the facial using a hand instrument.

4. *Proximal box.* Using a 169L carbide bur, place the proximal groove approximately 0.5 mm from the facial and gingival finish lines (Fig. 6-51). They should be a minimum of 3 mm long, and the axial walls of each groove should converge toward the occlusal surface. (Alternate method: A box may be used instead of a groove on the proximal surface if decay or an existing restoration makes it necessary. Refer to three-quarter partial veneer crown preparation for a mandibular premolar.)

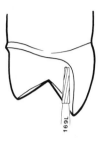

Fig. 6-51. Proximal groove: 169L carbide bur.

5. *Occlusal groove.* Using a 37 inverted cone carbide bur, join the proximal grooves by placing a groove on the inner incline of the facial cusp (Fig. 6-52). The groove is 0.5 to 1 mm deep and connects the proximal grooves. The groove should parallel the DEJ and be based in dentin. Do not place the groove at the expense of the facial cusp tip.

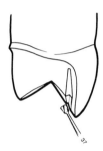

Fig. 6-52. Occlusal groove: 37 inverted cone.

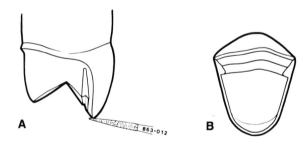

6. *Facial bevel.* Using a fine flame-shaped diamond, place a narrow bevel (<0.5 mm) on the labioocclusal finish line at a right angle to the path of insertion (Fig. 6-53).

Fig. 6-53. A, Facial bevel: 863-012 diamond. **B,** The facial bevel joins the proximal finish lines.

7. *Finishing the preparation.* Using a carbide finishing bur, round the line angles to ensure continuity of all finish lines (Fig. 6-54).

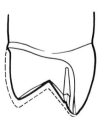

Fig. 6-54. Finish of preparation: carbide finishing bur.

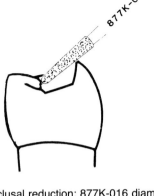

Fig. 6-55. Occlusal reduction: 877K-016 diamond.

Technique: Mandibular Premolar

Three-quarter crown preparation:
1. *Occlusal reduction* involves three steps.
   a. Using a tapered, round-ended diamond, reduce the occlusal surface to obtain 1.5 to 2 mm occlusal clearance. Maintain the basic anatomy of the tooth (Fig. 6-55).

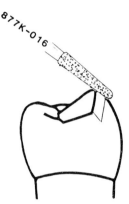

Fig. 6-56. Facial reduction 1 mm gingival to functional occlusal contacts: 877K-016 diamond.

   b. Using the same bur, reduce the outer incline of the functional cusp 1.0 mm gingival to functional occlusal contact with the opposing tooth (Fig. 6-56).

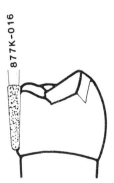

Fig. 6-57. Lingual reduction: 877K-106 diamond.

2. *Lingual reduction*. Using the same bur, reduce the lingual surface, creating a 0.5 mm chamfer at the cervical finish line. Extend the chamfer into the line angles (Fig. 6-57).

3. *Proximal surface reduction*. Using the 169L carbide bur, reduce the proximal surface by moving the bur from the lingual surface to the facial surface. Contact may be broken with the facial surface of the adjacent tooth at this time (Fig. 6-58). Using a narrow, round-end diamond, establish a light chamfer finish line on the interproximal surface.

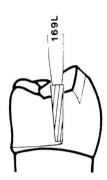

Fig. 6-58. Proximal reduction: 169L carbide bur.

4. *Proximal boxes*. Using a 169L carbide bur, place the proximal boxes facial to the central groove. The boxes are approximately 0.5 mm from the facial and gingival finish lines. The walls of the boxes are a minimum of 3 mm long, and the axial walls of the boxes should converge. However, the facial and lingual walls of each box diverge (Fig. 6-59).

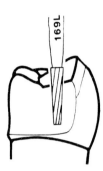

Fig. 6-59. Proximal boxes: 169L carbide bur.

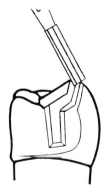

5. *Facial shoulder*. Using a 56 carbide bur, place the facial shoulder 0.5 mm occlusal to the facial finish line created during functional cusp reduction. The facial shoulder joins each of the proximal boxes (Fig. 6-60).

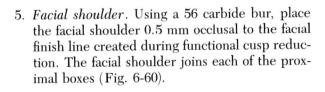

Fig. 6-60. Facial shoulder: 56 carbide bur.

6. *Reverse bevel.* Using a fine, flame-shaped diamond, refine the reverse bevel on the facial shoulder. It smoothly joins each of the proximal finish lines (Fig. 6-61).

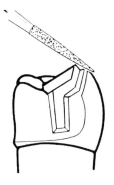

Fig. 6-61. Reverse facial bevel: 863-012 diamond.

7. *Finishing the preparation.* Using a round-ended, tapered carbide finishing bur, round all line angles to ensure the continuity of all finish lines (Fig. 6-62).

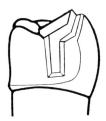

Fig. 6-62. Finish of preparation: carbide finishing bur.

Technique: Maxillary Molar

Seven-eights crown preparation:
1. *Occlusal reduction* has two steps.
   a. Using a round-ended, tapered diamond, reduce the inner incline of the mesial buccal cusp to obtain 1.5 mm occlusal clearance at the depth of the central groove and 1 mm at the cusp tip (Fig. 6-63).

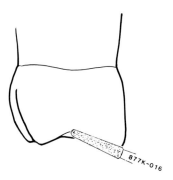

Fig. 6-63. Reduce buccal cusp 1.0 mm at tip and 1.5 mm at central groove: 877K-016 diamond.

   b. Reduce the remaining cusps to obtain 2 mm occlusal clearance (Fig. 6-64).

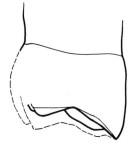

Fig. 6-64. Reduce lingual cusp 2.0 mm: 877K-016 diamond.

2. *Lingual reduction.* Using the same bur, reduce the lingual surface to develop a chamfer 0.5 mm in depth at the cervical finish line. Extend the chamfer into the line angles (Fig. 6-65).

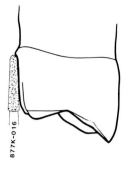

Fig. 6-65. Lingual reduction: 877-016 diamond.

3. *Proximal reduction* involves three steps.
   a. Using a 169L carbide bur, reduce the proximal surface by moving the bur from the lingual to the facial surface (Fig. 6-66).

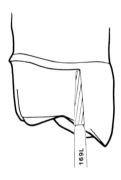

Fig. 6-66. Proximal reduction: 169L carbide bur.

   b. Using a narrow-diameter, round-ended tapered diamond, establish a light chamfer finish line on the mesial and distal interproximal surfaces (Fig. 6-67).
   c. Using a hatchet instrument from a facial direction, break the mesial proximal contact. Use a narrow tapered carbide bur to finish the flare.

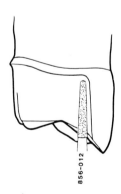

Fig. 6-67. Proximal chamfer: 856-012 diamond.

4. *Distofacial reduction.* Using a round-ended, tapered diamond, begin preparation of the facial surface at the facial groove and extend the preparation distally around the distofacial line angle, joining with the chamfer on the distal. Establish a 0.5 mm chamfer at the cervical finish line (Fig. 6-68).

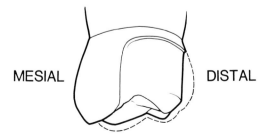

Fig. 6-68. Disto-facial reduction: 877K-106 diamond.

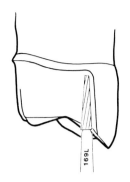

Fig. 6-69. Mesial box: 169L carbide bur.

5. *Mesial box*. Using a 169L carbide bur, place the mesial box facial to the central groove (Fig. 6-69). The box should be approximately 0.5 mm from the gingival and facial finish lines. The box is a minimum of 3 mm long, and the axial wall converges toward the occlusal surface (Fig. 6-70).

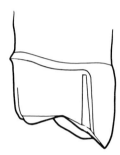

Fig. 6-70. The mesial box is 0.5 mm from the gingival and facial finish lines.

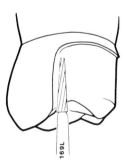

Fig. 6-71. Facial groove: 169L carbide bur.

6. *Facial groove*. Using a 169L bur, place a groove to the depth of the bur in the area of the midfacial groove. The groove is approximately 0.5 mm from the cervical finish line and the distofacial finish line. The groove is a minimum of 3 mm long, and the axial wall converges toward the occlusal surface. The mesial and distal walls of facial groove diverge toward the occlusal surface (Fig. 6-71 and 72).

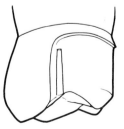

Fig. 6-72. The axial wall of the facial groove converges occlusally. The mesial and distal walls of the facial groove diverge occlusally.

7. *Occlusal groove*. Using a 37 inverted cone carbide bur, join the mesial box to the facial groove on the inner incline of the mesial facial cusp (Fig. 6-73).

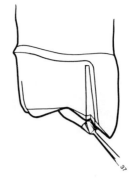

Fig. 6-73. Occlusal groove: 37 inverted cone.

8. *Facial bevel*. Using a fine flame-shaped diamond, place a narrow bevel (<0.5 mm) on the mesial facial cusp at approximately right angles to the path of insertion (Fig. 6-74 and 6-75).

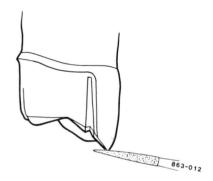

Fig. 6-74. Facial bevel: 863-012 diamond.

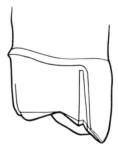

Fig. 6-75. The facial bevel joins the proximal and midfacial finish line.

9. *Finishing the preparation*. Using a tapered, round-ended carbide finishing bur, round the line angles to ensure the continuity of all finish lines (Fig. 6-76).

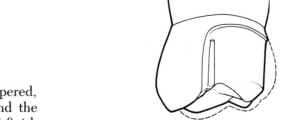

Fig. 6-76. Finish of the preparation: carbide finishing bur.

COMMON ERRORS

To achieve a satisfactory partial veneer crown restoration, it is important for the dentist to concentrate on detail and anticipate potential problems during each step of the preparation. The most common errors made in preparing a partial veneer crown are:

1. *Occlusal incisal reduction.*
   a. Insufficient reduction of the occluding surfaces resulting in a cast restoration that is less rigid and flexes under occlusal forces. In addition, inadequate occlusal clearance can lead to a perforation in the casting or to an overcontoured restoration with poor occlusion.
   b. Excessive reduction of the occlusal or incisal edge leads to an unnecessary display of metal, while decreasing retention and resistance form.

2. *Path of insertion.* The path of insertion for anterior partial veneer crowns is parallel to the incisal two thirds of the labial surface of the tooth rather than the long axis of the tooth. This maintains the esthetics of the labial surface while using maximum axial wall and groove length. Conversely, the path of insertion for posterior teeth usually parallels the long axis of the tooth to accommodate the parallelism of abutment teeth.

3. *Proximal reduction*
   a. Proximal extensions are approached from the lingual surface with small-diameter diamonds and with hand instruments to minimize facial display of metal.
   b. Proximal axial walls converge toward the lingual surface after proximal reduction to maintain labial surfaces intact (Fig. 6-77).
   c. The facial-lingual, as well as the mesodistal inclination of the path of insertion must be a constant reference during proximal reduction. This precaution will avoid excessive metal display and/or prevent suspension of the casting from seating due to adjacent tooth contours.

4. *Groove placement*
   a. Proximal grooves placed on anterior teeth are parallel to the incisal two thirds of the labial surface of the tooth rather than the long axis of the tooth. This allows grooves that are inclined lingually at the incisal surface, leaving the labioincisal corner intact (Fig. 6-78). Paralleling the grooves with the long axis of the tooth sacrifices the labioincisal corner and seriously compromises esthetics.
   b. Grooves or boxes are at least 3 mm in length.
   c. The base of the prepared groove or box is 0.5

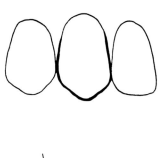

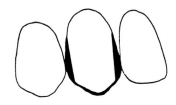
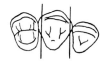

Fig. 6-77. A, Proximal walls converge toward the lingual to maintain the labial surface intact. **B,** Proximal walls without convergence toward the lingual produce excessive metal display.

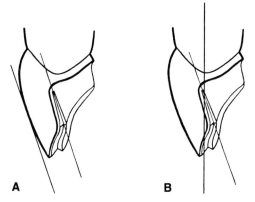

Fig. 6-78. A, Proximal grooves on anterior teeth parallel the incisal two-thirds of the labial surface. **B,** Proximal grooves on anterior teeth paralleling the long axis of the tooth sacrifices the labial-incisal corner.

mm coronal to the preparation finish line (Fig. 6-79).

    d. The grooves or boxes must draw with the rest of the preparation.

    e. Grooves must have a definite lingual wall to resist displacement (Fig. 6-80).

    f. Grooves must be placed facially enough to provide a bulk of metal to support the facial margin and yet not undermine the facial enamel. (Fig. 6-81).

4. *Incisal offset*

    a. The incisal offset is continuous with the proximal grooves or boxes to provide for maximum structural reinforcement of the facial veneering margin (Fig. 6-82).

    b. The incisal offset is placed without sacrificing or undermining the facial cusp of maxillary teeth (Fig. 6-83).

    c. The incisal offset may be unnecessary in certain circumstances on mandibular teeth where a facial step has been prepared for adequate occlusal clearance.

5. *Incisal or occlusal bevel*

    a. The narrow finishing bevel of approximately 0.5 mm placed on the labioincisal or labioocclusal surface of maxillary teeth is placed at right angles to the path of insertion to ensure esthetics. A slightly wider contrabevel can be placed on surfaces less critical to esthetics.

    b. On mandibular teeth where the facial cusp is the functional cusp, the occlusal bevel <u>does not</u> terminate where the maxillary tooth contacts during centric closure or eccentric movement.

Three-quarter crowns are enjoying a resurgence of popularity due to caries reduction, periodontal awareness, and improved pedogogic techniques. We genuinely hope this discussion will encourage the increased use of this conservative restoration.

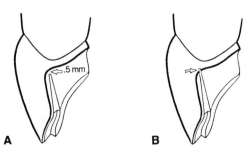

Fig. 6-79. A, The base of the prepared groove or box is 0.5 mm coronal to the finish line. **B,** The base of an incorrectly prepared groove extending below the finish line.

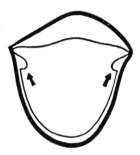

Fig. 6-80. Grooves with definite lingual walls resist displacement.

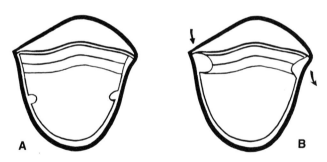

Fig. 6-81. A, Grooves incorrectly placed too far lingually to support facial margin. **B,** Grooves incorrectly placed. Left groove undermines facial enamel. Right groove has no definite lingual wall.

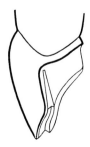

Fig. 6-82. Incisal offset is continuous with proximal grooves or boxes.

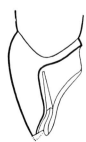

Fig. 6-83. Incisal offset incorrectly placed at expense of facial cusp.

BIBLIOGRAPHY

Beaudreau, D.E.: Atlas of fixed partial prosthesis, Springfield, IL, Charles C. Thomas, Published 1975, Chapter 4.

Cowger, G.T.: Retention, resistance, and esthetics of the anterior three-quarter crown, J.A.D.A. **62**:167, 1961.

Douglass, G.D.: Principles of preparation design in fixed prosthodontics, J. Acad. Gen. Dent. **21**:25, 1973.

Dykema, R.W., Goodacre, R.J., and Phillips, R.W.: Johnston's Modern practice in fixed prosthodontics, Philadelphia, 1986, W.B. Saunders Co.

Galun, E.A., Goodacre, C.J., Dykema, R.W., Moore, K.B. and Sowinski, L.L.: The contribution of a pinhole to the retention and resistance form of veneer crowns, J. Prosthet Dent. **56**:292, 1986.

Guyer, S.E.: Multiple preparations for fixed prosthodontics, J. Prosthet. Dent. **23**:529, 1970.

Ingraham, R., Bassett, R.W., and Koser, J.R.: An atlas of cast gold procedures, Buena Park, CA, 1969, Uni-Tro College Press.

Johnston, J.F., Phillips, R.W., and Dykema, R.W.: Modern practice in crown and bridge prosthodontics, Philadelphia, W.B. Saunders Co., 1971.

Kaufman, E.G., Coelho, D.H., and Colin, L.: Factors influencing the retention of cemented gold castings, J. Prosthet. Dent. **11**:487, 1961.

Kishimoto, M., Shillingburg, H.T., Jr., and Duncanson, M.G., Jr.: Influence of preparation features on retention and resistance. Part II: three-quarter crowns, J. Prosthet. Dent. **49**:188, 1983.

Kopp, E.N.: Partial veneer retainers, J. Prosthet. Dent. **23**:412, 1972.

Lorey, R.E., and Myers, G.E.: The retentive qualities of bridge retainers, J.A.D.A. **76**:568, 1968.

Peterka, C.: A modern three-quarter veneer crown, J.A.D.A. **27**:1175, 1940.

Potts, R.G. Shillingburg, H.T., and Duncanson, M.G., Jr.: Retention and resistance of preparations for cast restorations, J. Prosthet. Dent. **43**:303, 1980.

Shillingburg, H.T., and Fisher, D.W.: A partial veneer restoration, Austral. Dent. J. **17**:411, 1972.

Shillingburg, H.T., Hobo, S., and Fisher, D.W.: Preparations for cast gold restorations, Chicago, 1974, Quintessence Pub. Co.

Shooshan, E.D.: A pin-ledge casting technique—its application in periodontal splinting, Dent. Clin North Am. 189, 1960.

Thayer, K.E.: Fixed prosthodontics Yearbook. Chicago, 1984, Medical Publishers, Inc., Chapter 5.

Tjan, A.H., and Miller, G.D.: Biogeometric guide to groove placement on three-quarter crown preparations, J. Prosthet. Dent. **42**:405, 1979.

Tylman, S.D., and Malone, W.F.P.: Theory and practice of crown and fixed partial prosthodontics (Bridge), St. Louis, 1979, The C.V. Mosby Co., pp. 163-181.

Willey, R.E.: The preparation of abutments for veneer retainers, J.A.D.A. **53**:141, 1956.

SECTION D

Porcelain Jacket Crowns

David A. Kaiser, William F.P. Malone, Boleslaw Mazur, and Maria Lopez Howell

PORCELAIN JACKET CROWN (PJC)

Although the metal/ceramic (PFM) crown is extremely popular, the porcelain jacket crown (PJC) remains the most esthetic restoration for duplicating individual anterior teeth. Adequate tooth reduction is created to achieve space for the porcelain bulk required for strength of the restoration. The marginal adaptation is not comparable to cast restorations.

Pulpal and occlusal relationships are carefully examined before the PJC is prepared. Severe occlusal shear forces contraindicate PJC use, since porcelain can withstand compressive forces but is susceptible to fracture from shearing forces. Due to the reduction required for adequate porcelain strength, the size and position of the pulp is determined before selecting this type restoration.

Porcelain Jacket Preparation

The preparation sequence is: 1) incisal reduction, 2) axial reduction, 3) retention and resistance form, 4) marginal development and refinement.

Incisal reduction. The incisal reduction is performed in two stages. The initial reduction is perpendicular to the long axis of the tooth and 2 mm apical to the contemplated incisal edge of the finished restoration (Fig. 6-84). A line along the long axis and one marking the apical extent of the incisal reduction are valuable aids. The vertical line helps to align the diamond instrument during the proximal slices and avoid convergence of the proximal axial walls. The incisal reduction is not always (Fig. 6-84) extended to the adjacent teeth since the proximal slices remove these mesial and distal areas. It also avoids inadvertent contact with the adjacent teeth at this stage of preparation.

The incisal reduction is now completed. Initially, the reduction was performed in a flat plane perpendicular to the long axis of the tooth. It is now modified to a plane perpendicular to the inclination of the mandibular teeth, usually at a 45 degree angle to the long axis of the tooth in a normal occlusal relationship. This allows compressive forces that are tolerated by the porcelain (Fig. 6-85).

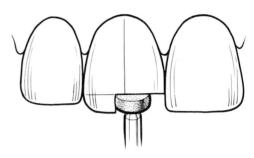

Fig. 6-84. Incisal reductions with a donut-shaped diamond to a predetermined level.

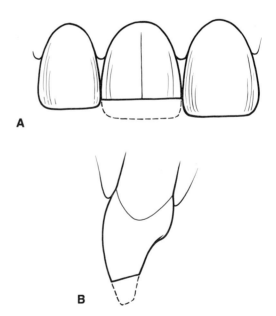

Fig. 6-85. A, Completed incisal reduction inclining from facial to lingual. **B,** The angle of the incisal edge is inclined at 17 degrees from facial to lingual surface.

Axial reduction. The axial reduction is accomplished in several stages. The mesial and distal areas are first reduced to a 2 to 5 degree taper without establishing a shoulder at this time. This initially isolates the tooth

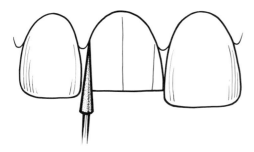

Fig. 6-86. Proximal reduction with thin needle-shaped diamond.

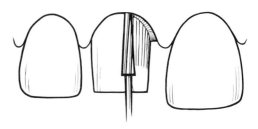

Fig. 6-88. Facial reduction is performed with a flat-ended diamond or a 700 carbide bur. Coarse diamonds are followed by multifluted carbide burs for refinement.

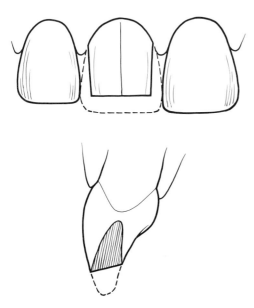

Fig. 6-87. The proximal reduction is completed from facial to lingual without attempting a gingival finish.

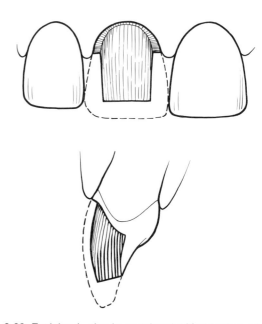

Fig. 6-89. Facial reduction is completed *without* refining the gingival finish line but anticipating support of the soft tissue.

and develops a taper. Pencil lines marking the taper required, along with the vertical axis line, are an aid. A long tapered diamond is carefully used. The lingual convergence of the anterior teeth is developed with these slices (Fig. 6-86). Figure 6-87 is a proximal view of initial incisal reduction and proximal slice.

The facial reduction is performed with a coarse, flat-ended diamond or No. 700 carbide bur to remove the labial surface while concomitantly establishing a preliminary shoulder. Smooth, controlled, sweeping motions are suggested to reduce refining procedures (Fig. 6-88). The incisal two-thirds of the facial surface should be inclined lingually to provide uniform porcelain and ensure suitable esthetics (Fig. 6-89). Flat facial surfaces are an obvious exception to these recommendations.

Retention and resistance form. The lingual surface of the tooth is reduced in two planes. First, a cingulum shoulder is placed with a flat-ended tapered diamond to create a 0.75 mm shoulder in the cingulum with a 2 to 5 degree taper. Alignment can be controlled by instituting the cingulum reduction at this time. It also prevents excessive reduction and maintains alignment of the preparation (Fig. 6-90).

The cingulum reduction is now completed. A flame or wheel shaped diamond is used to form to the lingual concavity of the anterior teeth. If the preparation is performed on a canine, this portion of the reduction commonly has two concave areas due to the canine lingual ridge, but these are not pronounced (Fig. 6-91 and 6-92). Lingual and proximal views illustrate the completed lingual surface (Fig. 6-93).

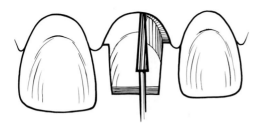

Fig. 6-90. The reduction of the cingulum to maintain vertical retention.

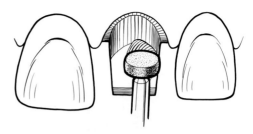

Fig. 6-92. The lingual reduction is completed with a donut-shaped diamond and is checked during protrusive movement.

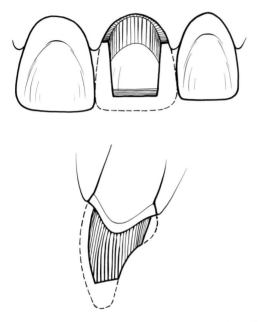

Fig. 6-91. Cingulum reduction is completed while maintaining the support of the interproximal soft tissue.

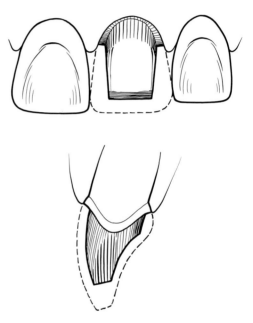

Fig. 6-93. Completed lingual surface reduction showing uniform reduction to accommodate protrusive excursions.

Marginal development and refinement. Margin continuity and uniformity is now completed. An end cutting bur held perpendicular to the shoulder is indicated for lowering margins. A sharp chisel is an excellent instrument for removal of undermined enamel and finishing the shoulder. The chisel also measures shoulder depth (Fig. 6-94).

The axial walls are smoothed to complete the preparation, while sharp line angles and point angles are rounded (Fig. 6-95). The labial gingival finish line is *rarely* supragingival, so special attention is directed to the soft tissue prior to subgingival tooth preparation (Fig. 6-96).

Appropriate treatment restorations are necessary to control gingival health. Figs. 6-97 and 6-98, with PJCs on the right maxillary central incisor lateral incisor and left maxillary central incisor, exemplify the esthetics and tissue health possible. This is accomplished

with diligent laboratory support. Fig. 6-99 illustrates the esthetics; Fig. 6-100 confirms the tissue response with an acceptable emergence profile.

Common Errors in Porcelain Jacket Crown Preparation

1. Excessive taper of proximal surfaces.
2. Insufficient tooth reduction on the facial surface.
3. Inadequate tooth reduction of the lingual surfaces for clearance and diminished strength for porcelain.
4. Variable shoulder width (No. 577 bur).
5. Shoulder not placed far enough apically (1 mm apical to tissue crest), but following contour of gingivae and <u>not</u> violating biologic width.
6. Undercuts at the axis gingival line angles.
7. Rough tooth preparations; remove irregularities with a sandpaper disc.

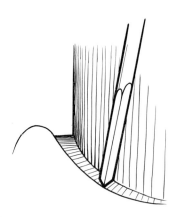

Fig. 6-94. Refinements are accomplished with a straight chisel removal of loose enamel rods.

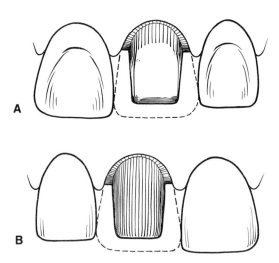

Fig. 6-95. Refined tooth preparation illustrating the **(A)** lingual surface and **(B)** the facial surface.

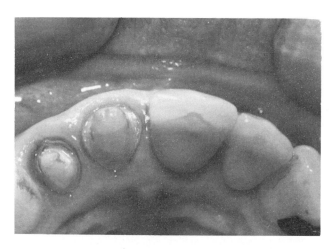

Fig. 6-96. Displaced porcelain jacket crowns on the right maxillary central and lateral incisor while a fracture of the incisal of the left central is evident. Note the inflammation in the intracrevicular space. Tissue management and heat-cured treatment restorations precede tooth preparations.

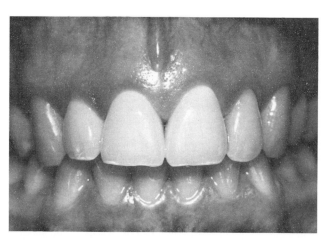

Fig. 6-97. Facial view of three porcelain jackets (Nos. 7, 8 & 9) with acceptable gingival health. The patient can assume partial credit because of meticulous oral hygiene.

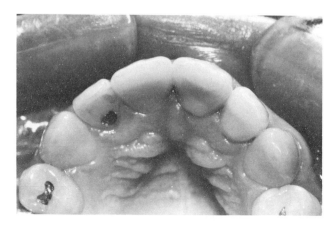

Fig. 6-98. Lingual view of Fig. 6-97 of exceptional laboratory support for contact areas and gingival margins.

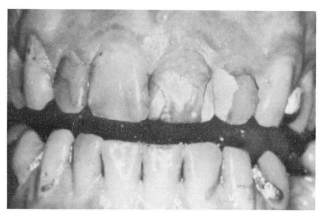

Fig. 6-99. A, Pretreatment for porcelain jacket crowns after caries control with glass ionomer restorations.

continued

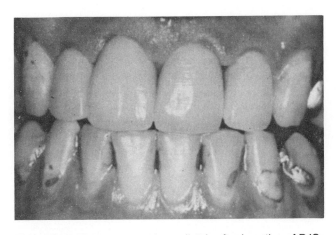

Fig. 6-99. B, Post treatment immediately after insertion of PJCs for four maxillary incisors while preserving the canines bilaterally. (Courtesy Col. H.F. Sawyer, Overland Park, IL.)

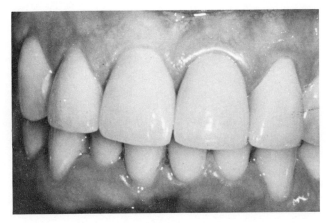

Fig. 6-100. Four porcelain jacket restorations after five years. Note the condition of the soft tissue.

BIBLIOGRAPHY

Adair, P.J., and Grossman, D.G.: The castable ceramic crown, Int. J. Periodont. Restor. Dent. 4(2):32-46, 1984.

Braze, B.: The Cerestore crown—is this the future of dental restorative veneering materials? II, Trends Tech. Contemp. Dent. Lab(3):14-20, 1984.

Chou, T.M., and Pameijer, C.H.: The application of microdentistry in fixed prosthodontics, J. Prosthet. Dent. 54(1):36-42, 1985.

Connor, M.A.: Porcelain, Cerestore and now, cast ceramic, Dent. Stud. 63(1):21-23, 1984.

Davies, T.: Clinical efficacy of all-ceramic crowns: the experience of a general practitioner, Compend. Contin. Educ. Dent. 6(10):742, 745-6, 748-9, 1985.

Donovan, T.E., Adisshian, S., Prince, J.: The platinum-bonded crown: a simplified technique, J. Prosthet. Dent. 51(2): 273-275, 1984.

Faull, T.W., Hesby, R.A., Pelleu, G.B., Jr., and Eastwood, G.W.: Marginal opening of single and twin platinum foil-bonded aluminous porcelain crowns, J. Prosthet. Dent. 53(1)29-33, 1985.

Jones, D.W.: Development of dental ceramics. An historical perspective, Dent. Clin. North Am. 29(4):621-644, 1985.

Munson, C.M.: Anterior crowns: principles and practice. 3. Preparation of vital teeth, Dent. Update 12(1):25-8, 30-1, 1985.

Neuhas, F.F.: Crown preparation. II. Quint. Int. 15(4):429-435, 1984.

Pasternack, S.G.: Compressive strengths of conventional, twin foil, and all-ceramic crowns (letter), J. Prosthet. Dent. 53(5):750, 1985.

Phil, G.K., and Brukl, C.E.: Compressive strengths of conventional, twin foil, and all-ceramic crowns, J. Prosthet. Dent. 52(2):215-220, 1984.

Piddock, V., Marquis, P.M., and Wilson, H.F.: The role of platinum matrix in porcelain jacket crowns, Br. Dent. J. 20: 157(8):275:80, 1984.

Piddock, V., Marquis, P.M., and Wilson, H.J.: Structure-property relationships of dental porcelains used in jacket crowns, Br. Dent. J. 20:157-:275:80, 1984.

Prince, J., Donovan, T.E., and Presswood, R.G.: The all-porcelain labial margin for ceramometal restorations: a new concept, J. Prosthet. Dent. 50(6):793-796, 1983.

Schmitt, S.M.: A two-die system for constructing porcelain jacket crowns, J. Prosthet. Dent. 51(2):195-198, 1984.

Shillingburg, H.T., Jr., and Kessler, J.C.: Recent developments in dental ceramics, Quint. Dent. Technol. 9(2):89-92, 1985.

Sozio, R.B., and Riley, E.J.: Esthetic considerations of the all ceramic crown, C.D.A.J. 12(4): 117-121, 1984.

Thomas, G.C.: Basic porcelain jacket crown ceramics. 2. Dent. Tech. 37(3):9-14, 16, 1984.

Thomas, G.D.: Basic porcelain jacket crown ceramics. 3. Dent. Tech. 37(4):6-12, 1984.

7

Jerry W. Nicholson, Ronald Highton, and
William F.P. Malone

ESTHETIC BONDING
(LAMINATES)

Societal pressure promotes a healthy and trim physique. Health centers, diet food stores, and markets for cosmetic enhancements are pandemic. The public is bombarded by media extolling the virtues of "the perfect smile." The dental profession is faced with specific esthetic demands and a rapid evolution of new but unproven techniques. Discretion should be exercised in selecting products and techniques that are not confirmed by independent, longitudinal studies. Although the direct bonding of porcelain veneers is relatively new, reports of success warrant its inclusion as a restorative treatment.

BONDING

The development of acid-etch technique 30 years ago introduced an aspect of molecular dentistry known as "bonding."[1] Phosphoric acid applied to tooth enamel created a surface of microscopic interstices for mechanically bonding unfilled resins. The prototype system using silica resins[2] was clinically deficient and was replaced with unfilled methacrylates that were less toxic, easily polished, and improved esthetically. However, due to a high polymerization shrinkage and a coefficient of thermal expansion that is higher than that of teeth, the marginal adaptation was compromised. The soft methacrylate surfaces were also subject to wear and discoloration. In the early 1960's, a new resin monomer system was developed by Bowen[2]—Bisphenol A Diglycidyl Methacrylate (Bis-GMA), using inorganic filler particles of quartz or heavy metal glass. The composite resin improved upon the properties of unfilled resin but was difficult to polish. Composite systems have now advanced to include blending of small particle and submicron fillers with visible light polymerization for dependable esthetics.

COMPARISON OF VENEER SYSTEMS

The improved resins have encouraged direct chairside application of composite resins to etched enamel surfaces. Advantages of direct composite veneers are:

1. Only one appointment is required.
2. The dentist directly controls form and color.

3. Cost to the patient is reduced.
4. Composite veneers are repairable.

The indirect porcelain technique, which involves laboratory fabrication of the veneers, compensates for the shortcomings of the direct composite resin technique:

1. The dentist may use the time saving and artistic skills of a ceramist.
2. Multiple units can be placed with less chair time.
3. Porcelain is the optimum material for color stability, esthetics, wear resistance, and tissue compatibility.

Processed materials other than porcelain have been suggested for the indirect technique: resins and composites processed at elevated pressures and/or temperatures (Dentacolor, Isosit, and Visio-Gem), castable hydroxyapatite,[3,4] and injectable ceramics (Dicor, Cerestore). The indirect resins have better physical properties than direct light-cure composites, but reduced bond strengths. One clinical research group reported a one year failure rate of 16 percent with this technique, compared to less than one percent for porcelain laminates.[5] The cast ceramics have the advantage of a waxup stage, excellent translucency, and possibly reduced plaque adherence.[6] Cast ceramics are technique sensitive, however, and offer limited improvement in physical or esthetic properties compared to porcelain. Cast apatite is being developed.

The choice of veneer materials and techniques depends on physical properties of the materials, bond strengths, enamel discoloration, experience of the dentist, and the number of units treated. A condensed comparison of clinical considerations (Table 7-1) is taken from the detailed description of veneer types in Table 7-2. Table 7-3 lists light-curing units.

PORCELAIN LAMINATES

Porcelain laminates are thin facings of ceramic porcelain affixed directly to teeth using a composite resin as bonding cement. Unlike composite veneers, which are directly fabricated on the patient's teeth, porcelain veneers are constructed on refractory dies made from elastomeric impressions. The inner surface of the porcelain veneer is treated with hydrofluoric acid, etching

Table 7-1. Veneer types[7]

Considerations	Direct resin	Indirect resin	Porcelain
Stength	Moderate	Moderate	High
Esthetics	Good-excellent	Good-excellent	Excellent
Coverage of dark color	Excellent (w/opaque)	Good	Good
Longevity potential	Fair-good	Fair-good	Good
Repair expectation	Low-moderate	Low-moderate	Low
Repair difficulty	Easy	Easy	Difficult
Indications	Dark discoloration	Routine	Routine
	Single teeth	Multiple preps	Multiple preps
	Good skills-color and contour		
	Bruxer-clencher	—	—
Contraindications	—	—	Bruxer-clencher
Cost to patient	⅓ Crown cost	½-⅔ Crown	⅔-1X crown
Laboratory cost	0	Varies	Varies

Table 7-2.

	Resin (direct)	Resin (indirect)	Procelain (indirect)
Representative successful brand names	DURAFILL • Kulzer, Inc. 10005 Muirlands Blvd., Unit G Irvine, CA 92718 (800) 854-4003 HELIOSIT • Vivadent USA, Inc. P.O. Box 304 Tonawonda, NY 14151 (800) 833-0022 PRISMA MICRO-FINE • Caulk-Dents-ply P.O. Box 359 Milford, DE 19963 (800) 532-2855 SILUX • 3M Co., Dental Products Lab. 260-28-09 St. Paul, MN 55144 (612) 733-1680 (Other brands of microfill are available)	DENTACOLOR • Kulzer, Inc. 10005 Muirlands Blvd., Unit G Irvine, CA 92718 (800) 854-4003 ISOSIT•N • Vivadent USA, Inc. P.O. Box 304 Tonawonda, NY 14151 (800) 833-0022 VISIO-GEM • Espe-Premier P.O. Box 111 Norristown, PA 19404 (800) 344-8235	CERINATE • Den-Mat Corp. P.O. Box 1729 Santa Maria, CA 93456 (800) 433-6628 CHAMELEON • Myron's Dental Lab. P.O. Box 1458 Kansas City, KS 68117 (800) 255-4620 PVS • S.S. White Dental Products 100 Holmdel Holmdel, NJ 07733 (201) 946-8000 PORCELITE • Kerr Co. Romulus, MI
Indications	1. Need to cover multiple color stains of dark striations. 2. Bruxer, clencher, abusive occlusal habits. 3. Patient with financial difficulty.	1. Typical, routine veneering needs for patients without deeply stained or striated teeth. 2. Dentist does not like to develop tooth anatomy. 3. Bruxer, clencher, abusive occlusal habits.	1. Typical, routine veneering needs for patients without deeply stained or striated teeth. 2. Dentist does not like to develop tooth anatomy.
Contraindications	1. Dentist does not like to develop tooth anatomy or does not have ability with color.	1. Difficult to cover dark stains & striations without placement of underlying opaquers before impression for veneers.	1. Bruxers, clenchers, abusvie occlusal habits. 2. Difficult to cover dark stains or striations without placement of underlying resin opaquers before impression for veneers.
Esthetic potential	Good-excellent if dentist has ability with color blending. Artistic dentist can produce excellent result.	Good-excellent with high-level laboratory support & correct patient selection.	Excellent with high-level laboratory support & correct patient selection.

Table 7-2. Continued

	Resin (direct)	Resin (indirect)	Procelain (indirect)
Expected longevity	Some brands in current generation of resins now observed 7-8 years. Should last at least 5-10 years with esthetic acceptability if placed correctly.	Observed for about 5 years. Should last 5-10 years with esthetic acceptability if laboratory constructs correctly & placed correctly.	Observed for only 2 years. Should last ±10 years with esthetic acceptability if laboratory constructs correctly & placed correctly.
Ease of placement	Preparation easy. Placement moderately difficult because dentist must to have "esthetic" sense for color & contour.	Preparation easy. Placement not difficult because veneer material is same as cementing medium & new polish can be placed on veneer if surface disturbed.	Preparation easy. Placement difficulties are: (1) veneer is fragile & can break, (2) selection of cement color, (3) loss of glaze through finishing.
Time required for <u>6</u> veneers after experience	Prep & place 1½-3 hours (up to 3 hr total time)	Prep ½-1 hour Seat 1-2 hours (up to 3 hr total time)	Prep ½-1 hour Seat 1-2 hours (up to 3 hr total time)
Frequency & location of clinical problems	Incisal edge fracture in ±10% of cases ±3 years into service. Discoloration on gingival & proximal margins at +3 years if not placed correctly. Can cause gingival irritation.	Infrequent incisal edge fracture ±3 years into service. Discoloration on gingival & proximal margins at +3 years if not placed correctly. Can cause gingival irritation.	Very little repair needed in 2 years of observation. Predict discoloration of gingival & proximal margins at 3+ years if not placed correctly. Can cause gingival irritation.
Repair difficulty	Simple. Remove defective portion down to enamel surface, etch, bond, & repair with resin.	Simple. Remove defective portion down to enamel surface, etch, bond, & repair with resin.	Difficult. Must replace veneer or patch with resin with esthetic difference between resin & porcelain.
Cost to patient	±⅓ crown cost	½-⅔ crown cost	⅔-1x crown cost
Laboratory cost to dentist	0	Up to $65/unit	±$65/unit

Christensen, R., Christensen, G. Newsletter: Clinical Research Assocaites: Veneers, Vol 10:4 April, 1986.

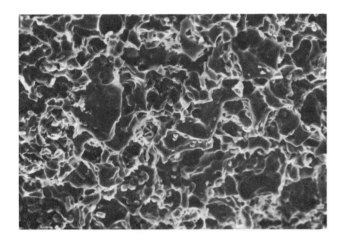

Fig. 7-1. Acid-etched (20 minutes), low-fusing Vita VMK 68 Porcelain (×500). (Courtesy Dr. Stewart Windeler, San Antonio, Tex.)

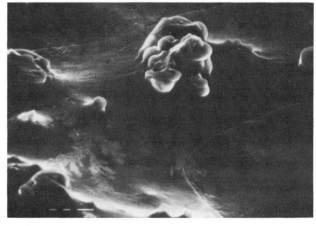

Fig. 7-2. Acid-etched (20 minutes), high-fusing Trubyte denture tooth (×500). (Courtesy Dr. Stewart Windeler, San Antonio, Tex.)

it frosty white and increasing the surface area with retentive irregularities for a mechanical bond to composite (Figs. 7-1 and 7-2). Addition of an organo-silane coupling agent to the etched surface prior to bonding chemically augments the mechanical bond to provide

ultimate bond strengths superior to etched enamel-composite and approaching the cohesive strength of porcelain.[8-10]

The first publication describing bonding of porcelain was in 1983,[11] but additional research studies to cor-

Table 7-3. Light-curing units*

Type	Product	Company	Features	Pros	Cons	Cost ($)†
Fiber optic	COE-LITE	COE	befg	Six curing times (10, 15, 20, 30, 40, 60 seconds)	Fiberoptic cord (corrugated)—difficult to clean, bulb not easily accessible.	600
	COMMAND	SYBRON/KERR	abe	Compact and durable, variable time settings (0-30 seconds)	No beeps at time intervals, bulb not easily accessible.	550
	MARATHON TWO	DEN-MAT	begh	Touch control on handle—easy to activate.	Bulb not easily accessible.	750
	PRISMA-LITE	L.D. CAULK	aeg	Durable	Trigger needs constant pressure for activation, bulb not easily accessible, power supply bulky.	595
Handpiece grip	HELIOLUX	VIVADENT	abcdefgh	Beeps at 20 seconds, bulb easy to replace, no fan (heat sink)—no noise.	Handle gets hot, handle cools down slowly.	670
	TRANSLUX CL	KULZER	abcdefgh	Automatic light shut off when returned to power supply, automatic fan shut off, beeps at 20 seconds, bulb easy to replace.	None	429
Pistol grip	ARISTOCRAT	HEALTHCO	abcdefg	Light made byy Demetron—similar to *VCL 300,* beeps at 10 seconds.	Trigger needs constant pressure for activation, no variable time settings.	515
	EFOS LITE	EFOS	bcdefg	Four curing tips (3, 8, 8, 15 mm) included in price. 3 mm tip for posterior composite, very quiet fan, three curing time settings (10, 20, 40 seconds) on handle, bulb easy to replace with clamp.	Fan stays on until switched off, cord a bit short, metal connector at base of curing tip overheats.	600
	VCL 300	DEMETRON	abcde	Variable time settings 5-65 seconds: automatic fan shut off, bulb easy to replace, four curing tips (3, 8, 11, 13 mm) priced separately; 3 mm tip for posterior composite; very well built.	Needs to be reactivated at specified time intervals; no beep at specified time.	675
	VISILUX II	3M	bcdefgh	Automatic fan shut off; beeps at 10 seconds; extra bulb provided.	Bulb difficult to grip; cord a bit short.	595

*Features:
a. Cord—Flexible and longer than 150 cm
b. Curing tip—7 to 12 mm in diameter
c. Curing tip—360° swivel
d. Curing tip—removable, 7 to 12 mm diameter autoclavable
e. Filter/screen—minimizes reflection of light to operator
f. On/off switch on handpiece
g. Timer beeps at specific time intervals
h. Timer recycles until shut off
†Check cost before purchase. Some light-curing units are offered with composites as an incentive.

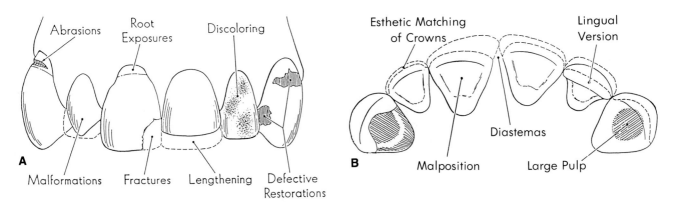

Fig. 7-3. Indications for veneers. **A,** Variety of clinical indications for esthetic bonding. **B,** Incisal view of laminate placement to improve alignment and esthetics.

relate with positive clinical results are sparse. The indirect porcelain technique is gaining acceptance. A survey in 1986 stated that 50 percent of U.S. dentists provide indirect veneers, and 41 percent of this group offer porcelain veneers.[12] Although new, the technique combines the durability, esthetics, and biocompatibility of porcelain; conservation, with facial intraenamel preparations approximately 0.5 mm in depth; and the reliability of the acid-etch composite bond. A research organization has stated that porcelain veneers will become an "accepted procedure" that promises "the highest esthetic potential to date for restoration of anterior tooth defects."[13]

TREATMENT PLANNING FOR LAMINATES
(Flow Sheet 1)

The dentist has a range of esthetic restorative procedures ranging from relatively simple to complex[14]:

1. Cosmetic contouring
2. Bleaching
3. Esthetic restorations
4. Bonding
5. Complete artificial crown
6. Orthodontics
7. Orthognathic surgery

Laminate bonding is indicated for a *combination* of mild-to-moderate anomalies of color, position, and form of the teeth. If the esthetic problem is limited to contour, cosmetic reshaping of the teeth might suffice; if limited to color or staining, consider bleaching. If the problem is localized to a specific portion of the tooth, consider a composite restoration. Teeth without sufficient enamel for bonding and/or with moderate-to-severe loss of coronal structure are crowned. Indications treatable by laminates include[15-17] (Fig. 7-3):

1. Stained/defective restorations
2. Diastema
3. Fractures

4. Attrition
5. Adolescent teeth (large pulps)
6. Discoloration
7. Malformations
8. Malpositions (slight)
9. Root exposure
10. Erosion/abrasion

Porcelain laminates are specifically useful for situations where ceramic-metal crowns are difficult, i.e., large adolescent pulps, occlusal limitations, or lower incisors.

Albers indicated that a tooth to be bonded should have at least 50 percent of its surface composed of etchable enamel.[17] Preferably, the peripheral margins are of enamel to conform to the "one millimeter circumferential principle" for long-term marginal integrity of the enamel-resin bond.[18] However, the veneer can be bonded to a sound composite or glass-ionomer restoration. Composite repair studies have revealed that a delayed resin-resin bond is formed, but with a reduced bond strength.[19] In vitro studies of layered composites have also demonstrated limited microleakage.[20] Glass-ionomer bases etched with phosphoric acid provide some micromechanical retention to composite and promote fluoride release.[21-25] Nonetheless, longitudinal success of the procelain laminate bonded to restorative materials instead of enamel is unknown.

CHOICE OF LAMINATE TECHNIQUE
(Flow Sheet 1)

The major treatment planning decision is often between the ceramic-metal crown and the indirect laminate. The esthetic advantages of the porcelain laminate are achievable with the porcelain-fused-to-metal crown. However, the conservative laminate avoids the complications associated with the technique for ceramic-metal crowns. The laminates:

1. Frequently do not require anesthetic and are less stressful to patients.

Flow Sheet 1 Treatment Planning for Porcelain Veneers

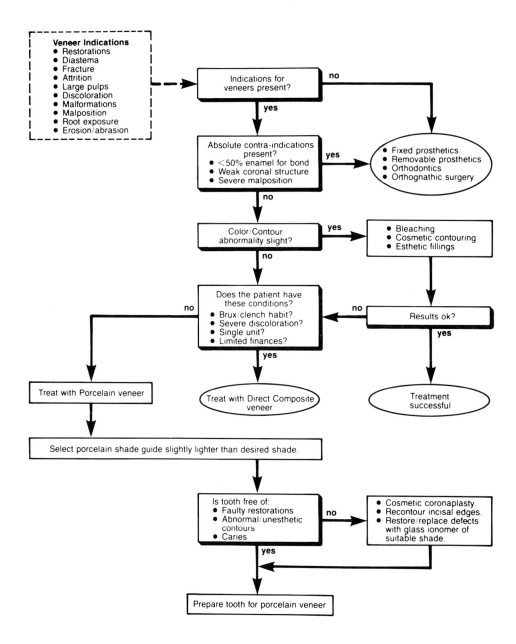

2. Do not usually involve dentin, averting pulp sensitivity.
3. Maintain natural contacts and incisal guidance.
4. Limit tissue-margin contact to facial.
5. Provide a polishable, nonsoluble luting agent at the margin.
6. Do not compress interproximal gingiva.
7. Eliminate metal collars and/or gingival metal display.
8. Do not usually require temporization.

Like porcelain crowns, laminates are extremely difficult to repair if fractured, and the quality of the laminate is dependent on laboratory expertise. Unlike complete ceramic-metal crowns, laminates can not be extrinsically characterized to modify color, and because of translucency of the laminate, the try-in shade is less predictable. Color modification of the laminate is only possible through selection of composite shades, opaque, and tints before curing. Compared to crown cementation, the placement of laminates involves technique-sensitive shading, etching, curing, and margination of the laminate (Fig. 7-4).

Currently, when a filling is insufficient, a PFM crown is the most frequent selection.[26] Further, some

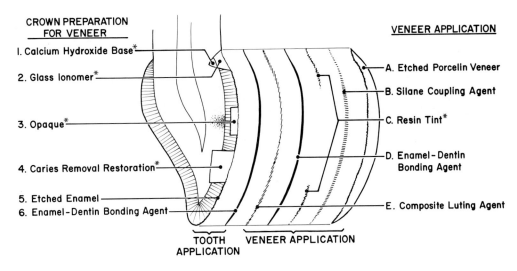

CROWN PREPARATION FOR VENEER

1. Calcium Hydroxide Base*
2. Glass Ionomer*
3. Opaque*
4. Caries Removal Restoration*
5. Etched Enamel
6. Enamel-Dentin Bonding Agent

VENEER APPLICATION

A. Etched Porcelin Veneer
B. Silane Coupling Agent
C. Resin Tint*
D. Enamel-Dentin Bonding Agent
E. Composite Luting Agent

TOOTH APPLICATION   VENEER APPLICATION

*Conditional on caries, contour, or color correction

Fig. 7-4. Tooth pretreatment *(left)* and laminating materials *(right)*.

third-party insurers regard laminates as elective esthetics and limit compensation.[12] Nonetheless, unless a tooth lacks etchable enamel or is structurally weak, laminates deserve consideration as a conservative approach with comparable esthetics.

PRELIMINARY TOOTH MODIFICATIONS
(Flow Sheet 1)

Before starting preparations, establish the desired shade. Correct preexisting restorations, defects, or contour anomalies (Fig. 7-4 and 7-7, A).

A shade is selected from a porcelain system that is one-half shade lighter than the desired shade.[27] This provides the dentist latitude and allows for a slight darkening attributable to increased translucency with polymerization of the composite luting agent. Since thin porcelain facings are translucent, an effort is made to remove isolated discolored areas of the crown with restorations or with thin opaqued composite veneers. Sound but discolored composite restorations may be resurfaced, while caries-suspicious restorations are replaced. Contour deficiencies greater than 1.0 mm resulting from caries, erosion, or attrition are restored with glass-ionomer cement of a suitable shade.[27,28] When a Class III is present, remove sufficient filling just prior to bonding to expose the enamel margins that are then etched and sealed with the bonding composite. The tooth crown should have a uniform contour to permit a uniform thickness of veneer and luting agent. The unequal polymerization shrinkage of varying thickness of composite luting agent induces stresses to the laminate.[31]

Unless incisal lengthening is desired, laminate in-

cisal margins terminate at the facioincisal angles (Fig. 7-7). Preliminary cosmetic contouring defines the esthetic alignment and incisal profile. Recontouring of rotated, tipped, or malpositioned tooth surfaces projecting labially from a uniform facial plane ensures restoration of harmonious facial contours.

After correcting defective restorations, contours, and color discrepancies, the tooth is ready for intraenamel preparation.

TOOTH PREPARATION FOR PORCELAIN VENEER
(Flow Sheet 2)

Advocates for eliminating intraenamel preparation cite "reversibility" of procedure and shortened chair time. There are several advantages for preparation[27]:
1. Suitable contour with decreased facial bulk.
2. Positive seating of laminate during cementation.
3. Reduced vulnerability to fracture with margination.
4. Increased laminate thickness for masking of stains.
5. Concealment of interproximal margins.
6. Reduction of tooth-laminate bond stress[29,30] (Fig. 7-6).

Because the "line of draw" for a porcelain laminate is from a facioincisal direction, the normal incisogingival convexity of the natural crown is maintained. The reduction varies with the marginal location, enamel thickness, tooth discoloration (masking depth), tooth-arch position, and functional requirements. The average enamel thickness at the center of a maxillary incisor is approximately 1.0 mm.[31] A *minimal* thickness of 0.5 mm for a porcelain veneer is readily accommodated.

Flow Sheet 2 Preparation for Porcelain Veneer

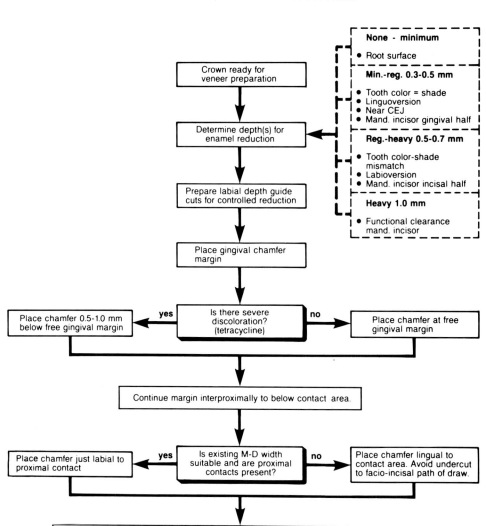

```
                              ┌─────────────────────────────┐
                              │ None - minimum              │
                              │ • Root surface              │
                              ├─────────────────────────────┤
  ┌──────────────────┐        │ Min.-reg. 0.3-0.5 mm        │
  │ Crown ready for  │        │ • Tooth color = shade       │
  │ veneer preparation│       │ • Linguoversion             │
  └──────────────────┘        │ • Near CEJ                  │
           │                  │ • Mand. incisor gingival half│
           ▼                  ├─────────────────────────────┤
  ┌──────────────────┐        │ Reg.-heavy 0.5-0.7 mm       │
  │ Determine depth(s)│◄──────│ • Tooth color-shade mismatch│
  │ for enamel reduction│     │ • Labioversion              │
  └──────────────────┘        │ • Mand. incisor incisal half│
           │                  ├─────────────────────────────┤
           ▼                  │ Heavy 1.0 mm                │
  ┌──────────────────┐        │ • Functional clearance      │
  │ Prepare labial depth│      │   mand. incisor            │
  │ guide cuts for     │       └─────────────────────────────┘
  │ controlled reduction│
  └──────────────────┘
           │
           ▼
  ┌──────────────────┐
  │ Place gingival   │
  │ chamfer margin   │
  └──────────────────┘
```

Crown ready for veneer preparation

Determine depth(s) for enamel reduction

Prepare labial depth guide cuts for controlled reduction

Place gingival chamfer margin

Place chamfer 0.5-1.0 mm below free gingival margin ←yes— Is there severe discoloration? (tetracycline) —no→ Place chamfer at free gingival margin

Continue margin interproximally to below contact area.

Place chamfer just labial to proximal contact ←yes— Is existing M-D width suitable and are proximal contacts present? —no→ Place chamfer lingual to contact area. Avoid undercut to facio-incisal path of draw.

Extend chamfer to incisal.
Complete uniform gross facial enamel reduction to peripheral margins and depth guides.

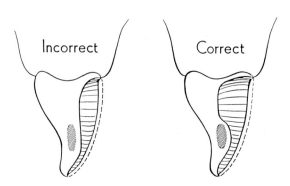

Incorrect   Correct

Fig. 7-5. Extension of lateral margins below contacts.

SEQUENCE OF TOOTH PREPARATION

Controlled reduction is possible with multiple depth wells or horizontal grooves prepared with various diameter ball diamonds or round carbide burs positioned so that the limiting shank is laid parallel against the enamel (Fig. 7-7, B to E). Bur depth wells are placed at the gingival in the mesiodistal center and at both proximal angles. Three more depth penetration indices are placed parallel to the gingival preparations at the midincisogingival surface in the same manner. If incisal reduction is required, a 1/2 round bur (0.07 mm) is used to notch the incisal edge in three more parallel positions (Fig. 7-7 E).

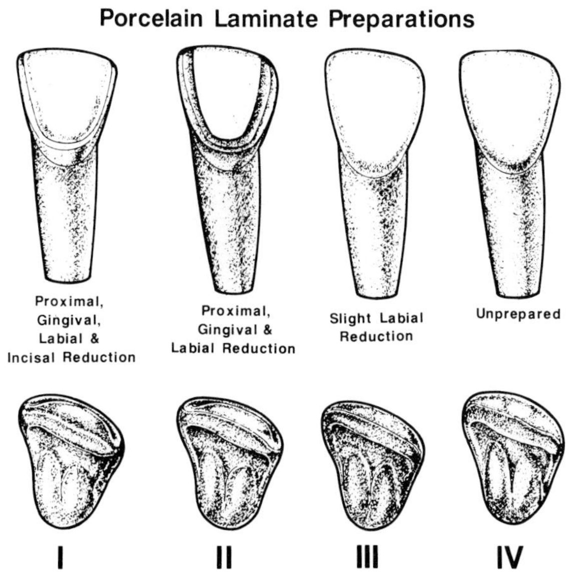

Porcelain Laminate Preparations

| Proximal, Gingival, Labial & Incisal Reduction | Proximal, Gingival & Labial Reduction | Slight Labial Reduction | Unprepared |

I   **II**   **III**   **IV**

Fig. 7-6. Recently, photoelastic studies of porcelain laminates fabricated for three differently prepared teeth and an unprepared tooth indicated that when the proximal, labial, and incisal surfaces were prepared, stress distribution to the laminate was acceptable. Therefore, to minimize the stress within the laminate and tooth, gingival, proximal, and incisal preparations are advisable. From Highton, R., and Taputo, A., J. Prosthet. Dent. 1987, In Press.

An anesthetic is not usually required, because most preparations are confined to the enamel. However, as the tooth preparation approaches the gingival and the enamel becomes thinner, sensitivity and/or tissue management may dictate anesthesia. Tissue retraction is recommended to dilate the intracrevicular space to directly observe the CEJ and to avoid inadvertent laceration of gingival tissue.

For the standard preparation, a gingival chamfer is placed at the height of the gingival crest unless severe discoloration mandates a subgingival margin to gain extra veneer thickness. A coarse tapered diamond or No. 8 round bur with the shank contacting the enamel surface (Figs. 7-7 C and 7-8, A and B) initiates the controlled depth chamfer.

The margin continues into the interproximal areas to the height of the labiopalatal or labiolingual contours. When the teeth are prepared in this manner, the finished laminate will not display "cement lines" viewed in profile (Figs. 7-5 and 7-8 C). If there are no restorations at the proximals, the preparation is extended just facial to the contact areas (Fig. 7-9). However, if there are existing restorations or an anomalous positioning of the teeth, contact is broken (Fig. 7-10). It is important to avoid mesial-distal undercuts that complicate seating the veneers.

If the existing tooth crown length is acceptable, the incisal margin is placed with a facioincisal bevel. The

incisal preparation may be altered to allow an "incisal wrap" of the laminate terminating on a lingual chamfer (Fig. 7-11) when:

1. The incisal thickness is too thin to support the veneer.
2. A lengthening of the incisal edge 1.0 to 2.0 mm is desired.
3. The facioincisal margin is visible and unesthetic.
4. Incisal enamel is structurally compromised (Fig. 7-12, A to D).
5. The incisal is subject to functional stress (mandibular incisors) (Fig. 7-11 B).

The facial surface is uniformly reduced with a fine diamond and water coolant to the peripheral margins and labial depth guides (Flow Sheet 3). The preparation is progressively refined and polished to remove contour irregularities, internal line angles, and bur striations to minimize stress to the thin porcelain veneer (Fig. 7-8, D to F). The sequential refinement restores the natural luster to the remaining enamel so that temporization is usually unnecessary.

If a dark intrinsic discoloration remains, a thin overlay of opaque composite resin may then be applied to partially mask the underlying stain. The surface is smoothed and made ready for the impression. Opaque added to the porcelain of the veneer and to the composite luting resin completes the color correction.

IMPRESSIONS

An impression material that allows fabrication of several replicate models (elastomeric impression material) is selected. Several types of trays are used for impressions. If preparation is limited to the maxillary anterior teeth, an anterior stock tray is adequate. However, an alginate impression is suggested during the appointment prior to preparation so that a custom tray may be fabricated to ensure uniform thickness of the impression material. The custom tray is extended 5 mm gingival from the gingival margin and covers half of the palatal surface, the adjacent unprepared teeth, and occlusal and/or incisal stops. When the lower anterior teeth are prepared, it is necessary to have a custom tray of the entire mandibular arch. An opposing model is also necessary to monitor the excursive movements.

TEMPORIZATION

Temporization is not usually needed because thermal shock and color or contour changes are minimal with veneer preparation. With limited exposure of dentin, a thin layer of dentin bonding agent can be applied before impressions. Temporary veneers under functional stress may be "spot welded" by etching a small spot of facial enamel for added retention. A polyethyl-methacrylate (Trim) or a microfilled com-

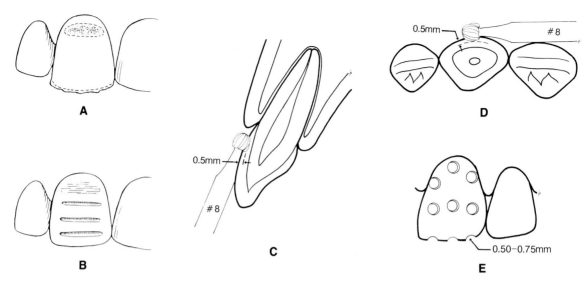

Fig. 7-7. A, Pretreatment tooth with gingival caries and irregular incisal edge. **B,** Tooth with caries removed and glass ionomer cement covering the dentin while the incisal edge has been equilibrated and horizontal depth grooves established (or place depth wells). **C,** Placement of 0.5 mm depth wells on the facial surface with No. 8 round bur. **D,** Initial placement of depth penetration gauges viewed incisally. **E,** Incisal depressions ½ round bur before intraenamel preparation.

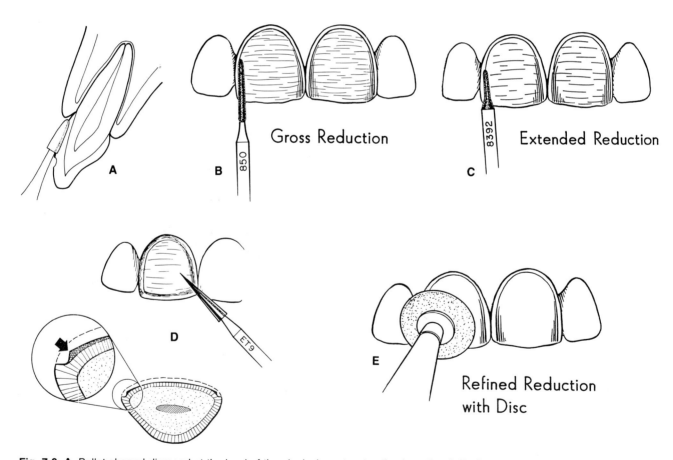

Fig. 7-8. A, Bullet-shaped diamond at the level of the gingival crest; retraction is optional. **B,** Gross reduction to limits of peripheral margins and depth glides. **C,** The peripheral reduction is performed maintaining the facial mesiodistal convexity. **D,** Round internal line angles remove diamond striations and polish enamel to a high gloss. **E,** Tooth preparation smoothed and polished with a cuttle fish sandpaper disc.

Continued.

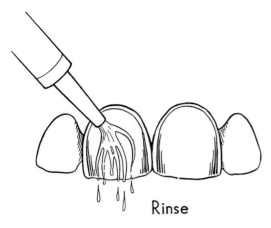

Fig. 7-8. F, Tooth preparations are thoroughly rinsed after refining the surfaces with a cuttle fish sand paper disc.

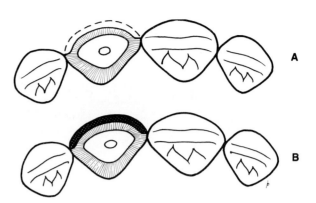

Fig. 7-11. A, Extension of preparation by establishing an incisal wrap with a lingual chamfer. **B,** Tooth preparation and clearance for mandibular incisor with normal arch position.

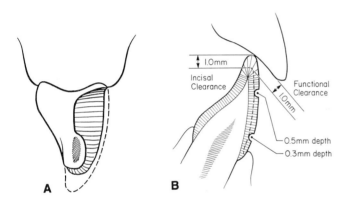

Fig. 7-9. The extent of labial and proximal reduction and laminate placement with the teeth in apposition (incisal view). **A,** Maintains existing contacts. **B,** Seated laminate.

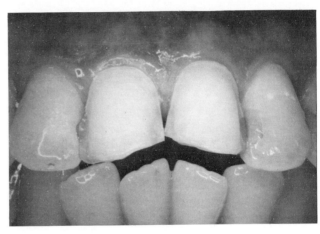

Fig. 7-12. A, Laminate tooth preparation for maxillary central incisors, including the incisal edge.

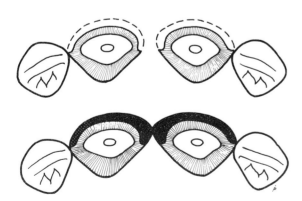

Fig. 7-10. The described preparation is for teeth in normal alignment; however, modifications for abnormal situations such as diastemas are appropriate. In these instances the proximal margins should be more palatally adjacent to the space so that the laminate is confluent with the prepared tooth. This precaution prevents lingual plaque accumulation.

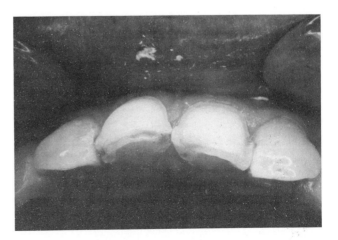

Fig. 7-12. B, Incisal view of laminate tooth preparation. Note the convexity mesiodistally and preservation of contact areas.

continued

Flow Sheet 3 Preparation for Porcelain Veneer

Gross facial reduction complete

↓

Facial free of localized spots of severe color/stain? — **no** → Reduce discolored enamel to accommodate thin, etch retained, shaded opaque.

yes ↓

Is the existing inciso-gingival tooth length acceptable? — **no** →

yes ↓

Is facio-lingual dimension at incisal edge sufficient for veneer support? — **no** →

yes ↓

Place facio-incisal bevel

Reduce Length	**Add length**
• Esthetics • Overbite • Thin incisal • Functional clearance Reduce incisal 1.0 mm short of desired length. Place linguo-incisal chamfer. Round incisal angles.	• Esthetics • Open bite • Attrition • Fracture Veneer may add 2.0 mm length. Place lingual chamfer 1.0-2.0 mm from incisal edge. Round incisal angles.

↓

Refine preparation with fine diamond or 12 bladed carbide to extend margins, round angles, and remove striations and roughness.

↓

Polish facial enamel to high gloss with super-fine diamonds and finishing discs to provide a normal enamel surface needing no temporization.

↓

Make an impression of veneer preparations using addition silicone or polyether elastomers. Block out open gingival embrasures. Place retraction cord if required. ← **no** — Does the patient have problem or concern for:
• Exposed dentin
• Sensitivity
• Opened contacts
• Abnormal contours
• Discolored teeth — **yes** → • Place 2 layers of dentin-enamel bonding agent
• Temporary composite or resin laminate spot etched to labial surface

↓

Prepare laboratory prescription for a shade slightly lighter than desired. Specify color, character, and contour modifications. Indicate whether heavy, moderate, slight, or no opaque is needed to mask partially discolored teeth. Color slides and study models may be helpful.

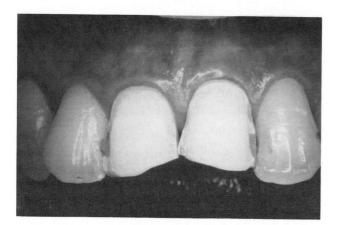

Fig. 7-12. C, Frosted appearance after etchant application. Contamination must be avoided.

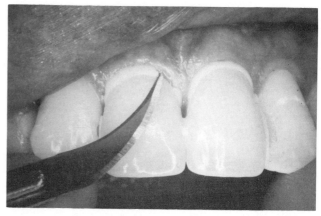

Fig. 7-12. D, After the porcelain laminate is bonded to the tooth, removal of excess composite with a Bard-Parker 12B Blade.

Flow Sheet 4 Try-in for the Porcelain Veneer

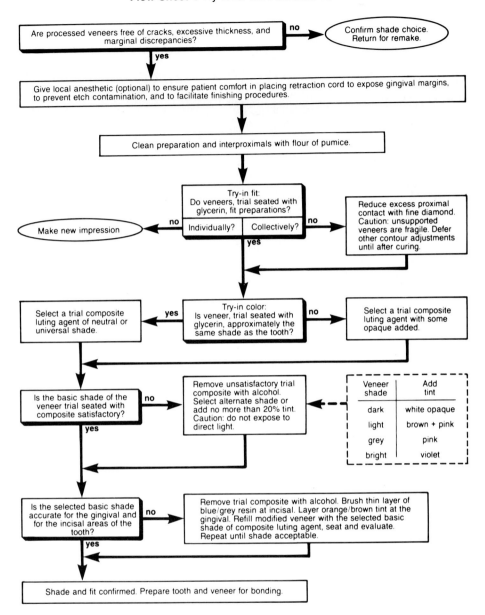

posite may be placed directly on the prepared unetched surface, finished, and polished. On the second visit, the temporary facing is easily removed with a scaler. Exercise care to avoid extending the resin beyond the prepared surface and injuring the gingiva.

TRY-IN OF THE PORCELAIN VENEER
(Flow Sheet 4)

The fabricated veneers are examined for fracture or excessive thickness. Color accuracy is verified at the try-in because the internal etching of the veneers reflects an overly white opaque appearance. Although optional, local anesthesia may (1) facilitate placing retraction cord (Fig. 7-13 A) to prevent contamination of the etched enamel during bonding and (2) allow

comfortable refinement of margins.

The preparations and interproximal embrasures are cleaned before veneers are placed. Each veneer is trial-seated with a water-soluble viscous media, glycerine or K-Y Jelly (Johnson & Johnson), for stabilization and assessment of color and fit. The veneers are seated simultaneously to check for displacement from bulky proximal contacts. Excess proximal contact is relieved with porcelain abrasive wheels. Adjustments not affecting placement are delayed until the fragile veneers have been affixed with light-cured composite.

Select one central veneer to test the basic shade of composite luting agent and the need for supplemental opaque or color tints. A neutral or universal composite shade for color confirmation is indicated if tooth color

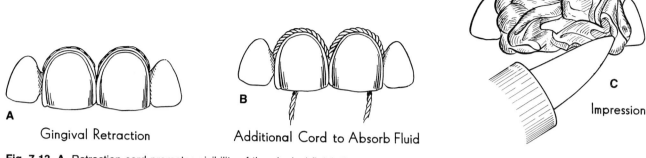

A

Gingival Retraction

B

Additional Cord to Absorb Fluid

C

Impression

Fig. 7-13. A, Retraction cord promotes visibility of the gingival finish line and avoids contamination. **B,** A second layer of retraction cord prevents contamination. **C,** Elastomeric impression materials are preferred. A custom tray is then seated with the heavy-bodied impression material over the light-bodied.

and shaded veneer are the same shade. If the discoloration of the underlying tooth is insufficiently masked by the veneer, select a basic shade with opaque added. Both chroma (color saturation) and value (lightness-darkness) can be adjusted with small increments of tint modifiers added to the basic shade of composite. Resin color modifiers can also be applied directly to the inner surface of the veneer to enhance a polychromatic effect.[32]

The trial veneer is placed on unetched enamel with the selected composite luting agent plus all other color enhancements that are needed. Direct illumination with the operatory light is avoided during the trial placements with light-cure resins. Repeated trials are possible because uncured resin can readily be removed from the veneer with application of or immersion in acetone or alcohol. At this point, consult with the patient for their approval or the need for additional modifications. With fit and color confirmed, the veneers are ready for bonding (Fig. 7-14, A to E).

BONDING THE PORCELAIN VENEER
(Flow Sheet 5)

The various materials "laminated" to the etched porcelain surface enhance the bond and modify color/opacity (See Fig. 7-4). The veneers are placed in a padded ultrasonic solution of acetone or alcohol to remove contaminates. The veneers are then rinsed, air dried, and arranged in left and right contralateral pairs, beginning with the centrals. A thin layer of silane coupling agent is brushed on the etched surface of the veneer and air dried for one minute. Some silanes require conditioning with phosphoric acid etchants. Silane coupling agents provide a significant chemical enhancement to the porcelain bond in vitro tests. If color modifiers were needed for characterization at the try-in, the tints are reapplied directly to the silanated veneers. A thin layer of light-cure enamel-dentin bonding or unfilled resin is applied

next but <u>not</u> light cured. The rationale for using dentin bonding agents at the porcelain-composite interface is based on studies of resin bonded to etched enamel. Low-viscosity bonding resins increased tensile bond strengths through surfactant action reducing trapped air and voids between the composite and etched enamel.[33] Dentin bonding agents have also improved the composite-enamel marginal seal and reduced marginal discoloration.[33]

The final steps for preparation and bonding of the veneers are:

1. Uniformly load the veneers with composite and cover to protect them from light polymerization. Several manufacturers produce customized composites with flowable viscosity and prepackaged shades with and without added opaque. Low-viscosity composites facilitate fast, low-stress placement. Higher-viscosity composites require rocking pressure and extra time to allow the composite to flow. Incisally wrapped veneers require first facial, then gingivally directed pressure for complete seating.

2. While maintaining a steady pressure on the veneer, slightly pull the interproximal matrix lingually to clear the proximal margins of excess composite. A short brush is used to clear all accessible margins (Fig. 7-15, A).

3. With the finger applying pressure and blocking light to the gingival half of the laminate, "tack" the veneer in place with a 20 second light exposure with a wide 15 mm curing light tip (Fig. 7-15 B, Table 7-2).

4. Repeat the removal of composite excess at the margins and cure the entire laminate for a total of 1.5 to 2.0 minutes, depending on thickness, color, and opacity of the laminate.

5. Check that no marginal excess is present interproximally that will interfere with seating the adjacent veneer. Composite flash is readily removed from the glazed porcelain or unetched enamel with carbide composite carvers, scalers, or surgical blades (Fig. 7-

Flow Sheeet 5 Bonding of the Porcelain Veneer

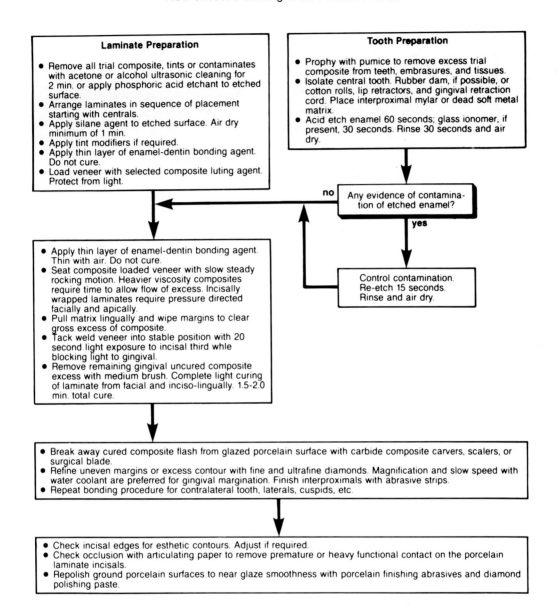

Laminate Preparation

- Remove all trial composite, tints or contaminates with acetone or alcohol ultrasonic cleaning for 2 min. or apply phosphoric acid etchant to etched surface.
- Arrange laminates in sequence of placement starting with centrals.
- Apply silane agent to etched surface. Air dry minimum of 1 min.
- Apply tint modifiers if required.
- Apply thin layer of enamel-dentin bonding agent. Do not cure.
- Load veneer with selected composite luting agent. Protect from light.

Tooth Preparation

- Prophy with pumice to remove excess trial composite from teeth, embrasures, and tissues.
- Isolate central tooth. Rubber dam, if possible, or cotton rolls, lip retractors, and gingival retraction cord. Place interproximal mylar or dead soft metal matrix.
- Acid etch enamel 60 seconds; glass ionomer, if present, 30 seconds. Rinse 30 seconds and air dry.

Any evidence of contamination of etched enamel?

no

yes

Control contamination.
Re-etch 15 seconds.
Rinse and air dry.

- Apply thin layer of enamel-dentin bonding agent. Thin with air. Do not cure.
- Seat composite loaded veneer with slow steady rocking motion. Heavier viscosity composites require time to allow flow of excess. Incisally wrapped laminates require pressure directed facially and apically.
- Pull matrix lingually and wipe margins to clear gross excess of composite.
- Tack weld veneer into stable position with 20 second light exposure to incisal third whle blocking light to gingival.
- Remove remaining gingival uncured composite excess with medium brush. Complete light curing of laminate from facial and inciso-lingually. 1.5-2.0 min. total cure.

- Break away cured composite flash from glazed porcelain surface with carbide composite carvers, scalers, or surgical blade.
- Refine uneven margins or excess contour with fine and ultrafine diamonds. Magnification and slow speed with water coolant are preferred for gingival margination. Finish interproximals with abrasive strips.
- Repeat bonding procedure for contralateral tooth, laterals, cuspids, etc.

- Check incisal edges for esthetic contours. Adjust if required.
- Check occlusion with articulating paper to remove premature or heavy functional contact on the porcelain laminate incisals.
- Repolish ground porcelain surfaces to near glaze smoothness with porcelain finishing abrasives and diamond polishing paste.

12 D). Repeat the bonding procedure for the contralateral tooth, working distally until all laminates are placed.

A sharp explorer and magnification aid in the inspection for, and removal of, composite flash and the refinement of porcelain margins to ensure a healthy gingiva. Use microfine and superfine finishing diamonds at slow speed with water spray to blend the margins. A smooth surface comparable to a glazed finish is achieved using flexible finishing discs[35] (3M Co., St. Paul, Minn.) or porcelain abrasive wheels[36] and finishing with a slurry polishing paste.[37] Equal

care is exercised to finish interproximal margins with thin strips ranging from medium to superfine grit.

Since porcelain is susceptible to stress fracture, the occlusion is adjusted in all excursions, especially for lengthened incisal edges (Fig. 7-15, C to E). Eliminate centric contacts at porcelain-enamel margins. Contours of incisal edges are shaped to conform to esthetic characterization. Surfaces that were modified by grinding are repolished with porcelain abrasives and slurry polishing paste (Fig. 7-16, A to U).

A color display of Figs. 7-16, A to U, is available at the end of the chapter as Fig. 7-17, A to S.

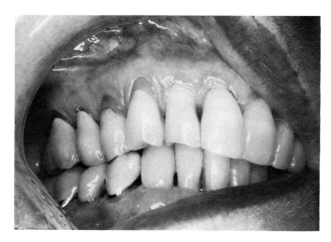

Fig. 7-14. A, Pretreatment view of the maxillary right lateral and canine. Note the occlusal attrition on the incisal edge and the periodontally compromised dentition.

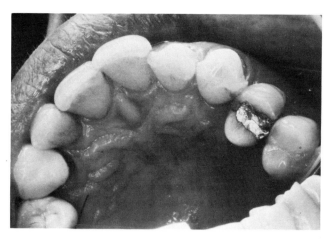

Fig. 7-14. B, Occlusal view of incisal tooth preparation and pronounced mesiodistal convexity.

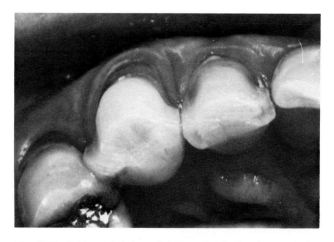

Fig. 7-14. C, Magnified view of B; the extended tooth preparation before application of opaques and glass ionomer cement. The exaggerated preparation is necessary because of the constricted cervix of the tooth.

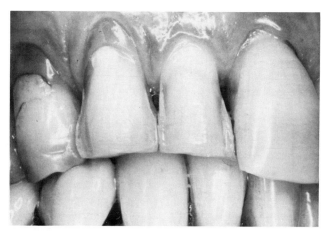

Fig. 7-14. D, Tooth preparation for porcelain laminate after placement of glass ionomer; smoothed and polished.

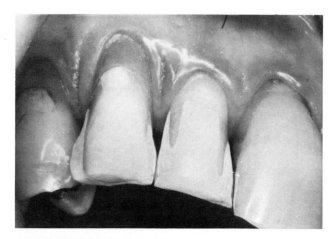

Fig. 7-14. E, Composite resin opaque modifiers and glass ionomer cement placed to ensure esthetics and allow the seating of a uniform porcelain laminate.

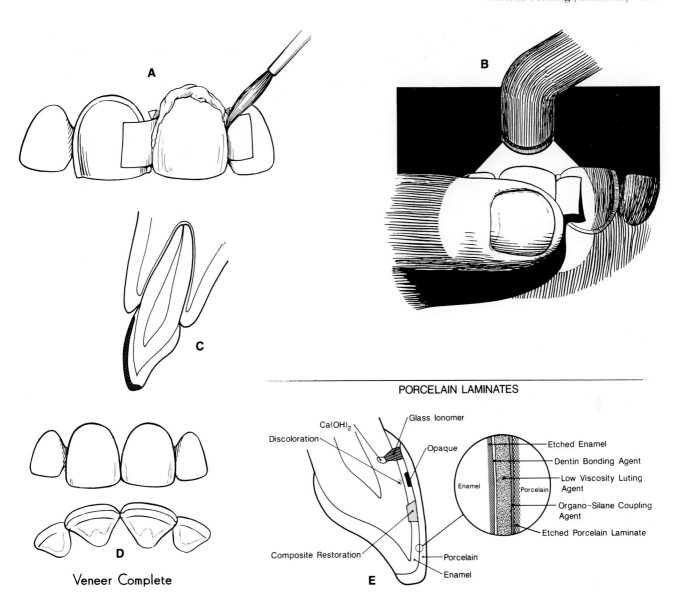

Fig. 7-15. A, Removal of flash from cavosurface angles. **B,** Light-activated composite resin bonded to the corrugated tooth surface of the porcelain laminate. **C,** Profile of the laminate in position. Note the relationship of the gingival tissue to the finish line of the laminate. **D,** Completed veneers without overcontouring. **E,** Laminate bonded to a tooth with various interfaces and rationale for bonding.

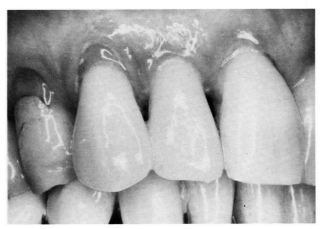

Fig. 7-15. F, Completed porcelain laminates terminating at the C,E,J. Note the restored incisal edge and smooth gingival transition disguising dark teeth.

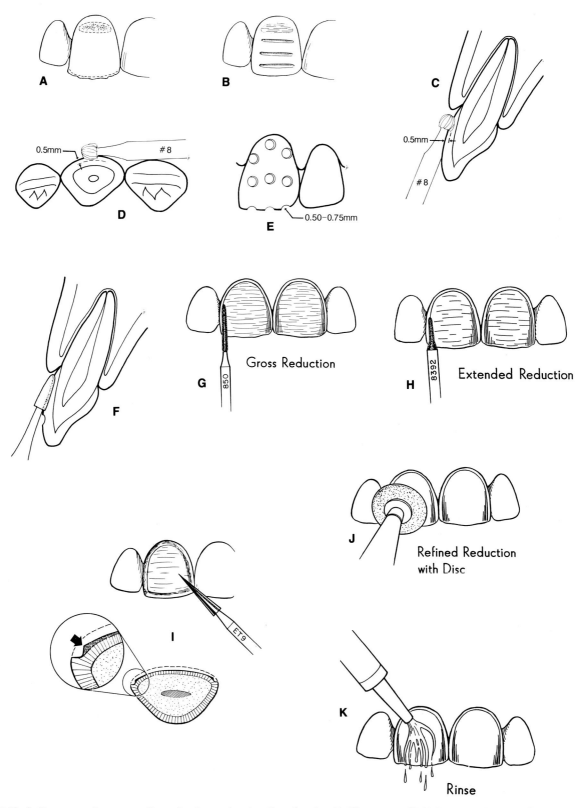

Fig. 7-16. A, Prepreparation: cosmetic contouring and restoration of caries. **B,** Placement of labial enamel depth guides. **C,** Placement of enamel depth guide using bur shank as control. **D,** Incisal view of enamel depth guides. **E,** Optional placement of the start of labial enamel depth guides. **F,** Gross labial reduction and gingival chamfer to depth guides. This can be accomplished with various diamonds. **G,** Gross reduction to peripheral chamfers and depth guides. **H,** Fine diamond to refine margins and smooth the preparation. **I,** Smooth multifluted carbide to blend and smooth internal line angles and remove striations. **J,** High polish restoring enamel luster to nearly normal appearance during laboratory fabrication of veneers. **K,** Thoroughly rinse the etched labial surface for a minimum of 30 seconds.

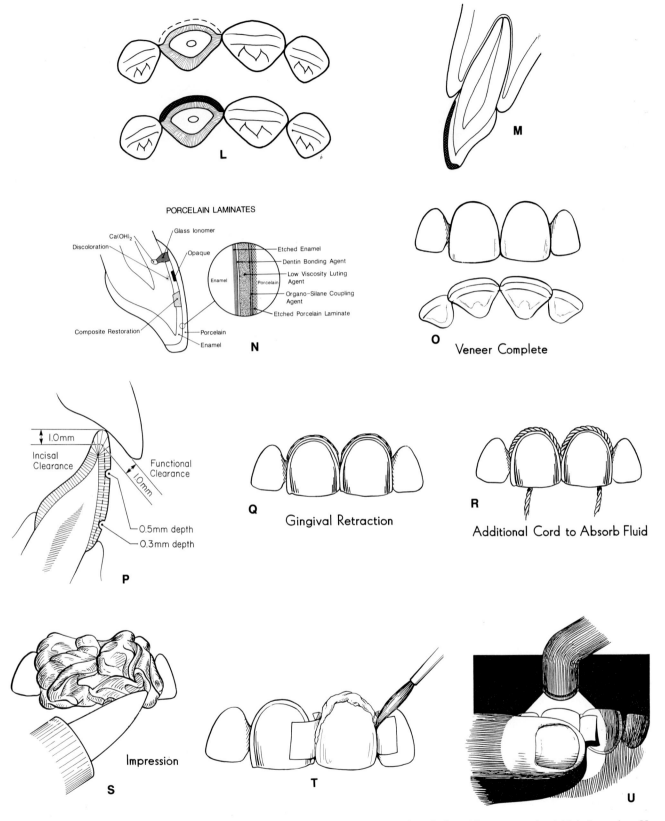

Fig. 7-16. L, Porcelain veneer preparation and restoration. Perceptively prepared teeth do not have excessive labial dimension. **M,** Porcelain veneer with incisal wrap to chamfer or butt joint. A lingual bevel creates a fragile porcelain margin. **N,** Abbreviated diagram of coronal preparation and laminate layers for the porcelain veneer. **O,** Completed laminate veneer illustrating smooth arch form. **P,** Tooth preparation for mandibular incisor. **Q,** Retraction is advised for visibility. **R,** Additional cord will absorb fluid. **S,** Elastomeric impressions with custom tray are advised. **T,** Removing excessive composite resin. **U,** Light-activated resins with mylar strips.

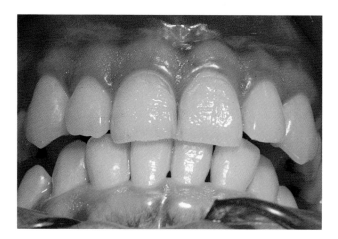

Fig. 7-17. A, Pretreatment "lemon sucker".

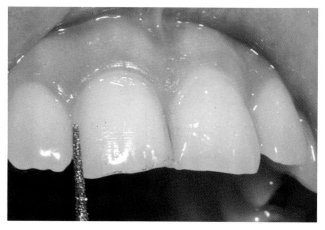

Fig. 7-17. B, Gross facial reduction with #5862-012 diamond or 850.

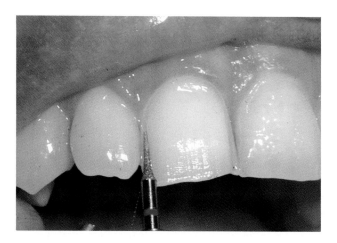

Fig. 7-17. C, Refined reduction to the contact areas with a No. 8392 diamond.

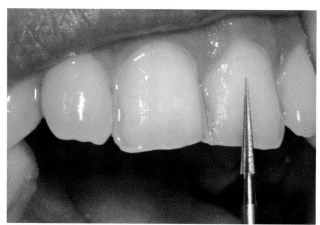

Fig. 7-17. D, Refining the facial surface with an E.T. No. 9.

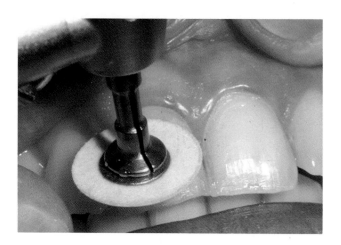

Fig. 7-17. E, Sandpaper disc to smooth and polish.

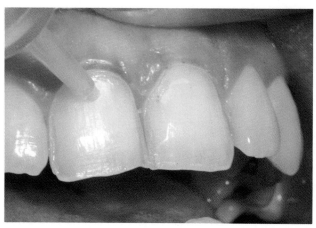

Fig. 7-17. F, Thoroughly rinsed ether water.

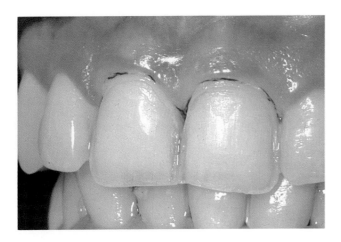

Fig. 7-17. G, Retraction cord to view the gingival margin.

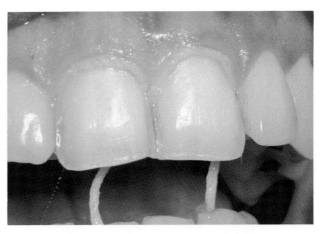

Fig. 7-17. H, Additional cord to absorb fluids.

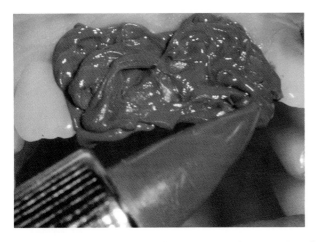

Fig. 7-17. I, Impression material (elastomeric before insertion of the custom tray (segments are adequate).

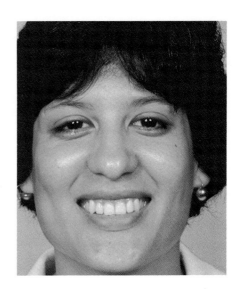

Fig. 7-17. J, Profile (pre-post comparison).

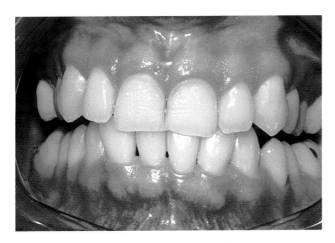

Fig. 7-17. K, Facial (pre-post comparison).

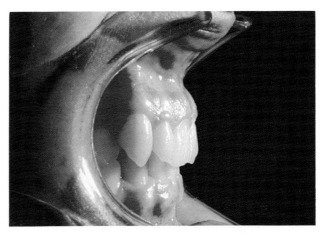

Fig. 7-17. L, Lateral (prepost comparison).

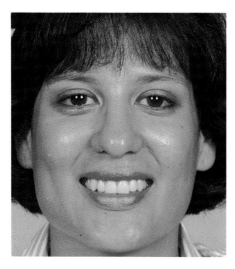

Fig. 7-17. M, Profile (Post treatment) with porcelain laminates.

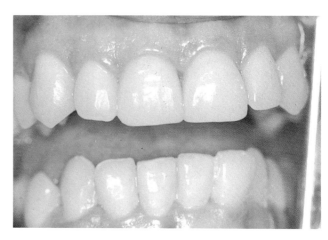

Fig. 7-17. N, Facial (post treatment) with porcelain laminates.

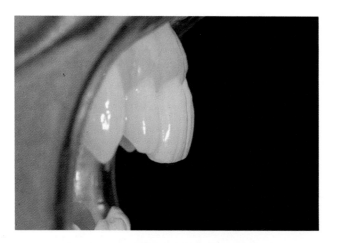

Fig. 7-17. O, Lateral (post treatment) with porcelain laminates. **A** through **O,** courtesy of Dr. Oscar Vargas, El Paso, Texas, Dr. Jerry Nicholson, San Antonio, Texas, Dr. William F.P. Malone, Alton, Ill.)

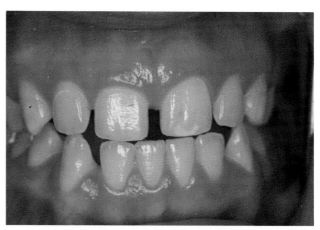

Fig. 7-17. P, Diasteman pretreatment (profile). (Courtesy Dr. Jack Griffin, Wood River, Ill.; Dr. William F.P. Malone, Alton, Ill.)

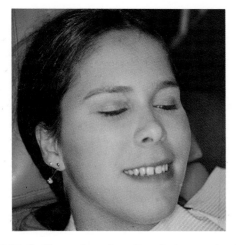

Fig. 7-17. Q, Closer view of maxillary incisors pretreatment.

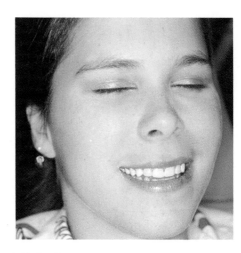

Fig. 7-17. R, Profile post treatment with free handed composite resin application.

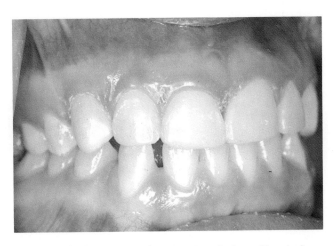

Fig. 7-17. S, Closer view of posttreatment of maxillary incisors with free handed composite resin application. (Courtesy Dr. Jack Griffin, Wood River, Ill.; Dr. William F.P. Malone, Alton, Ill.)

SELECTED REFERENCES

1. Bronocore, M.G.: A simple method of increasing the adhesion of acrylic filling materials to enamel surfaces, J. Dent. Res. **34**:849, 1955.
2. Bowen, R.L.: Properties of a silica-reinforced polymer for dental restoration, J.A.D.A. **66**:57, 1963.
3. Hobo, S., and Iwata, T.: A new laminate veneer technique using a castable apatite ceramic material. 1. Theoretical considerations, Quint. Int. **7**:451, 1985.
4. Hobo, S., and Iwata, T.: A new laminate veneer technique using a castable apatite ceramic material. 2. Practical procedures, Quint. Int. **8**:509, 1985.
5. Jordan, R.: Restorative Symposium, San Antonio, Tex., September 1986.
6. Chan, C., and Weber, H.: Plaque retention on teeth restored with full ceramic crowns: a comparative study, J. Prosthet. Dent. **56**:660, 1986.
7. Clinical Research Assoc. Newsletter **10**(5), April 1986.
8. Calamia, J., and Simonsen, R.: Effect of coupling agents on bond strength of etched porcelain, J. Dent. Res. (Abstr. 79) **63**:179, 1984.
9. Lee, J.G., Moore,B.K., Avery, D.R., and Hovijitra, S.T.: Bonding strengths of etched procelain discs and three different bonding agents, J. Dent. Child. **53**:409, 1986.
10. Lacy, A., Laluz, J., Watanabe, L., and Dellinges, M.: Effect of porcelain surface treatment on the bond to composite resin, J. Dent. Res. (Abstr. 1108) **66**:245, 1987.
11. Horn, H.: A new lamination: porcelain bonded to enamel, N. Y. Dent. J. **49**:401, 1983.
12. Dental Products: Report: Trends in Dentistry, December, 1986.
13. Clinical Research Associates: Porcelain veneers, CRA Newsletter, May 9(5):1, 1985.
14. Bonner, P.: Aesthetics give new lease on life, Dent. Today, June, 1986.
15. Nixon, R.: Use of porcelain laminate veneers enhances foreshortened, worn teeth, Dent. Today, October, 1984.
16. Nixon, R.: Using veneers expands practice, Dent. Today, May, 1986.
17. Albers, H.: Tooth-Colored Restoratives, ed. 7, Coatai, Calif. 1985, Alto Books, pp. 7-1 to 7-31.
18. Jordan, R.: Esthetic Composite Bonding, St. Louis, 1986, The C.V. Mosby Co., p. 28.
19. Miranda, F., Duncanson, M., and Dilts, W.: Interfacial bonding strengths of paired composite systems, J. Prosthet. Dent. **51**:29, 1984.
20. Chalkley, Y., and Chan, D.: Microleakage between light-cured composites and repairs, J. Prosthet. Dent. **56**:441, 1986.
21. Kidd, E.: Cavity sealing ability of composite and glass ionomer cement restorations, Br. Dent. J. **144**:139, 1978.
22. McLean, J., Prosser, H.J., and Wilson, A.D.: The use of glassionomer cements in bonding composite resins to dentine, Br. Dent. J. **158**:410, 1985.
23. Welsh, E.: Microleakage at the gingival wall with four class V anterior restorative materials, J. Prosthet. Dent. **54**:370, 1985.
24. Monteiro, S., Sigurjons, H., Swartz, M.L., Phillips, R.W., and Rhodes, B.F.: Evaluation of materials and techniques for restoration of erosion areas, J. Prosthet. Dent. **55**:434, 1986.
25. Swartz, M., Phillips, R., and Clark, H.: Long term F release from glass ionomer cements, J. Dent. Res. **63**:158, 1984.
26. Christensen, G.: The use of porcelain-fused metal restorations in current dental practice: a survey, J. Prosthet. Dent. **56**:1, 1986.
27. Albers, H.: Lecture—International Symposium on Laminate Systems in Dentistry, Philadelphia, October, 1986.
28. Nixon, R.: Clarifying concerns about porcelain veneers, Dent. Today, August, 1986.
29. Highton, R., Caputo, A., Matyas, J., and Tashima, B.: A photoelastic study of stresses on porcelain laminate preparations, J. Prosthet. Dent. (in press).
30. Highton, R., Caputo, A., Matyas, J., and Tashima, B.: Incisal load transfer by porcelain laminates, J. Dent. Res. **65**:806, 1986.
31. Schillingburg, H.T., and Grace: Thickness of enamel and dentin, J. S. Cal. Dent. Assoc. **41**:33, 1973.
32. Nixon, R.: Veneers and options to Aesthetics, Dent. Today **5**(5):24, 1986.
33. Asmussen, E.: Clinical relevance of physical, chemical, and bonding properties of composite resins, Oper. Dent. **10**:61, 1985.
34. Dumsha, T., and Biron, G.: Inhibition of marginal leakage with a dentin bonding agent, J. Dent. Res. **63**:1255, 1984.
35. Smith, G.A., and Wilson, N.H.E.: The surface finish of trimmed porcelain, Brit. Dent. J. **151**:222, 1981.
36. Schlessel, E.R., Newitter, D.A., Renner, R.P., and Gwinnett, A.J.: An evaluation of postadjustment polishing techniques for porcelain denture teeth, J. Prosthet. Dent. **43**:258, 1980.
37. Klausner, L.H., Cartwright, C.B., and Carbeneau, G.T.: Polished Goldstein, R.E.: Cosmetic contouring. In Esthetics in Dentistry, Philadelphia, 1976, Lippincott.

BIBLIOGRAPHY

Boksman, L., Jordan, R.E., and Skinner, D.H.: Alternative bleaching treatment for the non vital discoloured tooth, Compend. Cont. Ed. 28, **2**:471-478, 1984.

Boksman, L., Jordan, R.E., Suzuki, M., et al.: Etched porcelain labial veneers, Ontario Dentist. **62**:1, Jan. 1985.

Boksman, L., Jordan, R.E., Suzuki, M., et al.: Etched porcelain labial veneers, Ontario Dentist. **62**:1, Jan. 1985.

Carenza, F.: Glickman's Periodontology, Philadelphia, 1984, W.B. Saunders Co.

Cheung, W.S., Pulver, F., and Smith, D.C.: Custom-made veneers for permanent anterior teeth, J.A.D.A. **105**:1015, Dec. 1982.

Clinical Research Associates: Comparison of veneer types, CRA Newsletter **10**(4):1, 1986.

DeWet, F.A.: Polishing, Forum Esthetic Dent. **4**:12, 1986.

Garcia-Godoy, F., and Malone, W.F.P.: The effect of acid etching on two glass-ionomer lining cements, Quint. Int. **17**:621, Oct. 1986.

Garcia-Godoy, F., and Malone, W.F.P.: Acid penetration through fine calcium hydroxide liners, Texas State Dent. J. **103**:4-6, Oct. 1986.

Hobo, S., and Iwata, T.: A new laminate veneer technique using a castable apatite ceramic material. 1. Theoretical considerations, Quint. Int. **7**:451, 1985.

Hobo, S., and Iwata, T.: A new laminate veneer technique using a castable apatite ceramic material. 2. Practical procedures, Quint. Int. **8**:509, 1985.

Horn, H.: A new lamination, porcelain bonded to enamel, Dent. Clin. North Am. **27**:671, 1983.

Jordan, R.E., Suzuki, M., Boksman, L., and Skinner, D.H.: Labial resin veneer restorations using visible light cure composite materials, Alpha Omegan, (scientific issue) **74**:30-39, 1981.

Jordan, R.E., Suzuki, M., and Gwinnett, A.J.: Restoration of fractured and hypoplastic incisors by the acid etch resin technique: A three year report, J.A.D.A. **95**:795, 1977.

Jordan, R.E., Suzuki, M., Hunter, J.K., and Boksman, L.: Conservative treatment of tetracycline stained dentition, Alpha Omegan, (scientific issue) **74**:40-49, 1981.

Simonsen, R.J., and Calamia, J.R.: Tensile bond strength of etched porcelain, A.A.D.R. Abstracts. **1154**:297, 1983.

8

William F.P. Malone, Delmo J. Maroso, and Steven M. Morgano

RESIN-BONDED RETAINERS (MARYLAND BRIDGE)

Dentistry has experienced many advances in the past 30 years, i.e., ultraspeed tooth preparation with precision carbide and diamond burs, improved biomaterials, osseous integrated implants and panoramic radiographs, including computerized tomography with magnetic nuclear imagery. Nevertheless, the development of noninvasive microretentive techniques in restorative dentistry is a dramatic departure from traditional treatment.

The most recent imaginative approach in fixed partial dentures (FPD) is the composite resin-bonded metal retainer. The success of this technique depends upon the ability to etch specific high-modulus, nonprecious alloys. After eching, the metal framework can be bonded to enamel with a composite resin (Fig. 8-1). A thin, inconspicuous three-unit FPD can then be placed after the limited tooth reduction (Figs. 8-2 and 8-3). The attachment is composed of three strategic areas:

1. Etched enamel surface
2. Bonding resin
3. Etched metal surface

This prosthesis has been described facetiously as a cemented "Nesbit," a unilateral partial denture, or an adult space maintainer (Fig. 8-4). There is a certain element of truth in both contentions, but to dismiss the concept of conservatism, the potential of composite resin cements, and their appeal to patients could be described as anti-intellectual and socioeconomic irresponsibility.

ATTACHMENT

Acid etching of teeth was introduced by Buonocore.[1] Bowen (1962) developed the BIS-GMA composite resins.[2] Rochette suggested a perforated prosthesis for immobilizing periodontally compromised teeth using the acid etch technique and composite resins.[3] This procedure was improved and expanded by Howe and Denehy[4], but treatment was commonly restricted to younger patients with anterior "open bites."

Dunn and Reisbick[5] and Tanaka[6] were the first to successfully use micropores for retention of the resin to the casting. The procedure was refined by Thomp-

son et al.[7] with electrolytic etching of base metals. Simonsen et al.[8] then indicated that bond strength of the resin to cast metal substantially exceeded the strength of the bond between the resin and etched enamel.

Barrack[9] refined the tooth preparations to dramatically reduce the incidence of dislodgement and emphasized the advantages of the etched metal framework. Recent advances have simplified the treatment of the metal casting and have focused on the sensitivity of the bonding procedures (Figs. 8-5 and 8-6).

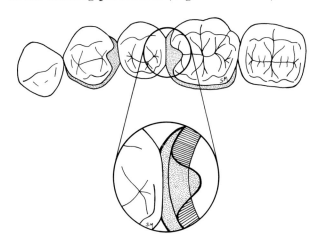

Fig. 8-1. "Wrap-around" is a crucial feature to the design because it enhances resistance to lingual displacement, increases the surface area of enamel bonding, and permits bonding to diversely directed enamel rods (inset).

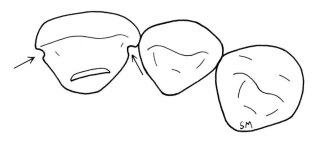

Fig. 8-2. "Wrap-around" is esthetically objectionable for an anterior abutment because of metal display. Perceptively placed proximal grooves (arrows) can be substituted for the "wrap-around" design. Note the cingulum rest seat.

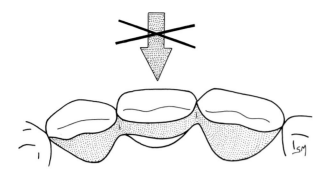

Fig. 8-3. Prepared proximal grooves offer resistance to lingual displacement of the RPD without facial metal display.

POSTERIOR MARYLAND BRIDGE

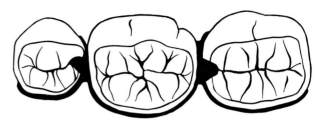

Fig. 8-4. A posterior resin-bonded prosthesis placed on untouched abutments illustrating an appropriately designed metal display.

	Group 1 Met-etch	Group 2 Electrolytic Etch	Group 3 Silicoated
Mean standard	11.85	16.556	24.29
Deviation	2.44	3.42	3.94

All a posteriori pair wise comparisons were significant at the 0.001 level using the Tukey multiple range test. Re, G., Kaiser, D.A., Malone, W.F.P., and Jones, Troy: J. Prosthet Dent in Press.

Fig. 8-5. Composite shear bond strengths (Mega Pascals) of three types of metal treatment for the tooth surface of the RBP.

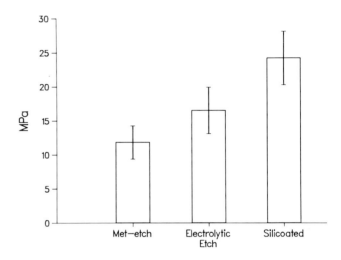

Re, G., Kaiser, D.A., Malone, W.F.P., and Jones, Troy: J. Prosthet Dent in Press.

Fig. 8-6. Retention in Mega Pascals to the tooth surface for the metal framework of the RBP.

INDICATIONS FOR RESIN-BONDED PROSTHESIS

Resin-bonded prostheses (RBP) have become more popular, especially for treating the medically compromised, indigent, and adolescent patients. This imaginative approach has become an alternative to conventional FPDs and RPDs because the RBPs are economical, conservative, and functional and do not irritate soft or hard tissue, i.e., as in replacement of mandibular incisors. The acid-etched, resin-bonded retainers are commonly esthetically appealing, but this can be attributed only to the more talented dental technicians.

Specific Indications

Resin-bonded prostheses are indicated for:
1. Retainers of FPD for abutments with sufficient enamel to etch for retention
2. Splinting of periodontally compromised teeth
3. Stabilizing dentitions after orthodontics
4. Medically compromised, indigent, and adolescent patients
5. Prolonged placement of interim prosthesis to augment surgical procedures, i.e., cranio-facial anomalies

Contraindications

1. Patients with an acknowledged sensitivity to base metal alloys

2. When the facial esthetics of abutments require improvement
3. Insufficient occlusal clearance to provide 2 to 3 mm vertical retention, e.g., abraded teeth
4. Inadequate enamel surfaces to bond, e.g., caries, existing restorations
5. Incisors with extremely thin faciolingual dimensions
6. Exceptionally demanding esthetics for adults

Advantages

The advantages are:
1. Noninvasive to dentin with lingual and proximal tooth preparation including occlusal rests
2. Conservative with undeniable patient appeal
3. Tissue tolerant because of supragingival margins without pulpal irritation
4. Unaltered casts without removable dies
5. Reduced cost with less chair time

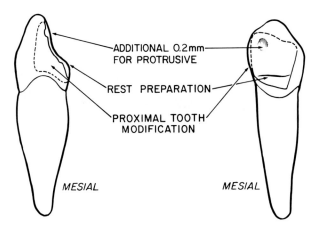

Fig. 8-7. Proximal (A) and lingual (B) surface preparation, including accommodation for protrusive movements.

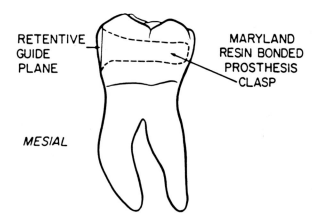

Fig. 8-8. Preparation of the lingual and proximal surfaces of a mandibular molar for clasps and retentive planes (0.6 mm).

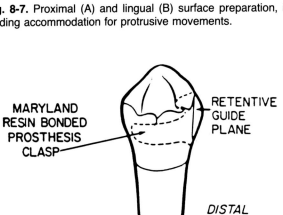

Fig. 8-9. Preparation of the lingual and proximal surfaces of a premolar with a 2 mm guide plane occlusogingivally.

Disadvantages

The disadvantages are:
1. Education is needed about concepts of micro-retention.
2. Demanding techniques and tooth preparation with discerning diagnosis
3. There is heavy dependence on the laboratory for the competent treatment of cast metals and selective waxing to avert overcontouring.
4. Plaque accumulation is prohibitive because design is outside the dimensions of the natural tooth, and bulky contours are intolerable for specific patients.
5. Patient expectations of esthetics are high, but routine results are fair to good—NOT outstanding.
6. Usually restricted to one (single pontic) tooth replacement
7. "Graying out" of teeth that are thin labiolingually at the incisal surfaces

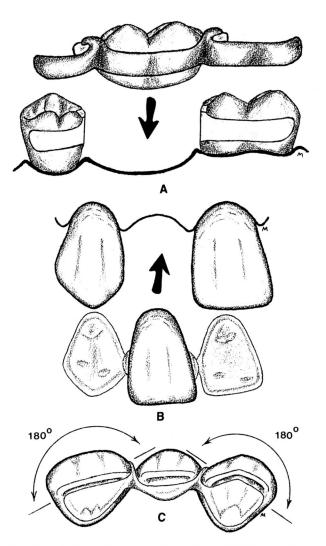

Fig. 8-10. A, Path of insertion of mandibular RBP in a rotational direction with one guide plane parallel or slightly undercut. **B,** Anterior RBP replacing a lateral incisal with proximal "wings," rotational insertion (undercut on distal of central), and maximum coverage of lingual surface. **C,** Incisal view of trial insertion of metal without porcelain to demonstrate both 180 degree and facial metal coverage.

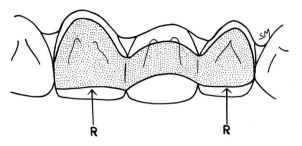

Fig. 8-11. Maximum lingual coverage for the retainers (R) or "wings" is fundamental. Outdated designs that do not provide maximum coverage are failure-prone.

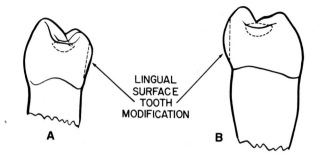

LINGUAL SURFACE TOOTH MODIFICATION

Fig. 8-12. Position of occlusal rests and the extent of lingual surface reduction on a premolar **A** and molar **B**.

FUNDAMENTAL PREPARATION CONSIDERATIONS

Although long-term supportive studies are unavailable, the success rate is impressive for RBPs that have the prescribed resistance and retention in the form of:

1. Nearly parallel opposing walls, i.e., 6 degree taper (Figs. 8-7 to 8-9)
2. A specific path of insertion (Fig. 8-10)
3. Sufficient occlusal clearance
4. Maximum coverage of virginal enamel (Fig. 8-11)
5. Vertical stops (Fig. 8-12)

The vertical path of insertion is developed in combination with the "wraparound 180 degree design" to prevent dislodgement of a rigid framework. High flexual stresses during function have sponsored suggestions by Caputo and Standlee[10] for minor box preparation of the occlusal rests and increased bulk (at least 0.6 mm) for the framework. So the natural contours of the abutment teeth are altered to accommodate the appropriate metal design (Fig. 8-13).

The fundamental considerations of the posterior RBP include:

1. Select axial reduction lingually at the height of contour (Fig. 8-14)
2. 1 mm deep occlusal rests inclined toward the center of the abutment teeth (Fig. 8-12)
3. 180 degree proximal "extensions" approximately 0.6 mm thick (Fig. 8-13)
4. A predesigned path of insertion
5. Facial-proximal retention on the posterior abutment

The fundamental considerations of the anterior RBP are:

1. Sufficient lingual surface clearance 0.6 to 0.8 mm for occlusion (1.0 mm is optimal) (Fig. 8-15)
2. Development of a cingulum rest
3. Creation of an incisogingival proximal surface path of insertion with an identifiable supragingival finish line about 1 mm from the crest of tissue

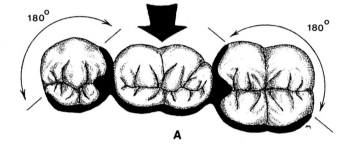

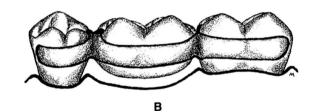

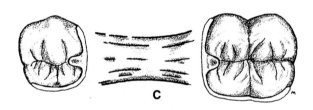

Fig. 8-13. A, Occlusal view of three-unit RBP demonstrating a 180 degree extention of the retentive clasps, the contour, and how lingual displacement prior to bonding should be impossible. **B,** Lingual "wraparound" and a sanitary pontic 3 mm above the tissue of the edentulous area. **C,** Position of the rests related to the height of the edentulous ridge.

4. Additional 0.2 mm to accommodate protrusive excursions of the mandible (Fig. 8-7)
5. Proximal-facial extensions for retention without a metal display (Fig. 8-16)
6. Possible rotational path of insertion with one proximal surface slightly undercut (Fig. 8-17)

All modifications should be consistent with the predesigned path of insertion.

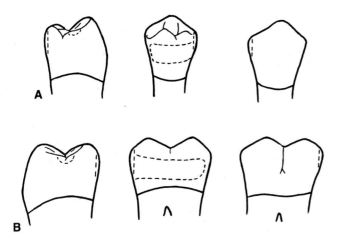

Fig. 8-14. Proximal, lingual surface preparation with the position of occlusal rests for vertical stops of the premolars **A,** and molars **B.**

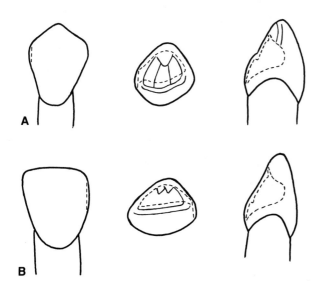

Fig. 8-15. A, Outline of the facial, lingual, and proximal tooth modification of the maxillary canine necessary for resistance to displacement. **B,** Outline of the facial, lingual, and proximal tooth modification of the maxillary central without excessive display of metal.

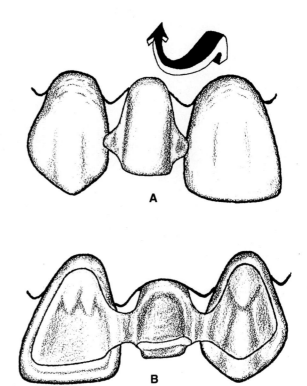

Fig. 8-16. Facial view **A,** of three-unit adhesive FPD illustrating the wings on the pontic engaging the proximal surfaces of the abutment teeth. **B,** This design and appropriate lingual surface coverage resists the lingual displacement of the RBP.

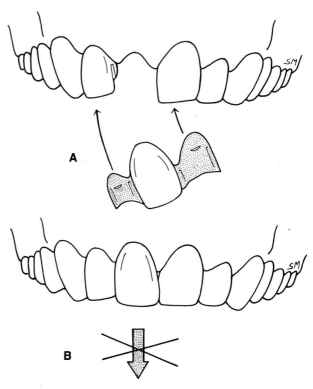

Fig. 8-17. A, Rotational or oblique path of insertion that allows the FPD to "snap" into place to resist displacement. **B,** The FPD resists displacement along other paths.

Aids in preparation include:
1. Rubber dam application with red or black pencil marks to identify preparation extensions
2. Interim impressions poured in colored casts to verify tooth preparation
3. Surveyed interim casts

Note: Electrosurgical tissue removal may be required at the interproximal surfaces adjacent to the edentulous areas prior to final impressions.

IMPRESSIONS

Elastomeric impressions are superior, and reversible hydrocolloid is less desirable for a final replica.

One cast is poured as a refractory cast, while the preparations for the second cast are outlined in red or black pencil on a diagnostic cast. This eliminates confusion between the laboratory and the dentist and results in a more accurate casting. An opposing complete arch cast and unilateral interocclusal records for the prepared side are required.

LABORATORY SERVICE

The RBP is waxed to correspond to the outline on the second cast, including the facial extensions. The pontic is almost universally a Stein pontic anteriorly and a sanitary pontic 3 mm superior to the tissue posteriorly. If the casting can be displaced lingually from the cast, the dentist must redesign the prosthesis, reprepare the abutments, and make another impression because the casting does not possess adequate retention and will fail (Figs. 8-13 to 8-17).

It has been suggested to return the casting with the porcelain (bisque bake) for a trial insertion.[8] This can be done with uncomplicated prostheses and by diligent technicians.

TRIAL INSERTION AND ETCHING

The first try-in is to:
1. Verify the complete seating of the prosthesis.
2. Test the resistance to lingual displacement.
3. Check the margins on each abutment.
4. Review the form of the substructure for the pontic.
5. Monitor the occlusal clearance during mandibular excursions.

The second try-in is to:
1. Review all the items for the first try-in.
2. Obtain agreement between patient and dentist that the prosthesis is suitable esthetically.

Return for metal conditioning:
1. Electrolytic etching.
2. Silicoating for a corrugated surface.
3. Met-etch in office-laboratory (Gresco Lab, Texas).

Note: The etched metal surface should remain uncontaminated, even though some authors claim this precaution is unnecessary.

The metal etching may be selective for each type of base metal, so universal treatment of different metals is usually discouraged.

BONDING

The prosthesis is returned in a plastic container to avoid contact with the treated metal surface.
A. Rubber dam application is imperative, and anesthesia is encouraged to ensure a cooperative patient.

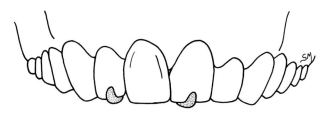

Fig. 8-18. Incisal rests are placed to ensure definitive seating during the bonding procedure. These rests are removed with rotary instruments after bonding, and the casting is smoothed and polished—without overheating, using a water spray.

B. The teeth to be bonded are pumiced to remove debris and the rubber dam inverted to prevent leakage.
C. Phosphoric acid (37 percent) etchant is applied to enamel for 30 to 60 seconds. When a light, frosty appearance has been accomplished, rinse with water for 30 seconds.
D. BIS-GMA composite resin cement is readied in the following sequence (asterisk preceding step indicates it is performed by assistant):
  1. Mix sealant (unfilled) resin.
  2. Apply sealant to tooth surface of metal retainers.
 *3. Mix cement composite resin.
  4. Apply sealant to etched enamel.
 *5. Place composite resin on prosthesis and hand to dentist.
 *6. Monitor isolated field.
  7. Insert prosthesis and apply constant pressure for 7 minutes.
 *8. Remove excess resin with a blunt instrument, particularly interproximally.

Incisal rests to ensure a repeatable path of insertion during trial insertions are removed with a water spray using a carbide bur in a high-velocity handpiece (Fig. 8-18). Instruct the patient to avoid premature pressure for 24 hours and to schedule a post insertion appointment to review the bonding and occlusion.

SEQUENCE OF TECHNIQUE AND COMMON PROBLEMS

A. Initial appointment
  1. Obtain radiographs to appraise periodontal profile and caries.
  2. Clean, pumice, and assess the facial surfaces of potential abutments.
  3. Review vertical length of potential abutments and occlusion.
  4. Make impressions for diagnostic casts and possible removable treatment partial for extraction site of anterior tooth.
  5. Discuss therapy and cost with patient.
  6. Record the appearance of teeth with shade guide.

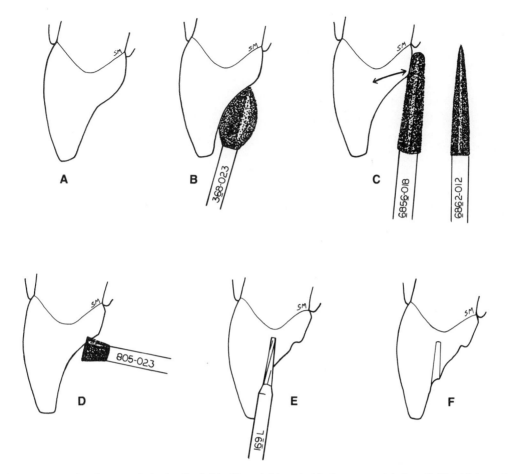

Fig. 8-19. Abutment preparation for an anterior tooth: **A,** Maxillary right central incisor—mesial view. **B,** Establish occlusal clearance with a football diamond to allow a casting thickness of at least 0.6 mm; a thickness of 1 mm is preferred. **C,** Reduce the height of contour of the cingulum with a large-diameter, round-end tapered diamond. Continue the reduction to the mesial surface (adjacent to the edentulous space) parallel to the planned path of insertion to permit maximal metal contact with the proximal enamel. Reduce the distolingual surface parallel to this planned path with a flame diamond short of the proximal contact with the contiguous tooth. **D,** Develop a cingulum rest seat (to resist gingival displacement of the FPD) with an inverted cone diamond stone. **E,** Place conservative proximal grooves, parallel to the planned path of insertion with a No. 169L carbide bur. These grooves are shallower, shorter, and more lingually placed than preparation of a classic three-quarter crown preparation. **F,** The completed preparation—entirely within enamel.

B. Second appointment
1. Mount diagnostic casts to reproduce interocclusal relationships and check for clearance.
2. Evaluate patient expectations of treatment.
3. Measure edentulous area to anticipate tooth modification of proximal surface.
4. Remove existing small, lingual restorations and replace with glass ionomer to be etched later as suggested by Godoy and Malone.[11]
5. Remove offending tooth, electrosurgically trim interproximal soft tissue, and apply Oringers solution of myrrh and benzoin three times.
6. Insert treatment restoration: fixed (acid-etched bonded denture or natural tooth) or removable treatment prosthesis to restore the patient's appearance.

C. Third appointment (after a suitable healing period)
1. Prepare the abutment teeth on the proximal and lingual surfaces with rests in the appropriate position (Fig. 8-19).
2. Make an interim impression to verify the retentive extension of the restoration.
3. Secure occlusal clearance by inserting a wax wafer to check the interocclusal space after preparation.
4. Make the final impression and paint the teeth with copalite as a temporary measure to avoid patient discomfort.
5. Review shade selection.

D. Fourth appointment
1. Try-in the casting with or without porcelain application and test for lingual displacement. Note: If the prosthesis can be displaced lin-

gually on the cast or intraorally, modify the tooth preparations and make new impressions or the prosthesis will *not* be successful.
  2. Review the margins of the casting, tissue contact of the pontic, and occlusion; characterize the porcelain pontic.
  3. Return to laboratory for refinement and metal treatment.
E. Fifth appointment
  1. Anesthesia is administered to reduce anxiety and salivary flow.
  2. A rubber dam is placed to isolate the field and avoid contamination.
  3. The assistant synchronizes the bonding by programming the duties of each attendant.
  4. Bonding is performed within 35 to 40 seconds from the start of the mixing to avoid an increase in the resin cement particle size. The majority of resin cements set in 90 seconds according to the manufacturer's directions, but additional working time is gained by refrigerating the cement before use. Other approaches have been suggested to improve the working time.

INTERIM VERSUS FINAL PROSTHESIS

The resin-bonded prosthesis has been considered an interim prosthesis, dentinally noninvasive, and somewhat reversible. However, because of various contingencies, an "adhesive bridge" can be bonded as a permanent restoration with shallow proximal grooves anteriorly and boxes posteriorly. This is particularly applicable for the aged, indigent, and medically compromised patients; RBP for adolescents or patients with periodontally compromised dentition are considered long-term or intermediate treatment.

The problem with an interim prosthesis is not usually the dentist or patient, but dental insurance administrators. They understandably do not provide funds for a second prosthesis within 5 to 7 years. Therefore, the adhesive bridge should be inserted with this understanding.

Causes of Failure

The common causes for dislodgement of the RBP are:
  1. Inappropriate patient selection
    a. Alignment of teeth results in a poor path of insertion
    b. Insufficient vertical length of the abutment teeth
    c. Inadequate virginal enamel for bonding
    d. History of metal sensitivity
    e. Thin labiolingual dimensions of abutments

  2. Incomplete tooth preparation
    a. Insufficient proximal and lingual surface reduction
    b. Incomplete or less than 180 degree extension of "wraparounds"
    c. Lack of accommodation to mandibular excursion, i.e., protrusive
  3. Bonding of the RBP
    a. Contamination
    b. Prolonged mixing
    c. Inappropriate luting agent

VERSATILE APPLICATIONS

Extensive periodontal splints to retain questionable teeth can be inexpensively accomplished with only slight tooth modifications rather than complete crown preparations (Fig. 8-20,A). Resin-bonded rest seats for RPDs are another diverse application in prosthodontics (Fig. 8-20,B).

SUMMARY AND CONCLUSIONS

The literature is replete with research on the microretentive, noninvasive techniques associated with the adhesive bridge. This innovative approach has been and continues to be misrepresented by inappropriate claims in texts and periodicals that overemphasize its simplicity. The reality is:
  A. Patient selection should be a discriminating procedure.
  B. Tooth preparation is arduous because of its intricate, demanding design, and vision is impaired by white-on-white surfaces.
  C. Bonding is a regimented procedure with a predetermined, coordinated effort between the dentist and assistant.
  D. Laboratory implementation requires informed, diligent technicians.
  E. Patient education as to the intent and limitations of the conservative procedure is necessary.

The adhesive FPD is a promising, imaginative treatment to augment traditional fixed prosthodontics. Research and education will silence objections, remedy mismanagement, and replace discouragement with enthusiasm. The RBP is primarily indicated for the adolescent, medically afflicted, indigent, and patients with a periodontally compromised dentition.

SELECTED REFERENCES
  1. Buonocore, M.G.: A simple method for increasing adhesion of acrylic resin filling materials to enamel, J. Dent. Res. **34**:849-853, 1955.
  2. Buonocore, M.G.: Retrospections on bonding, Dent. Clin. North Am. **25**(2):241-255, 1981.
  3. Rochette, A.L.: Attachment of a splint to enamel of lower anterior teeth, J. Prosthet. Dent. **30**(4):418-423, 1973.
  4. Howe, D.F. and Denehy, G.E.: Anterior fixed partial dentures

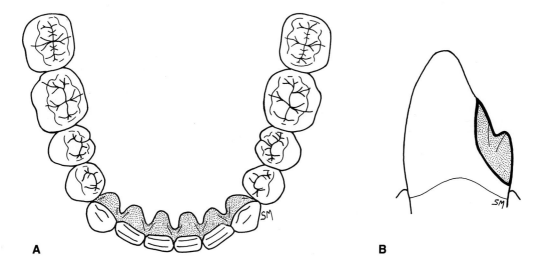

Fig. 8-20. Additional indications for the resin-bonded restoration include **A,** fixed splinting of periodontally compromised teeth or teeth that have been orthodontically repositioned and **B,** establishment of a cingulum rest seat to support an RPD on a tooth with unfavorable cingulum anatomy, e.g., a mandibular canine.

utilizing the acid-etch technique and a cast ... framework, J. Prosthet. Dent. **37:**28-31, 1977.

5. Dunn, B., Reisbick, M.H.: Adherence of ceramic coating on chromium-cobalt structures, J. Dent. Res. **55:**328, 1976.

6. Tanaka, T., Atsuta, M., Uchiyama, Y., and Kawashima, I.: Pitting corrosion for retaining acrylic resin facings, J. Prosthet. Dent. **42:**282, 1979.

7. Thompson, V.P., Livaditis, G.S., and Del-Castillo, E.: Resin bond to electrolytically etched nonprecious alloys for resin bonded prostheses, J. Dent. Res. (Special Issue A), (Abstr. No. 265), 1981.

8. Simonsen, R.J., Thompson, V., and Barrack, G.: Etched Cast Restorations: Clinical and Laboratory Techniques, Chicago, 1983, Quintessence Publishing Co.

9. Barrack, G.: Recent advances in etched cast restorations, J. Prosthet. Dent. **52:**619, 1984.

10. Caputo, A., and Standlee, P.: Biomechanics in Clinical Dentistry, Chicago, 1987, Quintessence Publishing Co., pp. 139-140.

11. Godoy, F., and Malone, W.F.P.: Effect of various etching times on two glass ionomer lining cements, Texas Dent. J. **104**(4):12, 1987.

BIBLIOGRAPHY

Bowen, R.L.: Synthesis of a silica-resin direct filling material, J. Dent. Res. **37:**90, 1958.

Brady, T., Doukoudakis, A., and Rasmussen, S.: Experimental comparison between perforated and etched-metal resin-bonded retainers, J. Prosthet. Dent. **54:**361, 1985.

Buonocore, M.G.: The use of adhesives in dentistry, Springfield, Ill., 1975, Charles C Thomas, Publisher.

De Castillo, E., and Thompson, V.P.: Electrolytically etched up alloys: resin bond and laboratory variables, J. Dent. Res. **61:**186, Special Issue (A).

Denehy, G.E.: Cast anterior bridges utilizing composite resin, Pediatr. Dent. **4:**44-47, 1982.

Doukoudakis, A., et al.: Direct bonded bridges, Oral Health **82:**29-31, 1982.

Eshleman, J.R., Moon, P.C., and Barnes, R.F.: Clinical evaluation of cast metal resin bonded anterior fixed partial dentures, J. Prosthet. Dent. **51:**761, 1984.

Gratton, D.R., Jordan, R.E., and Teteruck, W.R.: Resin-bonded bridges: the state of the art, Ont. Dent. **60:**9-19, 1983.

Highton, R., Caputo, A.A., and Matyas, J.: Retentive and stress characteristics for a magnetically retained partial denture, J. Dent. Res. **62:**680, 1983.

Janus, C.E. et al: The use of custom cast metal resin bonded cingulum rest seats under removable partial dentures, Compend. Cont. Ed. Dent. **6**(5):364, 1985.

Jordan, R.E., and Suzuki, M.: Temporary fixed partial dentures fabricated by means of acid-etch resin technique: a report of 86 cases followed up for three years, J.A.D.A. **96:**994-1001, 1981.

Leempael, P.J.B., Levensduur, en Nabehandelingen Van Kronen en Conventionele Bruggen in de Algemene Praktijk, Profechrift Nigmegen, 1987.

Livaditis, G.J.: Cast metal resin bonded retainers for posterior teeth, J.A.D.A. **101:**926, 1980.

Livaditis, G.J., and Thompson, V.P.: Etched castings: an improved retentive mechanism for resin-bonded retainers, J. Prosthet. Dent. **47:**52-58, 1982.

Malone, W.F.P., Godoy, F.G., Wolf, J., and Stewart, G.: Effect of various proportions of composite resin cement on bond strength of resin bonded prostheses. Submitted for Publication.

McLaughlin, G.: Composite bonding of etched metal anterior splints, Pediatr. Dent. **4:**38, 1982.

Nathanson, D., and Moin, K.: Metal-reinforced anterior tooth replacement using acid-etch composite resin technique, J. Prosthet. Dent. **43:**408-412, 1980.

Portnoy, L.: Constructing a composite pontic in a single visit, Dent. Surv. **49:**20-23, 1973.

Re, G., Kaiser, D.A., Malone, W.F.P., and Jones, Troy: Metal Conditioners for the resin bonded prosthesis, J. Prosthet. Dent. (in press).

Speiser, A.M., Levin, C.G., and Shulman, D.A.: In vitro comparison of bond strengths of three cements for resin bonded bridges, J. Dent. Res. **62:**462, 1983 (abstract).

Thayer, K.E., and Doukoudakis, A.: Acid-etch canine riser occlusal treatment, J. Prosthet. Dent. **46:**149, 1981.

Theobald, W.D., Duke, E.S., Norling, B.K., and Mayhew, R.D.: Bond strengths of various cements for resin bonded retainers, J. Dent. Res. **62:**458, 1983 (Abstract).

Thompson, V.P., and Livaditis, G.J.: Etched casting acid-etch composite bonded posterior bridges, Pediatr. Dent. **4:**38-43, 1982.

Young, K.C., Hussey, M., Gillespie, F.C., and Stephens, K.W.: In vitro studies of physical factors affecting adhesion of fissure sealant to enamel. In Silverstone, L.M., and Dragon, I.L., editors: Proceedings of the International Symposium on Acid Etch Technique, St. Paul, Minn., 1975, North Central Publishing, Sherry Co.

9

James D. Harrison and William J. Kelly, Jr.

TISSUE MANAGEMENT IN FIXED PROSTHODONTICS

There are several terms for the process of exposing margins when making impressions of prepared teeth. In this chapter, the term *tissue dilation* is synonymous with tissue retraction or displacement. Tissue management is the key factor in accurately duplicating subgingival margins.

In performing tissue dilation, the dentist must recognize the importance of using a regimented approach from diagnosis to cementation of the restorations. The gingival tissue should be healthy before restorative procedures begin, particularly with complete restorations that require a margin below the crest of the gingiva.[1]

TISSUE HEALTH

The rationale for tissue dilation does not originate with exposing gingival margins, since the health of the gingival tissues is crucial for success. Acceptable healthy gingival tissue is essential, as inflamed, redundant tissue is a liability to tissue dilation. Also, after impressions are made the tissue should be supported by appropriate treatment restorations on the newly prepared teeth (Fig. 9-1). Tissue shrinkage may occur after gingival margin placement or from irritation caused by treatment restorations.

In addition, patients receiving restorative procedures should be introduced to a regimented oral hygiene program. If gingival surgery was performed, the tissue should be mature before tooth preparation and tissue dilation. The healing of the gingival tissue after periodontal surgery varies, but a minimum of 3 to 5 weeks is recommended before preparation and tissue dilation.[2]

TISSUE DILATION

Classification

The classification for tissue dilation is as follows:
1. Mechanical—the tissue is displaced or dilated strictly by mechanical methods.
2. Mechanical-chemical—a cord is used for mechanically separating the tissue from the cavity margin and is impregnated with a chemical for hemostasis as impressions are made.
3. Surgical—a ribbon of gingival tissue is removed from the sulcus around the cavity margin with dental electrosurgery. This procedure creates a space in the tissue surrounding the tooth, controls seepage, and provides a trough for the impression material. Another method is gingitage—the literature has indicated successful exposure of the cavity margin with healing comparable to dental electrosurgery.[3] In this technique, special diamond stones remove the sulcus epithelium as the margins are finished beneath the crest of the gingiva (Fig. 9-2).

The cast metal preparations are constructed to minimize tissue laceration with subgingival margins. Tissue laceration can be reduced by avoiding subgingival margins and creating a sulcus space by dilation with the mechanical or mechanical-chemical method. The entire procedure is commonly repeated before making an additional impression. When using the surgical method, tissue dilation is not repeated. Only cleansing and spot coagulation to control bleeding in the created sulcus is necessary. Additionally, some dentists prefer to pack an astringent medicated cord into the surgical trough to control seepage.

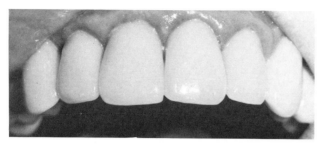

Fig. 9-1. Note healthy gingival tissue after placing treatment restorations.

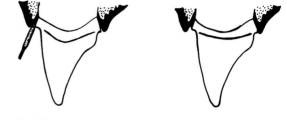

Fig. 9-2. Gingatage diamond refining margin and removing inner sulcur epithelium.

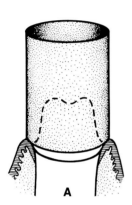
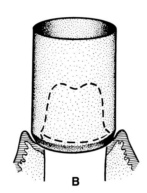

Fig. 9-3. A, Oversized copper band should be about 2.0 mm wider than the mesiodistal width of the tooth. **B,** The gingiva is trimmed and contoured inward to allow the band to just clear the preparation margin during the impression procedure.

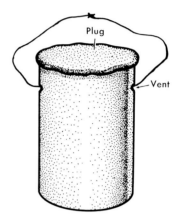

Fig. 9-4. Copper band with plug; vent with a loop of dental floss.

Elastomeric impression materials do not displace blood, saliva, debris, or tissue. The tissue therefore is displaced laterally, or a ribbon of tissue is removed to expose the cavity margin before the impressions. The tissue adjacent to the exposed cavity margin must also be reasonably dry and clean for accurate impressions.

Mechanical Tissue Dilation

Mechanical dilation is possible, but must be carefully performed to minimize trauma. Oversized copper bands are contoured to the gingiva and restricted toward the cavity margin when gently seated over the tooth (Fig. 9-3). A resin or compound plug is placed on the top for stability, and the band is vented for escape of excess elastomeric impression materials. A loop of dental floss is threaded through the vent to ease band removal after the impression material has set (Fig. 9-4).

The dentist must not exert excessive pressure on the band, or the tissue may be stripped from the tooth. Since tissue dilation can be accomplished effectively by other methods, mechanical dilation has limited application, but is a superb method to confirm gingival margins, ie., multiple abutment, full arch impressions with one or two questionable margins.

Mechanical Chemical Dilation

Mechanical chemical dilation consists of cords impregnated with chemicals that are eased into the intracrevicular space beneath the cavity margin without force (Fig. 9-5). The area must be kept dry but not dessicated if the hemostatic chemical in the cord is to have maximum effectiveness. After 5 to 10 minutes, the cord is gently removed and the sulcus surrounding the cavity margin is exposed and hemostasis maintained.

If bleeding is still evident, the crevice is repacked for an additional 5 minutes. If the area has been isolated with cotton rolls, the packed cord is damped before removal, as occasionally a dry cord adheres to the sealed capillaries and, on removal, causes bleeding. Subgingivally, the packing instrument is directed toward the area where the cord is already secure. Pushing away from the area previously retracted dislodges the cord.[4]

Cords impregnated with alum or aluminum chloride provide a styptic action to control seepage. Hemostatic agents like epinephrine are not recommended in patients with cardiac problems.[5-6]

Surgical Tissue Dilation

Continuous visualization of the subgingival margin is difficult for the dentist. Cords, chemicals, rubber

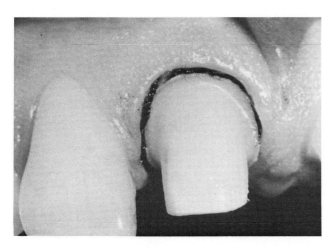

Fig. 9-5. Braided cord tucked into the gingival sulcus.

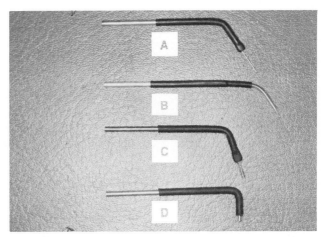

Fig. 9-6. Electrodes of choice. **A,** Straight wire. **B,** Varitip. **C,** Small continuous loop. **D,** A.P. 1½.

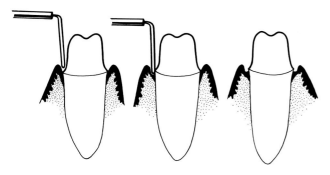

Fig. 9-7. A, Small loop electrode. **B,** Electrode in position beneath preparation margin. **C,** Subgingival tissue trough 0.3 to 0.5 mm beneath margin.

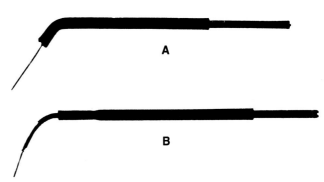

Fig. 9-8. A, Straight wire electrode. **B,** Varitip electrode.

or leather rings, copper, stainless steel and aluminum bands with other materials have been suggested for this purpose.[7-8] With refinement of dental electrosurgery, many of the problems of securing impressions of multiple abutment preparation can be alleviated.[9,10]

Electrosurgery requires profound local anesthesia. Odor is controlled by an outside ventilated oral evacuator system. Plastic suction tips are used, since momentary contact of an activated working electrode with a metal aspirator tip causes spot coagulation wherever the metal touches the tissue. For the same reason, plastic mounted mouth mirrors are indicated. The passive or indifferent plate is positioned under the patient's shoulder for biterminal application. Monoterminal application is rare.

CURRENTS AND ELECTRODE SELECTION

The current for subgingival margin exposure is acusection. Selection of electrodes varies, depending on the tooth and its arch position. These procedures can be performed without patient discomfort in a relatively bloodless field. With each electrode, the basics of electrosurgery are sustained. The working electrode

must be clean and without carbonization. In exacting marginal dilation, a carbonized electrode has a tendency to drag, tearing the tissue and causing bleeding. If a straight wire tip, varitip, or minute continuous-loop electrode is used, they should be cleaned between each application (Fig. 9-6).

The depth of tissue removal is determined by the morphology of the tissue and the biologic width. The tissue trough should extend about 0.3 to 0.5 mm below the margin of the cast restoration for definite margin detection in the impression and on the master dies. Fig. 9-7 illustrates a subgingival trough with a continuous-loop electrode. When using a continuous-loop there is usually a small amount of tissue left beneath the margin because of the shape of the loop. This tissue tag is removed using a single-wire or variable-tip electrode (Fig. 9-8). The variable-tip electrode wire can be adjusted to the desired length. Fig. 9-9 illustrates electrosurgical tissue dilation on a premolar tooth preparation using a continuous-loop electrode. The troughing procedure is pressureless, and if additional tissue refinement is required, a time lapse of at least 5 seconds is needed to dissipate heat.

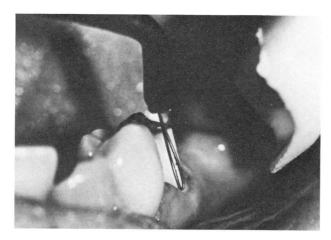

Fig. 9-9. A, Premolar veneer crown preparation before troughing.

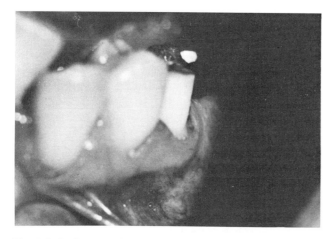

Fig. 9-9. B, Small loop electrode for tissue dilation.

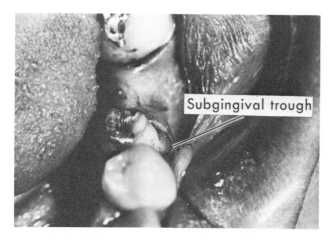

Fig. 9-9. C, Subgingival trough after electrosection.

Posner Electrode

With the AP 1½ electrode, the insulated portion of the electrode is directed around the tooth, removing the gingival sulcular epithelium (Fig. 9-10). The 1½ designation of the AP 1½ electrode indicates that the working tip extends 1½ mm beyond the insulation. This offers a precise, uniform 1½ mm sulcus depth incision. If less trough depth is desired, part of the tip is removed to create the desired depth at 0.5 mm, 0.75 mm, or 1.0 mm.

Electrode Tip

Variable-tip or straight-wire electrodes are popular. Tooth preparation with the desired margin is completed, and margins are terminated above the soft tissue. The single wire of the variable tip is adjusted to the desired subgingival depth, and the tooth is then circumscribed by repeated approaches around the tooth in segments. First the lingual subgingival trough; then the facial surface; and then the mesial and distal surfaces are established (Fig. 9-11). This prevents heat accumulation in the tissue. For most dentists, it is virtually impossible to circumscribe a tooth with one or two connecting passes. If a straight-wire electrode or the variable-tip electrode is used, the operator may find that the electrode is too fine to remove enough tissue to provide adequate bulk of impression material in the sulcus. This is especially true if the end of the working electrode is positioned parallel with the long axis of the tooth. By angling the working electrode at approximately 15 to 20 degrees and carrying the tip through the tissue until it rests against the tooth, a small wedge of tissue can be removed (Fig. 9-12). If bleeding occurs, it is usually interproximal and controlled with the same electrode using a coagulation current (Fig. 9-13 to Fig. 9-17).

Another method uses equal parts of hydrogen peroxide and water to arrest slight local hemorrhage. After the area is dry, the extended sulcus is debris free and the root and crown easily visualized. The margins can then be finished to the desired depth, the area again flushed with water and peroxide and the impressions secured.

In the anterior quadrants where the gingiva is especially thin, the angle of the working electrode is changed to be more nearly parallel to the long axis of the tooth. Again with the segmented approach, the sulcular epithelium is removed, and if a narrow facial-lingual sulcus has been created, the cord is placed before the impression to retract the tissue away from the tooth. It is axiomatic that the treatment restoration be suitably adapted to the existing margins without luting material impinging on the regenerating sulcular epithelium.

Dental impressions ideally extend 0.3 to 0.5 mm

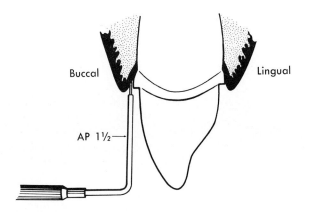

Fig. 9-10. Buccolingual view illustrating the use of AP 1½ for tissue dilation.

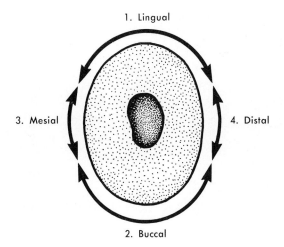

Fig. 9-11. Recommended sequence 1 to 4 to establish subgingival trough.

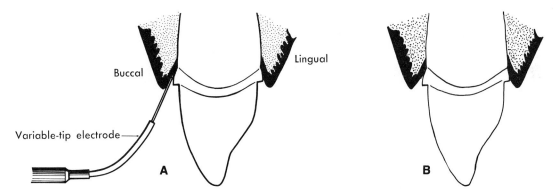

Fig. 9-12. A, Buccolingual view illustrating use of variable-tip electrode for tissue dilation. **B,** Subgingival tissue trough in buccal sulcus.

below the cavity margin to ensure accuracy. Electrosurgical removal of a ribbon of tissue around the cavity margin provides necessary space for adequate bulk of the elastic impression material.

After securing the final impression or impressions, tincture of myrrh and benzoin (Oringer's solution) is placed on the surgical area and air dried; this procedure is repeated three to five times before the treatment restoration is placed. Orabase may replace or supplement myrrh and benzoin in this procedure (Table 9-1). The tissue healing is rapid, and the subgingival trough heals in 5 to 7 days.[11] Table 9-2 lists the electrosurgical currents with indications. Fig. 9-18 provides an image of the tissue involvement of any electrode tip.

Discipline is imperative to the uneventful exposure of the cavity margin for making impressions for cast restorations. Tissue trauma, expenditure of time, and the shrinkage of tissue restricts traditional mechanical tissue dilation.

The mechanical-chemical method with cords can reduce trauma to the tissue but may produce a thin layer of impression material at the cavity margin once the cord is removed, since the tissue returns immediately to its original position. If a thin layer of impression material persists, marginal distortion of the individual dies results because of insufficient material in a critical area.

Dental electrosurgery provides a rapid, efficient method for tissue dilation, with adequate impression material in crucial areas. It does <u>not</u> cause significant shrinkage of the tissue or patient discomfort if appropriate post operative medication is used.

The key factors for successful electrosurgery are: profound anesthesia; appropriate current selection; a light stroke with a 5 second time interval between applications of the electrode; and maintaining the biologic width after tissue healing.

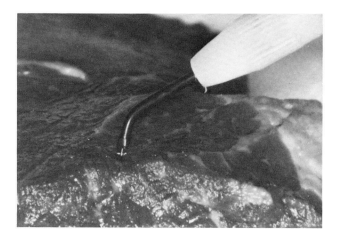

Fig. 9-13. Desiccation current.

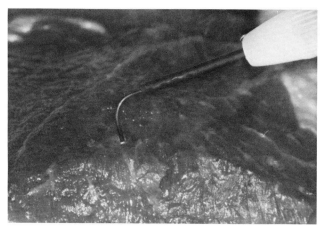

Fig. 9-14. A, Coagulation current—showing the use of a small ball electrode.

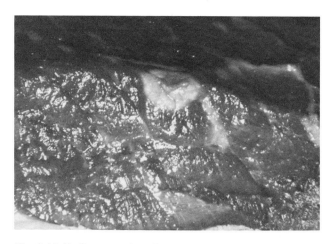

Fig. 9-14. B, Cross section where excessive coagulation current has been demonstrated.

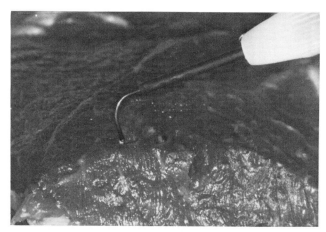

Fig. 9-15. Electrode remains above tissue.

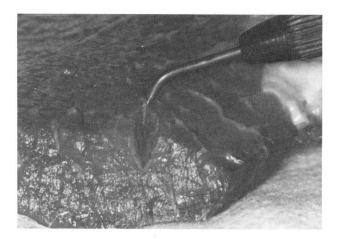

Fig. 9-16. A, Electrosection demonstrating a moderately deep incision.

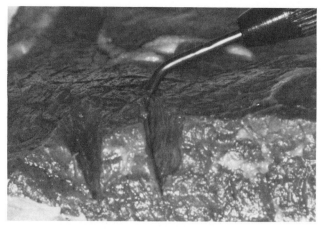

Fig. 9-16. B, Electrosection demonstrating two parallel deep incisions. Note the lack of coagulation at edges of the incision.

A
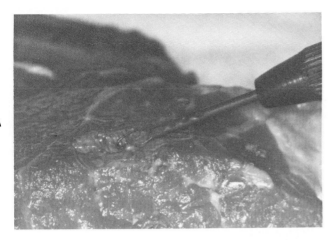
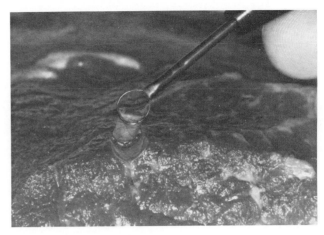
B

Fig. 9-17. A and **B,** Electrosection to plan tissues—large loop.

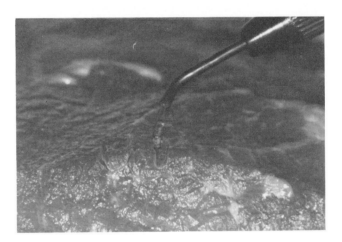

Fig. 9-17. C, Electrosection to plan tissue—narrow loop.

Table 9-1. Electrosurgical postoperative treatment

Product	Distributor	Active ingredient	Indication
Coracaine	Coralite Dental Products, Skokie, IL	Benzocaine	Superficial tissue displacement with Rx restorations or denture sores
Orabase	Hoyt Laboratory	Benzocaine	Multiple preparations within the intracrevicular space; dabbed on the tissue adjacent to treatment restorations
Ora 5	McHenry Laboratories, Colgate Palmolive, Needham, MA 02194	Iodine and copper sulfate, etc.	Routine restorative tissue management denture sores; 2 minutes on dried tissue
Oringer's solution	Local drug store	Mixture of 2 oz. of tincture of benzoin and 2 oz. myrrh	Routine electrosurgical use; apply repeatedly (3×) to dried surgical area
Coe-pak Tube 1 Tube 2	Coe Laboratories, Inc., Chicago, IL	Bithionol Chlorothymol	Minor oral surgery and periodontal procedures
Kirkland formula powder and liquid	Drug store or dental supply company	ZnO	Extensive periodontal or oral surgical procedures
Antibiotics	Drug store prescription—Systemic	V-cillin K, 250 mg of #20, q.i.d., for 5 days	Oral surgery and extensive periodontal surgery
	Topical	Triamcinolone acetonide ointment 17, 3× daily p.c. and at bedtime	

After Malone, W.F.P., and Kelly, W.: Electrosurgery in Dentistry, Dent. Clin. North Am. 26:851 1982

Table 9-2. Electrosurgical currents

Dessication (Fig. 9-13)

Monterminal current
1800° heat generation
Deeply penetrating
Not frequently used
When used: Fistulous tracts
Hemorrhage
Set machine on 6-coagulate.
  No indifferent plate.
  Setting is dessication does not occur.
  Plunged electrode in tissue.
  Use wire electrode.

Fulgeration (Fig. 9-15)

Monterminal current
Tip remains above tissue
  Current sparks to tissue and carbonizes the area along with dehydration.
When used: Fistulous tracts
Ulcerated surfaces
Papillomas
Undesirable tissue tags
Hemorrhage
Set machine on 2
Use same electrode as for dessication.
Activate electrode ⅛ inch above tissue.
Spray tissue surface with sparks in a circular motion until surface is blackened or carbonized.
Increase current if necessary.

Coagulation (Fig. 9-14)

Biterminal current
Use conductive plate.
Use conductive plate.
When used: Hemostasis
Coagulating ulcerative surfaces
To destroy necrotic tissue
To remove granulation tissue
Depth controlled by number of times the electrode contacts the tissue
Set machine on 3-5
  Use ball or bar electrode.

Electrosection (Fig. 9-16)

Biterminal current
Electrode held at right angles to cut surface.
Use tip of electrode.
Plan cut and carry through in one pressureless motion when possible.
When used: Cutting incisions Fig. 9-16
Gingival troughing Fig. 9-9
Planing tissue Fig. 9-17
Set machine on 2-4
  Low current = tissue adherence
  Too high = charring (browned surface)
  Settings vary with units, tissue resistance, size of electrode

---

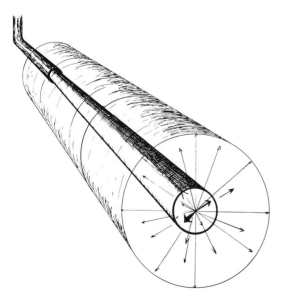

Fig. 9-18. Electrode tip with projected tissue involvement when activated. (Courtesy Dr. A.T. Young, Westchester, Ill.)

SELECTED REFERENCES

1. Porter, Z.C., and Malone, W.F.P.: Tissue Management, Littleton, Mass., 1982, P.S.G. Publishers.
2. Carranza, F.A.: Glickman Clinical Periodontology, ed. 6, Philadelphia, 1979, W.B. Saunders Co., pp. 788-789.
3. De Vitre, R., Golburt, R.B., and Maness, W.J.: Biometric comparison of bur and electrosurgical retraction method, J. Prosthetic Dent. 53(2):179-182, 1985.
4. Schillingburg, H.T., Hobo, S., and Whitsett, L.D.: Fundamentals of Fixed Prosthodontics, ed. 2, Chicago, Ill., 1981, Quintessence Publishing Co., pp. 200-203.
5. Harrison, James D.: Effect of retraction materials on the gingival sulcus epithelium, J. Prosthetic Dent. 11:514, May-June 1961.
6. Harrison, James D.: Current Therapy in Dentistry, Vol. I, St. Louis, 1964, The C.V. Mosby Co., pp. 193-195.
7. Tylman, Stanley D.: Theory and Practice of Crown and Fixed Partial Prosthodontics (bridge), ed. 6, St. Louis, 1978, The C.V. Mosby Co., pp. 403-410.
8. Johnston, John F., Phillips, Ralph W., and Dyjema, Roland W.: Modern Practice in Crown and Bridge Prosthodontics, ed. 3, Philadelphia, 1971, W.B. Saunders Co., pp. 183-190.
9. Kelly, W.J., and Harrison, J.D.: Tissue dilation during multiple case restorative procedures, Den. Clin. North Am. 26(4):759-780, 1982.
10. Oringer, M.J.: Electrosurgery in Dentistry, ed. 2, Philadelphia, 1975, W.B. Saunders Co., pp. 419-452.
11. Harrison, J.D., and Kelly, W.J.: Tissue response to electrosurgery. In Malone, W.F.P., editor: Electrosurgery in Dentistry, Springfield, Ill., 1975, Charles C Thomas, Publisher, pp. 186-206.

10

Ernst Schelb and Barry K. Norling

IMPRESSION MATERIALS AND TECHNIQUES

Historically, various materials have been used to make impressions for fixed prosthodontics. Early materials included rigid and semirigid compositions such as plaster, zinc oxide–eugenol, compound, and waxes; these materials still have limited uses in dentistry. However, current fixed prosthodontic impressions are the domain of the elastic materials, including reversible hydrocolloid and four types of synthetic elastomers.

IDEAL IMPRESSION MATERIAL

The fabrication of a casting requires an impression material that produces an accurate negative likeness of the oral tissues. The properties of the ideal impression are:

1. Complete plasticity before cure
2. Sufficient fluidity to record fine detail
3. The ability to wet the oral tissues
4. Dimensional accuracy
5. Dimensional stability
6. Complete elasticity after cure
7. Optimal stiffness

The material should be completely plastic both before and after curing so that the impression can be seated without undergoing elastic deformation and be recovered without distortion on removal of the impression. Both fluidity and the ability to wet the oral tissues are required to ensure that the impression replicates the fine details of the preparations. Dimensional accuracy implies absence of dimensional change (shrinkage) during curing. Dimensional stability is required so that the impression can be transported to the laboratory before pouring without dimensional changes. Removal from undercuts in the mouth, or removal of multiple dies or models should not produce any plastic deformation in the cured impression. The impression should be sufficiently flexible to permit ready removal over undercuts, but not so pliable that

it deforms under its weight or the weight of poured die material.

Although these properties relate to the crucial accuracy of the impression, other requirements of the impression exert an influence on clinical acceptability. The ideal material should:

1. Have an infinite shelf life
2. Need no armamentarium
3. Be nontoxic and nonirritating
4. Have acceptable odor, taste, and color
5. Have suitable working and setting times
6. Have strength to resist tearing
7. Be compatible with model and die materials
8. Be inexpensive
9. Be easy to dispense, proportion, and mix
10. Be easy to clean up
11. Facilitate visualization of the finish line
12. Permit multiple die pours
13. Facilitate the clinical identification of beginning and end of cure

Compatibility with model and die materials is commonly overlooked and include a number of factors. Hydrocolloid materials interfere with the setting of gypsum materials and produce a chalky surface with inferior detail. The elastomers exhibit varying degrees of compatibilities with different die stones evidenced by differences in fine detail. Epoxy die materials adhere strongly to all of the elastomers except the silicones.

None of the available elastic impression materials possess all of the ideal properties. In some cases, the deviations from the ideal of one property may influence the desirability of another. For example, high tear strength and elasticity are properties of the ideal material. The polysulfide materials exhibit poor elasticity and tend to distort on withdrawal from severe undercuts. However, these materials have high tear strength. The ability to be withdrawn from a severe undercut without tearing is a disadvantage, as tearing provides a warning that the material has experienced severe strain with accompanying plastic deformation. Specific deviations from ideal are addressed in the discussion of the elastic impression materials.

REVERSIBLE HYDROCOLLOID

Reversible hydrocolloid (synonyms: agar hydrocolloid, hydrocolloid, agar-agar) is a polysaccharide derived from seaweed. The material is supplied by the manufacturer as a preformed gel that is liquified before use. The forms available are bulk-packaged cylinders and unit packages, including collapsible tubes, carpules, and "sausages." Before use, the material is subjected to a controlled regimen with three water baths. The hydrocolloid conditioning includes a boiling water bath to liquify the hydrocolloid, a second bath for storing the material at 63 to 66 degrees Celsius and a bath for tempering the material at 44 to 46 degrees Celsius. A day's supply is first liquified by boiling and then transferred to the storage bath. Immediately before use, the material is placed in the tempering bath for about 10 minutes to reduce the temperature so that it is tolerated by the tissues.

The liquified hydrocolloid (sol) reverts to the gel upon cooling. Hence, the material is called "reversible" to distinguish it from alginate (irreversible) hydrocolloid, which gels by a chemical reaction. The alginates are incapable of sufficiently detailed reproduction for fixed prosthodontics, although they are routinely used for RPDs.

Trays for reversible hydrocolloid impressions have integral cooling water channels that accelerate gelation. Gelation occurs from the tray toward the tissues. The last portion of material to gel contacts the tissues, so any shrinkage accompanying gelation is compensated for. The hydrocolloids thus have excellent dimensional accuracy.

Because the material is approximately 85 percent water, however, dimensional stability is severely limited by evaporation. The agar hydrocolloids also undergo two other processes that limit dimensional stability. If the impression is immersed in water to avoid evaporation, the gel will imbibe water and swell; while attempts to avoid evaporation by wrapping the impressions in moist towels or storing them in humidors are of limited effectiveness. Even without alteration of water content, the forces that draw the agar molecules to form the gel continue to act after gelation, tending to force water with dissolved materials from the gel. This syneretic exudate is accompanied by shrinkage of the impression.

The combined effects of evaporation, imbibition, and syneresis are so deleterious that the impression must be poured immediately to avoid distortion. Brief exposure to water to remove blood and saliva or dipping in a "fixing" bath does not substantially alter the dimensional accuracy. A fixing bath is a dilute solution (2 percent) of potassium sulfate that compensates for the agar's tendency to retard the setting of gypsum model and die materials.

ELASTOMERIC IMPRESSION MATERIALS

The elastomeric impression materials include the polysulfide rubbers, condensation silicones, polyethers, and polyvinyl siloxanes. The chemical category is identified by the manufacturer on the package. In addition, the materials are also categorized as defined by the American Dental Association specification for elastomeric materials. While the technical details of the ADA specification are not covered here, certain classifications used in that specification should be understood to aid in material selection. The ADA specification categorizes all elastomers according to physical properties rather than chemistry. Limits on three critical properties—compression set, flow, and 24 hour dimensional change—define the type stated on the package.

The limits set are listed in Table 10-1. Compression set is related to the tendency of a material to remain deformed after a relatively rapid deformation. Type III materials experience more than twice the deformation of the other classes. Flow is related to the continuing deformation under long-term loads (as under the weight of the gypsum product before it sets). Type III materials may undergo four times the flow of materials in the other two classes. For dimensional change in 24 hours, type II materials are permitted twice the shrinkage of the other classes.

The significance of these classifications stems from the fact that impression materials of the same chemistry may be different depending on critical physical properties. For example, polysulfide elastomers are type I or type III, depending on the compression set. If large deformations are anticipated to result from withdrawal over exaggerated undercuts, a type I material experiences less distortion.

The specification also categorizes the materials according to four viscosities: very high, high, medium, and low. The selection of the appropriate viscosity depends on the specific impression method.

Table 10-1. ADA requirements for elastomeric impression materials*

Type	Maximum % compression set	Maximum % flow	Maximum % shrinkage (24 hr)
I	2.5	0.5	0.5
II	2.5	0.5	1.0
III	5.5	2.0	0.5

*Revised American Dental Association specification No. 19 for nonaqueous, elastomeric impression materials, J.A.D.A. **94:**733-741, 1977.

Polysulfide Rubber

The curing reaction of polysulfide rubber (synonyms: rubber base, mercaptan, thiokol rubber) involves the condensation of a thiol (-SH) terminated prepolymer by reaction with lead peroxide, copper hydroxide, or an organic peroxide and a sulfur coreactant to form disulfide linkages. The prepolymer contains more than two thiols per molecule to effect a cross-linked elastomer. The common reactant, lead peroxide, is dark brown, and produces a chocolate brown elastomer. Pastel green material results from substitution of copper hydroxide for lead peroxide. Virtually any desired color may be achieved by using an organic peroxide; however, excess organic peroxide evaporates after cure, decreasing dimensional stability.

Water and lead sulfide are byproducts of the curing reaction; water is also an accelerator. The elastomer is autoaccelerated, so once the cure reaction begins, it continues at an ever increasing rate. Water added intentionally or inadvertently (e.g., by absorption from humid air) speeds curing.

Loss of the water during the reaction and continuation of the curing reaction are the two principal limitations to dimensional stability of the polysulfide elastomers. The resulting dimensional changes are appreciable, so the impressions should be poured immediately after removal from the mouth. The polysulfides exhibit a slow elastic recovery when removed over deep undercuts. While it has been suggested that a programmed delay in pouring casts is advisable to allow for this recovery, the time required to position dowel pins or mix the gypsum product and the time required for the gypsum slurry to develop flow resistance are more than sufficient.

Condensation Silicone

The curing reaction of the condensation silicone (synonyms: silicone, polysiloxane) elastomers involves cross-linking of hydroxy (-OH) terminated linear poly(dimethylsiloxane) prepolymer with a trifunctional or tetrafunctional alkyl silicate or organo hydrogen siloxane. Both reactants are contained in the base paste. The reaction is catalyzed with an organometal compound, usually dibutyltin dilaurate. Regardless of the coreactant used with the prepolymer, a volatile byproduct is produced during the curing reaction. The byproduct is most commonly ethyl alcohol. Loss of the byproduct through evaporation accounts for most of the dimensional instability.

Because the accelerator is a true catalyst for the reaction, a wide latitude in base-catalyst ratios is permitted, and curing times may be adjusted over a broad range. However, the manufacturers' specified ranges should be followed to avoid complete failure of cure or uneven cure throughout the bulk of the impression.

Besides the viscosities common to the polysulfides, the condensation silicones are also supplied in an extremely high viscosity or putty material. These putties are used in the putty-wash techniques.

Polyether

The polyethers (synonym: epimine) cure through cross-linking of a difunctional epimine terminated prepolymer catalyzed by an alkyl benzene sulfonate catalyst. The reaction involves ring opening without formation of volatile byproducts. Thus, long-term dimensional stability is superior, although short-term (curing) dimensional changes approximate those of the polysulfides. The catalyst can be a sensitizer; patients who develop a sensitivity (allergic reaction) to the polyethers should avoid further contact.

The polyethers are not available in a complete range of viscosities. Regardless of brand, the original polyethers were the stiffest of the elastomers when cured, so the removal from undercuts was impeded, as was removal of the dies or casts. Some manufacturers supply a thinner that reduces the stiffness of the cured elastomer and prolongs the working and curing times. Unmodified, these materials have short working and curing times.

Recently introduced polyethers have been modified to greatly reduce the stiffness. These materials are identifiable by the addition of letters following the brand name (e.g., F for flexible). The newer materials are much easier to remove from undercuts and less traumatic for patients who are periodontally compromised. The reduced stiffness is not, however, an unmixed blessing. The flexible plastic trays used in the closed bite technique depend on the rigidity of the impression material to limit distortion. It is unclear whether the newer flexible polyethers are suitable for this technique. Because of their wettability, the polyethers are least likely to result in air bubble entrapment during pouring of the model or die; however, newer formulations are not quite as wettable as their predecessors.

Poly(vinylsiloxanes)

The backbone of the prepolymer of the addition silicones is a poly(dimethylsiloxane) (synonyms: addition silicones, vinyl(polysiloxanes). The materials are supplied as equal volumes of two prepolymers, one with terminal vinyl groups and the other with terminal hydrogens. A chloroplatinic acid ester catalyst catalyzes an addition reaction between terminal groups without volatile products. The equation elements are:

$$-N\begin{cases} CH_2 \\ | \\ CH_2 \end{cases}$$

Table 10-2. Comparison of elastomeric impression materials

	Polysulfide	Condensation silicone	Polyether	Poly(vinylsiloxane)
Representative brands	*Coe-Flex*	*Accoe*	*Impregum F*	*Express-H*
	Neo-Plex	*Cutter Sil*	*Permadyne*	*Mirror 3*
	Permlastic	*Xantopren*	*Polygel*	*Reprosil*
Working time	Medium-v. long	Short-medium	Short-medium	Short-medium
Curing time	Long	Medium-long	Medium	Short-long
Tear resistance	High	Low	Medium	Low
Stiffness	Medium-low	High-low	High[1]	Medium-high
Elastic recovery	Poor	Good	Fair	Excellent
Dimensional accuracy	Good	Fair	Good	Excellent
Dimensional stability	Fair	Poor	Good	Excellent
Flow after setting	High	Low	Low	Low
Esthetics (odor, taste, color)	Poor	Excellent	Fair	Excellent
Ease of cast pouring	Good	Fair	Excellent	Poor[2]
Time to cast pouring	Immediately	Immediately	1 Week	1 Week[3]
Shelf life	Fair	Poor	Excellent	Fair
Cost per impression	Medium	Low	Very high	High

1. Recently introduced polyethers are more flexible than the original materials and are rated medium.
2. Newer polyvinylsiloxanes identified as hydrophilic range in model pouring ease from equivalent to polyethers or polysulfides.
3. Polyvinylsiloxanes without hydrogen absorbers should not be poured immediately. Delays of 1 to 24 hours are recommended with stone dies; at least 24 hours with the slower-setting epoxy materials.

The poly(vinylsiloxanes) are characterized by excellent dimensional accuracy and long-term dimensional stability; however, they are inherently difficult to wet, making it difficult to pour a bubble-free cast. Newer materials have been modified for improved wettability and are appropriately identified.

Bubbles may also arise at the impression-elastomer interface because of hydrogen gas that evolves from the material during and after cure as the result of a side reaction not related to curing. For materials evolving hydrogen, delayed pouring from 1 to 24 hours may be required. Newer materials contain finely divided palladium as a hydrogen absorber and are poured immediately. This modification is not usually identified on the package but must be inferred from the pouring directions.

Early tray adhesives supplied with the poly(vinylsiloxanes) were ineffective. Acrylic trays required auxiliary retention (perforations). The newer adhesives are superior, but if problems with adhesion occur, perforations or a change of brand are indicated.

Working times vary from 2 to 4 minutes, although there are substantial differences among brands. Stiffness has been high, according to ADA test results. These results are skewed in comparison with other materials because of the lack of flow in the poly(vinylsiloxanes); any flow in the test makes the stiffness appear lower. The poly(vinylsiloxanes) are not as stiff as the original polyethers and consequently are not suited to the closed bite impression technique. However, newer materials have been specifically developed with increased stiffness for this technique. These stiffer poly(vinylsiloxanes) are the materials of choice for the closed bite technique (Table 10-2).

The polyvinylsiloxanes are supplied in the usual ranges of viscosities. Some brands exhibit shear thinning, so that the same viscosity material may be used for both tray loading and syringing.

TECHNIQUES

A variety of techniques have evolved over time. Selection of the specific technique depends on experience and an evaluation of an individual patient. Time, expense, and accuracy must all be considered in making the selection. In addition, the patient may dictate modifications in procedures. The following sections detail stepwise procedures. In all of the following technique steps, an asterisk indicates steps frequently delegated to the dental assistant. (Note: See Table 10-3 for impression technique guide.) As a general rule, an appropriate disinfection protocol should be followed after impression removal from the mouth.

Stock Tray

Synonyms: Putty wash
Mixing Method: Double mix and single mix
In the following description, the putty-wash technique is described. It should be recognized that stock trays can also be used with medium and heavy-bodied elastomers normally used with custom trays. The larger bulk of material normally required with a stock tray requires that the bulk material be precured, as in the putty-wash technique, or that the material not be subject to curing shrinkage. If a single mix technique is anticipated with a stock tray, the poly(vinylsiloxanes) are used.

Table 10-3. Impression technique guide

Tray	Mixing method	Impression material*	Sequence	Step(s)
Stock (putty wash)	Double	PVS, PS, CS	1	1-58
			2	Skip 59
			3	60--85
Stock (putty wash)	Single	PVS	1	1-5
			2	18-51
			3	6-8
			4	52-57
			5	Skip 58
			6	59-85
Custom	Single	PVS, PE, PS, CS	1	1-49
Closed bite	Single	PVS, PE	1	1-63
Double arch				
Copper tube	Single	PVS	1	1-33

*PVS = poly(vinylsiloxane); PS = polysulfide; CS = condensation silicone; PE = polyether.

Advantages:

1. Eliminates time and expense of fabricating custom tray.
2. Metal stock trays are rigid and are not susceptible to distortion.

Disadvantages:

1. More impression material is required.
2. Metal trays must be sterilized.

Technique:

1. Place patient in supine position.
2. Position operator at 9 o'clock position and assistant at 3 o'clock position.

Choosing correct tray:

3. Select tray type based on relative need for retention and personal preference (Fig. 10-1).
4. Select tray shape and size based on patient's arch shape and size.

Preparing stock tray for final impression:

5. Coat the tray evenly with adhesive on the inside and rim (Fig. 10-2).
   NOTE: If using stock tray technique (putty wash) with single mix method, refer to Stock Tray steps 18 through 52.
6. Mix the high-viscosity putty impression material according to manufacturer's instructions (Fig. 10-3).
7. Roll putty into elongated cylinder.
8. Insert into the stock impression tray.
9. Cover putty with the manufacturer's spacer (a sheet of polyethylene) (Fig. 10-4).
10. Insert and seat the tray with a rocking type motion.
11. Hold and wait until initial set (approximately 2 minutes).
12. Remove from the mouth with minimal sideward movement.
13. Wait and test for final set with the "clinical final set test," i.e., when a fingernail impression rebounds completely.

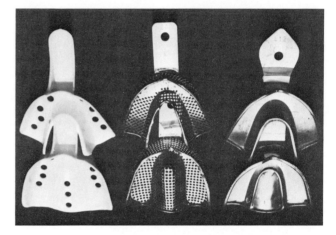

Fig. 10-1. Various type of trays are available: Plastic/perforated stock trays (left); Coe metal perforated trays (center); and Caulk's rim lock trays (right).

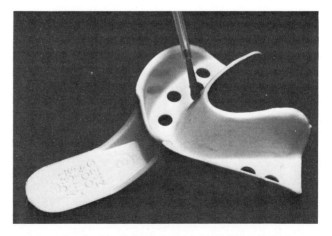

Fig. 10-2. Adhesives are necessary for most elastomers, and excessive amounts can distort the impression but are specific for each material.

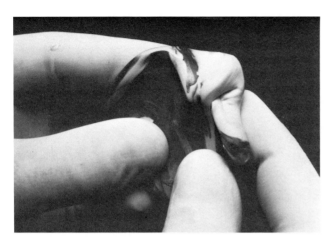

Fig. 10-3. The putty impression material is hard mixed with rapid finger movements. Some materials require glove removal.

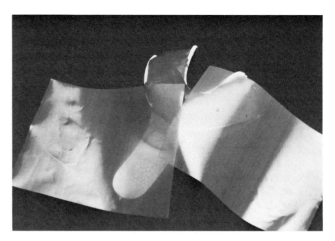

Fig. 10-4. A sheet of polyethylene over the putty impression.

14. Peel off the spacer.
15. Remove excess impression material with a sharp knife.
16. If additional relief is needed, remove more impression material (e.g., with a sharp hand instrument or acrylic bur).
17. Set tray aside.

Gingival displacement and management:

18. Isolate areas(s) to be impressed with cotton rolls and dry preparation(s) with short bursts of compressed air. The sulcus should be dry, but do not desiccate the dentin.
19. Choose a braided cord to prevent unwinding during placement.
20. Choose the diameter of cord(s) to push the tissue aside and physically enlarge the sulcular space by measuring the sulcus depth and width with a periodontal probe.
21. Note the subgingival areas of the finish line that need tissue displacement.
22. Cut approximately 1 to 1¼ inch of cord.
23. Choose a dull, blunted packing instrument with a width that fits comfortably into the sulcus.
24. Wrap the cord around the tooth and from the buccal, grasp the two ends with your thumb and forefinger.
25. Slide the cord down toward the sulcus.
26. Choose the mesiofacial or distal facial line angle to gently pack 1 mm of cord into the sulcus. This holds the cord in place to facilitate further sulcular displacement.
27. Continue packing the proximal sulcus and proceed toward the lingual, <u>not</u> facial surface.
28. Continue around the lingual toward the opposite proximal surface.
29. Control the buccal ends of the cord while pushing the cord with a hand instrument toward the tooth. Then roll it into the sulcus while pushing toward the already packed cord. This prevents the cord from being displaced. Observe the gingiva being displaced laterally from the tooth. Do not push the cord down apically; this strips the attached gingiva.
30. Determine the final length of the cord and allow 1 mm overlap plus 2 mm excess for uncomplicated removal.
31. Cut the cord with sharp scissors to prevent tugging on the cord.
32. Complete the packing at the facial surface. This varies according to the position of the finish line, supragingival or subgingival.
33. Evaluate tissue displacement; if you cannot see the finish line in a certain area(s), then additional cord(s) with increasing diameter is/are indicated.
34. Use alum (aluminum sulfate) to control seepage of fluids from the walls of the gingival sulcus. If the gingival sulcus is healthy and not lacerated, this medicament is sufficient.
35. Use epinephrine (8 percent) to control minor hemorrhage, but do not use on patients with lacerated tissue, cardiovascular disease, diabetes, or hyperthyroidism. Consult a current Physicians' Desk Reference (PDR) for drug contraindications.
36. If no medicaments are applied to the dry cord, then slightly moisten the cord with water. This will help prevent its sticking to the sulcular tissue upon removal.
37. If inflammation is present and seepage cannot be controlled, remove the cord and repeat steps 18 through 36 or use electrosection (acusection).
38. If inflammation is present and seepage cannot be controlled, then verify the temporary restoration's fit and surface texture. Cement the

provisional and allow gingival healing before making another impression.

39. Observe the finish line. If you cannot see all areas of the finish line, return to step 18. If you can see at least 0.5 mm below the finish line, continue.

40. Leave cord(s) in place for 8 to 10 minutes. While the cord is displacing the gingiva, it is compressing the blood vessels. Prolonged retention can cause belated gingival sloughing and migration.

41. Block out undercuts around the teeth in the arch with red rope wax. The tissue is dry but not dehydrated when applying the wax. This facilitates impression removal, reduces distortion, and averts tearing.

Prepare syringe:

42. Lubricate syringe "O"-ring lightly.

43. Trim tip. Open orifice to increase rate of flow or close orifice to decrease rate of flow. Orifice must be smooth and without cracks.

44. Measure arch length of tray to guide in dispensing the amount of elastomer (Fig. 10-5). RULE: Dispense one times the length of the tray for the low-viscosity elastomer (syringable).

Making final impression:

45. *Choose a large mixing pad, approximately 6 by 8 inches. Some brands of impression material have mixing devices that resemble a caulking gun and do not need a mixing pad. These dispense material by placing a replaceable cartridge and mixing tip into the gun and squeezing the trigger to express the material.

46. *Choose a spatula that is large enough to pick up the mixed impression material, yet sufficiently pliable to mix the material against the pad.

47. *Place the pad near the edge of a table about waist high.

48. *Mix the low-viscosity impression material according to manufacturer's instructions. First use a circular motion combining the two strands, (Fig. 10-6) then a figure eight motion (Fig. 10-7) to blend and flatten the mixture onto the mixing pad. Flattening the mixture and limiting the number of times you lift the spatula from the pad reduces the number of voids in the mixture.

49. *Mix according to manufacturer's instructions to obtain a streak-free mixture in less than 1 minute.

50. *Load the syringe by holding it at a slight angle while scraping the pad (Fig. 10-8). Wipe off excess at the tip with a paper towel, screw on the tip, and insert the plunger. Express a small

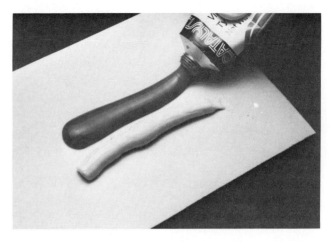

Fig. 10-5. Equal lengths of accelerator and base are common for the elastomeric impression materials.

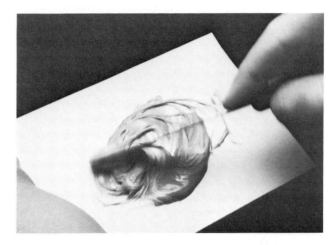

Fig. 10-6. Mixing the material in a circular motion with the *tip* of the spatula.

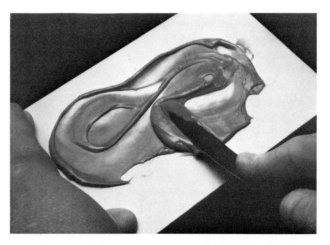

Fig. 10-7. Smooth blend of material with a figure eight motion using the *flat* surface of the spatula.

amount before handing to the dentist.

51. While the plunger is inserted into the syringe, the dentist initiates cord removal.

    NOTE: If using stock tray with single mix method, refer to section on stock tray, steps 6 through 8, and then continue with step 52.

52. Grasp the 2 mm excess of cord with forceps and slowly tease the top cord toward the occlusal with a gentle continuous pressure. Repeat for all cords.

53. Evaluate the retraction site for seepage, hemorrhage, or debris.

54. Quickly blow away seepage with short bursts of compressed air or dry with cotton pledgets.

55. If seepage cannot be controlled, see steps 34 through 38.

56. Syringe inaccessible areas first, e.g., distal lingual finish line.

57. Position the syringe so the elastomer is ahead of the tip's orifice (Figs. 10-9 and 10-10, A and B).

Insert tray:

    NOTE: For stock tray (putty wash) single mixing technique, skip to step 59.

58. *For stock tray (putty wash) double mixing technique, insert the low-viscosity impression material into the tray without overfilling the tray. Fill the inside slightly less than the depth of the external borders. Note that the excess flows to the back of the tongue or throat and causes discomfort. Skip to step 60.

59. *For stock tray (putty wash) single mixing technique, the unset high-viscosity impression material should already be in the tray, and the preparations syringed with low-viscosity impression material.

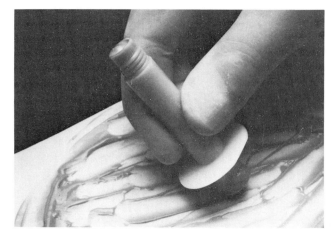

Fig. 10-8. Loading the syringe with swift, bold strokes.

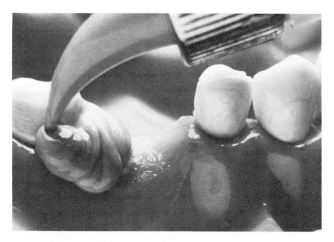

Fig. 10-9. The elastomer is placed in the most inaccessible areas first or an area where seepage has been a problem.

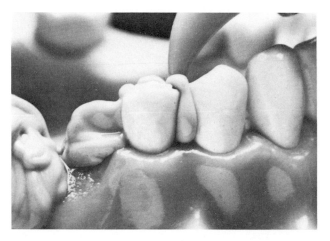

Fig. 10-10. A, A "soft ice cream" circular motion is usually effective.

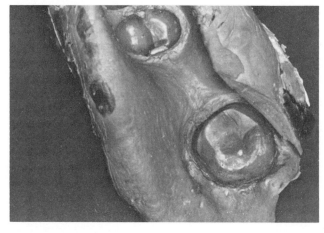

Fig. 10-10. B, Gingival margins of partial veneer crowns and distal margins of complete crowns are verified immediately in a polysulfide rubber base impression.

60. Spread the checks one at a time, first with the tray and then with an index finger.
61. Position the tray over the arch.
62. Seat from posterior to anterior, allowing the excess to extrude anteriorly.
63. Apply force in a vertical direction until further seating is impossible.
64. Evaluate final position and adjust tray quickly if necessary.

Evaluate final impression:
65. Stabilize the tray and wait the minimum time as suggested by the manufacturer to achieve the final set. Extended periods are usually advocated by researchers.
66. Perform "clinical final set test".

Remove tray:
67. Insert two fingers under each side of the tray to break the seal.
68. Remove the tray parallel to the preparation(s) path of withdrawal and transfer to assistant. This is crucial with cross arched impression.
69. Rinse impression with ambient water, and dry with short, small bursts of compressed air. Some elastomers are hydroscopic, so remove all the water.
70. Retraction cord(s) remaining in the impression material are removed carefully.
71. Check sulcus for residual impression material and remove any debris and clean the oral cavity.

Evaluate set impression:
72. Elastomeric material should be present 0.5 mm beyond visible finish line.
73. Note presence of bur marks, the junction of smooth root surface, and continuous finish line.
74. There should be no tray show-through in any areas of the impression, except at tissue stops.
75. There should be no shiny smooth areas; if present, they suggest moisture contamination.
76. There must be no voids present; if present, they suggest mixing problems or contamination. Disregard small voids in unimportant areas.
77. Review for tears (subtle undercuts to be "blocked out"). Polysulfides can distort without tearing, but sometimes reveal excessive distortion by a lightened color.
78. There should be no thin areas leaving the finish line unsupported. These areas distort under the weight of the stone.

Making working cast:
79. Position the dowel(s) into the impression. Insert one extra dowel pin on either side of the working dies. This ensures die removal despite errors during sectioning.
80. Check dowel(s) position(s) in impression for

parallelism and retention and add paper clips or orthodontic wire for retaining the second pour to the first. The Pindex System allows immediate pouring of impression.
81. Pour first layer of stone.
82. Wait for initial set of stone.
83. Lubricate die areas.
84. Bead and box impression.
85. Pour second layer of stone for the base.

Table 10-4. Time sequence for elastomeric double mix

Approximate time (minutes)	Assistant	Dentist
Putty		
0-0.5	Mix very high-viscosity material	Maintain isolated field
0.5-1.5	Load tray Position spacer(s) Hand to operator Remove cotton rolls Assist in seating tray	Seat tray
1.5-5	Clean up	Stabilize tray
5-	Remove spacer(s) Clean mouth and sulcus	Remove impression Trim and relieve impression Evaluate and set aside
Wash		
0-1	Mix low-viscosity material	Maintain isolated field
1-1.5	Load syringe	Remove retraction cord
1.5-2.5	Load tray Hand to operator Remove cotton rolls Assist in seating tray	Syringe low-viscosity material Seat tray
2.5-6	Clean up	Stabilize tray
6-	Rinse impression Clean mouth and sulcus	Remove impression Evaluate sulcus for debris Cement temporary restoration

Custom Tray

Synonyms: Acrylic tray
Mixing technique: Single
Advantages:
1. Less impression material is needed than with stock tray.
2. Because the trays are used only once, sterilization is not a problem.
3. A uniform thickness of impression material minimizes distortion resulting from curing shrinkage.
4. Precuring of the tray material is not required.

Disadvantages:
1. Construction of the custom tray is time consuming.

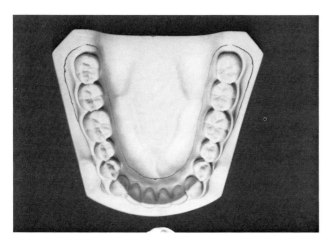

Fig. 10-11. Replica of diagnostic casts for custom tray construction.

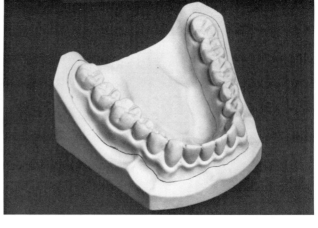

Fig. 10-12. Pencil line as a guide to periphery.

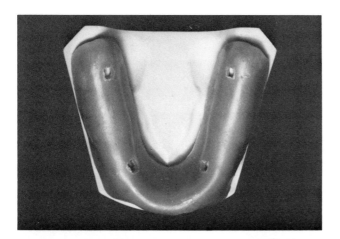

Fig. 10-13. Two or three millimeters of base plate wax for uniform thickness of impression material.

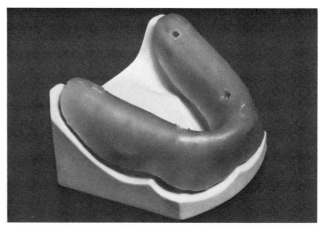

Fig. 10-14. Stops are incorporated in the wax for stability and patient comfort.

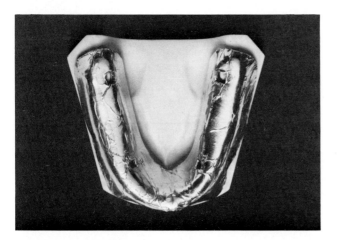

Fig. 10-15. Tinfoil is adapted to protect the wax during exothermic reaction of tray material.

2. The tray must "age" for 24 hours to minimize further distortion.
3. The monomer may be a sensitizer for some personnel.

Technique:
1. Soak replicas of the diagnostic casts in slurry water for 10 minutes.
2. Paint a layer of tinfoil substitute (or petroleum jelly) on the cast as a separating medium to prevent the resin from adhering to the cast.
3. Draw a pencil line on the cast as a guide in defining the tray extensions (Figs. 10-11 and 10-12).
4. Warm and adapt two sheets of base plate wax (total thickness, 2 mm) to the cast (Figs. 10-13 and 10-14). NOTE: for more rigid materials, polyethers and poly(vinylsiloxanes), 3 mm is required to facilitate removal from the mouth and removal of the replica cast.
5. Trim the excess wax to the pencil line with a knife.
6. Cover the wax with a thin tinfoil (or polyethylene) sheet to protect resin from wax during the exothermic cure (Figs. 10-15 and 10-16).

7. Remove wax to create four wide-spaced hard tissue stops at least 3 mm² and located on non-functional cusps (Figs. 10-9 and 10-10). Stops may be placed on firm tissue as a last resort.

8. Measure monomer (liquid) and polymer (powder) according to the manufacturer's recommended ratio.

9. Insert both (liquid first, then powder) into a suitable paper cup; most kits contain cups.

10. Mix according to manufacturer's recommendations.

11. Wait until doughy stage is reached, not sticky to the touch.

12. Form dough patty into a flattened shape approximately 4 mm thick.

13. Adapt flattened patty to tin-foiled diagnostic cast.

14. Trim excess to pencil line while resin is still doughy.

15. Use excess resin to form handle on the tray (Figs. 10-17, 10-18, and 10-19). This will help in removal from the mouth.

16. Moisten the unset tray surfaces with monomer (liquid) before joining.

17. Observe exothermic stage of curing acrylic resin.

18. Wait for the final set according to manufacturer's instructions (approximately 15 minutes).

19. Gently lift the tray from the cast.

20. Remove the wax spacer with the protector (Fig. 10-20).

21. Observe that all wax has been removed.

22. Trim and polish the tray using slow speed, continually checking for excessive heating of the acrylic resin.

23. Store at room temperature for 24 hours before making impression to minimize distortions. The adhesive can also be placed now.

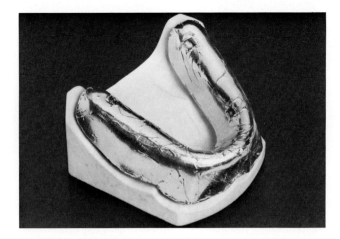

Fig. 10-16. Note the accommodation for the vestibule of the patient to avoid distention of the tissue.

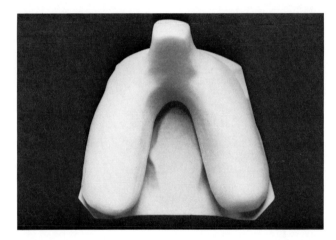

Fig. 10-17. Handle is positioned to avoid extended opening of the patient's mouth during impression and is more commonly used on the mandibular arch.

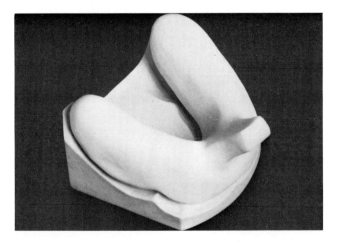

Fig. 10-18. The periphery is commonly *polished* to ensure smooth surfaces adjacent to patient's vestibules.

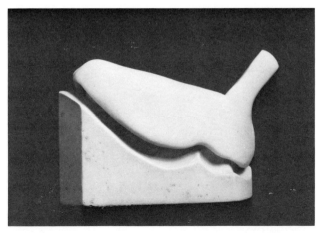

Fig. 10-19. Uniform thickness with confined margins ensures accuracy.

Gingival displacement and management:

24. See section on stock tray, steps 18 through 41.

Prepare syringe:

25. See section on stock tray, steps 42 through 44.

Making final impression:

26. Select medium to high-viscosity elastomer to line the tray.

27. Choose low-viscosity elastomer for syringing preparations.

28. *Provide two large mixing pads, approximately 6 by 8 inches. Some brands of impression material have mixing devices that resemble a caulking gun that do not need a mixing pad or spatula. These work by inserting a replaceable cartridge and mixing tip into the gun and squeezing the trigger to express the material into a tray or directly into the syringe.

29. *Obtain two spatulas that are shaped to manipulate the mixed impression material and pliable enough to mix the material against the pad.

30. *Place the pads near the edge of a table about waist high.

31. *Mix the low-viscosity impression material according to manufacturer's instructions. First use a circular motion combining the two strands, then a figure eight motion (Fig. 10-7) to blend and flatten the mixture. Flattening the mixture and limiting the number of times you lift the spatula from the pad reduces the number of voids in the mixture.

32. *Mix according to manufacturer's instructions, obtaining a streak-free mixture in less than 1 minute.

33. *Load the syringe by maintaining a slight angle while scraping the pad (Fig. 10-8). Wipe off excess at the tip with a paper towel, screw on the tip, and insert the plunger. Express a small amount before handing to the dentist.

34. *Mix the higher-viscosity impression material.

35. While the plunger is inserted into the syringe, the operator initiates cord removal.

36. Grasp the 2 mm excess of cord with forceps and remove the top cord slowly with a gentle continuous tug toward the occlusal. Do the same for all cords.

37. Evaluate tissue for seepage, hemorrhage, or debris.

38. Quickly blow away seepage with short bursts of compressed air or dry with cotton pledgets.

39. If seepage is evident, see section on stock tray, steps 34 through 38.

40. Syringe inaccessible areas first, i.e. distal lingual finish line.

41. Allow the elastomer to extrude ahead of the tip's orifice.

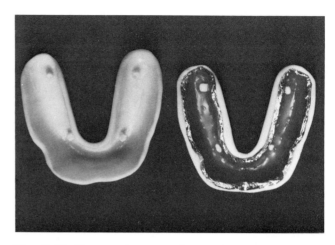

Fig. 10-20. The wax is removed, revealing the stops and a smooth surface extended to support the impression of the individual abutments.

Insert tray:

42. *Insert high-viscosity impression material into tray without overfilling the tray. Fill the inside slightly less than the depth of the outside borders. Note that the excess flows to the back of the tongue or throat and causes discomfort, and propels saliva under the tray causing bubbles. The patient is seated in an upright position to avoid this.

43. Spread the cheeks one at a time, first with the tray and then with your index finger.

44. Position the tray over the arch.

45. Seat from posterior to anterior, allowing excess to extrude in an anterior direction.

46. Continue seating in a vertical direction until the tray's stops prevent further progress.

47. Evaluate final position and adjust tray quickly if necessary.

Evaluate final impression:

48. See section on stock tray, steps 65 through 71.

Remove tray:

49. See section on stock tray, steps 72 to 76.

Evaluate set impression:

50. See section on stock tray, steps 77 through 87.

Closed Bite Double Arch Method

Synonyms: Dual quad tray, double arch, triple tray, Accu-bite, closed mouth impression

Minimum conditions:

1. The articulator must have a vertical dimension holding stop such as an incisal pin or other metal-to-metal contact. If the articulator's design does not provide for a positive stop, there must be sufficient natural teeth remaining to maintain vertical dimension. This approach is

Table 10-5. Time sequence for elastomeric single mix

Approximate time (min)	Assistant	Dentist
0-0.75	Mix low-viscosity material	Maintain isolated field
0.75-1.25	Load syringe	Remove retraction cord
1.25-2.0	Mix high-viscosity material	Syringe low-viscosity material
2.0-3.0	Load tray	Seat tray
	Hand to operator	
	Remove cotton rolls	
	Assist in seating tray	
3.0-6.0	Clean up	Stabilize tray
6.0-	Rinse impression	Remove impression
	Clean mouth and sulcus	Evaluate sulcus for debris
		Cement temporary restoration

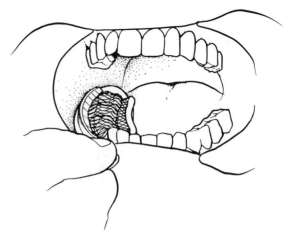

Fig. 10-21. Tray is inserted to determine the clearance laterally and distally.

limited to single castings in patients with suitable interdigitation.

2. There should be sufficient space distal to the terminal tooth in the arch to allow tray approximation.

Advantages:

1. The physical deformation of the mandible during opening is minimized.[1]
2. The shifting of teeth occuring during maximum intercuspation is captured.[2,3]
3. Less elastomeric impression material is needed so the patient is more comfortable.
4. Less gagging may occur.[4]

Disadvantages:

1. Tray is not rigid; depends on impression material for rigidity.
2. Is not a functionally generated technique, so it is limited to one casting per quadrant.
3. The distribution of the impression material is not uniform.

Technique[4,5]:

While waiting for anesthesia or after completion of tooth preparation:

1. *Evaluate the fit of the tray in patient's mouth.
2. Position the tray's crossbar distal to last tooth in arch (Fig. 10-21).
3. Instruct patient to close the mouth.
4. Observe the complete bilateral closure and the patient's comfort.
5. Adjust the tray, select new tray size, change brand, or modify technique.
6. Practice until patient is familiar with tasks.

Gingival displacement and management:

7. See section on stock tray, steps 18 through 41.

Prepare syringe:

8. See section on stock tray, steps 42 through 45.

Making final impression:

9. *Choose a large mixing pad, approximately 6 by 8 inches. Some brands of impression material have mixing devices resembling a caulking gun that do not need a mixing pad. These are activated by placing a replaceable cartridge and mixing tip into the gun and squeezing the trigger thus expressing the material.
10. *Select a spatula that is sufficiently large to elevate the mixed impression material, yet pliable enough to mix the material against the pad.
11. *Place the pad near the edge of a table about waist high.
12. *Mix the low-viscosity impression material according to manufacturer's instructions. First use a circular motion combining the two strands, then a smooth figure eight motion (Fig. 10-7) to blend and flatten the mixture onto the mixing pad. Flatten the mixture and limit the lifts of the spatula from the pad to reduce the number of voids in the mixture.
13. *Mix according to manufacturer's instructions to obtain a streak-free mixture within 1 minute.
14. *Load the syringe by maintaining it at a slight angle while scraping the pad (Fig. 10-8). Wipe off excess at the tip with a paper towel, screw on the tip, and insert the plunger. Express a small amount before handing to the dentist.
15. While the assistant is inserting the plunger into the syringe, initiate cord removal.
16. Grasp the 2 mm excess of cord with forceps and tease the top cord slowly with a gentle continuous pressure toward the occlusal. Repeat for all cords.
17. Evaluate site for seepage, hemorrhage, or debris.
18. Quickly remove seepage with short bursts of

compressed air or dry with cotton pledgets.

19. If seepage is uncontrolled, see section on stock tray, steps 34 through 38.
20. Syringe inaccessible areas first, i.e. distal lingual finish line; interproximal.
21. Allow the elastomer to extrude ahead of the tip's orifice.
22. *Mix the high-viscosity elastomer and "overfill" bilaterally.
23. Manually seat tray on maxillary arch.
24. For quadrant trays, position the crossbar distal to the last tooth in that arch.
25. Instruct patient to slowly close mouth.
26. Evaluate complete closure by observing the interdigitation (Fig. 10-22) on the opposite arch.
27. *Secure patient's comfort.

Evaluate final impression:

28. Wait the time suggested by the manufacturer to achieve the final set, plus 2 minutes.
29. Perform clinical final set test.

Tray removal:

30. Instruct the patient to open.
31. The impression adheres to one arch.
32. Place a finger on either side of the tray.
33. Remove with equal pressure bilaterally to minimize the distortion of the tray (Fig. 10-23).
34. Do not use the handle to remove tray.
35. *Remove residual impression material in sulcus or interproximal areas.
36. *Rinse impression with ambient water, and dry with short bursts of compressed air.
37. Retraction cord(s) in the impression material is/ are removed carefully.
38. Check sulcus for residual impression material. Remove debris and clean the oral cavity.

Pour die:

39. Trim excess impression material with a surgical knife.
40. *Vibrate the die stone and overfill the prepared tooth.
41. *Position dowel pin and allow stone to set.
42. *Place a bead of wax around the edges of the die to remove undercuts (Fig. 10-24).
43. *Lubricate the dowel pin and die stone with separating media.

Making working cast(s) and attaching to articulator:

44. *Box the impression (Fig. 10-25).
45. *Choose hinge articulator with incisal pin or vertical dimension stop (Fig. 10-26). (Recommended for neutroocclusion and one uncomplicated casting)
46. *Place sticky wax around circumference of tray.
47. *Cut a strip of boxing wax in half length-wise.
48. *Soften the wax uniformly over a gas flame.

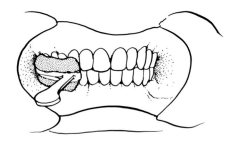

Fig. 10-22. Complete closure in centric closure position completely covering the mandibular tooth preparation.

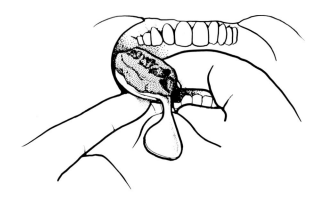

Fig. 10-23. Tray is removed with smooth, fluid movement.

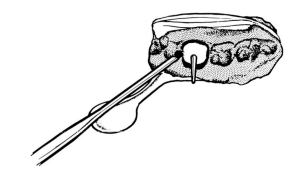

Fig. 10-24. Wax is used to "block out" undercuts surrounding the die.

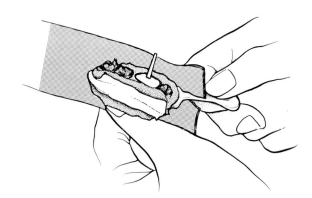

Fig. 10-25. The impression is boxed before pouring the adjacent and opposing teeth in stone.

49. *Adapt and box both upper and lower arches at one time.
50. *Seal the area at the junction of boxing wax and tray to prevent the stone from entering the opposite side of the impression.
51. *Cut small openings to accommodate the articulator so that correct positioning of the impression is possible.
52. *Position the tray, bisecting the interarticulator distance from top to bottom, parallel to the table top, and centered from side to side.
53. *Pour the opposing side (side without dies) first and close articulator arm into unset stone.
54. *Evaluate impression tray position and secure the dowel pins so they are not interfacing with the closure of the articulator arm on the working side.
55. *Wait 45 minutes for initial set of gypsum.
56. *Lubricate the die(s) with a separating media.
57. *Pour prepared side (with die) of impression with gypsum product.
58. *Close articulator arms until incisal pin contacts the lower arm (Fig. 10-27).
59. *Remove unset stone around tip of dowel pin(s) to facilitate removal.
60. *Place a rubber band around upper and lower arms of the articulator arm.
61. *Wait 45 minutes.

Removing impression tray from articulator:
62. *Remove rubber band and pull articulator arms apart slowly, separating the casts from the impression tray.
63. Evaluate casts and separate die(s) (Fig. 10-28).

Copper Band

The copper tube or band is used to salvage an impression of multiple preparations when there are only vague margins on one or two preparations that are not adequately replicated in the impression. The patient's condition, the extent of the aberration evaluated, and judgement determines whether the copper band technique saves time or whether a remake of the original impression is more appropriate. The steps for a copper band impression of a single prepared tooth are:

Fitting copper band to preparation:
1. Select copper band diameter by trial and error by deforming the tubes to semiellipsoidal cross section and trying in.
2. *Anneal selected tube by heating in flame and quenching in alcohol.
3. Mark approximate position of finish line with a sharp explorer tip.
4. Cut with scissors and smooth rough edges with carborundum stone.

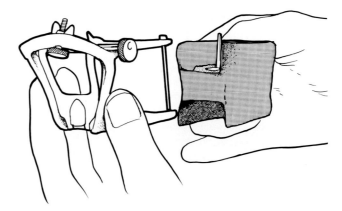

Fig. 10-26. A "verticulator" is another acceptable articulator for uncomplicated castings.

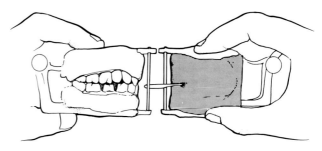

Fig. 10-27. Incisal pen should contact firmly upon centric closure position.

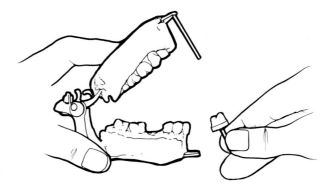

Fig. 10-28. The poured casts are checked for bubbles and other defects.

5. Evaluate fit; band should extend approximately 1 mm beyond finish line and produce minimal tissue blanching. Do not remove from preparation.
6. If fit is tight at finish line area, rock the tube gently from side to side. A space between finish line and copper band approximating the width of an explorer tip is optimum.
7. Cut orientation hole in top one-fifth of facial surface of tube.

Make compound plug:

8. Cover fingers with a light coat of petroleum jelly.
9. Gently heat red stick compound over a Bunsen burner flame; compress the warm mass with the lubricated fingers.
10. Evaluate viscosity and temperature; reheat or temper in a warm water bath if necessary.
11. Insert warm compound mass and fill approximately the top one-third of copper tube.
12. Seat and orient band onto preparation. Compress excess into hand lightly with lubricated finger. NOTE: The amount of compound is critical to the success of this step. The compound should just touch the occlusal surface.
13. *Cool tube with water.
14. Using Backus towel clamp, grasp top one-fifth of copper band and remove from mouth.
15. Evaluate preparation side of band. Only part of the occlusal surface should be impressed.
16. Relieve any excess by cutting. Slow speed with No. 6 or 8 carbide bur is suggested. Stop frequently to air cool or blow away debris.
17. Remove 0.2 mm of compound from the impressed occlusal surface. This creates a space for the heavy body polyvinylsiloxane.
18. Using a long shank No. 6 round carbide bur, drill a hole through the center of the compound plug. This will decrease hydraulic pressure to facilitate seating of the copper band.

Making impression:

19. Cut approximately four or five evenly distributed holes with a sharp No. 4 or No. 6 round carbide 2 to 3 mm above the bottom of the copper tube. Be careful not to heat the tube. These holes will retain the polyvinylsiloxane impression material and provide a suitable space at the finish line area. This additional space prevents marginal tearing.
20. Coat the internal surface sparingly with adhesive. Spot the internal surface; do not coat the entire area. The adhesive can occupy too much space in the finish line areas.
21. *Clean and isolate preparation.
22. *Prepare the syringe tip by securing a hole size approximating the diameter of the shank of a long shank bur. NOTE: some polyvinylsiloxane impression systems have an automixing device to facilitate the next two steps.
23. *Mix 1 inch of heavy-viscosity, but not putty, elastomeric impression material.
24. Inject the elastomeric into the copper band, filling the space completely from the compound to copper band edge.
25. Position fingers on top edge of band; orient and seat customized copper tube.

26. Evaluate tube position; if incorrect, reposition.
27. Stabilize band and compress excess into plug's hole with lubricated finger. Note excess expressed at gingival area.
28. Remove fingers; protect copper band from movement and await final set.
29. Grasp top one-fifth of impression with sharp Backus towel clamp and gently remove from tooth.

Evaluating impression and making die:

30. Evaluate impression; if the area needed is accurately impressed, proceed.
31. With a sharp surgical knife remove excess elastomeric.
32. *Using masking tape, box the impression, and pour in diestone.
33. *Trim diestone to form elongated tapered cylinder base for convenient manipulation during waxup.

The defective areas can be relieved on the original full arch impression and the waxing of the margin created from the copper band die and transferred to the relieved die for adjustment of proximal contacts and occlusion.

SELECTED REFERENCES

1. De Marco, T.J., and Paine, S.: Mandibular dimensional change, J. Prosthet. Dent. 32:482-485, 1974.
2. Regli, C., and Kelly, E.: The phenomenon of decreased mandibular arch width in opening movements, J. Prosthet. Dent. 17:49, 1967.
3. Goto, T.: An experimental study on the physiological mobility of a tooth, Shikawa Gakuho, 71:415-1444, 1971.
4. Pensler, A.V.: Variable impression technic for crown and bridge and restorations, Dent. Surv. 47(10):23-27, 1971.
5. Costello, W.J.: An efficient impression articulation technic, Dent. Surv. 53(12):44-45, 1977.
6. Wilson, E.G., and Werrin, S.R.: Double arch impressions for simplified restorative dentistry, J. Prosthet. Dent. 49:198-202, 1983.
7. Tylman, S.D., and Malone, W.F.P.: Theory and Practice of Fixed Prosthodontics, St. Louis, 1978, The C.V. Mosby Co.
8. Nayyar, Arun, and Thayer, K.E.: Accuracy of relined rubber base impressions (I.A.D.R. abstract), J. Prosthet. Dent. 37:714, 1977.

BIBLIOGRAPHY

Aiach, D., Malone, W.F.P., and Sandrik, James: Dimensional accuracy of epoxy resins and their compatibility with impression materials, J. Prosthet. Dent. 52:500, 1984.
Appleby, D.C., Cohen, S.R., Racowsky, L.P., and Mingledorff, E.B.: The combined reversible-hydrocolloid irreversible hydrocolloid impression system. Clinical application, J. Prosthet. Dent. 55:16, 1986.
Bombery, T.J., and Hatch, R.A.: Correction of defective impression by selective addition of impression material, J. Prosthet. Dent. 52:38, 1984.
Bomberg, T.J., Hatch, R.A., and Hoffman, W.: Impression material thickness in stock and custom trays, J. Prosthet. Dent. 54:170, 1985.

Ciesco, J.M., Malone, W.F.P., Sandrik, J.L., and Mazur, Boleslaw: A comparison of the accuracy and dimensional stability of five elastomeric impression materials, J. Prosthet. Dent. 45:89, 1981.

de Araujo, P.A., and Jorgensen, K.D.: Effect of material bulk and undercuts on accuracy of impressions, J. Prosthet. Dent. 54:791, 1985.

de Araujo, P.A., and Jorgensen, K.D.: Improved accuracy by re-heating addition-reaction-silicone impressions, J. Prosthet. Dent. 55:11, 1986.

Dirtoft, B.I., Jansson, J.F., and Abramson, N.H.: Using holography for measurement of in viro deformation in a complete maxillary denture, J. Prosthet. Dent. 54:843, 1985.

Eames, W.B., Sieweke, J.C., Wallace, S.W., and Rogers, L.B.: Elastomeric impression materials: effect of bulk on accuracy, J. Prosthet. Dent. 41:304, 1979.

Farah, J.W., Clark, A.E., and Ainpour, P.R.: Elastomeric impression materials, J. Oper. Dent. 6:15, 1981.

Fehling, A.W., Hesby, R.A., and Pelleu, G.B.: Dimensional stability of auto polymerizing acrylic resin impression trays, 55:592, 1986.

Langenwalter, E.M., Aquilino, S.A., Turner, K.A., Huber, L.R., and Leary, J.M.: The dimensional stability of elastomeric impression materials following disinfection, J. Prosthet. Dent. in Press, 1989.

Linke, B.A., Nicholls, J.I., and Faucher, R.R.: Distortion analysis of stone casts made from impression materials, J. Prosthet. Dent. 54:794, 1985.

Johnson, G.H., and Craig, R.G.: Accuracy of additional silicones as a function of technique, J. Prosthet. Dent. 55:196, 1986.

Johnson, G.H., and Craig, R.G.: Accuracy and bond strength of combination agar/alginate hydrocolloid impression materials, J. Prosthet. Dent. 55:1, 1986.

Nicholls, J.I.: The measure of distortion: theoretical considerations, J. Prosthet. Dent. 37:578, 1977.

Phillips, R., et al.: Report of Committee on Scientific Investigation of the American Academy of Restorative Dentistry, J. Prosthet. Dent. 55:754, 1986.

Sawyer, H.F., Birtles, J.T., Neiman, R., and Podshady, A.G.: Accuracy of casts produced from seven rubber base impression materials, J.A.D.A. 87:126, 1973.

Sawyer, H.F., Sandrik, J.L., and Neiman, R.: Accuracy of casts produced from alginate and hydrocolloid impression materials, J. Am. Dent. Assoc. 94:713, 1977.

Shillingburg, H.T., Hatch, R.A., Keenan, M.P., and Hemphill, M.W.: Impression materials and techniques used for cast restorations in eight states, J.A.D.A. 100:696, 1980.

Stackhouse, J.A., Harris, W.T., Mansour, R.M., and Von Hagen, S.: A study of bubbles in a rubber elastomer manipulated under clinic conditions, J. Prosthet. Dent. 57:591, 1987.

Stackhouse, J.A.: Relationship of syringe tip diameter to voids in elastomeric impression, J. Prosthet. Dent. 53:811-815, 1985.

Vermilyea, S.G., Powers, J.M., and Craig, R.G.: Polyether, polysulfide, and silicone rubber impression materials. 1. Quality of silver plated dies. J. Mich. Dent. Assoc. 57:371, 1975.

Vermilyea, S.G., Powers, J.M., and Craig, R.G.: Polyether, polysulfide, and silicone rubber impression materials. 2. Accuracy of silver plated dies. J. Mich. Dent. Assoc. 57:371, 1975.

11

Richard A. Hesby, Steven M. Morgano,
William F. P. Malone, John E. Flocken,
David A. Kaiser, and
Edmund Cavazos, Jr.

TREATMENT RESTORATIONS (Temporization)

Part I

Treatment Restorations: Temporaries

Treatment restorations protect the prepared teeth and simulate the form and function of the definitive restorations. Perceptive fabrication of a treatment restoration preserves the vitality of the pulp and secures patient comfort. A treatment restoration can also be a healing matrix for the surrounding gingival tissue and adjacent edentulous mucosa (Fig. 11-1).

THE PULP

A critical consideration when restoring vital teeth is the preservation of a healthy pulp. Hildebrand[1] has enumerated four irritants that affect the pulp: mechanical, thermal, chemical, and microbiologic. All forms of irritation can be inflicted during tooth preparation. The dentist must assess the recovery ability of a potential abutment and minimize the trauma to the tooth during and after preparation.[2] Coolants during tooth preparation and sedative medicaments placed within adequate provisional restorations usually encourage pulpal repair. One source of irritation is repeated dentinal exposure to oral fluids during fabrication of the FPD. Excessive exposure of prepared teeth to dessication results in increasing sensitivity at each successive appointment. Obtundants, insulators, and general sedative sealants are usually effective merely as interim measures. The programmed use of long-term treatment restorations should be weighted against predictable tissue inflammation,[3] dentinal hypersensitivity, patient inconvenience, and the risk of caries.

GINGIVAE

The gingival response to a restoration is closely related to the location and adequacy of the gingival finish line. Where and how the gingival termination is developed is of primary importance in minimizing gingival trauma. Injury to the attachment (junctional epithelium and connective tissue) directly affects the response of the soft tissue to the restoration. The gingivae, by general apposition around the teeth, protect against infection and contribute to arch stabilization.[4,5] Due to high vascularity, the gingivae heal readily, with occasional recession. However, the level of the gingival tissue after tooth preparation, tissue dilation, and placement of a treatment restoration can be predictable.[6,7,8]

The location of the gingival termination of the preparation supragingivally or intracrevicularly depends upon the clinical conditions. If intracrevicular margins are indicated, the exposure rate of the gingival margin depends upon 1) the age of the patient when the restoration is placed, 2) the nature and health of the gingiva, 3) projected oral hygiene, 4) occlusal relationships and arch position, and 5) liability of systemic diseases. With time, soft tissue commonly recedes. If the marginal exposure is esthetically objectionable after years of service, the restorations can be remade with minimal disruption.

Conversely, overextended and overcontoured treatment restorations can cause irreversible tissue damage. Hasty fabrication of a provisional prosthesis is usually responsible for adverse tissue responses during construction of an FPD.

TREATMENT RESTORATIONS: TEMPORIZATION

An interim covering after tooth preparation is necessary to preserve pulpal vitality and to ensure gingival health, patient comfort, and esthetics. There are three major causes of problems associated with treatment restorations:

1. The time required to fabricate adequate interim tooth coverage is underestimated by dentists.
2. Interim coverage is not always replaced by the cast restoration within a reasonable time.

255

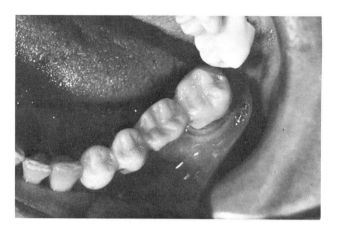

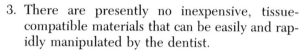

Fig. 11-1. Interim coverage perceptively fabricated performs as a healing matrix. (Courtesy Dr. Hanna Sweetnam, Joliet, Ill.)

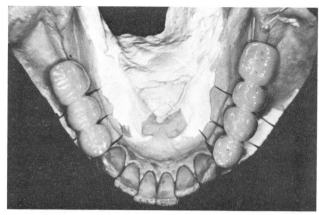

Fig. 11-2. Heat-polymerized treatment restoration fabricated on casts of prepared teeth to modify the occlusal plane of patient.

3. There are presently no inexpensive, tissue-compatible materials that can be easily and rapidly manipulated by the dentist.

Measures to combat these problems include fabrication of heat-processed interim restorations before tooth preparation, expanded appointments, and the coordination of appointment dates with laboratory services to accelerate insertion. Repeated patient visits to recement dislodged provisionals is inefficient and taxes the confidence of the patient.[9]

The eight requirements for treatment restorations are:

1. The pulp of the tooth must be insulated from adverse stimuli, including saliva leakage.
2. Arch position of the prepared teeth must be maintained to avoid extrusion and/or drifting of teeth and to preserve the accuracy of the master cast.
3. Treatment restorations should not impinge upon the gingival tissues.
4. Esthetics should be reasonable, particularly in the incisor and premolar areas.
5. A comfortable, functional occlusal relationship should be developed.
6. Interim coverage should possess sufficient inherent strength to withstand normal occlusal forces.
7. Treatment coverage should be designed with physiologic axial contours and open embrasures to allow the restoration to function as a healing matrix for the surrounding tissues.
8. Construction of treatment restorations should be within the realm of the average dentist, and they must be easily removed with minimal damage to the tooth and supportive structures.

Temporization is crucial, but universally demeaned because of its abbreviated existence. Nevertheless, the results of hastily fabricated treatment restorations commonly haunt the dentist and patient.

TYPES OF TREATMENT RESTORATION TECHNIQUES

Treatment restorations can be constructed as a single unit or as an FPD (splint) with or without edentulous areas (Fig. 11-2). They are composed of metal (precious and nonprecious) and nonmetallic materials.

Types of Techniques

1. Cast metal (precious and nonprecious)
2. Aluminum shell, copper band temporization
3. Preformed metal crowns
4. Cellulose acetate forms
5. Prefabricated polycarbonate forms
6. Heat-polymerized resin treatment restorations
7. Autopolymerizing resin-alginate impression technique
8. Vacuum-formed plastic (Omnivac) template technique
9. Postcrown technique

Various techniques are used to fabricate biologic interim restorations. Dentists commonly use the alginate direct impression technique, the popular "Omnivac" template approach, and preformed treatment restorations. The third technique is usually restricted to one or two units.

Fixed prosthodontics has improved treatment restorations from the hastily placed aluminum shell crowns to the contemporary indirect-direct efficient methods. The Omnivac system is an innovative method that elevates temporization to a healing matrix.

CAST METAL TREATMENT RESTORATIONS

Cast metal treatment restorations are used for patients with maladies difficult to diagnose, i.e., patients with gross maxillomandibular discrepancies (Fig. 11-3). The time lapse of treatment is commonly excessive; thus a cast metal provisional restoration allows evaluation of the occlusion, esthetics, periodontium, and

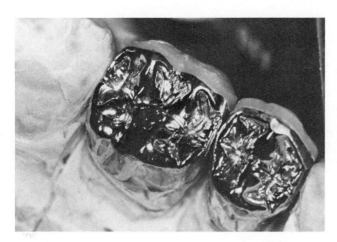

Fig. 11-3. Cast metal (reused gold) treatment restorations are fabricated for complex cases with long-standing occlusal problems.

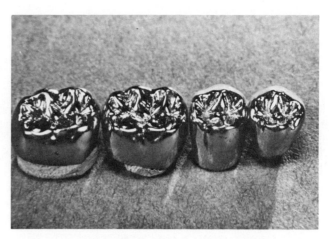

Fig. 11-4. Cast metal treatment restorations for re-establishment of occlusal vertical dimension. The occlusal surfaces are commonly frosted [sand blasted] to aid detection of prematurities.

TMJs and makes it possible to finalize the treatment plan without the liabilities of conventional temporaries. These treatment planning dilemmas are infrequent, and the use of a noble metal is somewhat pretentious but necessary. Nonprecious metals can be a rational alternative when a patient develops an idiosyncratic or allergic[10] tissue response to monomer-polymer products.

"Tap-off lugs" are routinely included to assist periodical removal of these costly cast treatment restorations. Nevertheless, cast metal treatment restorations can be truly a healing matrix for medically compromised patients.

Another indication for cast metal interim restorations is the maintenance of vertical dimension. Terminal molars are commonly restored before tooth reduction on anterior teeth. Nonprecious metal can be designated to retain the original vertical relationship. Highly polished axial surfaces for biocompatibility of metal and sandblasted (frosted) occlusal surfaces to aid occlusal determinations are fundamental (Fig. 11-4). Duplication of the pretreatment canine function can be accomplished in a similar manner.

Cast metal provisional restorations would be used more frequently if they were inexpensive. Commercial preformed metal crowns can be modified at the gingival and then cast. This method has merit for future cast metal healing matrixes. Even nonprecious cast metal treatment restorations are a luxury for routine fixed prosthodontics, but the enviable tissue response is undeniable.

ALUMINUM SHELL CROWNS

The use of the aluminum shell is restricted to premolars and molars. A shell of suitable diameter is selected and festooned to adapt to the preparation and height of the gingival crest. To secure the shell to the preparation, a luting media is placed into the shell. A resin mixture is placed within the shell for patients with a reduced interocclusal distance to enhance retention. The shell is then removed, trimmed for adequate occlusal relationships, and seated with a sedative cementing media. Aluminum shells do possess a consistency permitting short-term adaptation to a patient's occlusion but lack the rigidity for acceptable marginal strength and proximal contacts. With the advent of more tissue-tolerant products, aluminum shell crowns are rarely indicated but are available for emergencies such as trauma.

Copper band temporization is also unacceptable due to untoward tissue responses and poor occlusion. Copper bands can be used for an impression matrix but are undesirable for interim coverage.

PREFORMED COMMERCIAL METAL CROWNS

Preformed metal crowns are used primarily for the posterior teeth. Notable exceptions are the stainless steel crown forms adapted in pedodontics for fractured teeth. The preformed metal crown is a distinct improvement over its predecessor the aluminum shell crown or the copper band filled with a medicament. These newer products have improved occlusal and axial surfaces but still remain malleable to allow the shell to rapidly conform to the occlusion (Fig. 11-5, A). The cervical bands of some brands of preformed crowns are slightly constricted to favor a tolerable tissue relationship (Fig. 11-5, B). Although recession is common, irritation can be minimized by contouring the gingival margins. Selection of the size of the preformed crown is critical. The time-saving aspect of preformed products is their most attractive feature.

CELLULOSE ACETATE CROWN FORMS

The cellulose acetate crown form consists of a thin, soft, and transparent material. Sizes and shapes can

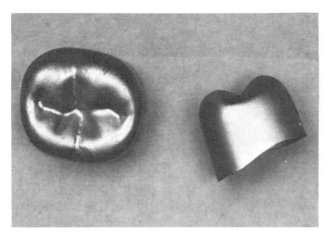

Fig. 11-5. A, Prefabricated anodized crowns that require a lining of acrylic resin followed by cementation with a sedative luting agent.

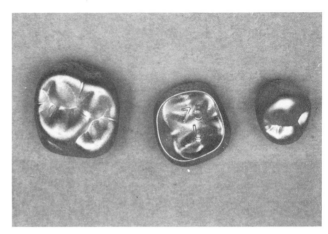

Fig. 11-5. B, Ion crown forms with constricted gingival margins and well-defined occlusal surfaces.

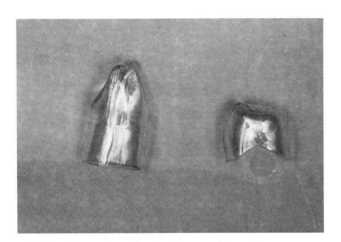

Fig. 11-6. Preformed celluoid crown forms. These forms must be removed after shaping the interim crowns.

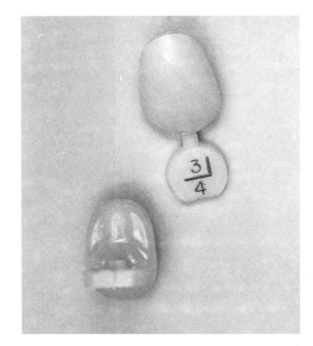

Fig. 11-7. Polycarbonate crowns for incisors, canines, and premolars.

be selected from a mold guide (Fig. 11-6). A selected crown form is trimmed and festooned to fit the preparation without impinging the soft tissue. The translucent matrix is then filled with a resin. There are three popular resins in use:

1. Polymethyl methacrylate, e.g., "Temporary Bridge Resin" (Caulk)
2. Vinyl polyethyl methacrylate, e.g., "Trim" (Bosworth)
3. Epimine (Ethyl imine derivative) resin, e.g., "Scutan" (Premeir)

Autopolymerizing polymethyl methacrylate is the most commonly used resin. It is relatively inexpensive and easily manipulated. The primary disadvantages of this material are the exothermic heat of polymerization, especially in bulky pontic areas, and potential pulpal and mucosal irritation from the free monomer. Color stability is adequate when compared to other autopolymerizing resins, but discoloration will still occur.

Vinyl polyethyl methacrylate is a less commonly used resin. The major problem with this resin has been poor color stability.[11] The restoration invariably becomes significantly darker with time.

The epimine resin (ethyl imine derivative) will produce considerably less exothermic heat during polymerization.[12] The material has been reported to produce better marginal adaptation when compared to three other resins.[13] Epimine plastic is not commonly used because it is expensive, has poor resistance to abrasion, and discolors more than other resins.[14]

The material is selected and mixed according to the

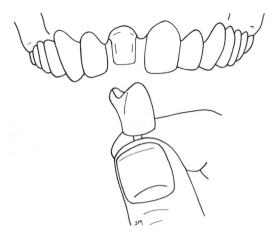

Fig. 11-8. A preformed polycarbonate crown is selected.

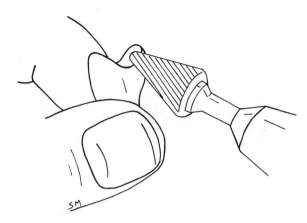

Fig. 11-9. The gingival margin of the preformed crown is adjusted to approximate the finish line of the tooth preparation.

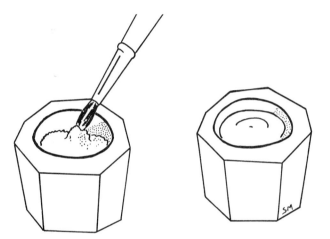

Fig. 11-10. A small amount of tooth-colored autopolymerizing acrylic resin is picked up with a sable brush.

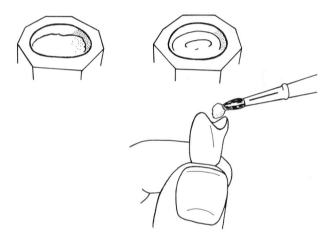

Fig. 11-11. The acrylic resin is added in increments, to avoid trapping air, until the crown is filled.

manufacturer's directions. The form is filled and gently pressed upon the lubricated preparation while the excess is removed. The crown matrix is repeatedly removed and reseated during the latter stages of polymerization to minimize distortion and to ensure removal after the resin is set. The cellulose shell is peeled off after the material has set. The occlusion is adjusted, and the treatment restoration is trimmed and polished. Cementation medium depends upon the specific clinical conditions.

PREFABRICATED POLYCARBONATE CROWNS

The polycarbonate crown form can provide excellent coverage for anterior teeth (Fig. 11-7). An appropriate preformed crown is selected to establish proximal contact (Fig. 11-8). The gingival margin of the preformed crown is adjusted to approximate the gingival termination of the tooth preparation (Fig. 11-9). The monomer and polymer for a tooth-colored

acrylic resin are placed in separate dappen dishes, and a small amount of resin is picked up with a sable brush (Fig. 11-10). The acrylic resin is added in increments, to avoid trapping air, until the crown is filled (Fig. 11-11).

The filled polycarbonate crown is seated onto the lubricated tooth preparation. The crown is reseated repeatedly to prevent excess resin from setting into proximal undercuts (Fig. 11-12). Because of the limited volume of resin lining the crown form, the heat of polymerization is not a problem.

After the resin has set, a cone-shaped laboratory bur is used to remove excess resin, eliminate overextensions, and develop the emergence profile (Fig. 11-13). The fit of the gingival margin is then evaluated clinically. The crown should not extend apical to the finish line of the tooth preparation (Fig. 11-14). Overextended or untrimmed gingival margins can cause unfavorable tissue responses.

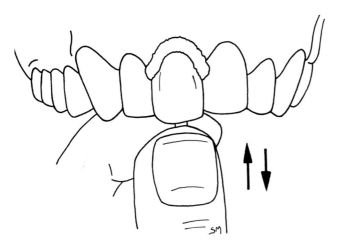

Fig. 11-12. The polycarbonate crown is seated onto the lubricated tooth preparation. The crown is pumped up and down to prevent excess resin from setting into the proximal undercuts.

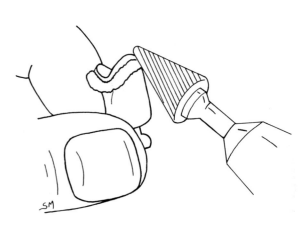

Fig. 11-13. A cone-shaped laboratory bur is used to remove excess resin, eliminate overextensions, and develop the emergence profile.

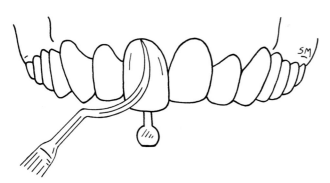

Fig. 11-14. The fit of the gingival margin is carefully evaluated. The crown must *not* extend apical to the finish line of the tooth preparation.

The incisal edge and lingual surface of the crown are adjusted for optimum esthetics and occlusion. The crown is then highly polished with a Burlew wheel, followed by flour of pumice (Fig. 11-15, A). The finished provisional crown is cemented with a temporary sedative luting agent (Fig. 11-15, B). The polycarbonate crown form <u>remains</u> on the tooth preparation as an integral component of the provisional restoration, whereas the cellulose crown form is <u>removed</u> before cementation of the treatment restoration.

HEAT-POLYMERIZED RESINS FOR TREATMENT FPDs

Crowns prepared in the laboratory on diagnostic casts are indicated with multiple preparations if alternate methods are impractical (Fig. 11-16). Mock tooth preparations are performed on a second set of diagnostic casts. The technician or dentist formulates the desired occlusion and contact areas in wax on the mounted casts. Centric occlusal stops can be estab-

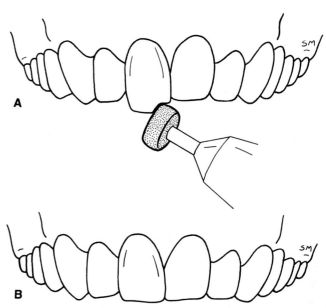

Fig. 11-15. A, The incisal edge and lingual surface of the crown are adjusted. The crown is then highly polished with a Burlew wheel, followed by flour of pumice. **B,** The finished provisional crown is cemented with a temporary luting agent.

lished in metal if prolonged wear of the treatment prosthesis is anticipated (Fig. 11-17).

The wax is removed and heat-polymerized temporaries are fabricated. If these provisional restorations are fabricated on simulated preparations, they must be relined before cementation. The technique is similar to relining a polycarbonate form.

Plastic denture teeth can be used to fabricate esthetically pleasing, functional treatment restorations. A wide variety of shades and molds render this technique adaptable for most pontic areas.[15] Using plastic

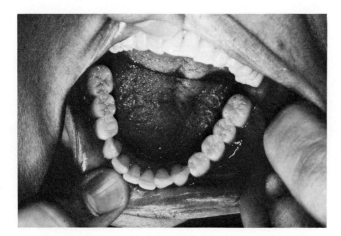

Fig. 11-16. Bilateral heat-polymerized treatment prostheses for occlusal plane restoration.

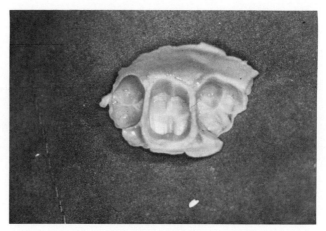

Fig. 11-18. An autopolymerized interim restoration for a maxillary first molar from a prepreparation alginate impression. Buccal flute is retained on the facial surface to ensure healthy tissue.

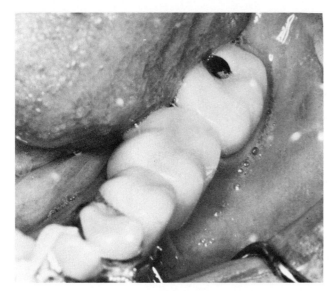

Fig. 11-17. A, Heat-polymerized, metal reinforced treatment restoration with metal centric stop for prolonged wear.

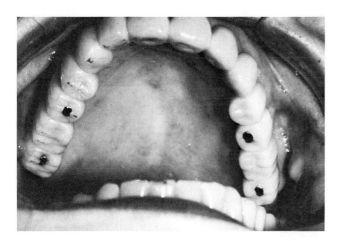

Fig. 11-17. B, Heat-polymerized metal reinforced full arch maxillary splint with positive metal occlusal stops prior to placement of cast super-structure.

teeth to construct treatment restorations before tooth preparation is a practical method for developing esthetics and a satisfactory occlusal plane.

Laboratory expenses and the time needed by the dentist to prepare secondary diagnostic casts may be prohibitive for a three-tooth prosthesis, but the heat-polymerized resin technique will often save chairtime with extensive restorative dentistry.

AUTOPOLYMERIZING RESIN-ALGINATE IMPRESSION TECHNIQUE

An alginate impression of the teeth is made during the appointment for preparations but before tooth reduction. The borders and interproximal extensions of the alginate impression are trimmed, and the impression is placed in a damp environment to control distortion. After preparations are complete, a mixture of acrylic resin is placed in the section of the alginate impression corresponding to the crown preparations. The tooth preparations are lubricated and the alginate impression with the resin is then replaced in the mouth. A small amount of the acrylic resin is kept in the hand to judge the progress of the set. The impression is removed when the resin reaches a doughy stage—just before achieving a rigid state. Care is taken to prevent the heat of polymerization from damaging the mucosa or dental pulps. The resin restoration is then removed from the alginate impression (Fig. 11-18) and reinserted into the mouth to check occlusion and trim the margins. By this time polymerization has progressed to initial stages of rigidity, and the treatment matrix can be finished, polished, and cemented. The alginate impression technique is suitable for fabricating single-tooth temporary crowns and short-span provisional FPDs (Fig. 11-19). Similar methods use a strong pliable wax or impression putty instead of alginate.[16]

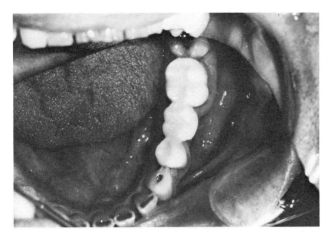

Fig. 11-19. Three-unit mandibular interim FPD directly fabricated from a prerestorative alginate impression. Note the buccal flute on the first molar.

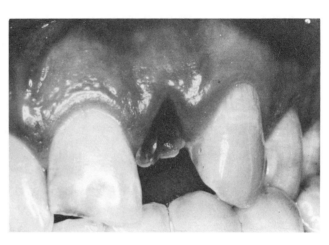

Fig. 11-20. A, Trauma to the maxillary anterior incisors resulting in a linear fracture of tooth No 10. (Courtesy Dr. T.E. Yuhas, Palos Heights, Ill.)

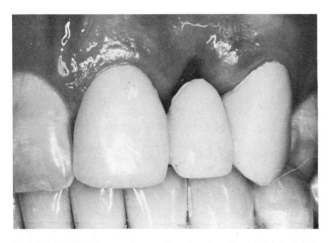

Fig. 11-20. B, Three-unit maxillary treatment prosthesis fabricated with the plastic template method and autopolymerizing acrylic resin. Note the interproximal embrasures without pontic-tissue contact.

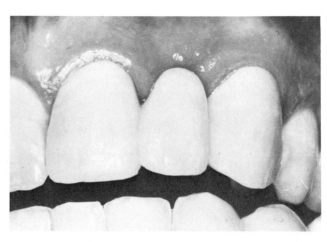

Fig. 11-20. C, Three-unit maxillary porcelain-fused-to-metal FPD.

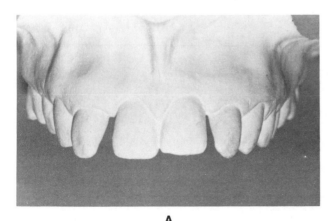

A

Fig. 11-21. A, Pretreatment diagnostic cast for patient to receive six-unit maxillary anterior prosthesis after removal of laterals.

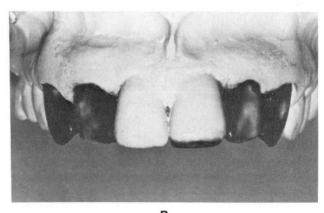

B

Fig. 11-21. B, Diagnostic cast modified with wax to improve esthetics. *Continued*

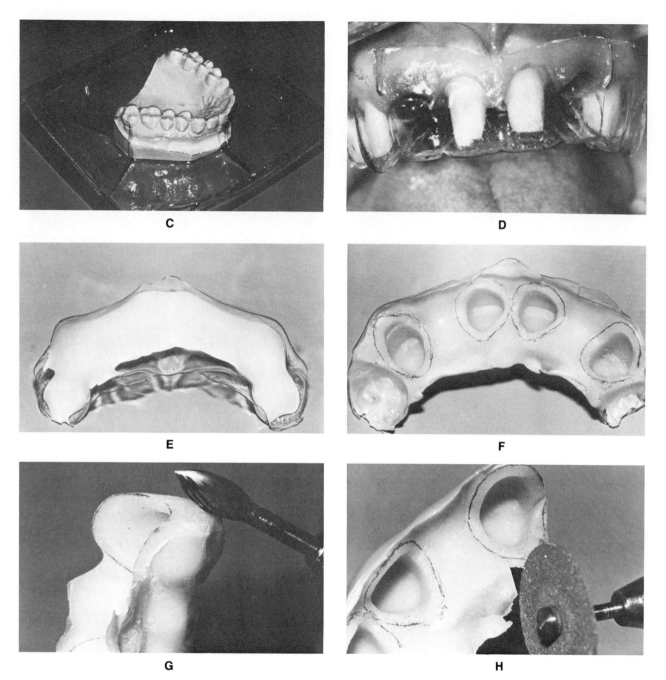

Fig. 11-21. C, Replica cast from impression with vacuum-formed plastic shell to form template. **D,** Preliminary tooth preparation after removal of maxillary lateral incisors illustrating intraoral adaptation of template. **E,** Autopolymerizing resin placed in template and gently seated when the sheen leaves the surface. The vacuum-formed shell is removed repeatedly to avoid entrapment in subtle undercuts. **F,** Provisional splint with gingival margins marked in pencil. **G,** Acrylic bur establishes contours while maintaining marginal integrity. **H,** Trimming flash perpendicular to gingival finish line. Embrasure areas are magnified to ensure easy cleaning.

Continued

VACUUM-FORMED PLASTIC TEMPLATE (OMNIVAC) TECHNIQUE

The plastic template technique is a versatile, innovative, and uncomplicated approach to temporization (Fig. 11-20). A translucent vacuum-formed template is commonly used to construct direct anterior (Fig. 11-21) or posterior (Figs. 11-22 to 11-30) provisional crowns and FPDs that are esthetic and functional.[17]

A thermal vacuum machine is used to adapt a plastic sheet over a stone duplicate of the diagnostic waxup. The vacuum-formed matrix is tried intraorally after tooth preparation to verify sufficient tooth reduction (Fig. 11-22). A suitable shade of autopolymerizing tooth-colored acrylic resin is selected. A sprinkle tech-

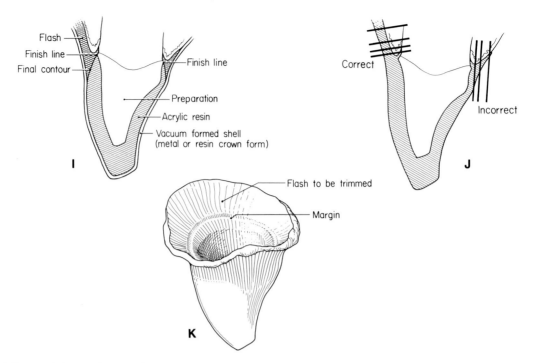

Fig. 11-21 I, Proximal view to illustrate the template seated on the prepared tooth. **J,** Contouring the template requires patience and time. The initial trimming is performed to eliminate flash before establishing contours. **K,** Flash removal to the finish line is required to prevent overextended margins that cause tissue recession. (From Dent. Clin. North Am. **29:**403 1985.)

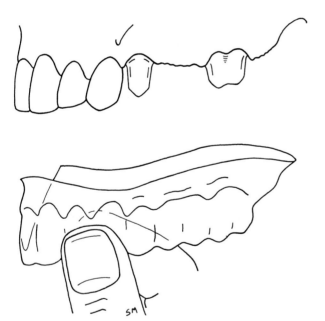

Fig. 11-22. The vacuum-formed matrix is tried intraorally to verify sufficient posterior tooth reduction.

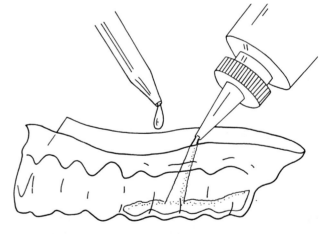

Fig. 11-23. Autopolymerizing tooth-colored acrylic resin is added in increments, using a sprinkle technique, until the area of the FPD is filled.

nique is used to fill the template in the area of the provisional restoration (Fig. 11-23).

Once the resin loses its glossy surface, the filled matrix is seated onto the lubricated tooth preparations. The matrix is pumped up and down to prevent the resin from setting into undercuts (Fig. 11-24). When the resin becomes warm (not hot), especially

in the pontic area, the restoration is copiously irrigated with cold water as it is periodically removed and reseated. Failure to control the exothermic heat of polymerization can result in disastrous injury to the dental pulps and oral mucosa.

After the resin has completely set, the matrix is removed and the finish lines of the tooth preparations are outlined in pencil (Fig. 11-25). The restoration is trimmed with a cone-shaped laboratory bur (Fig. 11-26). Embrasures are developed with a sandpaper disc (Fig. 11-27), and the lingual or palatal surface of the pontic is contoured with a long, tapered laboratory

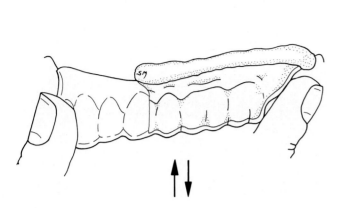

Fig. 11-24. Once the resin loses its glossy surface, the filled matrix is seated onto the lubricated tooth preparations. The matrix is pumped up and down to prevent the resin from setting into undercuts. Care is taken to prevent tissue trauma from the exothermic heat of polymerization.

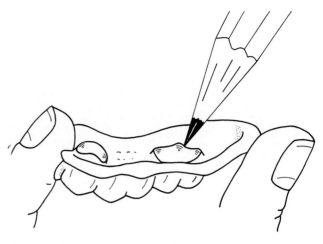

Fig. 11-25. After the resin is completely set, the matrix is removed and the finish lines of the tooth preparations are outlined in pencil.

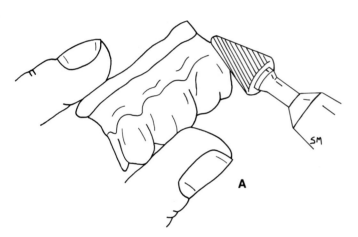

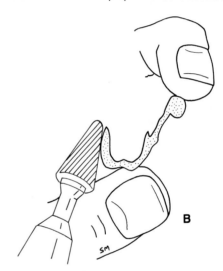

Fig. 11-26. A, Cone-shaped laboratory bur is used to remove excess resin, develop the emergence profiles, and eliminate overextension. **B,** The bur is angled to maintain an adequate bulk of resin in the gingival areas.

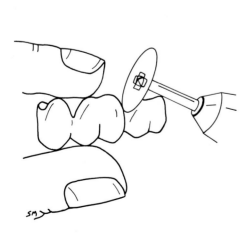

Fig. 11-27. Broad embrasures are developed with a sandpaper disc (medium cuttle).

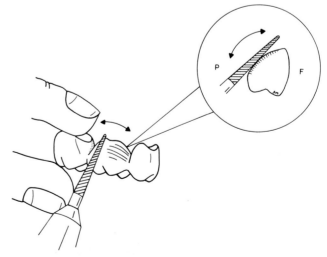

Fig. 11-28. Palatal surface of the pontic is contoured to mimic form planned for the definitive FPD. A convex tissue-contacting surface is the most hygienic.

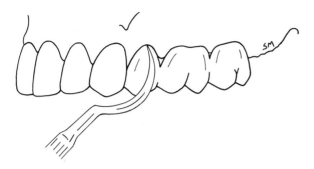

Fig. 11-29. The marginal adaptation of the treatment FPD is evaluated clinically, and the occlusion adjusted.

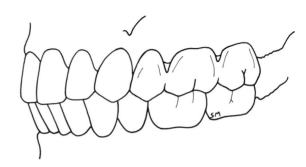

Fig. 11-30. The treatment FPD is highly polished and seated with temporary cement. Note that this patient had all first premolars previously removed for orthodontic treatment.

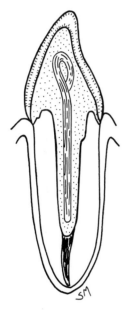

Fig. 11-31. A mandibular canine prepared for post and core. A polycarbonate crown is filled with acrylic resin and adapted to fit the post preparation. Note that a wire (a paper clip) is used for reinforcement.

bur. The pontic should mimic the planned design of the definitive pontic. A convex tissue surface is the most hygienic (Fig. 11-28).

The marginal adaptation of the provisional FPD is evaluated clinically for overextensions, underextensions, and overhangs (Fig. 11-29). Overextensions and overhangs are removed. Underextensions are corrected using additional resin carried to place with a sable brush. The occlusion is adjusted as indicated, and the esthetic contours are finalized. The completed provisional FPD is highly polished and then seated with a temporary cement (Fig. 11-30).

POSTCROWN TECHNIQUE

Interim crowns for endodontically treated teeth are arduous to prepare. If the tooth is part of an FPD, the temporary restorative measures are even more involved. Single-treatment restorations on endodonti-

cally treated teeth in a critical arch position require additional coronal radicular stabilization.

A wire (paper clip) or a nonprecious metal post is adapted to the canal. The seleted polycarbonate crown form is then filled with an acrylic resin and placed over the post, including a portion of the radicular surface of the tooth. The crown form must be pumped up and down to prevent resin from locking into undercuts during polymerization. After sufficient polymerization has occurred, the crown is removed with the temporary post set within the resin. Care must be exercised to trim the root coverage area to encourage a favorable tissue response. The entire assembly of makeshift post extension and crown form is cemented with a weak adhesive (Fig. 11-31). Esthetics and gingival tissue healing dictate this interim restoration.

RADIOPAQUE TREATMENT RESTORATIONS

The majority of treatment restorations are acrylic resins. Unfortunately, resins are radiolucent and cannot be detected on radiographs. Treatment restorations can be dislodged during mastication, trauma, and parafunctional habits. Accidental inhalation becomes a real danger, e.g., during sleeping hours. Although accidentally swallowed dental materials are usually passed without incidence, they can be lodged in the digestive tract or even aspirated, so the need for a radiopaque resin is real if a chest radiograph is recommended.[18]

The first patent for a radiopaque dental resin was issued almost a quarter of a century ago; however, an acceptable denture resin has not yet been formulated. Apparently, nontoxic, radiopaque denture resins with acceptable color, stability, and strength are difficult to manufacture.

Education is the patient's greatest protection. The use of polycarboxylate cements for interim coverage is popular because the greater adhesion provides increased stability, particularly in long-span treatment prostheses. Patients must be warned to discontinue wearing a treatment restoration that is fractured or previously dislodged.

LIMITATIONS OF TEMPORIZATION

Interim coverage is unsuitable for a variety of reasons. Dentists are aware of the inadequacies of "temporaries" when compared to perceptively constructed treatment restorations. The limitations of temporization are:

1. *Lack of inherent strength.* Temporaries fracture in long-span coverage in patients with bruxism habits or a reduced interocclusal clearance. If the bulk is increased, the patient's discomfort is evident.
2. *Poor marginal adaptation.* This inherent deficiency is difficult to improve upon. Temporization infers "adequate" margins at best.
3. *Color instability.* This is apparent when temporary restorations are placed for an inordinate length of time.
4. *Poor wear properties.* Teeth will drift or torque if the patient places heavy occlusal stress upon the interim coverage.
5. *Detectable odor emission.* This is undeniable despite the dentist's close attention to sufficient embrasure spaces. Resins, particularly autopolymerizing types, are porous.
6. *Inadequate bonding characteristics.* Few cements currently secure an adequate interface relationship with resins. Eugenol-bearing sedative cements are notorious for incompatibility with methyl methacrylate resins.
7. *Poor tissue response to irritation.* Mild or moderate tissue irritation is always present. Certain techniques are merely less irritating than other techniques.
8. *Arduous cement removal.* Cement in the proximal gingival cuff and the apex of the embrasure areas resists dislodgement. Operator concentration reduces the incidence of redundant cement, but rarely is all of the luting media removed after placement of interim coverage.
9. *Time expenditure for fabrication can be prohibitive.* The short term of the interim coverage encourages hastily fabricated temporaries—*not* treatment restorations.

PROVISIONAL SPLINTS

Provisional splints imply an adroitly designed, heat-polymerized resin used as a durable therapeutic restoration. They are usually employed in conjunction with advanced periodontal treatment (Fig. 11-32) or complex restorative dentistry (Fig. 11-33). The limitations of autopolymerizing splints have been graphically illustrated.[19]

Heat-processed provisional splints primarily pro-

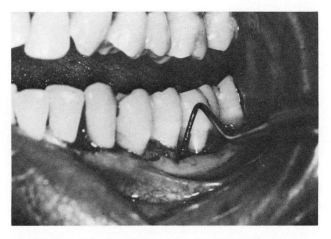

Fig. 11-32. A, Periodontal surgery and concomitant placement of a provisional splint. Osseous defect is on the distal surface of a mandibular second premolar.

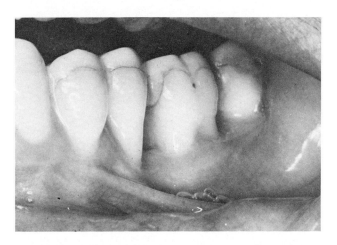

Fig. 11-32. B, Provisional splint retained until healing of the osseous defect is completed.

vide the opportunity to:

1. Reestablish a physiologic crown contour[20] (Fig. 11-34).
2. Develop adequate embrasure areas before replacement with a definitive restoration.[21]
3. Establish a satisfactory occlusion if there is a disparity between the maxilla and mandible[22,23] (Fig. 11-35).
4. Formulate a template for desirable esthetics (Fig. 11-36).
5. Permit periodic removal to assess surgical recovery.

The varying capacities of patient recovery are the subjective factors that are so difficult to assess.[24] Dr. J. E. Flocken describes in Part II a unique indirect method of fabricating treatment restorations that addresses many of the deficiencies of temporaries. Various methods and materials are available for the fabrication of interim coverage for prepared teeth. Hasty

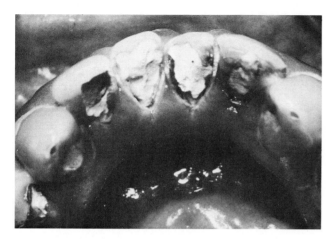

Fig. 11-33. A, Nearly insurmountable restorative problem, but with crown lengthening, endodontics, coronal radicular stabilization, and heat-processed treatment interim provisional splint, preservation of the incisors is possible.

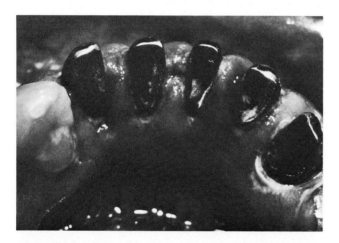

Fig. 11-33. B, Multiple endodontics with cast posts and cores prior to the crown lengthening.

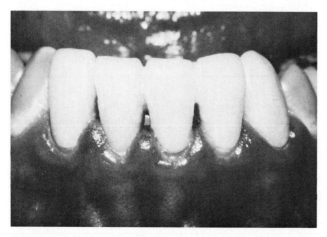

Fig. 11-33. C, Splinted treatment restorations on cores after crown lengthening to encourage healing of soft tissue. Note marginal gingivae and open embrasures. (Courtesy Dr. Ilze Eglitis, Albany, N.Y.)

fabrications result in predictable disappointment for the patient and the dentist. Knowledge of innovative techniques and materials ensures successful treatment restorations.

Part II

Treatment Restorations: A Healing Matrix

TERMINOLOGY

It is unfortunate for dentistry that the word "temporary" has been used to describe an exacting interim restoration. Treatment restorations are designed to benefit prepared teeth, surrounding gingivae, and the occlusion.

IRRITATION

The concept of "temporaries" implies a capricious design. It has become commonplace for temporaries to provide minimal protection to the operative site. Hastily fabricated temporaries result in unfavorable axial contours with inadequate marginal adaptation and gingival irritation. The major shortcoming of the "temporary" concept is failure to remove excessive sedative cement within the gingival crevice.

HEALING MATRIX

To establish a climate for favorable tissue response, the restoration is gently removed after the sedative cement has set. This permits: 1) removal of cement within the gingival crevice; 2) identification of margins for trimming the treatment restoration; 3) clearing of the embrasures; and 4) removal of cement on the outer axial surfaces of the treatment restorations.

SPECIFIC TECHNIQUE

The dental literature is replete with more than 100 references on temporary coverage. Unfortunately, certain techniques can initiate gingival irritation and recession. An indirect technique for fabricating a treatment restoration is recommended and is described in detail. The advantages of an indirect technique are:

1. Superior marginal adaptation.[25]
2. Minimal pulpal or mucosal irritation from free resin monomer.
3. No thermal shock to the dental pulp or oral mucosa from the exothermic heat of polymerization.
4. Stronger, denser, less porous restoration, since polymerization occurs under 30 psi.
5. Less chair time involved, since the work is accomplished in the dental laboratory by an auxiliary.
6. Greater comfort for the patient.

SEQUENCE OF FABRICATION

Before the appointment for preparations, the diagnostic casts are modified with wax to increase the

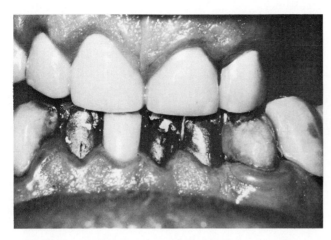

Fig. 11-34. A, Patient with reduced interarch distance with fractured veneer crowns.

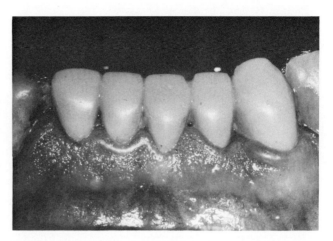

Fig. 11-34. B, Treatment restoration replacing fractured veneer crowns. Note the embrasure areas prior to periodontal surgery.

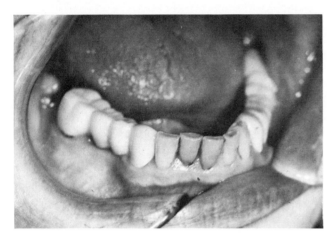

Fig. 11-35. A, Bilateral treatment restoration placed to program a modification in vertical dimension of occlusion.

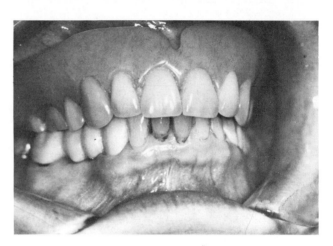

Fig. 11-35. B, Patient input and comfort preestablished before cast restorations are seated.

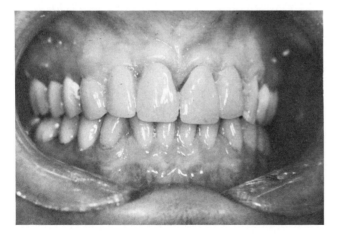

Fig. 11-36. "Epimine" resin provisional splint (prior to relining) establishes esthetics.

contour of the gingival third buccally and lingually of the teeth scheduled for complete crowns. This permits sufficient plastic material in the gingival area of the treatment restoration for polishing. Treatment restorations can be fabricated by the dental assistant or laboratory technician in the interim between the completion of tooth preparation, gingival dilation, and the final impression.

TECHNIQUE

A. Review the diagnostic data when the patient arrives. The corrected cast is then water soaked to remove entrapped air and to facilitate removal of the cast from the alginate overimpression. If vacuum-forming equipment is available for a clear plastic template, this alternative method provides a matrix for fabricating the treatment restoration and is a guide for tooth preparation. An alginate overimpression is carefully made of the diagnostic casts by the dental auxiliary. The borders of this impression are trimmed, interproximal extensions removed, and the impression stored in a humidor.

B. After tooth preparation, an initial impression is used as a cleanup procedure and for constructing the treatment restoration. This impression identifies the margins and confirms the draw of multiple preparations. The cleanup impression is accomplished with:
   1. A full-arch hydrocolloid impression.
   2. A full-arch alginate impression in which alginate material is rolled into the gingival crevice with finger pressure.
   3. A combination of hydrocolloid injected into the gingival crevice with an alginate covering impression.[26] Three precautions are necessary:
      a. The interval of time between insertion of the hydrocolloid and placement of the alginate covering impression must be short.
      b. Approximately ⅛ inch less water within the measuring cup is used to make a thicker alginate that acts as a plunger to drive the hydrocolloid into the gingival crevice.
      c. The surface of the alginate must remain untouched to stabilize the water-powder ratio.
C. Pour the cleanup impression of the preparations in impression plaster or model plaster mixed with slurry water to accelerate the set. The cast is gently separated from the impression by air pressure after the initial set.
D. Trim the cast with the mesial and distal ends at right angles to the line of the teeth. Wherever possible, cut the cast in the middle of an unprepared tooth. The edentulous posterior reproduction is also trimmed at a right angle. The cast is curetted in areas of intracrevicular tooth preparation to expose margins. All positive blebs on the cast that will prevent seating of the overimpression are removed. If a vacuum-formed plastic template is used, verify that it seats completely on the cast.
E. Apply a liquid tin foil substitute (diluted by 50 percent with water) to the cast. Blow off excess liquid but do not allow the coating to dry.
F. Proceed immediately to place 2 or 3 drops of resin monomer into the crevice and sift in resin polymer. Utilize vibration to prevent air entrapment. If the mix is too thick add additional monomer.
G. Dry the overimpression well. Mix a sufficient quantity of autopolymerizing resin in a dappen dish to a heavy liquid consistency.
H. Vibrate the fluid resin into the prepared areas within the overimpression (template). Fill the pontic areas and approximately two-thirds of the

abutment areas. Avoid excess resin in the impression of the adjacent unprepared teeth.
I. Carefully reseat the cast into the overimpression. Excessive pressure produces a subocclusal restoration; insufficient pressure results in supraocclusion.
J. Secure the cast and impression assembly with a rubber band without squeezing the cast into the impression.
K. Place the assembly in warm water (110 degrees Fahrenheit) in a pressure pot under 30 pounds of pressure for 15 minutes. Use only approved safe pressure pot equipment and assemble the pressure pot correctly. The higher the pressure, the denser the treatment restoration.
L. Remove the assembly from the pressure pot. Separate the cast with the treatment restoration from the overimpression.
M. Fill in any voids in the restoration. Wet with monomer, then sift in polymer, and replace in the pressure pot for 10 to 15 minutes.
N. Remove the treatment restoration from the cast with the point of a knife.
O. Trim and polish the treatment restoration. Test fit the treatment restoration in the mouth, and adjust the occlusion and the interproximal areas.
P. Cementation requires special procedures. Dry the treatment restoration thoroughly and place a sedative luting agent for cementation.
Q. As a sedative dressing, use a modified zinc-oxide and eugenol cement along with a neosporin ointment. Neosporin ointment contains neomycin, a fungicide, and bacitracin, a bacteriostatic agent. Place approximately ⅛ inch of neosporin ointment on the mixing pad; add 4 or 5 drops of liquid, mix and add enough powder to produce a "mashed-potato" consistency. Line the inner aspects of the treatment restoration and seat with normal occlusal loading. Allow the cement to set 4 or 5 minutes. The consistency of the sedative cement is adjusted with the neosporin ointment to achieve this 4 or 5 minute setting time.
R. When the initial set has occurred, use a pair of Backhaus towel forceps with a cotton wood stick (Dixon Manufacturing) as a fulcrum to remove the treatment restoration. The sedative cement lining also serves as an excellent impression material for further identification of the margins. Remove excessive cement from the treatment restoration and the gingival crevices (Fig. 11-37).
S. Recement the treatment restoration by reactivating the sedative cement. Dry the cement surface and apply a thin coat of modified eu-

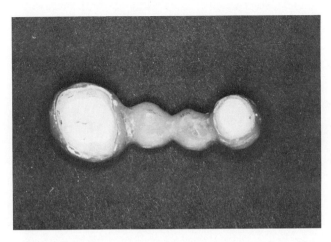

Fig. 11-37. Trimmed interim FPD removed after being seated with a zinc-oxide and eugenol sedative cement; it is then re-seated.

genol liquid. The prepared teeth are lightly dried and the treatment restoration is replaced. The cleaned, recemented restoration requires only limited adjustment.

SELECTED REFERENCES

1. Hildebrand, G.Y.: Studies in Dental Prosthodontics, Stockholm, 1937, Ableebolaget Fahlcrantz Bactrycheri, Vol. 1.
2. Collett, H.A.: Protection of the dental pulp in construction of fixed partial denture prostheses, J. Prosthet. Dent. 31:637-646, 1974.
3. Garvin, P., Malone, W.F.P., Toto, P., and Mazur, B.: Effect of self-curing acrylic resin treatment restorations on the crevicular fluid volume, J. Prosthet. Dent. 47:284-289, 1982.
4. Hagerman, D.A., and Arnim, S.S.: The relation of new knowledge of the gingiva to crown and bridge procedures, J. Prosthet. Dent. 5:538, 1955.
5. Cran, J.A.: Development of the gingival sulcus, Aust. Dent. J., 11(5):322-328, 1966.
6. Coelho, D.H., and Brisman, A.S.: Gingival recession with modeling plastic copper band impressions, J. Prosthet. Dent. 31:647, 1974.
7. Harrison, J.P.: Effect of retraction materials on the gingival sulcus epithelium, J. Prosthet. Dent. 11:514-521, 1961.
8. Daughlin, J.W.: The emphasis is on electrosurgery, Am. Acad. Gen. Dent. J. 18:25-28, 1973.
9. Bassett, R.W., Ingraham, R., and Koser, J.R.: An Atlas of Cast Gold Procedures, Buena Park, Calif., 1964, Uni-Tro College Press, Chapter 1.
10. Giunta, J.L., Grauer, I., and Zablotsky, N.: Allergic contact stomatitis caused by acrylic resin, J. Prosthet. Dent. 42:188-190, 1979.
11. Krug, R.S.: Temporary resin crowns and bridges, Dent. Clin. North Am. 19:313-320, 1975.
12. Braden, M., and Clarke, R.L.: An ethylene imine derivative as a temporary crown and bridge material, J. Dent. Res. 50:536, 1971.
13. Robinson, F.B., and Havijitia, S.: Marginal fit of direct temporary crowns, J. Prosthet. Dent. 47:390-392, 1982.
14. Crispin, B.J., and Caputo, A.: Color stability of temporary restorative materials, J. Prosthet. Dent. 42:27-33, 1979.
15. Tonn, J.H., and Cook, J.A.: Esthetic temporary crowns from plastic denture teeth, J. Mich. Dent. Assoc. 53:118-120, 1971.
16. Fritts, R.W., and Thayer, K.E.: Fabrication of temporary crowns and fixed partial dentures, J. Prosthet. Dent.,
30(2):151-155, 1973.
17. Sotera, A.J.: A direct technique for fabricating acrylic resin temporary crowns using the Omnivac, J. Prosthet. Dent. 29:577-580, 1973.
18. Monar, E.J.: Why temporary restorations should be opaque, J. Calif. Dent. Assoc. 35:12-15, 1972.
19. Loomar, D.A.: Provisional crown and bridge, J. N. J. Dent. Soc. 41(3):10-12, 1969.
20. Deferick, D.R.: The processed provisional splint in periodontal prosthesis, J. Prosthet. Dent. 33:553-558, 1975.
21. Kazis, H., and Kazis, A.: Complete Mouth Rehabilitation, Philadelphia, 1956, Lea and Febiger Publisher, p. 365.
22. Malone, W.F.P.: The occlusal epidemic: profile of confusion, Ill. State Dent. J. 39:(10):643-652, 1970.
23. Myers, G.E.: Textbook of Crown and Bridge Prosthodontics, St. Louis, 1969, The C.V. Mosby Co., pp. 184-189.
24. Yuodelis, R.A., and Faucher, R.: Provisional restorations: an integrated approach to periodontics and restorative dentistry, Dent. Clin. North Am. 24:285-303, 1980.
25. Crispin, B.J., Watson, J.F., and Caputo, A.A.: The marginal accuracy of treatment restorations: a comparative analysis, J. Prosthet. Dent. 44:283-290, 1980.
26. Appleby, D.C., Pameijer, C.H., and Boffa, J.: The combined reversible hydrocolloid/irreversible hydrocolloid impression system, J. Prosthet. Dent. 44:27-35, 1980.

BIBLIOGRAPHY

Amsterdam, M.: Provisional splinting: principles and techniques, Dent. Clin. North Am., pp. 72-99, March 1959.

Antonoff, S.J., and Levine, H.: Fabricating an acrylic resin temporary fixed prosthesis for an allergic patient, J. Prosthet. Dent. 45:678-679, 1981.

Breeding, L.C.: Indirect temporary acrylic restorations for fixed prosthodontics, J.A.D.A. 105:1026-1027, 1982.

Clements, W.G.: Predictable anterior determinants, J. Prosth. Dent. 49:40-45, 1983.

Davidoff, S.F.: Heat-processed acrylic resin provisional restorations: an in-office procedure, J. Prosthet. Dent. 48:673-675, 1982.

Fiasconaro, J.E. and Sherman, H.: Vacuum-formed prosthesis. I. A temporary fixed bridge or splint, J.A.D.A. 76:74-78, 1968.

Gegauff, A.G., and Pryor, H.G.: Fracture toughness of provisional resins for fixed prosthodontics, J. Prosthet. Dent. 58:23, 1987.

Grossman, L.I.: Pulp reaction to the insertion of self-curing acrylic resin filling materials, J.A.D.A. 46:265-269, 1953.

Hunter, R.N.: Construction of accurate acrylic resin provisional restorations, J. Prosthet. Dent. 50:520-521, 1983.

Jordan, R.D., Zakaraisen, K., and Turner, K.A.: Temporization of an extensively fractured anterior tooth, J. Prosthet. Dent. 47:182-184, 1982.

Kaiser, D.A.: Accurate acrylic resin temporary restorations, J. Prosthet. Dent. 39:158-161, 1978.

Kaiser, D.A., and Cavazos, E.: Temporization techniques in fixed prosthodontics, Dent. Clin. North Am. 29:403-412, 1985.

Langenwalter EM, Jordan R.D.: Fabrication of a provisional complete denture J. Prosthet. Dent. 58:246, 1987.

LaBarre, E.E.: Fabrication of separate adjacent provisional restorations, J. Prosthet. Dent. 49:631-632, 1983.

Langeland, K., and Langeland, L.: Pulp reactions to crown preparation, impression, temporary crown fixation, and permanent cementation, J. Prosthet. Dent. 15:129-143, 1965.

MacEntee, M.I., Bartlett, S.O., and Loadholt, C.B.: A histologic evaluation of tissue response to three currently used temporary acrylic resin crowns, J. Prosthet. Dent. 39:42-46, 1978.

Matheney, J.L.: Temporary reversible post and core restoration for multirooted teeth, J. Prosthet. Dent. 52:338-340, 1984.

Miller, S.D.: The anterior fixed provisional restoration: a direct method, J. Prosthet. Dent. 50:516-519, 1983.

Moskowitz, M.E., Loft, G.H., and Reynolds, J.M.: Using irreversible hydrocolloid to evaluate preparations and fabricate temporary immediate provisional restoration, J. Prosthet. Dent. 51:330-333, 1984.

Nayyar, A., and Edwards, W.S.: Fabrication of a single anterior intermediate restoration, J. Prosthet. Dent. 39:574-577, 1978.

Nayyar, A., and Edwards, W.S.: Fabrication of a single posterior intermediate restoration, J. Prosthet. Dent. 39:688-691, 1978.

Newitter, D.A.: Predictable diastema reduction with filled resin: diagnostic wax-up, J. Prosthet. Dent. 55:293-296, 1986.

Samani, S.I.A., and Harris, W.T.: Provisional restorations for traumatically injured teeth requiring endodontic treatment, J. Prosthet. Dent. 44:36-39, 1980.

Schneider, R.L.: Using clear polypropylene splints in the fabrication of anterior porcelain fused-to-metal fixed restorations, Quint. Dent. Technol. 11:92, 1987.

Troendle, K.B., Canales, M.L., and Richardson, J.T.: Temporary replacement of missing maxillary incisor, J. Prosthet. Dent. 55:277, 1986.

Webb, E.L., and Murrary, H.V.: Temporization of severely fractured vital anterior teeth, J. Prosthet. Dent. 54:198-200, 1985.

Wood, M., Halpern, B.G., and Lamb, M.F.: Visible light-cured composite resins: an alternative for anterior provisional restorations, J. Prosthet. Dent. 51:192-194, 1984.

12

Yvonne Balthazar, La Deane Fattore,
Timothy O. Hart, and
William F.P. Malone

INTEROCCLUSAL RECORDS

Diagnosis and treatment of the patient for fixed prosthodontics requires the dentist to create a duplicate model of the patient's intraoral relationships (Fig. 12-1). This goal is accomplished by:

1. Accurate elastomeric impressions
2. Durable, and stable working models
3. Repeatable registration of interocclusal relationships
4. Mounting of the patient's models on an appropriate articulator

There are two basic categories of interocclusal registrations: centric and eccentric interocclusal records. These are further categorized as follows:

1. Centric registrations
   a. Centric occlusion records
   b. Centric relation records
2. Eccentric registrations
   a. Lateral excursive records (lateral "checkbites")
   b. Protrusive records (protrusive "checkbite")

These registrations are accomplished with various materials and techniques.

INTEROCCLUSAL REGISTRATION MATERIALS
Characteristics of Ideal Interocclusal Bite Registration Medium

The general requirements of an ideal material for registration of interocclusal records are:

1. Limited resistance before setting to avoid displacing the teeth or mandible during closure.
2. Rigid or resilient after setting.
3. Minimal dimensional change after setting.
4. Accurate record of the incisal and occlusal surface of the teeth.
5. Easy to manipulate.
6. No adverse effects on the tissues involved in the recording procedures.
7. The interocclusal record is verifiable.

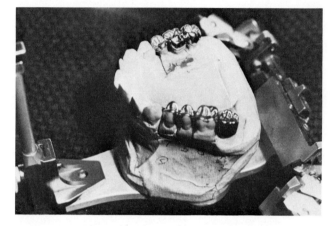

Fig. 12-1. Maxillary member of Denar 4 demonstrating bilateral castings with complete crowns on the terminal molars and three-quarter crowns anteriorly.

Plaster

Impression plaster is basically plaster of Paris to which modifiers have been added. These modifiers accelerate setting time and decrease setting expansion. Records of impression plaster are accurate, rigid after setting, and do not distort with extended storage. However, impression plaster is difficult to handle because the material is fluid and unmanagable prior to setting. The final interocclusal record is brittle.

Waxes

Thermoplastic waxes are frequently used for interocclusal registrations as records or as carriers for registrations (Fig. 12-2). Wax is widely accepted as an interocclusal recording material due to its ease of manipulation. However, studies have demonstrated that wax interocclusal records are inaccurate, unstable, and inconsistent because they can interfere with passive and active mandibular movement.

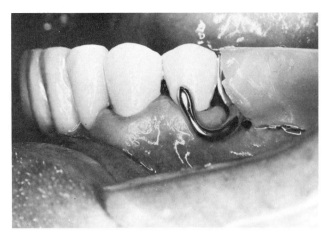

Fig. 12-2A. Wax reinforced with the RPD skeleton ensures the stability of the interocclusal record.

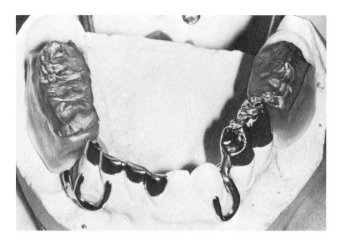

Fig. 12-2B. Aluwax is a common interocclusal record with an RPD because of its ease of manipulation.

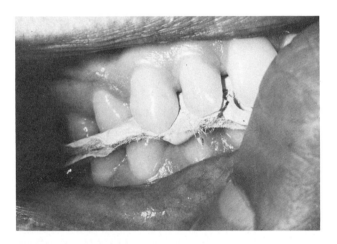

Fig. 12-3. Interocclusal record of zinc oxide eugenol paste on a carrier.

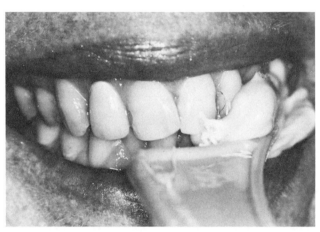

Fig. 12-4. Polyether interocclusal record with a carrier obtained on the prepared side so the contralateral side can be secured visually.

Zinc Oxide–Eugenol Pastes

Zinc oxide–eugenol (ZOE) paste is an effective interocclusal registration material (Fig. 12-3). The advantages of ZOE paste include:

1. Fluidity before setting. Fluidity is a critical quality of an interocclusal registration material because it ensures minimal interference with mandibular closure during record-making procedures.
2. Adhesion to its carrier.
3. Rigidity and inelasticity after final set.
4. Accuracy in recording occlusal and incisal surfaces of the teeth.
5. High degree of repeatability.

Despite the popularity of ZOE for interocclusal registrations, disadvantages exist. They are: 1) lengthy setting time, 2) significant brittleness, and 3) the accuracy of the registration material may surpass the accuracy of the casts, resulting in improper fit.

Silicone Elastomers

Two types of silicone elastomers are available as interocclusal registration materials: condensation silicone and addition silicone. Currently, addition silicone has gained acceptance because it is more stable than condensation silicone. The advantages of silicone interocclusal registration materials are:

1. Accuracy
2. Stability after setting
3. Minimal resistance to closure
4. Does not require a carrier

One major disadvantage of silicone is resistance to compression of the set material, which contributes to difficulty in the seating of plaster casts.

Polyether Elastomers

Polyether impression materials were introduced to dentistry in the early 1970s. Polyether interocclusal registration material consists of the basic impression

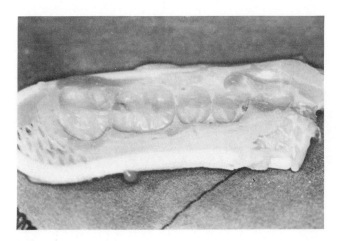

Fig. 12-5. Polyether interocclusal record with carrier trimmed to include only the cusp tips for the "prepared" side. The resiliency of the material will distort the mounting if it is beyond the greater convexity of the tooth.

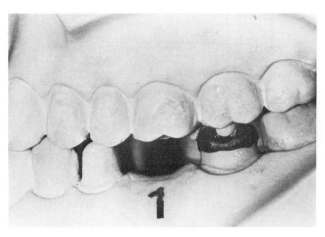

Fig. 12-6. Acrylic "bonnet" placed on the posterior abutment for a three-unit FPD. The term inal molar maintains the vertical dimension. (courtesy, Dr. E. Schelb, San Antonio, Tex.)

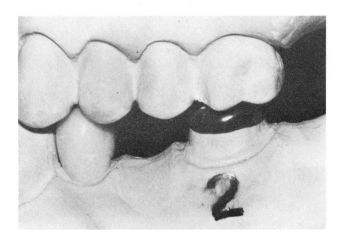

Fig. 12-7. Acrylic "bonnet" to maintain the vertical dimension. This procedure is more critical if the posterior abutment is also the terminal teeth in the arch. (courtesy, Dr. E. Schelb, San Antonio, Tex.)

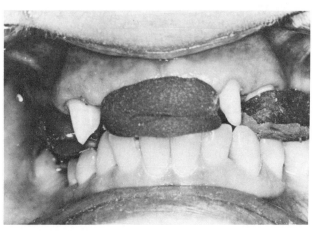

Fig. 12-8. Acrylic interoccusal record stabilized with a polyether. The combining of materials is common.

material augmented by plasticizers and fillers (Fig. 12-4). The advantages of this material as an interocclusal registration material are:

1. Accuracy
2. Stability after polymerization and during storage
3. Fluidity and minimal resistance to closure
4. Polyether can be used without a carrier

Disadvantages are that resiliency (Fig. 12-5) and accuracy may exceed the accuracy of plaster casts. Both of these factors can interfere with the placement of plaster casts into the recording medium during mounting procedures. The records are trimmed to remove excess material and preserve <u>only</u> the teeth indentations, avoiding distortions.

Acrylic Resins

Acrylic resin can be used as an interocclusal registration material. The most frequent application of acrylic resin for interocclusal records is in the fabrication of single-stop centric occlusion records (Figs. 12-6 and 12-7). Acrylic resin is both accurate and rigid after setting (Fig. 12-8). Disadvantages of acrylic resin as an interocclusal registration material include: 1) dimensional instability of some commercial formulations due to continued polymerization resulting in shrinkage and 2) the strength and rigidity of the material can damage plaster casts and dies during articulator mounting.

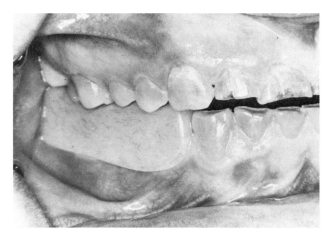

Fig. 12-9A. Stabilized bite plane for a patient with dentinogenesis imperfecta. Difficult treatment warrants refined interim procedures to ensure success. The restoration of vertical dimension is necessary for this young patient.

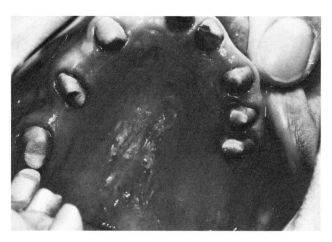

Fig. 12-9B. Coping tooth supported prostheses require stabilized bite rims constructed prior to tooth preparation to duplicate the vertical dimension.

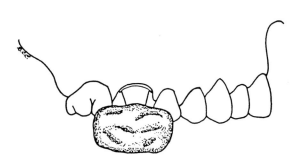

Fig. 12-10. Shape the material over the prepared surface of the tooth.

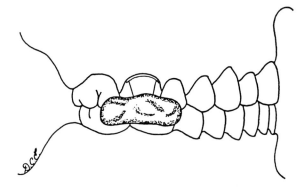

Fig. 12-11. Instruct the patient to close to the normal interocclusal position.

Stabilized Bite Rims

Stabilized rims may be constructed on replicas of the diagnostic casts. The rims are transferred to the mouth and the centric closure position recorded. Stabilized rims are indicated for positioning the casts prior to the formulation of the treatment plan and tooth preparation (Fig. 12-9, A and B).

CENTRIC REGISTRATIONS
Centric Occlusion

Centric occlusion is defined as that maxillomandibular relationship that is dictated by the maximum interdigitation of the existing dentition.[5] Therefore, for a centric occlusion to exist, the patient must exhibit at least three interocclusal points of contact. Clinically, these contacts are distributed in the form of two posterior and one anterior interdigitation. Direct intercuspation is indicated in the fabrication of single crowns or FPDs with an occlusal position and tooth form within normal physiologic limits. This includes the following:

1. The patient does not exhibit signs or symptoms of craniomandibular disorders.
2. The indicated fixed prosthodontic restorations do not interfere with the stable tripodization of centric occlusion.
3. Change in restorative vertical dimension is not anticipated.
4. The patient's centric relation is coincident with the centric occlusion.

The most accurate and frequently utilized centric occlusion registration is hand articulation of the patient's casts. However, clinical situations occasionally arise when interdigitation of the patient's interocclusal relationship is unstable. This occurs when the distalmost molar is prepared as the abutment for a three to five-unit posterior FPD. When this condition occurs, the dentist must ensure the stability and the repeatability of the patient's interocclusal relationship. Stability is

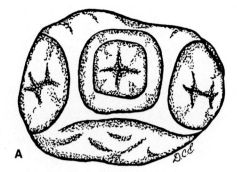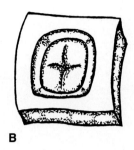

Fig. 12-12. Trim the record to provide minimal contact with the embrasures and axial surfaces of the unprepared teeth. **A,** Relationship with excess material. **B,** Trimmed to seat on casts.

accomplished by supplementing the maximum inter-cuspation with an interocclusal record or occlusal stop. The technique for an interocclusal stop is:

1. Prepare an appropriate portion of the interocclusal material according to the manufacturer's instructions. Interocclusal registration materials that are used for this technique include polyether, silicone, and acrylic resin.
2. Shape the material over the prepared surface of the tooth, avoiding flow of the material over the unrestored occlusal surfaces of the adjacent teeth (Fig. 12-10).
3. Instruct the patient to close the teeth to the normal interocclusal position, and allow the material to set (Fig. 12-11).
4. Before using the interocclusal record for cast articulation, trim the record to provide minimal contact with the embrasures and axial surfaces of the unprepared teeth (Fig. 12-12).

Centric Relation

Unlike centric occlusion, centric relation is a maxillomandibular relationship that is not influenced by the intercuspation of the patient's dentition. Although there are numerous definitions of centric relation, the indications and requirements of centric relation registrations remain consistent. The requirements of a centric relation registration are:

1. Because a centric relation record is obtained at an opened vertical dimension, a facebow is indicated in relating the maxillary model to the upper member of the articulator.
2. The interocclusal registration material must be passive so that it does not interfere with clinical positioning of the mandible.
3. The registration of centric relation must be repeatable.
4. The centric relation registration should record a position from which the patient can make eccentric mandibular movements.

Clinically Accepted Techniques

Numerous techniques and recommendations describe the most desirable method of positioning the mandible for centric relation registration.

Mandibular guidance considerations. Guidance of the mandible into the interocclusal registration material can be accomplished by the dentist, by the patient, or by both. An active centric relation record is an interocclusal registration that is directed by the patient's neuromuscular effort. A passive centric relation record is an interocclusal registration in which the dentist is responsible for guiding the mandible and its subsequent centric position. Passively recorded registrations were reported as more consistent and repeatable.[8] The three recommended passive centric relation guidance techniques available are:

1. *Chin point guidance.* The patient's mandible is guided in an arcing motion to the terminal hinge position. During this manipulation, posteriorly directed force is placed gently against the chin (Fig. 12-13). The mandible is then manipulated into a passive interocclusal registration medium.
2. *Dawson's bimanual manipulation.* The dentist approaches the patient from behind and places the thumbs lightly over the mandibular symphysis and the fingers along the inferior border of the mandible (Figs. 12-14 and 12-15). The mandible is then manipulated into a retruded position. When the mandible is moving freely in an arc around its terminal hinge axis, firm pressure is applied to seat the condyles posterosuperiorly in the glenoid fossae (Fig. 12-16). An upward lifting force is applied on the inferior border of the mandible by the fingers of each hand. A downward distally directed force is applied to the symphysis by the thumbs. The mandible is then guided into the interocclusal registration medium.
3. *Tongue-to-palate.* The patient is requested to touch the tongue to the posterior border of the hard palate (Fig. 12-17). The patient is then re-

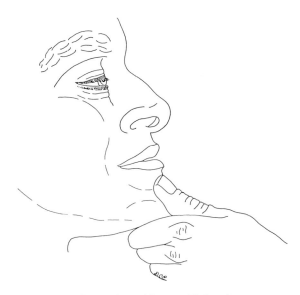

Fig. 12-13. Chin point guidance with thumb pressure.

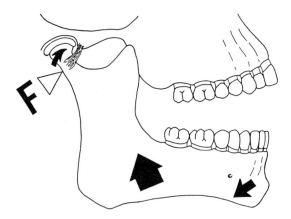

Fig. 12-16. The downward force of the thumbs and upward force of the fingers helps to seat the condyles in the glenoid fossa.

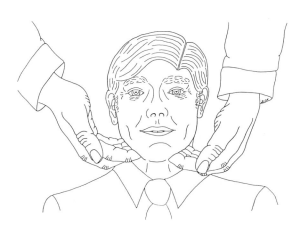

Fig. 12-14. Dawson's bimanual manipulation: forces directed upward by the fingers along the inferior border of the mandible.

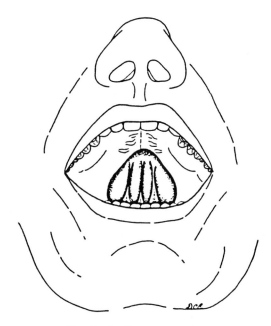

Fig. 12-17. Tongue to palate.

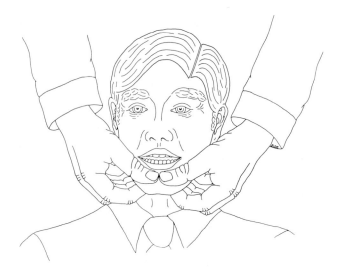

Fig. 12-15. With the thumbs in position, the mandible is guided into a retruded position.

quested to hold the tongue in place while carefully elevating the mandible until the interocclusal recording medium is engaged.

Registration techniques. The vertical dimension at which a centric relation record is made is determined by the thickness of the carrier, the thickness of the interocclusal material, or by a specific occlusal stop. Accordingly, the two most common techniques for controlling the vertical dimension of a centric relation record are the bite wafer technique and the anterior stop (Lucia Jig) technique.

Overall armamentarium

Piece of tin foil (½ by 1 inch)

Acrylic powder and monomer

Mixing cup and cement spatula

Articulating Paper

Straight handpiece and acrylic bur

Commercial bite wafers or baseplate wax for fabricating bite wafers

Bard Parker blade and handle

Bite registration paste

Air syringe

Mounting stone or plaster

Plaster bowl and plaster spatula

Articulating forceps

Rubber band (1 mm thick)

Articulator mounting stand

Bite wafer technique. Most of the stable interocclusal materials are capable of sustaining a specific shape before the initial setting reaction. This is desirable because a primary requirement of a registration material is that it be passive upon introduction to the teeth. It then becomes necessary to support the interocclusal registration material with a carrier, much as it is necessary to use an impression tray during impressions (Fig. 12-4). The most common technique is a thermoplastic bite wafer made from baseplate wax or a similar material. The dentist obtains centric relation record using a warm wax wafer. After verification of the record, the mild indentations in the wax are "washed" with a more accurate material (typically ZOE paste) and the recording is repeated. The resulting interocclusal record represents a stable laminate consisting of the thermoplastic wafer and a wash of paste or elastomer.

Anterior stop technique. The anterior stop centric relation record is accomplished with an anterior deprogramming appliance. This technique involves an anterior acrylic jig that is fabricated before the interocclusal record. This jig deprograms the influence of the posterior dentition by creating a platform that the incisal edge of the mandibular central incisor contacts. This provides posterior space for the interocclusal material and the carrier.

Fabrication of the anterior jig (discluder)

1. Burnish a small piece of foil over the lingual surfaces and incisal edge of the maxillary centrals on the cast (Fig. 12-18).
2. Mix 2 ml of acrylic monomer and 4 ml of acrylic powder in a mixing cup. When it reaches the doughy stage, apply it to the foil on the cast and mold it to a gently sloping ramp. Allow the acrylic to set.
3. Remove the jig from the cast and seat it on the patient anterior teeth (Fig. 12-19 A). Instruct the patient to "close on your back teeth" (Fig. 12-19, B and C). Observe the interocclusal dis-

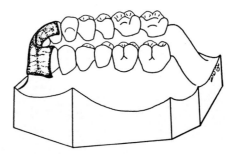

Fig. 12-18. Burnish a small piece of foil over the lingual surfaces and incisal edges of the maxillary central incisors on the cast.

tance between the most posterior teeth.

4. Adjust the jig by marking with articulating paper and grinding the marks until the posterior teeth are within 1 mm of interocclusal distance (Fig. 12-19 D). This clearance can be tested by interposing a 1 mm thick rubberband held in articulating forceps.
5. Leave the jig in place while preparing the wax wafer.

Preparation of wax wafer and centric relation record

1. Heat a wax wafer in the water bath for 1 minute and press the warmed bite wafer to the occlusals of the maxillary teeth with the jig in place (Figs. 12-20 and 12-21).
2. Remove the wafer (leaving the jig) and refine the shape to the patient's arch form. Reheat the trimmed wafer and replace it on the maxillary teeth.
3. While guiding the mandible, instruct the patient to "close on your back teeth" until the lower anterior teeth touch the anterior jig (Fig. 12-22). Wait 30 seconds, and then remove the wafer and run it under cold water. Using the Bard Parker blade, remove excess wax from the area surrounding cusp tip indentations (Fig. 12-23). Replace the wax record in the mouth and confirm the centric relation indentations.
4. Remove the wafer and apply a thin layer of ZOE bite registration paste to the lower cusp indentations of the wafer (Fig. 12-24). Position the bite wafer on the maxillary teeth and lightly guide the patient's lower jaw to closure. Allow the paste to set. Remove and inspect the centric relation record (Fig. 12-24 D).

ECCENTRIC REGISTRATIONS

The purpose of eccentric interocclusal registrations or "check-bites" is to assist the dentist in setting the articulator fossa elements on a semiadjustable articulator. There are two types of eccentric registrations: lateral-excursive records (lateral check bites) and protrusive records.

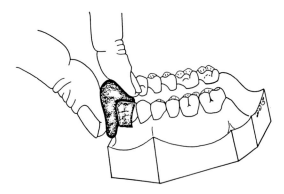

Fig. 12-19. A, Acrylic in its doughy stage is molded to the foil, forming a deprogrammer with a gently sloping ramp.

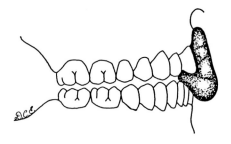

Fig. 12-19. C, Adjust the jig until the posterior teeth are within 1 mm of the interocclusal distance.

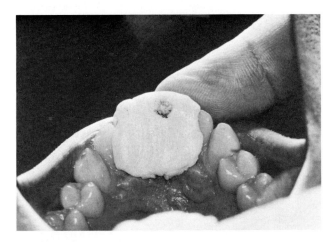

Fig. 12-19. B, Ramp seated intraorally and marked with articulating paper.

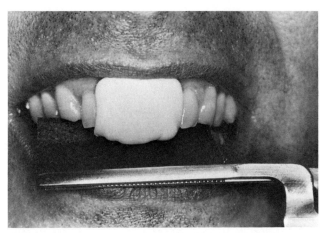

Fig. 12-19. D, Final intraoral adjustments concomitant with centric closure.

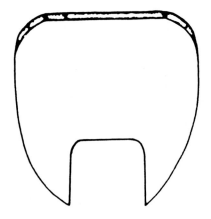

Fig. 12-20. Trimmed baseplate with anterior segment removed.

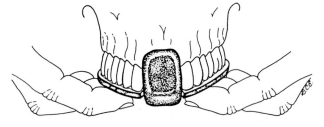

Fig. 12-21. Adapt the warmed wax wafer to the occlusal surfaces of the maxillary teeth with the jig in place.

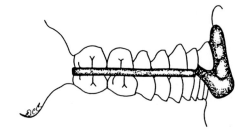

Fig. 12-22. While guiding the mandible, instruct the patient to "close on your back teeth" until the mandibular teeth touch the anterior jig.

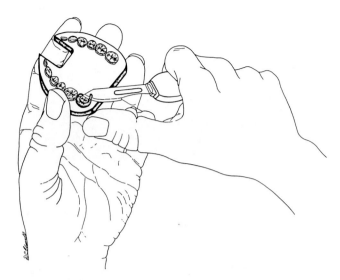

Fig. 12-23. Remove excess wax from the area surrounding the cusp tip indentations.

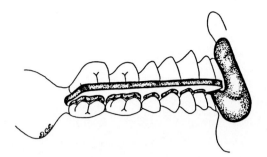

Fig. 12-24. B, This is replaced into the mouth.

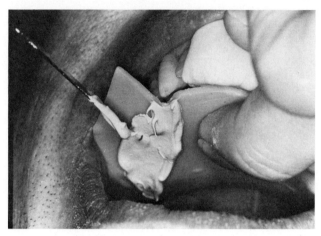

Fig. 12-24. C, Additional registration paste is added to stabilize the waxed wafer.

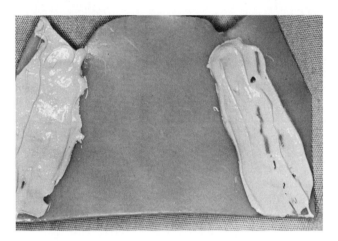

Fig. 12-24. A, A thin layer of registration paste applied to the mandibular cusp tip indentations of the record.

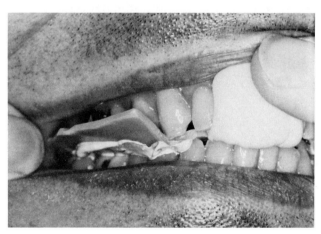

Fig. 12-24. D, Stabilized wax wafer with the Lucia jig anteriorly.

Lateral Check-Bites

Lateral check-bites are used to set the condylar elements of an arcon semiadjustable articulator. The registration records the lateral excursive maxillomandibular relationship and is performed without occlusal contact. The record usually consists of a carrier or wax wafer and an interocclusal recording material of ZOE wash. The technique is:

1. Before the lateral interocclusal registration is fabricated, the patient's casts are mounted on an arcon articulator using the appropriate facebow and centric relation record.
2. Arbitrarily set the superior walls of the fossae to an angle of 30 degrees and the medial walls to 15 degrees. If an articulator having fixed progressive sideshift is used, set the immediate sideshift to 1 mm.

3. Manipulate the mandibular member of the articulator into left lateral excursion so that the left mandibular canine is edge to edge with the left maxillary canine. Open the incisal pin to create a 2 mm space between the incisal edges of the canines (Fig. 12-25). Make a pencil mark at the point on the incisal table that the incisal pin contacts when the casts are in this edge-to-edge lateral excursion position.

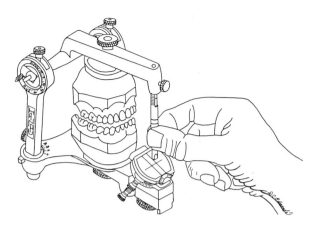

Fig. 12-25. Manipulate the mandibular member of the articulator into a lateral excursion so that the mandibular canine is edge to edge with the maxillary canine. Open the incisal pin to create a 2 mm space between the incisal edges of the canines.

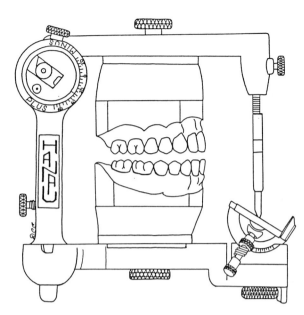

Fig. 12-27. Move the maxillary cast into a protrusive position with the incisors in an end-to-end relationship. Open the incisal pin to create a 2 mm interincisal space. Note that the condyle is set at 30 degrees.

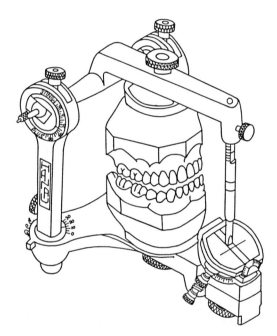

Fig. 12-26. Move the maxillary cast into a protrusive position with the incisors in an end-to-end relationship. Note the position of the incisal guide pin. It is 2 mm behind the solid line that represents the CR position.

4. Soften the wax wafer and place it on the lower cast; move the upper member to the previously determined lateral excursion as indicated by the pencil mark on the incisal guide table. Close the articulator until the incisal guide pin touches the surface of the incisal table. Chill the wax wafer to remove it from the cast without distortion.

5. While the patient is present, soften the wafer slightly in a water bath. Place the wafer against the upper teeth and have the patient move into left lateral excursion until the lower teeth locate

the indentations in the wax made by the mandibular cast. Have the patient bite firmly into the wax. Reline the preregistered lateral check-bite record with bite registration paste, then place it against the maxillary teeth and have the patient move into the lateral position. The bite paste fills the voids in the record between the arbitrary articulator setting and the patient's condylar inclinations.

6. After the paste sets, trim the lateral check-bite so only shallow cuspal imprints remain. Seat it on the mandibular cast and place the maxillary cast over it. Loosen the horizontal and medial condylar housing walls of the right condylar housing. Set them to allow the horizontal and medial walls to just contact the condyle. Tighten the walls and remove the record.

7. Repeat this procedure using right lateral excursion to set the left condylar housings.

Protrusive Check-Bites

When a nonarcon articulator is anticipated, a protrusive interocclusal record is indicated. Protrusive excursive record fabrication is similar to the lateral interocclusal records, but only one record is necessary. The procedure is:

1. The horizontal condylar inclinations of a nonarcon articulator are arbitrarily set at 30 degrees.

2. Move the upper cast into a protrusive position with the incisors in an end-to-end relation. The

incisal guide pin is placed in the center track of the incisal table. Open the incisal pin to create a 2 mm interincisal space and mark the incisal table accordingly (Figs. 12-26 and 12-27).

3. Soften the wax wafer and preregister it on the articulator, using the incisal table marking as a guide. Cool the wafer and remove it from the articulated casts.

4. With the patient present, soften the wafer and place it against the maxillary teeth and have the patient protrude the mandible until the lower teeth find the indentations. Then ask the patient to bite firmly into the indentations.

5. Reline the preregistered protrusive record with registration paste and refine the record in the mouth.

6. Seat the trimmed protrusive check-bite on the mandibular cast and place the maxillary cast over it. Loosen the horizontal condylar inclination locking nuts and manipulate them until the maxillary casts seat into the refined indentations of the check-bite. Finally, tighten the condylar inclination locking nuts.

MOUNTING OF CASTS

After the clinical interocclusal records are made, the mandibular cast is mounted to the maxillary cast on the articulator. The following procedures should be used:

1. The casts are carefully inspected, and any bubbles or artifacts removed from the occlusal and axial surfaces of the teeth.

2. The relationship between soft tissue areas of the cast and the interocclusal record is evaluated. The points of interference between the record and the plaster of these areas are relieved before mounting.

3. The articulator is inverted and the interocclusal record is seated on the occlusal surface of the maxillary cast. The mandibular cast is related to the maxillary cast with the record.

4. The articulator is closed to ensure that the lower mounting ring does not contact the base of the mandibular cast.

5. Place the plaster onto the mandibular cast and the mounting ring and then close the articulator.

SELECTED REFERENCES

1. Pipia, R.N., Interocclusal records. Tylman's Theory of Fixed Prosthodontics 7th Tylman, S.D., and Malone, W.F.P. St. Louis, 1978, The C.V. Mosby Co.
2. Clark, G.T., Carter, M.C.: Electromyographic study of human jaw-clenching muscle endurance, fatigue and recovery at various isometric force levels. Arch Oral Biol. 30:563, 1985.
3. Van Sickels, J.E., Rugh, J.D., Chu, G.W., and Lemke, R.R.: Electromyographic relaxed mandibular position in long-faced subjects. J. Pros. Dent. 54:578, 1985.

4. Hobo, S., Iwata, T.: Reproducibility of mandibular centricity in three demensions. J. Pros. Dent. 53:649, 1985.
5. Ash, M.: Occlusal adjustment: An appraisal. J. Mich. Dent. Assoc. 110:743, 1985.

BIBLIOGRAPHY

Balthazar-Hart, Y., Sandrik, J., Malone, W.F., et al.: Accuracy and dimensional stability of four interocclusal recording materials, J. Prosth. Dent. 45:586, 1981.

Berman, M.: Accurate interocclusal records, J. Prosth. Dent. 10:620, 1960.

Calagna, L.J., Silverman, S.I., and Garfinkel, L.: Influence of neuromuscular conditioning on centric relation registrations, J. Prosth. Dent. 30:598, 1973.

Dawson, P.E.: Evaluation, Diagnosis, and Treatment of Occlusal Problems, 1974, St. Louis, The C.V. Mosby Co., p. 58.

Douglass, Gordon: The cast restoration-why is it high? J. Prosth. Dent. 34:491, 1975.

Englehardt, J.P.: A 2 micron polycarbonate sheet, Quintessence Journal of Dental Technology 3:1, 1976.

Fattore, LaDeane, Malone, W.F., Sandrik, J.L., et al.: Clinical evaluation of the accuracy of interocclusal recording materials, J. Prosth. Dent. 51:152, 1984.

Helkimo, M., Ingerval, B., and Carlsson, G.E.: Comparison of different methods in active and passive recording of the retruded position of the mandible, Scand. J. Dent. Res. 81:265, 1973.

Ingerval, B., Helkimo, M., and Carlsson, G.E.: Recording of the retruded position of the mandible with application of varying external pressure to the lower jaw in man, Arch. Oral Biol. 16:1165, 1971.

Kabeenel, J.L.: Effect of clinical procedures on mandibular position, J. Prosth. Dent. 14:266, 1964.

Kantor, M.E., Silverman, S.I., and Garfinkel, L.: Centric relation recording techniques—a comparative investigation, J. Prosth. Dent. 18:379, 1972.

Lassila, V., and McCabe, J.F.: Properties of interocclusal registration materials, J. Prosth. Dent. 53:100, 1985.

Lucia, V.O.: A technique for recording centric relation, J. Prosth. Dent. 14:492-505, May 1964.

Lundeen, H.: Centric relation records: the effect of muscle action, J. Prosth. Dent. 31:244, 1974.

Lundquist, D.O., and Fiebiger, G.E.: Registrations for relating the mandibular cast to the maxillary cast based on Kennedy's classification system, J. Prosth. Dent. 35:371, 1976.

Millstein, P.L., Clark, R.E., and Kronman, J.H.: Accuracy of wax interocclusal registrations, J. Prosth. Dent. 19:40, 1973.

Millstein, P.L., and Clark, R.E.: Determination of accuracy of laminated wax interocclusal wafers, J. Prosth. Dent. 50:327, 1983.

Millstein, P.L., Clark, R.E., and Kronman, J.H.: Determination of the accuracy of wax interocclusal registrations, J. Prosth. Dent. 15:189, 1971.

Millstein, P.L., and Clark, R.E.: Differential accuracy of silicone-body and self-curing resin interocclusal records and associated weight loss, J. Prosth. Dent. 46:380, 1981.

Millstein, P.L., Clark, R.E., and Myerson, R.L.: Differential accuracy of the silicone-body interocclusal records and associated weight loss due to volatiles, J. Prosth. Dent. 33:649, 1975.

Millstein, P.L.: A simplified method for recording selected occlusal positions, Quint. Internat. 9:879, 1981.

Mohamed, S.E., and Christesen, L.V.: Mandibular reference positions, J. Oral Rehab. 12:355, 1985.

Postol, I.M.: Interocclusal registration at the vertical dimension of occlusion using acrylic resin copings, J. Prosth. Dent. 48:1, 1982.

Pruden, W.H.: The role of study casts in diagnosis and treatment planning, J. Prosth. Dent. 10:707-710, July 1960.

Shillingburg, H.T., Hobo, S., and Whitsett, L.D.: Mounting the Mandibular cast, Fundamentals of Fixed Prosthodontics, Chicago, 1981, Quintessence Publishing Co., p. 291.

Simon, R., and Nicholls, J.: Variability of passively recorded C.R., J. Prosth. Dent. **44:**21, 1980.

Sindledecker, L.: Effect of different centric relation registrations on the pantographic representation of centric relation, J. Prosth. Dent. **46:**271, 1981.

Skurnik, Harry. Accurate interocclusal records, J. Prosth. Dent. **21:**154, 1968.

Strohaver, R.A.: A comparison of articulation mountings made with centric relation and myocentric position records, J. Prosth. Dent. **18:**379, 1971.

Teo, C.S., and Wise, M.D.: Comparison of retruded axis articulation mountings with and without applied muscular force, J. Oral Rehab. **19:**207, 1981.

Thayer, K.E.: Interocclusal records and cast articulation, Fixed Prosthodontics Chicago, 1984, Year Book Medical Publishers, p. 134.

Tylman, S., Malone, W.F.P., and Pipia, R.N.: Methods of recording interocclusal relationships, Tylman's Theory and Practice of Fixed Prosthodontics, ed. 7, St. Louis, 1978, The C.V. Mosby Co.

Urstein, M., Fitzig, S., Cardash, Z., et al.: A method of recording the interocclusal relationship of the teeth, Dent. Med. **3:**13, 1985.

Williamson, J., Steinke, R., Morse, M., Swiff, G.: Centric relation-comparison of muscle determined position and operator guidance, Am. J. Orthod. **18:**78, 1980.

Wirth, C.G.: Interocclusal centric relation records for articulator mounted casts, Dent. Clin. North Am. **1531:**627, 1971.

13

**Steven M. Morgano, William F.P. Malone,
Delmo J. Maroso, D.A. Kaiser,
and John Sobieralski**

LABORATORY SUPPORT FOR FIXED PROSTHODONTICS

MASTER CASTS WITH REMOVABLE DIES

One method of fabricating removable dies requires the alignment of dowel pins before pouring the final impression. The time required to set up the pins delays the pouring of the impression, which can be detrimental for some impression materials, e.g. hydrocolloid. The pins can inhibit the flow of the stone and predispose to bubble formation.

Contemporary techniques that permit pin placement after the master cast is separated from the impression are more convenient. The Pindex System (Whaledent International, New York, N.Y.) (Fig. 13-1) is a versatile, innovative method.

THE PINDEX SYSTEM

Advantages of this system are:
1. The final impression is poured without delay and without the disadvantage of pins suspended in the impression.
2. The removable sections are planned with the finished master cast rather than with the impression.
3. All pins are placed parallel to one another so that the entire master cast with pins can be removed from the secondary base in one piece. Dies can then be sectioned from the underside of the base—reducing the chances of damaging the stone at the finish lines.
4. Double pinning with parallel pins for each die improves accuracy and stability.

Preparing the Master Cast

Pour the final impression with vaccuum-mixed die stone. Retrieve the master cast from the impression after the stone sets (Fig. 13-2) and reduce it to form a horseshoe. The buccolingual width of the base of the horseshoe is 15 to 18 mm, and there should be a

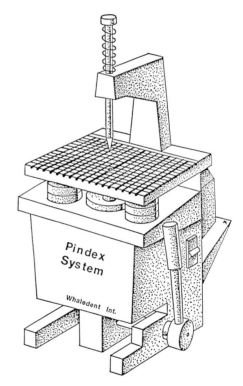

Fig. 13-1. The Pindex drill manufactured by Whaledent International, New York, N.Y.

15 mm thickness at the base of the cast between the gingival margins of the preparations and the inferior border (Fig. 13-3).

Pin placement. Reduce the undersurface of the cast so that it is perfectly flat. The manufacturer supplies a "flat surface grinder" to flatten the base. Drill two holes for each removable section as far apart as possible to provide space for the pins and sleeves. This ensures the stability of the dies (Fig. 13-4 A).

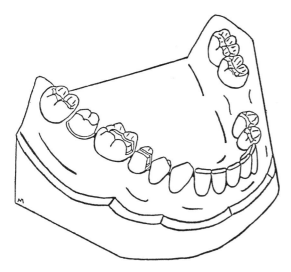

Fig. 13-2. The master cast is retrieved from the impression.

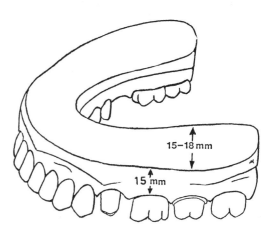

Fig. 13-3. The cast is ground to form a horseshoe.

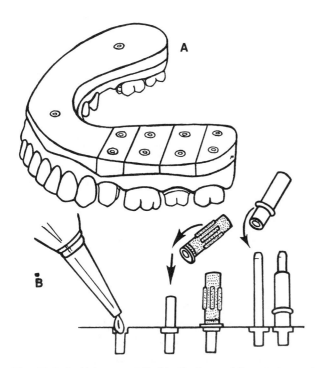

Fig. 13-4. A, Holes are drilled in the base of the master cast-two holes for each removable section. **B,** Pins are cemented in the prepared holes. The white sleeves are placed over the long pins, and the gray sleeves are placed over the short pins.

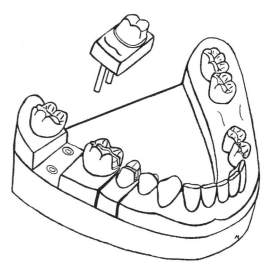

Fig. 13-5. Dies are sectioned with a die saw. Two widely separated parallel pins produce a stable removable die that can be accurately seated. [Courtesy Dr. D.J. Maroso, Alton, Ill. Fig. 13-1-5].

Cement pins in the prepared holes with low-viscosity cyanoacrylate cement. The short index pins are cemented in the lingual holes first, followed by the long pins in the buccal holes. Wipe away any excess cement immediately. Place the white sleeves over the long pins and the gray sleeves over the short pins (Fig. 13-4 B).

The secondary base. Place a strip of carding wax over the extensions of the long pins and over the openings of the gray sleeves (covering the short pins). Box the pinned master cast, paint plaster separator on the base, and pour a secondary base with cast stone. The manufacturer supplies a rubber base-former that also can be used to produce the secondary base.

Removable dies. Trim the secondary base on the model trimmer after the stone sets. The entire master cast can be removed from the secondary base in one piece. Dies are sectioned with a die saw (Fig. 13-5). Trim each die carefully to expose the finish line. Clean the stone grindings from the dies, pins, base, and pin holes, and reseat the dies. The master cast is now ready to be mounted.

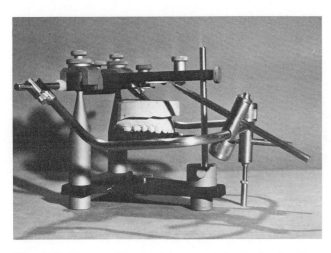

Fig. 13-6. The maxillary cast is mounted with the face-bow record.

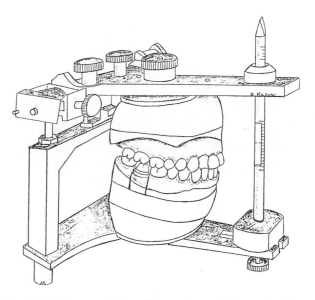

Fig. 13-7. The mounted maxillary and mandibular casts. (Courtesy Dr. D.J. Maroso, Alton, Ill.)

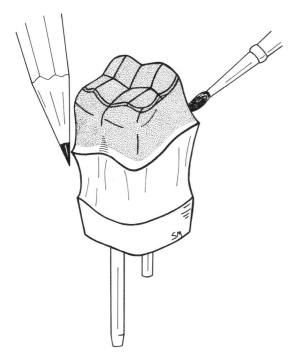

Fig. 13-8. The finish line is delineated with a sharp, red wax pencil, and die relief is painted on the preparation 0.5 to 1 mm short of the finish line.

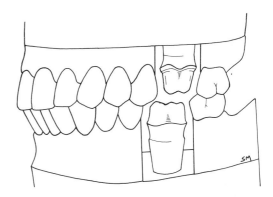

Fig. 13-9. Mounted maxillary and mandibular master casts. First molars have been prepared for cast restorations with the original position of the cusp tips preserved.

Mounting the Casts

Index and mount the maxillary cast with the face-bow record (Fig. 13-6). After the mounting stone sets, relate the indexed mandibular cast to the mounted maxillary cast. If there are sufficient unprepared teeth to produce a stable maxillomandibular relationship in centric occlusion, relate the mandibular cast to this position and lute it with wooden dowels or blades and sticky wax. Holding the casts together with rubber bands is unreliable and not recommended. An interocclusal record is often required to accurately relate the mandibular cast (see Chapter 12). Invert the articulator and mount the mandibular cast (Fig. 13-7).

Developing the Wax Patterns

Die preparation. Prepare the dies for waxing after the master casts have been mounted. Delineate the finish lines with a sharp, red wax pencil, and paint die relief onto the preparations 0.5 to 1 mm short of the finish lines (Fig. 13-8). Three coats of TRU-FIT (George Taub Products & Fusion Co., Inc., Jersey City, N.J.) will produce a thickness of relief of approximately 35 to 40 microns. The finish lines can be sealed with a small amount of low-viscosity cyanoacrylate applied with a cotton tip applicator. Remove excess cyanoacrylate immediately with compressed air.

Wax pattern fabrication—posterior teeth. Biomechanically designed tooth preparations maintain the original position of all cusp tips, facilitating the development of a functional occlusion (Fig. 13-9). Dip

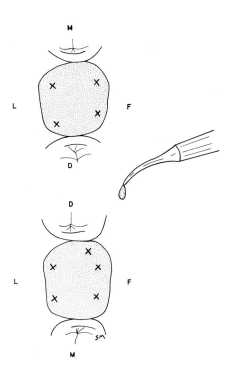

Fig. 13-10. Desired position of the cusp tips (marked with an "X"). Occlusal view of the maxillary and mandibular first molars shown in Fig. 13-9.

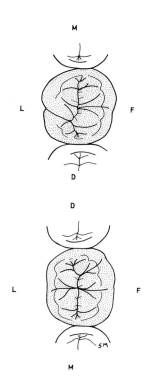

Fig. 13-12. Completed occlusal surfaces for the first molars.

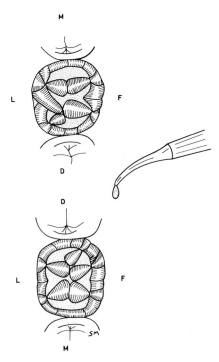

Fig. 13-11. Wax is systematically added to form the functional occlusal design (See Chapter 14).

the prepared, lubricated die into molten wax to coat the entire preparation, or flow hot wax onto the die with a No. 7 wax spatula. Seat the dies onto the master casts and establish preliminary axial contours in wax.

Place wax cones representing the cusp tips with a wax dropping instrument (Fig. 13-10). Place functional (stamp) cusps first, followed by the nonfunctional cusps. Close the articulator after each cone placement to monitor the centric-occlusal position of each cusp tip. Move the articulator into eccentric positions to ensure that cusps pass between one another without interference.

Add wax gradually to form the buccal, lingual, mesial, and distal cusp ridges and the proximal marginal ridges (Fig. 13-11). Evaluate centric and eccentric occlusion with each wax addition. Flow wax between the ridges to complete the anatomic form and carve the supplemental grooves (Fig. 13-12). Check the occlusal contacts with zinc stearate powder and adjust as indicated (see Chapter 14) for desired occlusal contacts.

Check the occlusion with 0.0005 inch shim stock (Artus Corp. Englewood, NJ 07631). Cusps on the wax patterns and on the stone teeth must all hold shim stock (Fig. 13-13).

Refine the axial contours to simulate normal anatomic contours. Proximal surfaces are flat or slightly concave occlusogingivally and form a triangular embrasure (Fig. 13-14). The proximal contact is in the occlusal third of the crown—except between the first

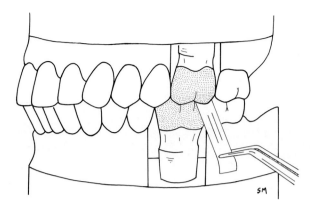

Fig. 13-13. Cusps on the wax patterns and on the stone teeth must all hold shim stock.

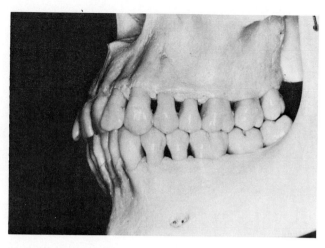

Fig. 13-14. Proximal surfaces are flat or slightly concave occlusogingivally and join at the contact to form a triangular embrasure.

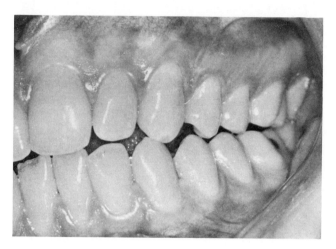

Fig. 13-15. Facial surfaces are flat as they emerge from the gingival sulcus.

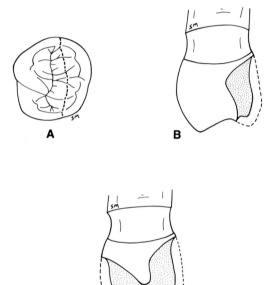

Fig. 13-16. A, Wax is cut away *(dotted line)* for the ceramic veneer after the contours and occlusion are finalized. **B,** Proximal view of cut-back for a maxillary first molar with a metal occlusal surface. **C,** Proximal view of cut-back for a maxillary first molar with a ceramic occlusal surface. Note the marginal ridge is supported with metal.

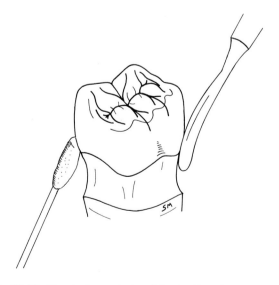

Fig. 13-17. Marginal wax is burnished with a beaver-tail burnisher. The buccal flute, so carefully placed in the preparation, is reproduced in the wax-up. A cotton tip applicator soaked in die lubricant polishes the wax.

and second maxillary molars where the contact may be in the middle third. Facial and lingual axial surfaces are also flat occlusogingivally (Fig. 13-15), and all marginal ridges are of equal occlusogingival height.

Cut away wax where ceramic veneers are planned (Fig. 13-16) and readapt the wax to the finish lines. Burnish the marginal wax with a beaver-tail burnisher and smooth and polish all surfaces with a cotton tip applicator soaked in die lubricant (Fig. 13-17). Wash the wax patterns with a liquid detergent solution to remove excess lubricant.

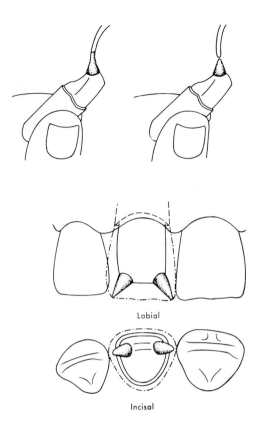

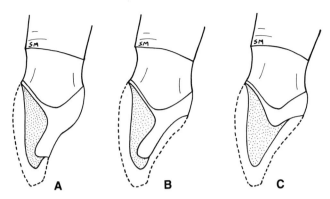

Fig. 13-20. Three distinct cut-backs for the anterior metal ceramic crown. **A,** Proximal and occlusal contact in metal. **B,** Proximal contact in metal and occlusal contact in porcelain. **C,** Proximal and occlusal contact in porcelain.

Fig. 13-18. Wax cones determine the position of the incisal corners.

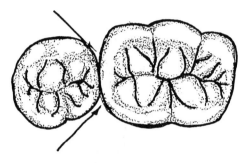

Fig. 13-21. Facial and lingual extensions for mesioocclusal casting on the mandibular first molar.

Place the patterns back on the master casts to verify proximal and occlusal contacts. Make final corrections as indicated. The patterns are now prepared for investing.

Wax pattern fabrication—anterior teeth. Anterior wax patterns are developed in a similar manner. Wax cones determine the position of the incisal corners (Fig. 13-18). Functional and esthetic morphology is then developed—consistent with the desired anterior guidance (Fig. 13-19). Gingival and incisal embrasures, incisal edge position, occlusal relationships, axial contours, and esthetic form are definitively established in wax, then the wax is removed for the ceramic veneer. Three distinct types of cut-back are commonly employed for anterior teeth (Fig. 13-20).

After cut-back, the wax pattern is prepared for investing. The inlay-onlay preparation will be used to illustrate appropriate spruing techniques.

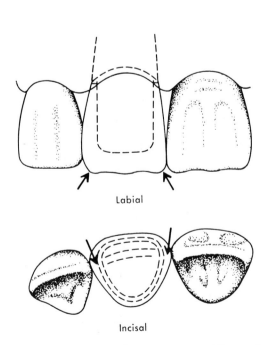

Fig. 13-19. The position of the wax cones and the contiguous and opposing teeth guide the development of anatomic contours and the anterior guidance.

INLAY-ONLAY SPRUING

Preparation

Establish the contact area with the adjacent tooth (No. 29) and draw vertical lines with a sharp pencil held at a 45 degree angle (Fig. 13-21). These lines

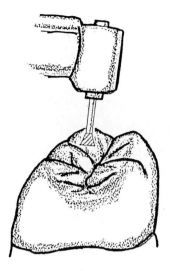

Fig. 13-22. Tooth preparation is started in the central pit with a No. 34 inverted cone.

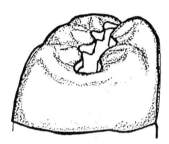

Fig. 13-23. Occlusal outline is determined by occlusal topography, caries, and occlusion.

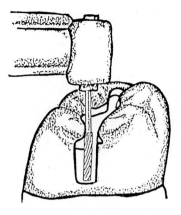

Fig. 13-24. The proximal step is developed to include the contact area with the final extensions dependant upon caries.

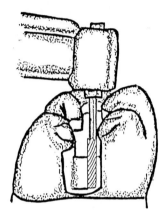

Fig. 13-25. The axial wall is slightly convex, reflecting axial contour of the natural tooth.

represent the final extension of the box preparation and are equidistant into a self-cleansing buccal and lingual area. Generally, lingual flares are overextended, while buccal flares are underextended. This procedure assumes greater importance when the tooth is rotated.

Initial penetration is accomplished with a No. 34 inverted cone bur in the central pit (Fig. 13-22). The vertical dimension of the cutting surface of the bur is 1.0 mm. The depth of the cut is more easily determined visually. It also readily forms a flat pulpal floor. Final pulpal floor depth will be 1.5 to 2.0 mm. The pulpal wall is extended for the length of the central groove at a depth of 2 mm. Slight extensions are carried into all primary grooves.

The occlusal outline form is extended using a No. 56 and No. 169 bur to eliminate undercuts created by the No. 34 bur. The No. 169 bur in a vertical position allows for occlusal divergence. The occlusal outline represents a smooth, continuous flow into the groove extensions and dovetail in the distal pit (Fig. 13-23). The pulpal wall remains flat during the extensions in outline form, and the distal dovetail does not encroach

upon the marginal ridge. Clinically, the pulpal floor is positioned to the ideal depth. The remaining caries are removed, and the bases reestablish a flat pulpal wall.

A No. 56 or No. 256 bur is used to begin the proximal box formation. The pulpal-axial wall is approximately 2.5 to 3.0 mm in height (assuming appropriate pulpal floor depth). Contact is broken and separation is achieved. A matrix band can be placed around No. 29 to prevent damage to the distal surface during box preparation of No. 30. Do not extend the buccolingual dimension of the box to the initial vertical pencil marks. The flare from the bow provides this final extension (Fig. 13-24).

Maintain a slight convexity to the axial wall of the preparation corresponding to the axial contour of the uncut tooth. Failure to maintain this slight convexity results in vague interior line angles to the box form and an uneven width to the gingival wall (Fig. 13-25). The gingival wall is uniformly 1.0 mm in width. The axial wall forms a slight obtuse angle with the gingival wall, i.e. the axial wall converges slightly. All other walls of the preparation diverge to receive the casting.

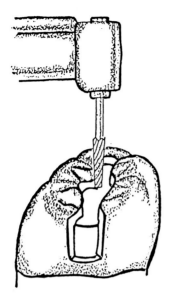

Fig. 13-26. A No. 699L or No. 169 carbide bur is directed to smooth and define the internal line angles.

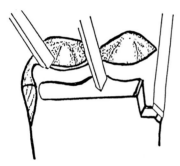

Fig. 13-27. Internal line angles are developed with hand instruments. Sharp hand instruments accomplish bevels.

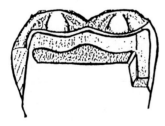

Fig. 13-28. The proximal flare is performed with No. 169L carbide burs.

A No. 69 bur is used to smooth the walls of the preparation and further define internal line angles of the box. Hold the bur vertical to the path of draw of the preparation. The taper to the bur provides sufficient divergence to the cavity wall (Fig. 13-26).

Gingival bevel, occlusal bevel, sharpness, and detail to the entire preparation are accomplished using sharp

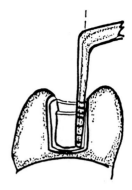

Fig. 13-29. Divergence is assessed with a periodontal probe.

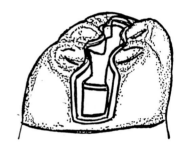

Fig. 13-30. A smooth continuous outline form.

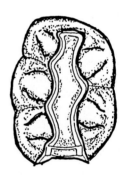

Fig. 13-31. Nearly parallel walls.

hand instruments. Clinically, gingival and occlusal bevels are placed with small flame-tipped diamond points, i.e. the 8874 (Fig. 13-27). The proximal flares to self-cleansing buccal and lingual surfaces are performed with hand instrumentation and the 169L carbide (Fig. 13-28).

The periodontal probe is invaluable in determining divergence of cut walls, axis of draw, and of undercuts. The shank of the instrument is observed to determine angulation after placement on a cut surface (Fig. 13-29). The final preparation exhibits a smooth, continuous occlusal outline form with a slight beveling (Fig. 13-30).

The box exhibits opposite near-parallel walls with a flare to the self-cleansing areas. The gingival wall is a uniform depth with a 45 degree gingival bevel (Fig. 13-31). Internal line angles are sharply defined. The

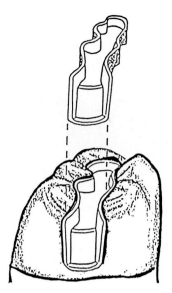

Fig. 13-32. A continuous bevel.

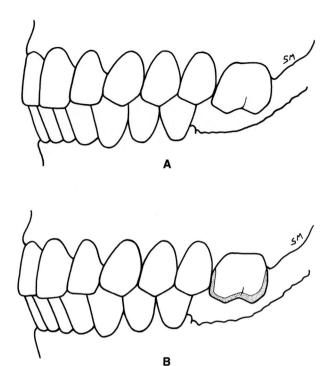

axial wall is slightly convex. The pulpal floor is flat with sharply defined pulpal axial angles. A continuous definite bevel occurs occlusally and gingivally (Fig. 13-32).

The use of an onlay-inlay (Fig. 13-33) to correct the occlusal plane is misguided because of limited vertical length. Pulpal integrity, biologic width, and furcation involvment are additional restrictions that are only partially resolved with endodontics, cast restorations, and crown lengthening including osseous recontouring. Extraction should be performed if supraeruption exceeds 3mm.

Spruing and Investing of Inlays and Crowns

The importance of spruing an inlay or crown is obvious; yet the governing principles are frequently misunderstood and the finished casting is unsuccessful. The purpose of the sprue is to gain a portal through which the molten gold enters the mold cavity and to create a reservoir of molten metal from which the casting can draw as it cools and shrinks. There are seven rules for spruing:

1. Use a short, thick sprue rather than a long, thin one. When molten metal cools, the outer surface cools fastest and solidifies first, forming a shell of solid metal around a molten center. As the metal continues to cool, this shell increases in thickness and then the inner section finally solidifies. A thin section will solidify while there is still molten metal at the center of a thicker section. If the sprue is thinner than the casting, it will solidify completely while the thicker part of the casting is still partly molten. Thus no more metal can be supplied from the sprue as the

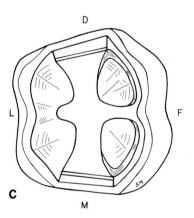

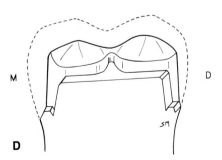

Fig. 13-33. A, An onlay only *minimally* alters occlusal relationships. The supraerupted maxillary first molar produces an unfavorable plane of occlusion for a mandibular RPD. **B,** An onlay only reproduces the original occlusal plane discrepancy; thus, a complete coverage artificial crown is indicated. **C,** Occlusal view of a mandibular onlay preparation. **D,** Facial view of MOD onlay preparation. *Continued.*

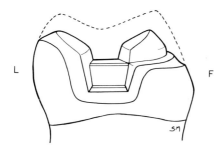

Fig. 13-33, cont'd. E, Proximal view highlighting the facial hood-erpendicular surfaces.

metal shrinks, creating voids in the metal or "shrink spot porosity" (Fig. 13-34).

2. Attach the sprue to the bulkiest part of the pattern (Fig. 13-35).
3. Never feed a bulky section through a thin section (Fig. 13-36).
4. Attach the sprue to the pattern so that the gold entering the mold will not be directed against a perpendicular surface. (Fig. 13-37).
5. Attach the sprue securely, but do not plunge the hot sprue deeply into wax. This may distort the pattern and the distortion may go unnoticed until the casting is completed and does not fit on the die or tooth (Fig. 13-38).
6. Never use a "bottleneck" sprue. If a bur shank is used, do not use the tapered part of the shank unless you build up the shank with wax. If you build up the shank with wax, be sure the wax is smooth (Fig. 13-39).
7. Firmly secure the sprue to the pattern to ensure stability during investment so that the pattern is not dislodged from the sprue. (Fig. 13-39).

SOLDERING
Preceramic Soldering

The FPD is waxed to complete contour and occlusion. Provision is made for the connector in the wax patterns. Two flat, parallel soldering plates with a 0.3 mm gap are developed to maintain physiologic facial, lingual, and gingival embrasure form. The solder gap is as uniform as possible to minimize distortion due to uneven contraction of the solder (Fig. 13-40).

Wax is cut away from the patterns where porcelain is planned, without altering the soldering plates (Fig. 13-41). An alternative design is to establish a deep rest preparation (Fig. 13-42 A) which increases the surface area of solder contact and improves the strength of the connector. This connector design avoids encroaching on the gingival embrasure when the available area for the solder joint is unusually short occlusogingivally. Provision is made in the tooth preparation for the rest seat (Fig. 13-42, B).

The wax patterns are invested, cast, and divested. After fitting the castings to the master dies, the sol-

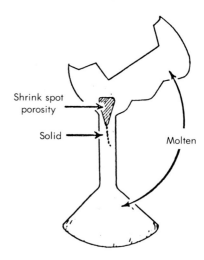

Fig. 13-34. Shrink spot porosity (wrong).

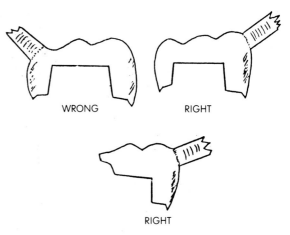

Fig. 13-35. Locate the bulkiest portion.

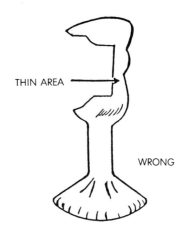

Fig. 13-36. Locate the thin areas.

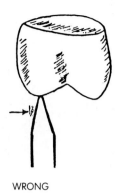

WRONG

Fig. 13-37. Avoid perpendicular surfaces.

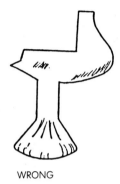

WRONG

Fig. 13-38. Avoid distorting pattern with hot sprue.

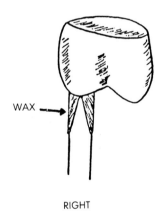

WAX →

RIGHT

Fig. 13-39. Constricted sprue; abrupt or gradual sprues are discouraged.

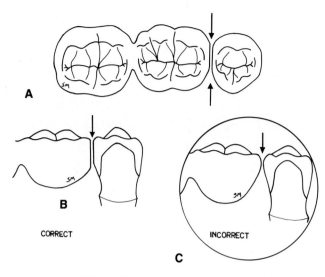

A

B   CORRECT

C   INCORRECT

Fig. 13-40. A, FPD with 3 mm gap between flat parallel plates. **B,** Flat surfaces. **C,** Point contact is discouraged.

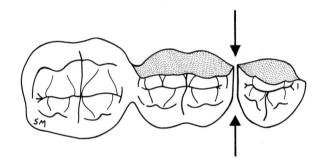

Fig. 13-41. Wax removal for porcelain maintaining flat parallel walls.

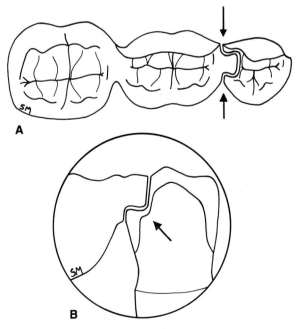

A

B

Fig. 13-42. A, Deep rest from pontic to abutment. **B,** Space allowed in tooth preparation for deep rest seat.

dering plates are finished with a rubber wheel. The castings are then tried intraorally and indexed for soldering. Indexing can be accomplished with impression plaster or with chemically activated acrylic resin (DuraLay, Reliance Dental Mfg. Co., Worth, IL). The dimensional accuracy of impression plaster is considered superior to resin and produces consistent results.

After indexing, the castings are firmly luted to the plaster with sticky wax, and the FPD is invested in high-heat soldering investment. All margins must be completely covered with investment. After one hour, the sticky wax is softened with hot water and the index is carefully removed from the set investment. Hot water is used to flush off wax residue. The investment block is trimmed and funneled with a No. 25 Bard Parker blade from the facial and the lingual surface to provide access for solder placement and direct the flame of the soldering torch to the connector area (Fig. 13-43).

If Dura Lay was used as an indexing medium, the resin must be eliminated in a burn-out oven. The invested castings are brought from room temperature to 900 degrees Fahrenheit and heat soaked until all traces of resin are eliminated. This usually takes 60 minutes. The resin burn-out is an additional step not required when plaster is used as an index, and the prolonged heating necessary to eliminate the Dura Lay increases the potential for oxide formation, which inhibits solder flow. After complete purging of the resin, the invested castings can be removed from the oven for fluxing and soldering.

When plaster is used for an index, the castings are prefluxed and placed in a room temperature burn-out oven and brought to 900 degrees Fahrenheit to preheat the assembly. Prolonged heat soaking is not necessary.

The preheated investment block is placed on the soldering block. The high-fusing preceramic solder recommended by the alloy manufacturer is coated with flux and placed within the joint space. The investment and castings are rapidly heated with the reducing portion of the flame from a single orifice gas-oxygen torch. The flame is directed from the opposite side where the solder was placed. When the solder flows, the flame is removed immediately.

The invested prosthesis is bench cooled, divested, and the connector is evaluated for completeness.

Postceramic Soldering

After the porcelain has been characterized and glazed, the castings are indexed intraorally. The castings are firmly luted to the plaster index, and all exposed porcelain is covered with sticky wax to prevent contact with the soldering investment.

The FPD is invested in low-heat soldering investment to cover all margins. After a one hour set, the investment is flushed with hot water, the index is removed, and the invested prosthesis is cleaned of residual wax.

The investment block is trimmed—exposing as much porcelain and metal as possible to permit controlled heating and cooling of the metal and porcelain. Excess investment can restrict heat conduction and produce nonuniform thermal changes in the metal or porcelain, which predisposes to porcelain cracking.

The investment is placed in a room temperature burn-out oven and brought to 900 degrees Fahrenheit to desiccate the investment. When steam does not

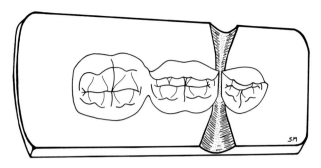

Fig. 13-43. Invested FPD illustrating funneled area for flame direction.

condense on a mouth mirror held over the investment, water elimination is complete.

The investment is removed from the oven and allowed to bench cool. The joint is fluxed, and low-fusing solder that has been coated with flux is added to the joint space from the lingual. Use a strip of solder at least twice the size of the proposed solder joint. The flux is added to a prosthesis that is warm (not hot) to prevent flux from spattering and staining the ceramic. Commonly, .650 solder is used for postceramic soldering, but the alloy manufacturer's recommendations should be followed.

The investment block is placed in front of the muffle of a vacuum porcelain oven set at 900 degrees Fahrenheit and preheated for 10 minutes. The investment block is then placed in the oven, and the temperature is raised at a rate of 75 degrees Fahrenheit per minute, under vacuum. When the solder flows, the soldering block is removed. The oven may have to be raised as high as 1,600 degrees Fahrenheit, depending on the fusing temperature of the solder.

The FPD is bench cooled. Restricted or rapid cooling can create a porcelain–metal thermal mismatch with stress concentration and porcelain cracking. The prosthesis is divested and the connector is evaluated for completeness.

Once the FPD has been postceramic soldered, the porcelain cannot be refired. Since the firing temperature of the porcelain is higher than the fusing temperature of the solder, reglazing the porcelain will melt the solder.

PRESCRIPTION WRITING FOR DENTAL LABORATORIES IN FIXED PROSTHODONTICS

The laboratory technican encourages as much input as possible for a successful prosthesis. Explicit drawings are indicated to avoid misconceptions or costly remakes. The following drawings by the dentist are suggested for open, continual communication:

1. Gingival marginal designs (Fig. 13-44).
2. Pontic design, i.e. anterior (Fig. 13-45); posterior (Fig. 13-46 and 13-47).

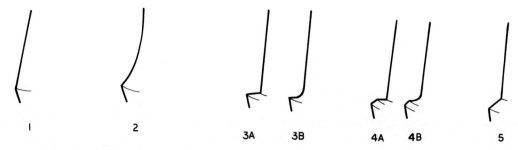

Fig. 13-44. Gingival marginal designs depending upon clinical conditions. 1, Knife edge. 2, Chamfer. 3A, Shoulder with sharp internal line angle. 3B, Shoulder with rounded internal line angle. 4A, Beveled shoulder with sharp internal line angle. 4B, Beveled shoulder with rounded internal line angle. 5, Vesel (sloped shoulder).

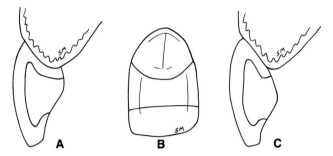

Fig. 13-45. Anterior pontic designs, "Stein pontic" is recommended. A, Ridge lap-mesial views. B, Ridge lap-lingual view. C, Modified ridge lap (Stein style).

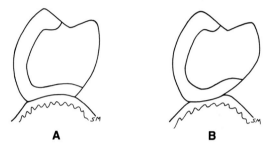

Fig. 13-46. Posterior pontic design ("Stein" is suggested for tissue). A, Ridge lap-mesial view. B, Modified ridge lap (stein style)-mesial view.

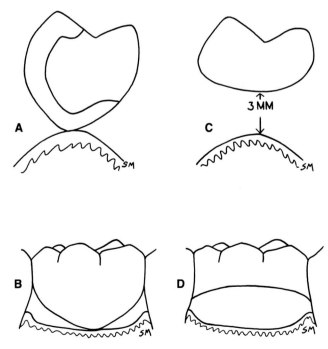

Fig. 13-47. A to **D,** Posterior pontic design; sanitary pontic (3 mm) is the most hygienic. A, Bullet pontic-mesial view. B, Bullet pontic-buccal view. C, Sanitary pontic-mesial view. D, Sanitary pontic-buccal view.

3. Metal posterior surfaces dictated by occlusion and esthetics (Fig. 13-48).
4. Metal anterior surfaces (Figs. 13-49 to 13-52).
5. Fixed-removable rests and guide planes that are already placed within the tooth preparation are emphasized in drawings so the laboratory will use a surveyor during waxing for .010 retentive areas (Figs. 13-53 to 13-57).
6. Special articulation instructions.
7. Shade selection.
8. The dentist's signature and license number.
9. Date of submitting patient's working casts or impression with interocclusal records.
10. Date of case returned for try-in or completion.
11. For increased comprehension:
    a. Modified and original diagnostic casts.
    b. Impressions with poured casts.
    c. Dissected dies.
    d. 2 × 2 slides or color prints and, in rare cases, appointments for patient to have shade selection confirmed by the ceramist.
12. Telephone communication between the dentist and dental technician is common and necessary.

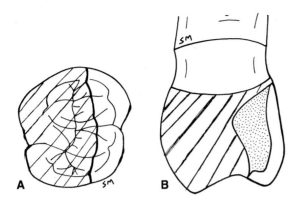

Fig. 13-48. Metal coverage is suggested for stamp cusps to allow occlusal modification. Patient's wishes can subjugate professional recommendations. **A,** Porcelain coverage over the occlusal one third of the facial surface. **B,** Porcelain extended proximally to ensure esthetics.

The expectations of patients are high, even though the limitations of the artificial teeth are obvious. Prosthodontists replace and do not create teeth. It requires 14 years to complete the natural dentition—not weeks, and patients should be reminded of this. However, through research, dedication, and diligence the dental profession can restore function and esthetics, and prevent the need for complete denture service.

It is the ultimate fulfillment for the dentist to have a patient smile who couldn't or wouldn't because of an unsightly smile. This accomplishment is worth the anguish, frustration, and industry associated with successful prosthodontics.

However, the role of the dental technician is often minimized. Without a team effort, prosthodontics is rarely satisfactory. A coordinated approach with refined communication is a primary premise to realizing goals and practical expectations.

BIBLIOGRAPHY

Burch, J.G., and Miller, J.B.: Evaluating crown contours of a wax pattern, J. Prosthet. Dent. **30:**454-458, 1973.

Campagni, W.V., Preston, J.D., and Reisbeck, M.N.: Measurement of paint-on die spacers used for casting relief, J. Prosthet. Dent. **47:**606-611, 1982.

Eames, W.B., O'Neal, S.J., Monteiro, J., et al.: Techniques to improve the seating of castings, J.A.D.A. **96:**432-437, 1978.

Eames, W.B.: The casting misfit/how to cope, J. Prosthet. Dent. **45:**283-285, 1981.

Fukui, H., Lacy, A.M., and Jendersen, M.D.: Effectiveness of hardening films on die stone, J. Prosthet. Dent. **44:**57-63, 1980.

Hembree, J.H., and Cooper, E.W.: Effect of die relief on retention of cast crowns and inlays, Oper. Dent. **4:**104-107, 1979.

Letzner, Heinz: Esthetics in combination prostheses, Quin. Dent. Technol. **11:**97, 1987.

Marker, V.A., Miller, A.W., Miller, B.H., and Swepston, J.H.: Factors affecting the retention and fit of gold castings, J. Prosthet. Dent. **57:**425-430, 1987.

Myers, M., and Hembree, J.H.: Relative accuracy of four removable die systems, J. Prosthet. Dent. **48:**163-165, 1982.

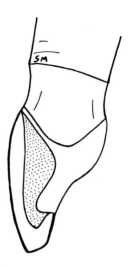

Fig. 13-49. Anterior metal-ceramic crown with met8l centric occlusal contact and metal proximal contact.

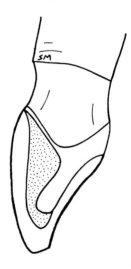

Fig. 13-50. Anterior metal-ceramic crown with metal proximal contact areas but ceramic "centric stops."

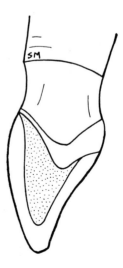

Fig. 13-51. Anterior metal-ceramic crown with both ceramic centric and proximal contact.

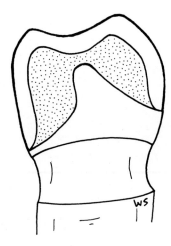

Fig. 13-52. Metal-ceramic crown with ceramic occlusal.

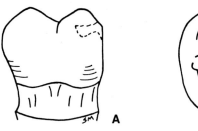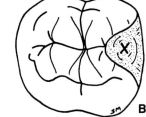

Fig. 13-53. A, All metal molar crown with mesial guiding plane. **B,** Mesial rest seat.

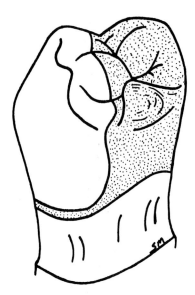

Fig. 13-54. Premolar metal-ceramic crown for RPD abutment with metal occlusal surface, distal guiding plane, and occlusal rest seat.

Seals, R.R., and Stratton, R.J.: Surveyed crowns: a key for integrating fixed and removable prosthodontics, Quint. Dent. Technol. **11**:43, 1987.

Tanquist, R.A.: Die trimming: a guide to physiologic contour, J. Prosthet. Dent. **48**:485-489, 1982.

Yuodelis, R.A., Weaver, J.D., and Sapkos, S.: Facial and lingual contours of artificial complete crown restorations and their effects on the periodontium, J. Prosthet. Dent. **29**:61-66, 1973.

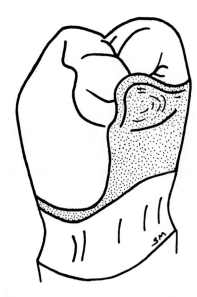

Fig. 13-55. Premolar metal-ceramic crown for RPD abutment with ceramic occlusal surface and metal distal guiding plane and occlusal rest seat.

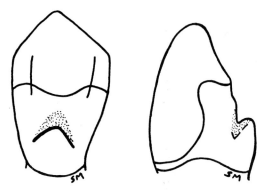

Fig. 13-56. Canine metal-ceramic crown with inverted "V" cingulum rest seat in metal.

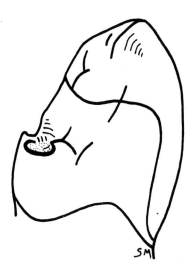

Fig. 13-57. Canine metal-ceramic crown with mesial circular rest seat in metal for RPI clasp assembly.

14

OCCLUSION

Lee M. Jameson, Steven M. Morgano,
David L. Tay, and William F.P. Malone

OCCLUSION FOR NATURAL TEETH

Occlusion is the integrated relationship of the teeth, periodontium, temporomandibular joints, and neuromusculature, not merely the interdigitation of teeth. Few topics generate as much controversy and emotionalism as occlusion. This "confusion with occlusion"[1] exists because:

1. Success of occlusal treatment has been subjective and not documented with clinical research.
2. A singular concept of occlusion cannot be applied to all patients.[2]
3. Occlusion is often equated with instrumentation (articulators) without sufficient attention to the biologic principles.

Clinical Success

The doctrine of clinical "success" is commonly cited as proof of the validity of a method of occlusion treatment. Vague cause-and-effect relationships are assumed, which minimize the biologic uniqueness of the patient.

Realistically, there is a complex interaction of many components of the masticatory system. Changes in one component affect the entire system. Treatment depends on integrated knowledge of all factors that influence the harmony between form and function. Clinical success is not a substitute for controlled scientific experimentation.

Concept of Tolerances
Individualizing occlusal treatment

The science of occlusion is individual centered.[2] The dentist should recognize a wide range of normal and differentiate the appropriateness of occlusal treatment.[3]

Adaptive tolerances vary for specific occlusal conditions of individual patients. It is this wide range of adaptation that allows successful treatment with diverse occlusal theories.

The rationale for occlusal treatment is preserve, restore, and maintain a state of orthofunction, i.e., harmony between occlusal morphology and neuromuscular function within the adaptive range.[4] Exceeding

a patient's capacity to adapt commonly results in abnormal function. Two conceptual goals guide the treatment of occlusion:

1. Restorations are designed to conform to the functional tolerances of the patient.[4]
2. A specific occlusion should be individually determined.[2]

Biologic Control of Mastication

Definition. Mastication is a highly coordinated neuromuscular function manifested as a cyclical learned pattern modified by sensory feedback.

The passive components in the biologic control of occlusion include the occlusal surfaces of the teeth and the anatomy of the temporomandibular joints; the active components are neuromuscular and include joint receptors, spindle mechanisms, periodontal ligament receptors, and other oral receptors.

A key component of occlusion is the neuromusculature. Discrepancies in occlusal relationships are commonly expressed as myalgia or muscle pain.[5]

Biologic Load Transmission

Role of tooth contacts in mastication. The literature is replete with references to artificially created occlusions but contains few studies of occlusal contacts of the natural dentition.[6-9] Cusp-fossa occlusal contacts, i.e., cusps contacting at three simultaneous areas on the opposing tooth (Fig. 14-21), are not normally found in the natural dentition. Natural tooth contacts can violate occlusal theories concerning horizontal incline forces but are well tolerated by individuals.

During mastication, tooth gliding contacts occur while the mandible is entering and leaving centric occlusion (Figs. 14-1 and 14-2). These contacts are of short duration and low magnitude when compared to the forces generated in centric occlusion. These contacts are not beneficial and are at best tolerated.

Eccentric occlusal relations, e.g., group function or canine disclusion, (Fig. 14-20, B and C) and occlusal schemes, e.g., cusp fossa occlusal contacts, are commonly used in prosthodontics to avoid undesirable eccentric contacts. Chewing (Fig. 14-3) does not

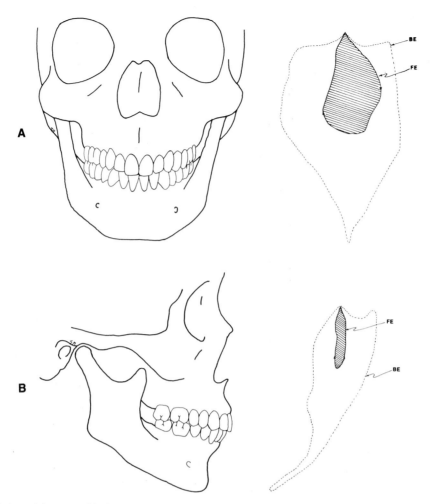

Fig. 14-1. A, Frontal view of the central incisor area during adult chewing (soft food) comparing the fundamental area (FE) and border area (BE). **B,** Sagittal view comparing the functional chewing area (FE) of an adult to the border area (BE).

evoke a patient's adaptive mechanism unless the occlusion has been unfavorably altered, e.g., restorations in premature occlusal contact, occlusal interferences, supraerupted teeth, reduced periodontal support, or parafunctional habits.

Importance of stable centric occlusion. Centric occlusion, or maximum intercuspal position, is the termination of the chewing cycle (Figs. 14-1 to 14-3) and the functional position of stability for the stomatognathic system. It is not located on a border pathway (Fig. 14-1 and 14-2). **It is desirable to preserve and reinforce it rather than contribute to its loss or create a new position.**[10]

Centric relation is a border position, i.e., a terminal hinge position (Fig. 14-4). It is a clinical concept rather than a biologic entity.[11] Historically it evolved as a transferable horizontal axis of mandibular rotation that facilitated the development of replicable interocclusal records at an open vertical dimension. Maximum intercuspation with the condyles in centric relation is not required for all patients needing occlusal therapy.[12]

This simple hinge rotation (Fig. 14-4) occurs at centric relation when the mandible is retruded by the dentist. Functional jaw movement studies have shown that this gnathologic hinge-axis type movement is unobserved during mastication or other functional activity.[13,14] Centric relation is used by the dentist when the centric occlusal position is dysfunctional or cannot be preserved (e.g., in complete oral rehabilitation or in complete denture service). It is usually recommended that the occlusal scheme permit freedom of movement for the mandible, rather than "locking" the mandible in the terminal hinge position.[15,16]

The anterior superior condylar position obtained by bimanual manipulation[17,18] or with an anterior stop[19,20] may be more a physiologic position than the most retruded position obtained by chin-point guidance. A repeatable condylar position is significant in that it facilitates precision.[10]

The clinical manipulation of the mandible allows the dentist to record and transfer to an articulator a terminal hinge axis. This procedure, together with a cen-

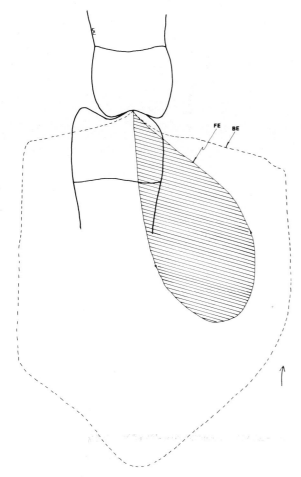

Fig. 14-2. Frontal view of the first molar area during adult chewing comparing the functional area (FE) and the border area (BE). Laterotrusive (working) side.

tric relation interocclusal record, allows the patient's dental casts to be related on an articulator for occlusal analysis. Accurate transfer of the terminal arc of closure also compensates for minute changes in vertical dimension on an articulator during the fabrication of FPDs or RPDs.

The temporomandibular joint and human jaw function. The TMJ is a freely movable articulation involving the condyle and the squamotemporal bone. It is a true synovial joint. The articular disc (Fig. 14-6) completely separates the fluid-filled joint space into superior (arthrodial) and inferior (ginglymoid) compartments.

The dense fibrous tissue of the articular disc is biconcave and avascular, with innervation only in peripheral areas. The central portion is thinnest, with a thicker anterior and posterior lip. Only the anterolateral aspects of the condyle, the central portion of the disc, and corresponding areas of the articular eminence are loaded at maximum intercuspation.[21,22] Slight opening and closing jaw movements shift the areas of loading.[23] Thus, this relatively illfitting sy-

novial articulator permits the simultaneous sliding, spinning, and rolling characteristic of complex jaw movement (Figs. 14-7, A and B).

This slackness of the condyles in their fossa results in a direct lateral jaw movement referred to as the Bennett movement or immediate side shift (Fig. 14-7, C). The reported prevalence of this lateral movement varies from 30 percent[24] to 86 percent[25] of the population, with a mean dimension ranging from 0.3 mm[26] to 1.0 mm.[27]

The temporomandibular joint has two positions at opposite extremes of habitual joint movement where the opposing articular surfaces become congruent, preventing further movement.[28] These positions are close-packed positions[28] (Fig. 14-8), i.e., border positions. Repeated use of these extreme close-packed positions is outside the normal range of function.

Anterior guidance. Anterior guidance is the dynamic relationship of the mandibular anterior teeth to the lingual contours of the maxillary anterior teeth (Fig. 14-9). The anterior teeth are capable of protecting the posterior teeth during eccentric movements by virtue of their periodontal proprioceptive feedback and a lever system so that less force is exerted on the anterior teeth.[29-32]

When the posterior teeth of a patient are lost prematurely, the anterior guidance is overloaded. Loss of the stability of the posterior occlusion eventually exceeds physiologic tolerances and manifests as:

1. Mobile teeth with possible bone loss
2. Muscle pain
3. Overloading of the temporomandibular joints
4. Decreased masticatory efficiency

Guidelines for Developing a Functional Restored Occlusion

Guidelines to occlusal waxing. Laboratory wax addition techniques have been developed to restore a patient's occlusion using crowns or an FPD (Fig. 14-10, A). Two common techniques are the cusp marginal ridge (developed by Everett V. Payne and refined as a multicolor teaching technique by Harry L. Lundeen; Fig. 14-19) and cusp fossa (developed by Peter K. Thomas; Fig. 14-21) occlusal schemes. The cusp fossa technique is a one-tooth to one-tooth (Fig. 14-21, A) scheme and is commonly only used when restoring several contiguous teeth and the teeth opposing them.

In cooperation and communication with the dental laboratory technician, the dentist should use the following guidelines to ensure the development of a biologic occlusion:

1. The occlusal plane from anterior to posterior should be without dramatic steps and with the cusp tips at the same height. Single restorations would fit into the patient's existing occlusal plane.

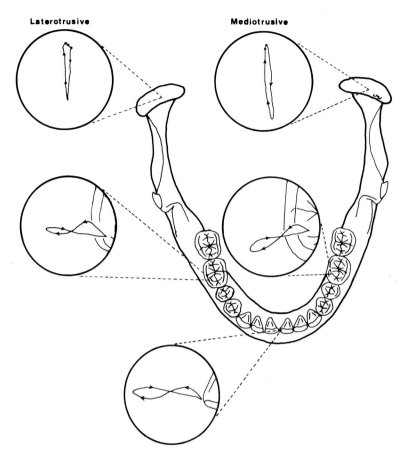

Fig. 14-3. Composite horizontal view adult functional chewing at condyles (laterotrusive-working and mediotrusive-balancing), first molars and anterior at central incisors.

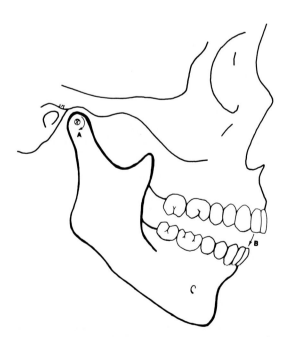

Fig. 14-4. Sagittal view showing pure hinge movement of the mandible. **A,** Rotation about a horizontal axis through the condyles. **B,** Opening movement at the incisors.

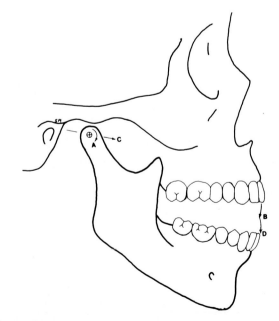

Fig. 14-5. Sagittal view showing hinge and translatory movement of the mandible. **A,** Rotation about a horizontal axis through the condyles. **B,** Opening movement of the condyle. **C,** Translatory movement at the incisors.

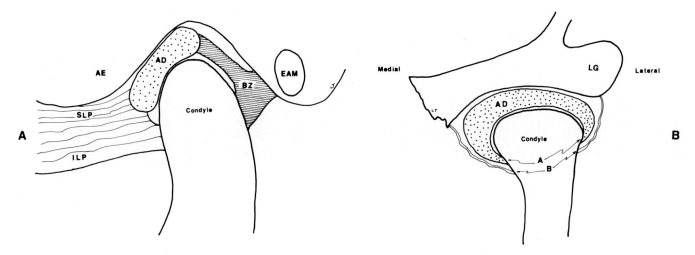

Fig. 14-6. A, Sagittal view of temporomandibular joint at maximum intercuspation. AE = articulator eminence, AD = articular disc, BZ = bilaminar zone, EAM = external auditory meatus, ILP = interior belly of the lateral pterygoid muscle, SLP = superior belly of the lateral pterygoid muscle. **B,** Frontal view of the temporomandibular joint at maximum intercuspation. A = lateral and medial disc attachments, B = attachments of the capsule to the lateral and medial poles of the condyle, AD = articular disc, LG = lateral lip of the glenoid fossa.

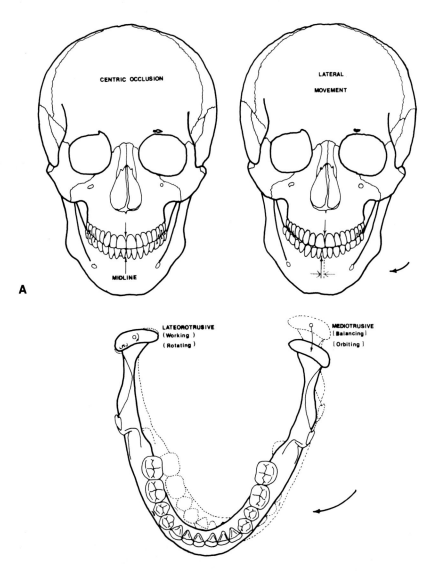

Fig. 14-7. A, Frontal and horizontal view of a lateral mandibular movement from centric occlusion.

Continued.

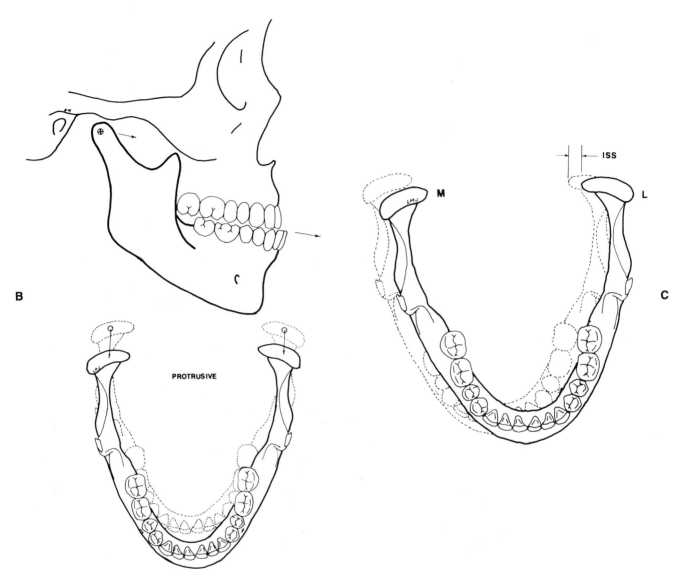

Fig. 14-7. B, Sagittal and horizontal view of a straight protrusive mandibular movement from centric occlusion. **C,** Bennett movement or immediate side shift (ISS) of mandible on the laterotrusive (working) side. L = laterotrusive condyle, M = mediotrusive condyle.

2. Marginal ridges are of equal height (Fig. 14-10, B).
3. Proximal contours (Fig. 14-10, B) should be supportive but not intrusive of the gingival space.
4. Intracrevicular margins prepared below the CEJ are restored without overcontouring,[33] and supragingival crown contours to avoid deflective bulges hindering oral hygiene.[34]
5. Whenever possible, establish cross-tooth stabilization, i.e., centric contact of guiding and supporting cusps (Fig. 14-11).
6. Restored occlusion should avoid eccentric irritations, i.e., mediotrusive-balancing and laterotrusive-working interferences (Figs. 14-12, A and B).

Articulator selection. The purpose of an articulator is to facilitate fabrication of restorations outside of the patient's mouth. Registrations recorded from the patient are used to program the articulator. The movements of an articulator are mechanical, so articulators cannot reproduce human mandibular movements. Even a fully adjustable articulator (Fig. 14-13) can only reproduce border movements.

Three basic registrations are acquired from the patient and transferred to the articulator:

1. Facebow, to relate the maxillae to the hinge axis
2. Maxillomandibular record to relate the mandibular cast to the maxillary cast
3. Eccentric registrations, to program the condylar controls of the articulator

Eccentric registration. Eccentric registrations do not record function but transfer the boundaries (i.e.,

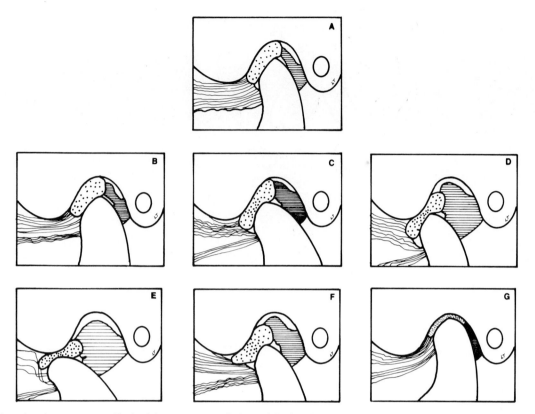

Fig. 14-8. Functional temporomandibular joint movement during adult chewing, sagittal view. **A,** Maximum intercuspation. **B,** Postural (clinical rest) position. **C,** Opening rotation phase. **D,** Translatory phase. **E,** Functional anterior close-packed position (FACP). **F,** Closure phase. **G,** Functional posterior close-packed position.

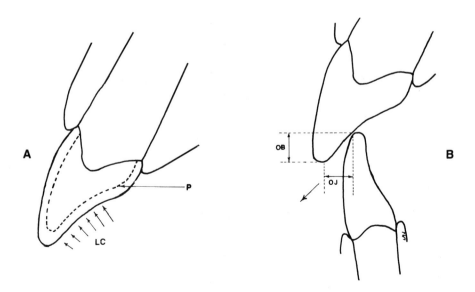

Fig. 14-9. A, Mesial view showing outline *(dotted line)* of a preparation on a maxillary central incisor (P) and the lingual concavity (LC) of anterior guidance. **B,** Relationship of maxillary and mandibular anterior teeth illustrating the vertical (overbite = OB) and horizontal (overjet = OJ) components of anterior guidance.

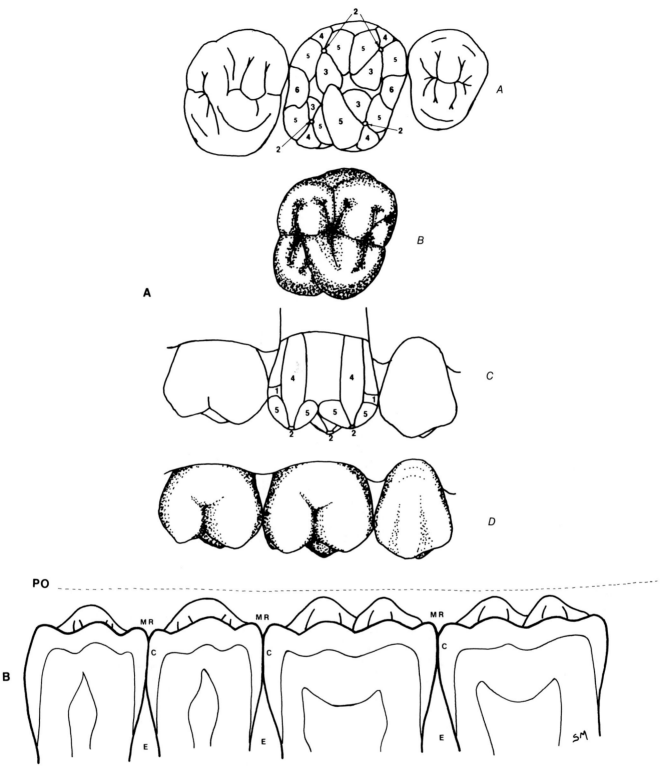

Fig. 14-10. A, Developing a functional occlusion using the wax addition technique. *A,* Sequence of occlusal anatomy development: 1, contact bars (C only), 2, buccal and lingual cusp cones, 3, triangular ridges of the buccal and lingual cusp, 4, buccal and lingual contour ridges, 5, mesial and distal cusp ridges of buccal and lingual cusps, and 6, marginal ridges. *B,* Completed crown showing occlusal anatomy of maxillary first molar. *C,* Buccal view showing proximal contact and buccal contour ridges: 1, contact bars, 2, buccal cusp cones, 4, buccal and lingual contour ridges and 5, mesial and distal buccal cusp ridges. *D,* Buccal view showing complete crown contours maxillary right first molar. **B,** Marginal ridges are of equal height with a smooth occlusal plane. Proximal contours are flat occluso + gingivally and do *not* intrude on the gingival space.

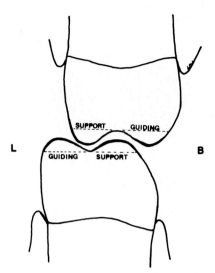

Fig. 14-11. Frontal view of first molar area showing guiding and support cusps.

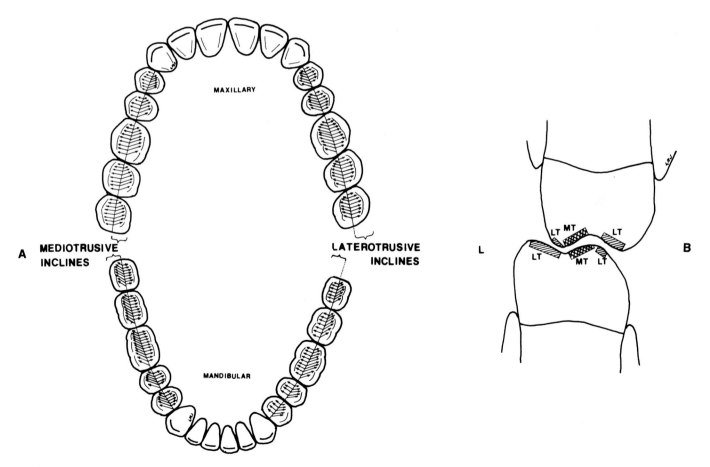

Fig. 14-12. A, Horizontal view showing laterotrusive (working) inclines and mediotrusive (balancing) inclines of both maxillary and mandibular arches. **B,** Frontal view of the first molar area showing laterotrusive (LT) and mediotrusive (MT) inclines.

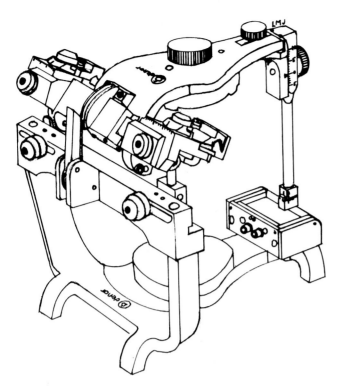

Fig. 14-13. Eccentric fully adjustable Denar Model 5A articulator (Denar Corporation, Anaheim, CA).

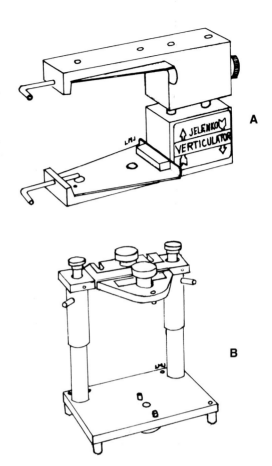

Fig. 14-14. Noneccentric articulators. **A,** The Verticulator (Jelenko Pennwalt, New Rochelle, NY). **B,** Corelator (Denare Corporation, Anaheim, CA).

border positions) within which functional movements can occur (Figs. 14-1 and 14-2). Even "functional chew-in techniques"[35] do not record "chewing" but merely lateral movements.

Treatment positions. The treatment position dictates whether an eccentric movement articulator (semiadjustable or fully adjustable) is required or a noneccentric movement articulator (e.g., Verticulator and Corelator; Fig. 14-14) is adequate.

If centric occlusion is the only treatment position, the precise endpoint of that position must be accurately maintained by the articulating device. One that opens and closes at 90 degrees to the occlusal plane (e.g., Verticulator and Corelator, Fig. 14-14) or a simple hinge type (Fig. 14-15) is adequate. Since centric occlusion is *not* a border position, it is not related to border pathways, and a facebow transfer is unnecessary. Eccentric pathways may be registered with an occlusal index (e.g., a functionally generated path), or the restoration is adjusted directly intra orally after fabrication.

A simple hinge articulator can perpetuate or precipitate occlusal interferences on cuspal inclines[36] (Fig. 14-15). If centric relation is the treatment position, a joint-oriented technique such as a hinge axis recording is necessary to transfer this end-point border position. The hinge axis is the common reference between the patient and the articulator. The eccentric pathways can be dynamically registered with the pan-tographic, engraving techniques or positionally recorded with eccentric "check bites."

Mechanical determinants of occlusion. Traditional determinants of occlusion have inferred a correlation between craniomandibular anatomic specification (e.g., the angle of the eminentia) and the occlusal surfaces of the teeth (e.g., cusp height, fossa depth, and ridge groove direction.)[25] *Neither* the temporomandibular joints, the teeth, the anterior guidance nor the neuromusculature has been scientifically proven to be the predominant occlusal determinant. As a result, theories of occlusion, using each one of these or various combinations as the dominant factors, have been proposed as guidelines for restoring a patient's occlusion.

The only advantage of the traditional determinants is their relation to *mechanical* articulator movements. No existing articulator can produce exactly the mandibular movements; this is not the primary objective. The purpose of an articulator is to facilitate the fabrication of restorations that encourage favorable occlusal contacts without loss of stability.

Positive/negative error. A positive surface error (Fig. 14-16) occurs when the condylar inclination on

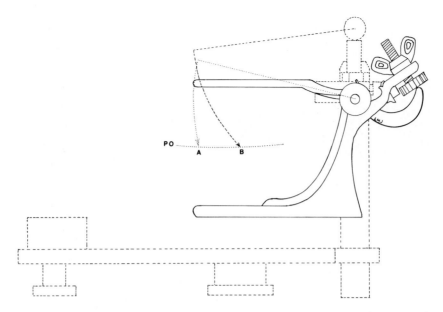

Fig. 14-15. Comparison of the arc of closure between a noneccentric simple hinge articulator and an eccentric semiadjustable arcon type articulator. A crown or bridge fabricated on the simple hinge type will necessitate considerable adjustment of the crown or bridge in the patient's mouth. PO = plane of occlusion, A = arc of closure at the first molar area for the simple hinge type, B = arc of closure for the arcon type articulator.

the articulator is set at a greater angle than the patient's condylar angle and results in deflective positive contact on the occlusal surface of the restoration in eccentric position. A negative occlusal surface error is one that results when the condylar guide is set with an angle *less* than the patient's inclines. The results are a negative feature, such as a groove or fossa that is wider than required. While negative error is preferable to positive error, excessive negative error can result in reduced occlusal efficiency and instability of centric occlusion. If a patient has a naturally occurring canine disclusion, (Fig. 14-20, B) the resulting disclusion of the posterior teeth is an example of controlled compensation. This allows the dentist to use simpler articulators, since the vertical component of the anterior guidance separates the posterior teeth in eccentric positions and deemphasizes the influence of ridge and groove directions and cusp height.

Articulator selection. The articulator errors may be negligible on a fully adjustable articulator (Fig. 14-13) or clinically significant on a simple hinge articulator (Fig. 14-15). The articulator that is selected should be based on:

1. Treatment position (centric relation versus the preexisting centric occlusion).
2. Type of dentistry the patient requires, i.e., edentulous, partially edentulous, or dentate.
3. Complexity of restorative dentistry.
4. The anterior guidance of the patient and whether it is duplicated.
5. Whether the vertical dimension of occlusion requires alteration (a hinge axis registration to

relate this common border reference position from the patient to the articulator).
6. The mandibular immediate side shift (Fig. 14-7, C).
7. The eccentric occlusal prescription, i.e., cross-arch balance versus group function versus canine disclusion.
8. Occlusal morphology, i.e., cusp to fossa, freedom in centric.
9. Technique used, e.g., a functionally generated path can supplement the capabilities of a semiadjustable articulator.
10. Teaching considerations (arcon versus non arcon Figs. 14-17 and 14-18).
11. Economic and time constraints.
12. The skill of the dentist in the mechanical and biologic aspects of occlusion.
13. The dentist's preference for a particular instrument.

"Normal occlusion" implies not only the centric closure position, but also the full range of functional mandibular movements. The importance of occlusion is self-evident. However, the technical aspects of restoring an occlusion, especially the limitations of treatment with atypical occlusal relationships, have received insufficient emphasis in dental research.[37]

The patient's chewing behavior should be respected. For a patient with a wide range of freedom during lateral excursions of the mandible, it would be undesirable to develop an occlusion that restricts movement. The effect of dental restorations upon the balanced equilibrium of the neuromuscular complex

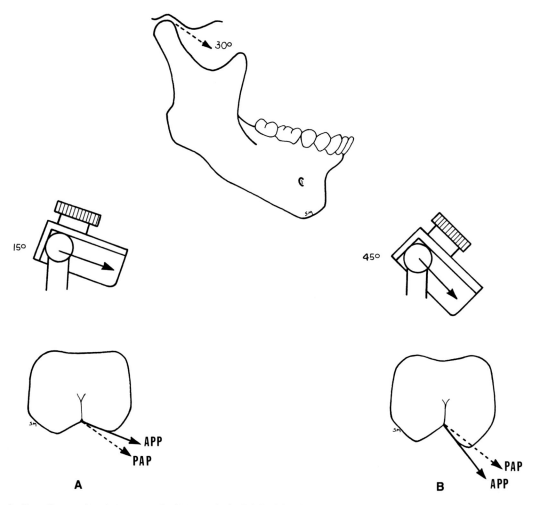

Fig. 14-16. A, Negative occlusal error—articulator path *(solid line)* is shallower than the patient's path *(dotted line)*. **B,** Positive occlusal error—the articulator path *(solid line)* is steeper than the patient's path *(dotted line)*.

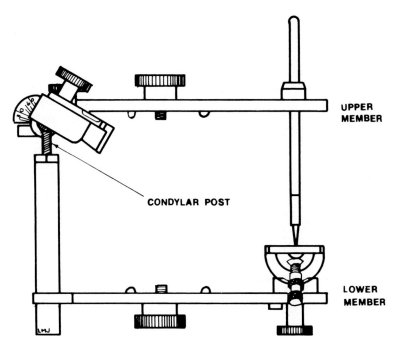

Fig. 14-17. Eccentric semiadjustable arcon articulator by Whip Mix (Whip Mix Corporation, Louisville, KY). Condylar sphere is attached to the lower member of the articulator, while the mechanical fossa is part of the upper member (similar to the anatomy of the human skull).

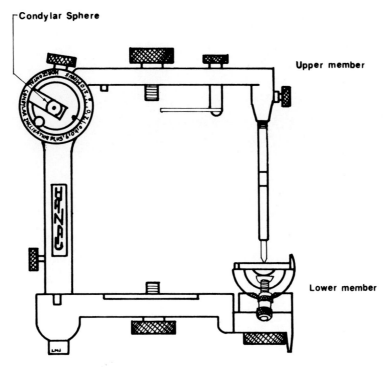

Fig. 14-18. Eccentric semiadjustable nonarcon articulator by Teledyne Hanau (Teledyne Hanau, Buffalo, NY). Condylar sphere is attached to the upper member of the articulator, while the mechanical fossa is part of the lower member of the articulator.

is undeniable. Occlusal harmony is preserved by conservative restorative dentistry that maintains the vertical dimension and the periodontal health of the dentition. An articulator is merely an instrument to relate the maxillary and mandibular casts of the patient for study and preliminary occlusal therapy. Understanding the limitations of articulators and their effects on patient treatment is essential.

Restorative dentistry can fail, however, and some patients continue to lose teeth in spite of the most refined interdisciplinary treatment. But early recognition of clinical symptoms and propitious recall systems can prolong the serviceability of teeth and avert complete edentulism for the majority of patients.[38]

DIFFERENTIATION BETWEEN NATURAL, FIXED, AND REMOVABLE OCCLUSION

Occlusion with artificial teeth differs from a natural occlusion. The goals of occlusal reconstruction with fixed prosthodontics are not identical to the goals of occlusal reconstruction with removable prosthodontics. In this section, the differences between the occlusal schemes recommended for prosthodontics are compared with a natural dentition. Suggestions are presented for occlusal rehabilitation when fixed and removable prosthodontics are integrated and when fixed prosthodontics is supported by osseointegrated implants.

Natural Dentition

A healthy, natural Angle Class I occlusion is characterized by simultaneous, equalized contact of all teeth (anterior and posterior) in maximum intercuspation (centric occlusion). Centric occlusion is generally *not* coincidental with the terminal arc of closure (centric relation).[39] Usually, the centric occlusal contact is a cusp-marginal ridge relationship (Fig. 14-19).[40]

In a straight protrusion, the anterior incisor teeth disclude all posterior teeth (Fig. 14-20, A). In a lateral excursion, the working canine may disclude posterior teeth on the working side (canine disclusion; Fig. 14-20, B), or may permit posterior teeth on the working side to occlude simultaneously (group function; Fig. 14-20, C). Frequently, there is a combination of canine disclusion and group function in the same patient.

Tooth contact on the nonworking side in a lateral excursion is undesirable, since it may interfere with patient comfort and mastication. Nonworking contacts have been associated with periodontal disease in the natural dentition.[41]

Fixed Prosthodontics

An occlusion restored with fixed prosthodontics often differs from a natural occlusion. When the majority of the occlusal surfaces are restored with fixed restorations, the patient's identical, preexisting centric oc-

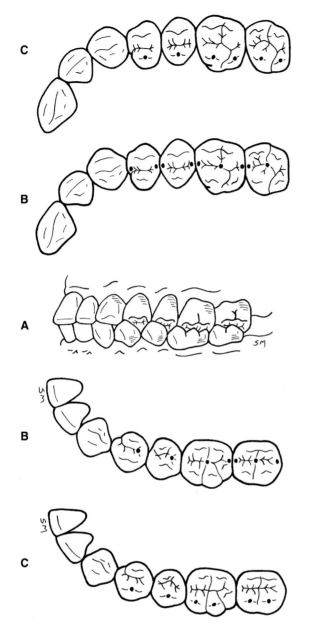

Fig. 14-19. A, A cusp-marginal ridge occlusion. **B,** Marginal ridge and fossa contacts in centric occlusion. **C,** Cusp contacts in centric occlusion.

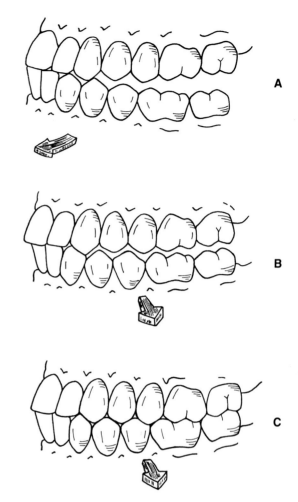

Fig. 14-20. A, Straight protrusion—anterior teeth disclude posterior teeth. **B,** Canine disclusion—the canine discludes the posterior teeth in a lateral working position. **C,** Group function—simultaneous contact of the canine and the posterior teeth on the working side in a lateral excursion.

clusal position cannot be preserved. Therefore, the restored centric occlusion is planned to coincide with centric relation—a repeatable position.[42] All interceptive occlusal contacts along the terminal arc of closure on teeth not receiving artificial crowns are eliminated with selective grinding. The restored centric occlusion is a simultaneous, equalized contact of all teeth (anterior and posterior) coincidental with centric relation.

The location of centric occlusal contacts is selected by the dentist. Frequently, a cusp-fossa occlusion is prescribed (Fig. 14-21) to enhance stability and re-

duce interproximal food impaction.[43] Occlusal tables are narrowed to maintain forces within the confines of the root system and to minimize nonworking contacts.[44]

The anterior teeth disclude posterior teeth in straight protrusion. Lateral working positions may be canine disclusion or group function (Fig. 14-22). Group function is prescribed when a canine is compromised and cannot support the entire eccentric load, e.g., moderate alveolar bone loss about the canine or previous apicoectomy. Nonworking contacts are eliminated in lateral excursions (Fig. 14-23).

Removable Partial Prosthodontics

When a removable partial denture (RPD) restores posterior teeth and is tooth-supported, the occlusion is similar to a fixed partial denture (FPD). When posterior teeth are restored with an extension base (Ken-

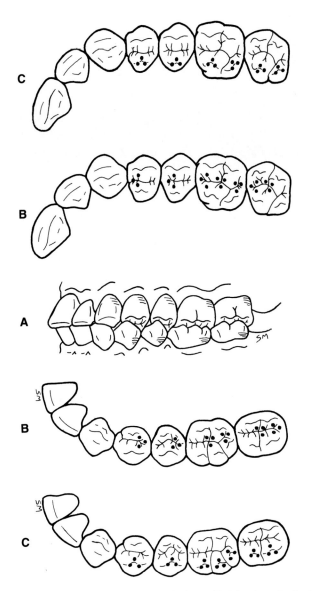

Fig. 14-21. A, A cusp fossa-occlusion with tripod contacts. **B,** Fossa contacts in centric occlusion. **C,** Cusp contacts in centric occlusion.

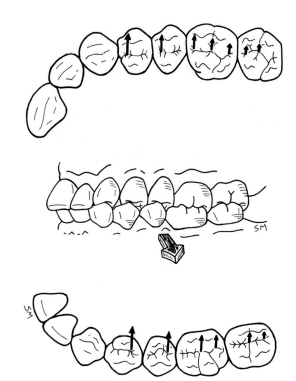

Fig. 14-22. Cusp pathways on the working side in a lateral excursion, starting from a cusp-fossa relationship. Cusps will travel the same paths in group function (with posterior tooth contact) or in canine disclusion (with *no* posterior tooth contact).

nedy Class I or Class II) RPD, special consideration is given to the occlusion.

With an extension base RPD, it is essential that all teeth (natural and artificial) occlude in centric occlusion with simultaneous, equalized contact. An exception is the mandibular RPD that occludes with a maxillary complete denture—where no centric contact on the anterior teeth is recommended. When most or all of the posterior teeth are artificially restored, centric occlusion coincides with centric relation or possesses a smooth movement from centric relation occlusion to centric occlusion.

Working, nonworking, and protrusive contacts on the artificial posterior teeth are avoided to control nonvertical forces on the abutment teeth.[45] Thus, whenever possible, eccentric occlusal loads are borne by the natural teeth—with the disclusion of the artificial teeth. A notable exception is the mandibular RPD that occludes with a maxillary complete denture—where posterior tooth contact is advisable in eccentric positions.

Detrimental forces to the abutment teeth and residual ridges can be minimized with favorable buccolingual placement of the artificial posterior teeth[46] (Fig. 14-24) and a short, narrow occlusal table.[47] Substituting premolars for molars is effective in maintaining a narrow and short occlusal table. Good cuspal anatomy with sluiceways is important for efficient mastication, which will reduce the forces required to comminute food.[48]

Complete Denture Prosthodontics

Since a complete denture rests upon displaceable mucosa, the occlusion plays a significant role in enhancing or counteracting the support, retention, and stability of the denture base. A harmonious occlusion firmly seats the denture, whereas a single interceptive occlusal contact disturbs the position of the denture base on the mucosa—and promotes instability, poor retention, tissue trauma, soreness, and accelerated bone resorption.

The desired centric occlusion is a simultaneous, nondeflective, bilateral contact of all posterior teeth

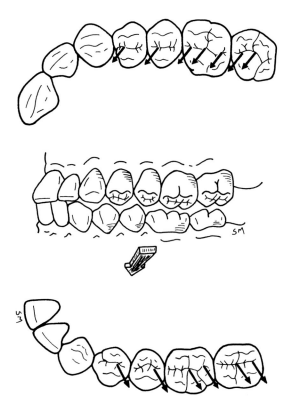

Fig. 14-23. Cusp pathways on the nonworking side in a lateral excursion.

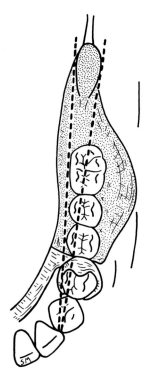

Fig. 14-24. An excellent guide to the buccolingual placement of mandibular artificial posterior teeth is a triangle *(dotted lines)* suggested by Pound.[46] Where practical, the lingual cusps of all posterior teeth are located within a triangle that extends from the mesial contact on the canine to the buccal and lingual sides of the retromolar pad. Note that the occlusal table is short and narrow and the denture base is broad.

in centric relation with no contact of the anterior teeth.[49] Since bone resorption is more rapid in the anterior portions of the edentulous ridges,[50,51] the posterior teeth should not be discluded by the anterior teeth in eccentric positions.

While a nondeflective occlusion can be obtained with zero degree (cuspless) posterior teeth set to a flat plane, this type of occlusal scheme places constraints on the arrangement of the anterior teeth, since a zero anterior guidance (no vertical overlap of the anterior teeth) is desired. If significant vertical overlap of the anterior teeth is dictated by esthetics, phonetics, or the position of natural mandibular anterior teeth, deflective forces can occur in eccentric positions with a flat posterior occlusion. Whenever there is vertical overlap of the anterior teeth, a cuspated occlusal scheme is recommended to distribute nonvertical forces (Fig. 14-25). Cuspated teeth can be set with posterior tooth contact in protrusion (Fig. 14-25, B) and cross-arch contacts in lateral excursions (Fig. 14-25, C)—all in concert with the incisal and canine guidance.

There are guidelines for occlusal rehabilitation when integrating fixed and removable prosthodontics. Because of the fundamental differences between a fixed and a removable occlusion, confusion can occur when a patient requires fixed and removable prosthodontics.

An Extension Base RPD that Occludes with Fixed Restorations

Diagnosis and treatment planning. Preliminary jaw relation records are made and diagnostic casts are mounted on a semiadjustable articulator. The height of the occlusal plane[52,53] and length of the occlusal table are determined (Fig. 14-26). A trial setup for the RPD is arranged. A short, narrow occlusal table for the RPD is preferred, and the teeth are placed in the most advantageous buccolingual position (Fig. 14-24). The fixed restorations are planned with a diagnostic waxup to occlude with the stock denture teeth (Fig. 14-27). Whenever possible, natural anterior teeth disclude all posterior teeth in straight protrusion (Fig. 14-28), and all teeth on the extension base are discluded in lateral excursions.

Treatment procedures. The record base with the trial setup for the RPD represents the desired occlusal plane and serves as an excellent guide for occlusal reduction during tooth preparation for artificial crowns. After tooth preparation, the master cast with removable dies is mounted on the programmed semiadjustable articulator with the trial setup for the RPD (Fig. 14-29). The occlusal surfaces for the fixed res-

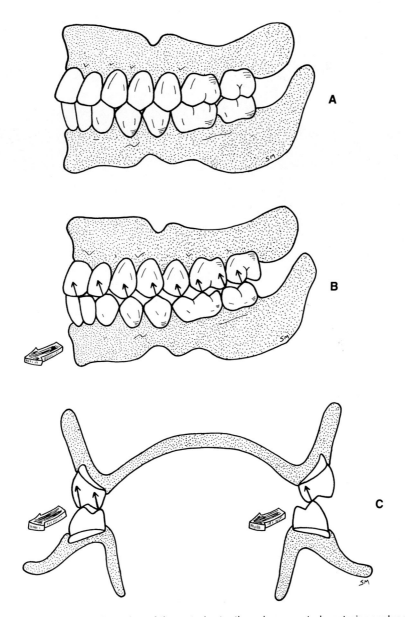

Fig. 14-25. A, Complete dentures with vertical overlap of the anterior teeth and a cuspated posterior occlusal arrangement. Anterior teeth do *not* have centric occlusal contacts. **B,** Simultaneous contact of posterior teeth in straight protrusion distributes stresses over as wide an area as possible. **C,** Cross-arch contacts in lateral excursions mitigate stress concentration on the working side.

torations are waxed to occlude as planned with the trial setup for the RPD. The fixed restorations are completed. Metal occlusal surfaces are preferred for the cast restorations. If porcelain occlusal surfaces are required for esthetics, the *occluding RPD teeth must also be porcelain*.

After trial seating of the completed fixed restorations, the RPD is fabricated. Acrylic resin posterior teeth (the exact mold used in the trial setup) are set to occlude with the metal occlusal surfaces of the fixed restorations. This is a simple procedure, since the fixed restorations were waxed to occlude with the stock teeth.

Some authorities have recommended metal occlusal surfaces on the RPD to better coordinate with the fixed occlusal surfaces.[54-56] Modern economic realities often preclude the fabrication of a customized metal occlusion for the RPD. Acrylic resin teeth are acceptable in most instances and produce excellent results when the fixed restorations are preplanned to occlude with the selected mold.

After the wax try-in, the RPD is processed. The final occlusal adjustment is performed on the articulator after a clinical remount. Centric occlusal contacts are verified on the articulator and intraorally with 0.0005 inch shim stock.

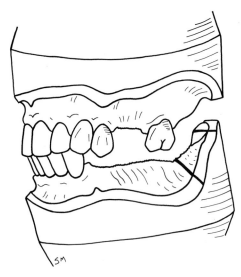

Fig. 14-26. Mounted diagnostic casts. A maxillary FPD that occludes with a mandibular RPD is planned. Note that the maxillary posterior teeth are supraerupted. The preferred height of the occlusal plane is marked (one-half to two-thirds the height of the retromolar pad). The occlusal table should *not* extend past the abrupt upward slope of the residual ridge (marked on the cast).

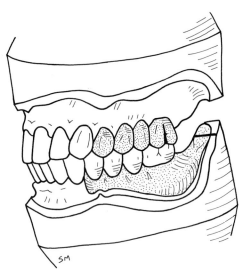

Fig. 14-27. Establishing the desired occlusal scheme begins with a trial setup of the mandibular teeth *followed by* a diagnostic waxup for the maxillary FPD.

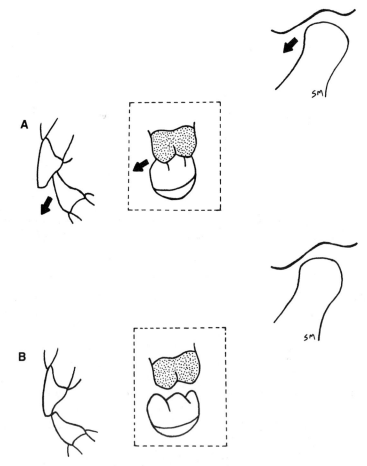

Fig. 14-28. A, Simultaneous contact of anterior and posterior teeth in centric occlusion when a maxillary FPD occludes with a mandibular extension base RPD. **B,** Disclusion of posterior teeth by natural anterior teeth in straight protrusion.

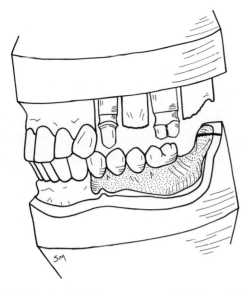

Fig. 14-29. Mounted maxillary master cast with mandibular trial setup. Maxillary FPD will be fabricated to occlude harmoniously with the mandibular stock teeth.

Figs. 14-30 and 14-31 demonstrate a completed occlusal rehabilitation where fixed and removable partial prosthodontics are integrated.

Problems and common errors. Most problems originate at the treatment planning stage. Often the planning for the RPD is *postponed* until after the fixed restorations are definitively seated! A common error is to arbitrarily wax the fixed restorations without regard to the occlusal scheme for the RPD. This can produce an unfavorable plane of occlusion (Fig. 14-32). With capricious placement of cusps and fossae in the cast restorations, the establishment of centric occlusal contacts in the finalized occlusion is arduous, and results are often disappointing.

Finally, regardless of how carefully the occlusion is executed, occlusal harmony is lost in the presence of ridge resorption. Broad denture base coverage (Fig. 14-30), resulting from a two-stage impression technique (such as the altered cast technique) in the mandible, is the best deterrent to accelerated ridge resorption and promotes longevity to the planned occlusal scheme.

Maxillary Complete Denture that Occludes with Fixed Restorations

Diagnosis and treatment planning. A record base with an occlusion rim is fabricated for the maxillary diagnostic cast. Jaw relation records are made, and the maxillary and mandibular diagnostic casts are mounted on a semiadjustable articulator at the desired vertical dimension of occlusion. The interarch clearance, especially in the region of the maxillary tuberosities, and the plane of occlusion are assessed. Preprosthetic surgery may be indicated to restore ac-

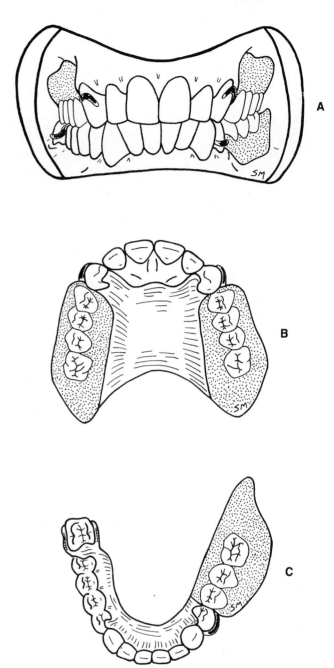

Fig. 14-30. A, Complete mouth reconstruction where fixed and removable prosthodontics have been integrated. **B,** Maxillary arch. Six anterior teeth are restored with complete crowns. All posterior teeth are replaced with the RPD. Note the narrow occlusal tables. Broad palatal coverage with the chromium cobalt denture base offers resistance to the forces of occlusion. **C,** Mandibular arch. The FPD extends from No. 21 to No. 31, with No. 23 to No. 26 and No. 28 to No. 30 replaced with pontics. The posterior pontics on the FPD are all premolars to maintain a narrow occlusal table in harmony with the maxillary RPD. The left posterior teeth are replaced by the mandibular RPD, with a short, narrow occlusal table and broad denture base coverage.

ceptable interarch clearance and improve the plane of occlusion.

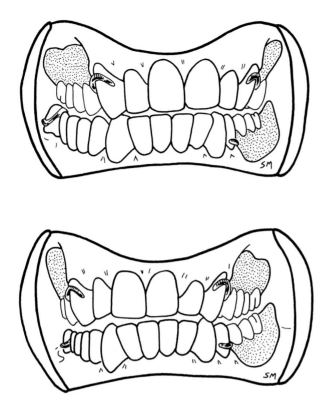

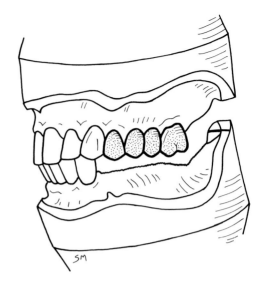

Fig. 14-32. Maxillary FPD was fabricated *without* a mandibular diagnostic setup. The occlusal plane is inferior to the lower border of the retromolar pad—well below the desired position (one-half to two-thirds the height of the retromolar pad).

Fig. 14-31. Same patient as in Fig. 14-30. The canines disclude all posterior teeth in right and left lateral excursions.

A diagnostic setup of the maxillary denture teeth is accomplished. Maxillary anterior teeth are not placed in contact with the natural mandibular anterior teeth. Selective grinding of the mandibular anterior teeth will often improve the anterior guidance.

The anterior guidance is dictated by esthetics, phonetics, and the position of the mandibular anterior teeth and is rarely compatible with zero degree posterior teeth. Therefore, anatomic posterior teeth are usually indicated for the trial setup.

The fixed restorations are planned with a diagnostic waxup. Posterior teeth not receiving cast restorations may require selective grinding. Any areas of the stone teeth that are recontoured on the diagnostic cast are marked in red.

The completed diagnostic occlusal scheme includes bilateral, simultaneous, nondeflective contact of all posterior teeth in centric relation with no contact of the anterior teeth (Fig. 14-33, *A*). In a straight protrusion, the posterior teeth maintain simultaneous contact—preferably for the full height of the cusps (Fig. 14-33, *B*). In lateral excursions, cross-arch contact of all posterior teeth is recommended consistent with the lateral (canine) guidance (Fig. 14-25, *C*).

Treatment procedures. The maxillary trial setup is evaluated clinically for esthetics and phonetics. It is important that the anterior arrangement be verified at this time, since any alteration of the anterior guidance may require modification of the posterior occlusion.[57]

The natural mandibular teeth are recontoured intraorally where indicated on the diagnostic cast. After tooth preparation for cast restorations, the mandibular master cast with removable dies is mounted with the maxillary diagnostic setup on the semiadjustable articulator at the established vertical dimension of occlusion.

The fixed restorations are waxed as planned to occlude with the maxillary setup. The restorative material on the occlusal surfaces of the fixed and removable prostheses must be compatible. A metal occlusion on the fixed restorations with acrylic resin artificial teeth on the complete denture is recommended. When fixed restorations are completed with porcelain occlusal surfaces, they must occlude with porcelain denture teeth. Porcelain denture teeth are not recommended in occlusion with natural enamel nor metal restorative material.[58] After the fixed restorations are completed and provisionally seated, the complete denture is fabricated.

Setting of the artificial teeth for the maxillary denture is facilitated because of the customized mandibular occlusion. At the wax try-in appointment for the complete denture, centric relation is verified. Since esthetics and phonetics were evaluated previously, the anterior tooth arrangement should be acceptable to the patient and the dentist.

After the denture is processed, the occlusion is refined on the articulator with a clinical remount. The

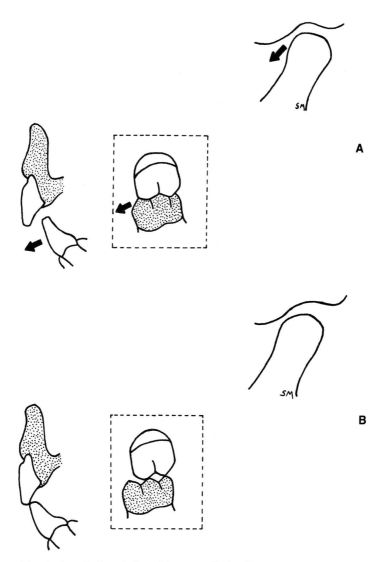

Fig. 14-33. A, A maxillary complete denture that occludes with a mandibular fixed prosthesis. There is simultaneous contact of all posterior teeth in centric occlusion with *no* contact of the anterior teeth. Note the vertical and horizontal overlap of the anterior teeth. **B,** In straight protrusion, the posterior teeth maintain simultaneous contact as the anterior teeth are brought into contact.

final occlusion is evaluated on the articulator and intraorally with 0.0005 inch shim stock for balanced contacts in centric occlusion, straight protrusion, and lateral excursions.

Problems and common errors. Most problems result from hasty planning. Often, the mandibular fixed restorations are completed on an unmounted mandibular cast, completely ignoring the maxillary arch. Without the anterior guidance and posterior maxillary trial setup to influence the mandibular occlusal morphology, a rational occlusal scheme cannot be expected. When the maxillary complete denture is finally inserted, the occlusion is often compromised, and the patient complains that the denture is loose! In an attempt to alleviate the complaint, the dentist may choose to rebase or reline the complete denture.

Rebasing will not correct the occlusal disharmony, and the complaint of "looseness" remains.

Occlusal Rehabilitation with Fixed Prosthodontics Supported by Osseointegrated Implants

The essential feature of an osseointegrated implant is the intimate adaptation of bone to the implant—without connective tissue encapsulation.[59] Conversely, a natural tooth is attached to bone by highly differentiated connective tissue—the periodontal ligament. This periodontal ligament is responsible for the major proprioceptive input controlling masticatory function,[60] and acts as a "shock absorber" of occlusal stress.[61] It is the periodontal ligament that regulates osteogenesis and cementogenesis and allows alterations in tooth position.[61]

Since the bone-implant interface has no connective tissue shock absorber, excessive impact forces can result in early failure of the implant. There is no periodontal ligament to provide its sensory input and to allow adaptation to slight occlusal discrepancies.

Because of anatomic limitations, five or six implant fixtures are placed in the anterior portions of the edentulous arch—usually no further distally than the premolar region. The fixed prosthesis will contain one to three cantilevered pontics bilaterally.

The nature of the osseointegrated implant with the design of the prosthesis mandates a disciplined approach when establishing occlusal relationships.[62,63]

Centric occlusion coincides with centric relation at a physiologic vertical dimension of occlusion. All teeth (anterior and posterior) occlude simultaneously in centric relation. With cantilevered pontics, anterior forces are better tolerated, and the anterior teeth should disclude the posterior teeth in eccentric positions. An exception to this occlusal arrangement is the mandibular FPD supported by an osseointegrated implant that occludes with a complete denture.

Anteriorly directed forces are not well tolerated by a complete denture. Therefore, the recommended centric occlusion is a bilateral, simultaneous contact of the posterior teeth without anterior tooth contact. If the anterior arrangement will permit a zero anterior guidance, zero degree posterior teeth may be set to a flat occlused plane. If vertical overlap of the anterior teeth is required, anatomic posterior teeth are recommended with balanced contacts in eccentric positions (Fig. 14-25).

Authorities on the osseointegrated prosthesis recommend the exclusive use of acrylic resin artificial teeth—to substitute for the missing periodontal ligament shock absorbers.[64] The occlusal refinements are accomplished on an adjustable or semiadjustable articulator with a clinical remount. The definitive occlusal contacts are verified on the articulator and intraorally with 0.0005 inch shim stock.

SELECTED REFERENCES

1. Malone, W.F.: The occlusal epidemic-profile of confusion, Ill. Dent. J. **39**:643, October 1970.
2. Brecker, S.C.: Clinical Procedures in Occlusal Rehabilitation, ed. 2, Philadelphia, 1966, W.B. Saunders Co.
3. Moyers, R.E.: Development of Occlusion, Dent. Clin. North Am 13:3, 523, July 1969.
4. Krogh-Poulsen, W.G., and Olsson, A.: Occlusal disharmonies and dysfunction of the stomatognathio system, Dent. Clin. North Am., November 1966.
5. Bell, W.E.: Temporomandibular Disorders: Classification/Diagnosis/Management, ed. 2, Chicago, 1986, Year Book Medical Publishers, pp. 219.
6. Ross, I.F.: Occlusal contacts of the natural teeth, J. Prosthet. Dent. **32**:6,660, December 1974.
7. Ross, I.F.: Incisal guidance of natural teeth in adults, J. Prosthet. Dent. **31**:2, February 1974.
8. Pameijer, J.H.N., Glickman, I., and Roeber, F.W.: Intraoral occlusal telemetry. II. Registration of tooth contacts in chewing and swallowing by intraoral electronic telemetry, J. Prosthet. Dent. **19**:151, 1968.
9. Pameijer, J.H.N., Glickman, I., and Roeber, F.W.: Intraoral occlusal telemetry. III. Tooth contacts in chewing, swallowing, and bruxism, J. Periodontol. **40**:253, 1968.
10. Celenza, F.V., and Nasedkin, J.N.: Position paper. In Occlusion—the State of the Art, Chicago, 1978, Quintessence Publishing Co., p. 31.
11. Tay, D.: The role of close-packed positions in the pathogenesis of temporomandibular joint internal derangements, Ann. Acad. Med. **15**(3):419, July 1986.
12. Guichet, N.F.: An introduction to clinical management of orofacial pain TMJ dysfunction, etiology, diagnosis, protocol for treatment, A Position paper, Copyright by N.F. Guichet, Anaheim, Calif., 1982, p. 27.
13. Gibbs, C.H., and Lundeen, H.L.: Jaw movements and forces during chewing and swallowing and their clinical significance. In Wright, John: Advances in Occlusion, 1982, Littleton, PSG, Inc.
14. Grab, H., and Zander, H.A.: Tooth contact patterns in mastication, J. Prosthet. Dent. **13**:1055, 1963.
15. Schuyler, C.H.: An evaluation of incisal guidance and its influence in restorative dentistry, J. Prosthet. Dent. **9**:3,374, May-June, 1959.
16. Schuyler, C.H.: The function and importance of incisal guidance in oral rehabilitation, J. Prosthet. Dent. **13**:1011, 1963.
17. Dawson, P.E.: Evaluation, Diagnosis, and Treation of Occlusal Problems, St. Louis, 1974, The C.V. Mosby Co., p. 58.
18. Shillingburg, H.T., Jr., Hobo, S., and Whitsett, L.D.: Fundamentals of Fixed Prosthodontics, ed. 2, Chicago, 1981, Quintessence Publishing Co., p. 260.
19. Williamson, E.H., Steinke, R.M., Morse, P.K., and Swift, T.R.: Centric relation-comparison of muscle determined position and operator guidance, Am. J. Orthod. **77**:133, 1980.
20. Woelfel, J.B.: New device for accurately recording centric relation, J. Prosthet. Dent. **56**(6):716, December 1986.
21. Mohl, N.D.: Functional anatomy of the temporomandibular joint. In Laskin, D., Greenfield, W., Gale, E. et al., The president's conference on the examination diagnosis and management of temporomandibular disorders, Chicago ADA, 1983.
22. Kopp, S.: Topographical distribution of sulphated glycosaminogylcans in the surface layers of the human temporomandibular joint, J. Oral Pathol. **7**:283, 1978.
23. DuBrul, E.L.: The craniomandibular articulation. In Sicher's Oral Anatomy, ed. 8, St. Louis, 1988, Ishiyaku EuroAmerica.
24. Bellanti, N., and Martin, K.: The significance of articulator capability. II. The prevalence of immediate side shift, J. Prosthet. Dent. **42**(3):255, September 1979.
25. Aull, A.E.: Condylar determinants of occlusal patterns, J. Prosthet. Dent. **15**:826, September 1965.
26. Bellanti, N., and Martin, K.: The significance of articulator capability. II. The prevalence of immediate side shift, J. Prosthet. Dent. **42**(3):255, September 1979.
27. Lundeen, H.L., and Wirth, C.G.: Condylar movement patterns engraved in plastic blocks, J. Prosthet. Dent. **30**:866, December 1973.
28. Williams, P.L., and Warnick, R.: Arthrology. In: Gray's anatomy, Edinburgh, 1980, Churchill Livingston, p. 420.
29. Sassouni, V.S.: A classification of skeletal facial types, Am. J. Orthod. **55**:109, February 1969.
30. DiPietro, G.J., and Moergel, J.R., Jr.: Significance of the Frankfort–mandibular plane angle to prosthodontics, J. Prosthet. Dent. **36**(6):624, December 1976.
31. DiPietro, G.J.: A study of occlusion as related to the Frank-

fort–mandibular plane angle, J. Prosthet. Dent. 38(4):453, October 1977.

32. Proffit, W.R., Fields, H.W., and Nixon, W.L.: Occlusal forces in normal and long-face adults, J. Dent. Res. 62(5):566, May 1983.
33. Weisgold, A.: Coronal forms of the full crown restoration—their clinical application, Chicago, 1981, Quintessence Publishing Co.
34. Jameson, L.M., and Malone, W.F.: Crown contours and gingival response, J. Prosthet. Dent. 47(6):620, June 1982.
35. Meyer, F.S.: The generated path technique in reconstructive dentistry. II. Fixed partial dentures, J. Prosthet. Dent. 9(3):432, May-June 1959.
36. Ash, M.M., and Ramfjord, S.P.: An Introduction to Functional Occlusion, Philadelphia, 1982, W.B. Saunders Co.
37. Tylman, S.D., and Malone, W.F.P.: Tylman's Theory and Practice of Fixed Prosthodontics, St. Louis, 1978, The C.V. Mosby Co.
38. Malone, W.F.P., Jameson, L.M., and Porter, Z.C.: Tooth preparation for periodontally compromised dentitions, Ill. State Dent. J. 53:228, July-August 1984.
39. Posselt, U.: Range of movement of the mandible, J.A.D.A. 56:10-13, 1958.
40. Shillingburg, H.T., Jr., Hobo, S., and Whitsett, L.D.: Fundamentals of Fixed Prosthodontics, ed. 2, Chicago, 1981, Quintessence Publishing Co., p. 307.
41. Youdelis, R.A., and Mann, W.V., Jr.: The prevalence and possible role of nonworking contacts in periodontal disease, Periodontics 3:219-223, 1965.
42. Lucia, V.O.: The fundamentals of oral physiology and their practical application in the securing and reproducing of records to be used in restorative dentistry, J. Prosthet. Dent. 3:213-231, 1953.
43. Thomas, P.K.: Syllabus on full mouth waxing technique for rehabilitation, San Diego, Instant Printing Services, 1967.
44. Malone, W.F.P., Mazur, B., Tylman, S.D., and Sawyer, H.P.: Biomechanical considerations of tooth preparation for fixed prosthodontics. In Tylman, S.D., and Malone, W.F.P.: Tylman's Theory and Practice of Fixed Prosthodontics, ed. 7, St. Louis, 1978, The C.V. Mosby Co., pp. 101-103.
45. Colman, A.J.: Occlusal requirements for removable partial dentures, J. Prosthet. Dent. 17:155-162, 1967.
46. Pound, E.: Aesthtic dentures and their phonetic values, J. Prosthet. Dent. 1:98-111, 1951.
47. Frechett, A.R.: Partial denture planning and special reference to stress distribution, J. Prosthet. Dent. 1:710-726, 1951.
48. Miller, E.L.: Removable Partial Prosthodontics, Baltimore, 1972, The Williams and Wilkins Co., p. 152.
49. DeVan, M.M.: Delivery and after care. In Sharry, J.J.: Complete Denture Prosthodontics, ed. 3. New York, 1974, McGraw-Hill Book Co., p. 278.
50. Tallgren, A.: The continuing reduction of the residual alveolar ridges in complete denture wearers: a mixed-longitudinal study covering 25 years, J. Prosthet. Dent. 27:120-132, 1972.
51. Kelly, E.: Changes caused by a mandibular removable partial denture opposing a maxillary complete denture, J. Prosthet. Dent. 27:140-150, 1972.
52. Ismail, Y.H., and Bowman, J.F.: Position of the occlusal plane in natural and artificial teeth, J. Prosthet. Dent. 20:405-411, 1968.
53. Lundquist, D.O., and Luther, W.W.: Occlusal plane determinations, J. Prosthet. Dent. 23:489-498, 1970.
54. Schultz, A.W.: Comfort and chewing efficiency in dentures, J. Prosthet. Dent. 1:38-48, 1951.
55. Eich, F.A.: The role of removable partial denture in the destruction of the natural dentition, Dent. Clin. North Am. pp. 717-731, 1962.
56. Wallace, D.H.: The use of gold occlusal surfaces in complete and partial dentures, J. Prosthet. Dent. 14:326-333, 1964.
57. Jordan, L.G.: Arrangement of anatomic-type artificial teeth into balanced occlusion, J. Prosthet. Dent. 39:484-494, 1978.
58. Monasky, G.E., and Taylor, D.F.: Studies on the wear of porcelain, enamel, and gold, J. Prosthet. Dent. 25:299-306, 1971.
59. Branmark, P.-I.: Introduction to osseointegration. In Branmark, P.-I., Zarb, G.A., and Albrektsson, T.: Tissue-Integrated Prostheses: Osseointegration in Clinical Dentistry, Chicago, 1985, Quintessence Publishing Co., p. 11.
60. Crum, R.J., and Loiselle, R.J.: Oral perception and proprioception: a review of the literature and its significance to prosthodontics, J. Prosthet. Dent. 28:215-230, 1972.
61. Zarb, G.A., and Albrektsson, T.: Nature of implant attachments. In Branemark, P.I., Zarb, G.A., and Albrektsson, T.: Tissue-Integrated Prostheses: Osseointegration in Clinical Dentistry, Chicago, 1985, Quintessence Publishing Co., pp. 89-91.
62. Adell, R.: Long-term treatment results. In Branemark, P.-I., Zarb, G.A., and Albrektsson, T.: Tissue-Integrated Prostheses: Osseointegration in Clinical Dentistry, Chicago, 1985, Quintessence Publishing Co., pp. 176-177.
63. Zarb, G.A., and Jansson, T.: Prosthodontic procedures. In Branemark, P.-I., Zarb, G.A., and Albrektsson, T.: Tissue-Integrated Prostheses: Osseointegration in Clinical Dentistry, Chicago, 1985, Quintessence Publishing Co., p. 248.
64. Skalak, R.: Aspects of biomechanical considerations. In Branemark, P.-I., Zarb, G.A., and Albrektsson, T.: Tissue-Integrated Prostheses: Osseointegration in Clinical Dentistry, Chicago, 1985, Quintessence Publishing Co., pp. 126-128.

BIBLIOGRAPHY

Atwood, D.A.: A critique of research of the posterior limit of mandibular position, J. Prosthet. Dent. 20:21-36, 1968.

Brecker, S.C.: Practical oral rehabilitation, J. Prosthet. Dent. 10:1001-1008, 1959.

Cohen, L.A.: Two techniques for interocclusal records, J. Prosthet. Dent. 13:438-443, 1963.

Culpepper, W.D., and Moulton, P.S.: Considerations in fixed prosthodontics, Dent. Clin. North Am. 23:21-35, January, 1979.

Firtell, D.N., Finzen, F.C., and Holmes, J.B.: The effect of clinical remount procedures on the comfort and success of complete dentures, J. Prosthet. Dent. 57:53-57, 1987.

Halpern, G.C., Halpern, A.R., and Norling, B.K.: Minimizing intraoral occlusal adjustments, J. Prosthet. Dent. pp. 448-450, 1982.

Lauritzen, A.G., and Wolford, L.W.: Occlusal relationships: the split-cast method for articulator techniques, J. Prosthet. Dent. 14:256-265, 1965.

Lucia, V.O.: Remounting procedures for completion of full-mouth rehabilitation, J. Prosthet. Dent. 30:679-684, 1973.

Preston, J.D.: Preventing ceramic failures when integrating fixed and removable prostheses, Dent. Clin. North Am. 23:37-52, January, 1979.

Pound, E.: Accurate protrusive registrations for patients edentulous in one or both jaws, J. Prosthet. Dent. 50:584, 1983.

Roedema, W.H.: Relationship between the width of the occlusal table and pressures under dentures during function, J. Prosthet. Dent. 36:24-34, 1976.

Stuart, C.E.: Good occlusion for natural teeth, J. Prosthet. Dent. 14:716-724, 1964.

Walker, P.M.: Remounting multiple castings prior to final cementation, J. Prosthet. Dent. 14:145-148, 1981.

Walker, P.M.: A technique for the adjustment of castings in a remount procedure, J. Prosthet. Dent. 46:263-270, 1981.

15

J. Marvin Reynolds

OCCLUSAL ADJUSTMENT

The science of occlusion encompasses more than mere interrelationships of teeth. It involves the stomatognathic system in health and disease. Occlusion is a physical, neuromuscular, and psychologic phenomenon. Comprehension of the interdependence of the teeth, the periodontium, the musculature of the head and neck and the temporomandibular articulation is needed. It is fundamental to understand the relationships between essential determinants in normal and abnormal functions.[1]

There is a mutual relationship between the contact of teeth, the position of the condyles, and the muscular activity associated with the mandible. The teeth control conditioned reflex activities more than innate reflexes. Therefore, interferences are probably less damaging during learned functional activities.[1] Tooth contact occurs during closing action of the mandibular muscles. The occlusal contact results in sensory feedback to the central nervous system.[2] The information either reinforces or modifies the neural information (engram) that is responsible for the next analogous activity. Each occlusal contact originates from neuromuscular activity, and the contact releases neuromuscular activity. Thus, dentists can potentially modify muscular activity by dental procedures that alter the occluding surface of a tooth.

OCCLUSAL TERMINOLOGY

The following definitions are used:

Arch segments

   Incisor segment. The part of the dental arch containing the incisor teeth.

   Canine segment. The part of the dental arch containing the canine and the adjacent teeth.

   Posterior segment. The part of the dental arch containing the premolars and molars.

Deflective occlusal contact. Tooth contact that deflects or has the potential to deflect condylar movement.

Dysfunction. State of functional disharmony in which the forces developed during function result in pathologic changes in the tissues or in some functional disturbances.

Interceptive occlusal contact. Initial tooth contact that stops or prevents joint tooth stabilization of the mandible.

Intercuspal position (IP). Occlusal position of maximum intercuspation; focal apex (terminal point) of all mandibular movements with a cranial component; occlusal position that has the most cranial location.

Laterotrusive contact. Contact occurring on the side of the mandible in laterotrusion. Synonym: working contact.

Laterotrusive side. Side of the mandible that has moved away from the medial plane and is located lateral to intercuspal position. Synonym: working side.

Mediotrusive contact. Contact occurring on the side of the mandible in mediotrusion. Synonym: balancing contact, nonworking contact.

Mesiotrusive side. Side of the mandible that has moved toward the median plane and is located medial to intercuspal position. Synonym: balancing side, nonworking side, idling side.

Orthofunction. State of functional harmony in which the forces developed during function are kept within the adaptive physiologic range and all tissues maintain a state of physical health.

Retruded contact position (RCP). Initial occlusal contact position when the mandible is retruded.

Shear cusps. Cusps not involved in intercuspal-position contacts; cusps not involved in fossae or marginal ridge contact.

Support cusps. Cusps that occlude in intercuspal position; cusps that occlude in fossae or on marginal ridges.

Terminal hinge position (THP). The position of the mandible when it is located in the hinge position of the envelope of motion.

CONCEPTS OF OCCLUSION

The concepts of occlusion can be analyzed in the following manner:

Interarch relationship
1. Intercuspal position at retruded mandibular position
2. Intercuspal position at retruded mandibular position and the uppermost condylar position
3. Intercuspal position not at retruded mandibular position or uppermost condylar position

Excursive tooth guidance
1. Maximum guidance (bilateral balance)
2. Segment guidance (working-side balance or group function)
3. Minimum guidance (posterior disclusion with canine guidance)

Occlusal morphology
1. Natural anatomy
2. Modified anatomy
3. Flat anatomy

Intertooth relationship
1. Cusp to ridge
2. Cusp to fossa
3. Cusp to embrasure
4. Cusp to plane
5. Plane to plane

Anterior guidance
1. Critical
2. Insignificant

The outline permits 270 possible combinations or plans. Is one plan significantly better? If so, under what circumstances? It is presently doubtful that one plan is scientifically proven to be superior.

The temporomandibular joint permits movement to gain a mechanical advantage through the principle of levers. A lever system must have an effective fulcrum. Joint stabilization is also necessary to ensure reciprocal muscular activity during dental treatment.

During mastication, the fulcrum may shift to the bolus of food. However, the teeth should not be the principal fulcrum during empty-mouth closures or contact movements.

The force vectors in the temporomandibular joints guide the condyles up and forward during shortening of the closing muscles and then move the condyles back along the articular eminences. The most effective braced position of the mandible exists when the condyle-disc assembly is uppermost against the articular eminences.[3]

The teeth permit the condyles to travel to the upper limits in the joint compartments and allow the closing muscles to shorten through contraction. This infers that the intercuspal position of the teeth relates to vertical and horizontal factors[4] of the joints and muscles. The teeth and temporomandibular joints are considered as one functional unit called the articular triad.[5] When the intercuspal position of the teeth is not integrated with a positioning of the joints that is favorable to the musculature, the occlusion can cause microtrauma in the joint-muscle system, the tooth-periodontal attachment apparatus, or the tooth.

Centric relation has been defined as the most retruded position of the mandible.[6] The most posterior position of the mandible can station the condyles posteriorly and inferiorly in relation to the articular eminence. Centric relation is a border position. Border limits do not normally involve functional movements but are terminal intraborder movements.[7] Intraborder movements should reach border positions without interference from the teeth.

Another dimension can be added to the centric relation-intercuspal position relation. It is the uppermost position of the condyles in the glenoid fossae. The uppermost condylar position averages 0.54 mm above and 0.18 mm in front of the rearmost condylar position.[7a] Therefore, to permit complete freedom of movement of the condyles in the temporomandibular joint, the intercuspal position occurs when the condyle-disc complex is braced uppermost against the posterior slope of the articular eminence. The retruded contact position and intercuspal position are similar in more patients than is usually acknowledged. During hinge closure, a given point on a mandibular tooth will arc up and forward at an angle of about 45 degrees.[8,9] This means that approximately 1 mm of anterior tooth movement occurs with each 1 mm of vertical closure without bodily change of the condyle relative to the articular eminence. Therefore, a slide from RCP to IP where the vertical and horizontal components are equal could occur interorally with limited forward movement of the condyles.

When a slide from retruded contact position to intercuspal position is observed, the vertical component is considered with the forward component. When each component is similar, the condyles are mainly rotating during the slide (Fig. 15-1). Any bodily displacement of the condyles is rarely more than 0.1 to 0.2 mm. When the anterior component of a slide predominates, the condyles are pulled forward (Fig. 15-2). If the slide is less than a millimeter, dysfunction is unlikely. If the vertical component predominates, the closure is commonly pivoting around a posterior interfering tooth, and the condyles are deflected down and back (Fig. 15-3) with a higher incident of dysfunction.

A slide from retruded contact position to intercuspal

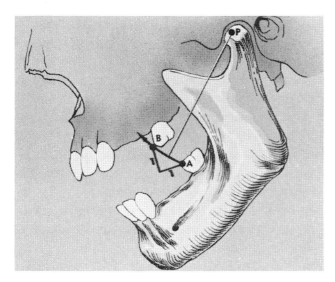

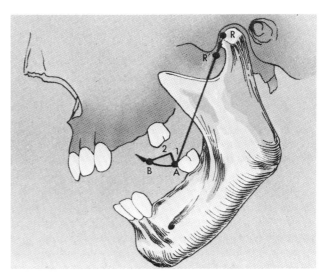

Fig. 15-1. Normal closure of mandible about its axis, P, will move cuspal elements of mandibular teeth up and forward along an arc, AB, at an angle of about 45 degrees. For each unit of vertical closure, cusp moves forward about the same without bodily change of condyle. This applies for most dentitions in the premolar and first molar area.

Fig. 15-2. This demonstrates a slide from RCP to IP (arc AB) where the occlusal elements of the mandibular teeth move forward more than vertically. When this occurs, condyle must move down and forward during closure, R to R'.

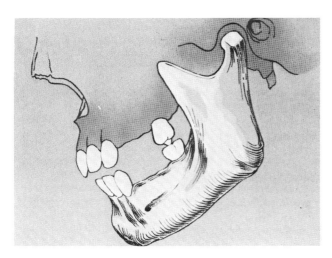

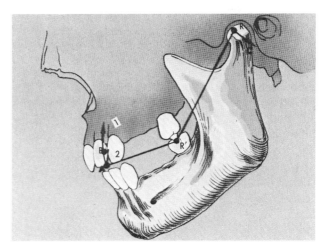

Fig. 15-3. A, Mandible closes on maxillary cusp that is in supraclusion. **B,** As closure continues, axis may shift from condyle, R, to contact on tooth, R'. Condyle is probably twisted down and back toward **C.** This will result in a slide frm RCP to IP in which the vertical component predominates. The condyle probably pivots downward from its seated position as IP is attained.

position needs to be correlated with its magnitude, the vertical and anterior components of the slide, the movement of the condyles from RCP to IP, and the functional status of the musculature.

Empty-mouth excursive tooth guidance is another occlusal consideration. How many teeth are needed in the guidance and where should they be located? Do certain forms of group guidance have an advantage over minimal guidance?

Williamson et al.[10-13] at the Medical College of Georgia have demonstrated that fewer mandibular elevator muscles are EMG active with canine guidance than with group function. The exact reason is not known,

but it appears that nature has a design preference for canine and incisor excursive guidance. This writer has observed that a majority of occlusal related MPD pain patients have open anterior teeth relations in IP or poor anterior guidance.

It is difficult to maintain constant occlusal and condylar relations because the type and rate of change are different for each individual. There are subtle changes in the occluding surfaces of teeth from attrition, alterations in tooth positions, differences in the thickness of the disc, and the decrease in the transjoint distance through remodeling associated with aging.

When the occlusal surfaces of teeth contact each

other, wear occurs.[14] Wear results from the nature of the material and the area and frequency of contact. Group function and bilateral balance increase the number of teeth in contact and also expand the range of movement during contact. Either situation increases the range of movement where contact is possible, with greater potential for wear of the teeth.

When multitooth guidance occurs, wear may be uneven among the teeth. Posterior teeth travel shorter distances than anterior teeth for each degree of lateral rotation. Different materials may be involved, and the slower-wearing tooth may eventually develop a deflective contact.

When more than one pair of teeth in the posterior segment provides guidance a deflective contact frequently develops on the most posterior tooth. This results from uneven wear or from an effective loss of vertical height through the joints. The more distal the contact, the greater the disharmony. Joint height decreases with the degenerative processes associated with aging.[6]

The relationship of the articular triad remains stable longer if wear is minimized. To accomplish this, intercuspal position is developed as a dead stop without a slide and with the condyles in their uppermost braced position. The guidance occurs in the canine or incisor segment between a minimum number of teeth, and outside the normal cyclic movements used in expression.

As long as the mandible is tripoded (both temporomandibular joints and one pair of occluding teeth), joint-tooth stabilization is insured. As more and more teeth participate in guidance, legs are added to the system and the articular triad is eventually lost. A stable joint-tooth relationship is also lost. The result is the creation of a fulcrum on a tooth. The consequence is a muscle-tooth stabilization of the mandible that can cause an imbalance in muscle activity and muscular dysfunction.

As teeth develop flat occluding surfaces, wear is accelerated, and occlusal stability is reduced. Wear can be reduced and horizontal forces minimized when the contact area is small and restricted to the central part of the teeth.

A sectional study of articulated casts from ideal dentitions demonstrated space between the opposing surfaces of teeth in the intercuspal position. The contacts were between spheroid surfaces with a limited incline plane effect. The combined area of contact was minimal and estimated to total about 4 to 5 mm. Each contact was surrounded by space. The space created by well-developed supplemental and developmental grooves appeared critical for a well-organized and stress-free stable occlusion (Fig. 15-4).

Another aspect of stable, unworn dentitions is the

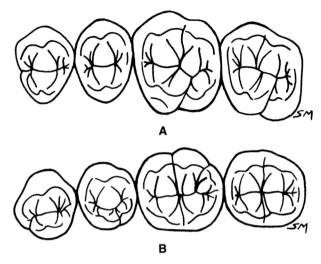

Fig. 15-4. A, Maxillary posterior teeth of caries-free dentition. **B,** Mandibular posterior teeth of caries-free dentition. Note numerous developmental and supplemental grooves creating a variety of spheroid ridges and the absence of flat planes.

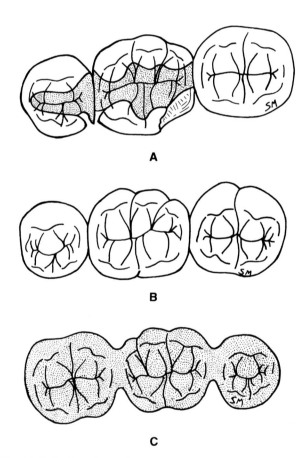

Fig. 15-5. A, Mandibular first molar has fractured lingual cusp and a carious MODB amalgam restoration. Second premolar has a fractured disto-occlusal amalgam restoration. **B,** Finished new restoration of that in **A.** Second premolar has a disto-occlusal amalgam, and first molar has complete veneer crown. **C,** Three-unit mandibular posterior bridge prior to cementation.

continued

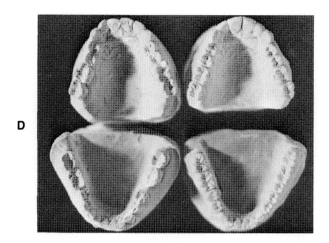

D

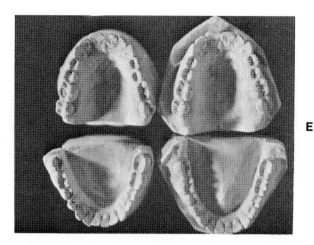

E

Fig. 15-5. D, Before and after casts where all teeth were restored except mandibular six anteriors. Two maxillary lateral incisors and mandibular left first molar were restored with three-unit bridges. All other restorations were either all metal or ceramometal-veneer crowns. **E,** Before and after casts of dentition where occlusion was altered by seleccted grinding. Notice that natural occlusal anatomy was recreated in each restorative procedure.

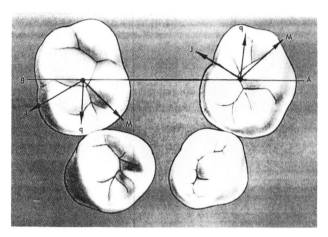

Fig. 15-6. Representation of opposing maxillary and mandibular teeth for maxillary ML cusp on the mandibular molar and mandibular DF cusp on the maxillary molar. Line AB represents frontal plane in area of IP tooth contact. Lines L represent laterotrusive paths of opposing cusps. Lines M represent mediotrusive paths and lines P protrusive. Notice that all excursive movements of mandibular teeth have an anterior component and all excursive movements of maxillary teeth have an apparent posterior component.

reciprocal arrangement of opposing elevations and depressions. This arrangement provides escape routes for cusps in excursive movements and a mechanism for developing a definite intercuspal position. When restoring teeth with a Class II or Class III relationship, a suitable plan is to create optimal anatomy of maxillary teeth and modify mandibular tooth anatomy to provide a reciprocal relationship of ridges and grooves.

Natural anatomy is recommended for the occlusal surfaces of teeth, and it should be reestablished in clinical procedures unless lateral guidance is created

between posterior teeth (Fig. 15-5). If an error is made, it should be with more ridges and grooves, avoiding flat surfaces.

The intercuspal position contacts are correlated with a specific excursive guidance. From centric relation the mandibular teeth have an anterior component to excursive movement paths (Fig. 15-6). Lower support cusps are thus occluded more mesially than in disclusion for a balanced articulation. The reverse is true for maxillary support cusps, since maxillary teeth have an apparent posterior component to excursive paths from retruded position (Fig. 15-7).

Specifically, in bilateral balance the lower support cusps are shaped and positioned in IP so guidance can exist on the distal surfaces of the upper teeth. The upper support cusps are positioned in IP so guidance can exist on the mesial part of lower teeth. From these locations of intercuspal-position contacts, the mesial parts of lower support cusps slide against the distal cusp slopes of upper teeth in excursive movements. Distal surfaces of upper cusps slide against mesial cusp slopes of lower teeth (Fig. 15-7 A).

For a group function (unilateral balance), the mandibular support cusps are positioned to occlude in intercuspal position on maxillary marginal ridges. From this location the upper marginal ridges and distal cusp slopes of the upper facial cusps provide guiding surfaces in laterotrusive movements. The lingual embrasures provide space for disclusion during mediotrusive movements of the lower support cusps. Both opposing marginal ridges may have intercuspal position contacts in this guidance, but the contact on the distal marginal ridge increases contact in mediotrusive movements. The upper support cusps are occluded in intercuspal position on lower marginal ridges when cross-tooth laterotrusive guidance is desired; otherwise the upper support cusps occlude in lower distal fossae. The molars normally have a cusp occluding in the opposing central fossa to function harmoniously with other cusps (Fig. 15-7 B).

A cusp-to-fossa occlusion in intercuspal positions predominates in anterior guidance and posterior disclusion. This means mandibular support cusps occlude on the mesial surfaces of maxillary teeth. The embrasures provide space for disocclusion of the posterior cusps during laterotrusive and mediotrusive movements. The organization of the second cusp placement on molars in the opposing central fossa and the associated ridge and groove directions are precisely organized to ensure disclusion of these cusps in excursive movements. Sharp secondary anatomy creates space for disclusion of IP contacts along excursive paths (Fig. 15-7 C).

An occlusion may appear acceptible on initial examination or with unmounted casts. The arch form is satisfactory and the teeth occlude well. However, unless the final closure of the teeth is integrated with a favorable positioning of the joints to the musculature, the occlusion can be predisposed to dysfunction.

Proper occlusion permits joint-tooth stabilization of the mandible without splinting, twisting, or hyperactivity of the musculature. The condyle-disc assembly is permitted to function on the posterior slopes of the articular eminences without deflective contacts.

AN OPTIMUM OCCLUSAL PLAN

The features of an occlusal plan that promote orthofunction, remain mechanically stable, feel comfortable, and look pleasing are as follow:

Anterior segments

Occlusal component:

1. The maxillary anterior teeth overlap the mandibular anterior teeth in intercuspal position.
2. The anterior teeth contact in the intercuspal position during empty-mouth power closures.
3. The coupled anterior teeth remain free of contact during normal movements of the mandible associated with speech and expression.

Esthetic component:

1. The incisal edges of the maxillary anterior teeth form a convex downward curve similar in outline to the lower lip in smiling (Fig. 15-8).
2. The V of the incisal embrasures between maxillary anterior teeth is progressively wider from central incisor to first premolar (Fig. 15-9).
3. The length, tilt, and position of the maxillary anterior teeth permit a comfortable seal of the lips with closure into IP.

Posterior segments

Occlusal component:

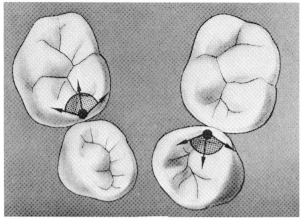

A

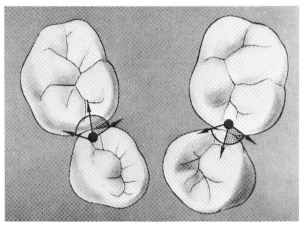

B

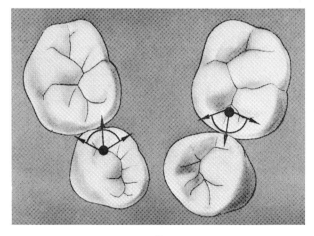

C

Fig. 15-7. Preferred general location for intercuspal-position contacts when balanced occlusion is desired. Adjacent cuspal inclines (shaded areas) provide bulk for excursive tooth contact. **B,** Preferred general location for intercuspal-position contact when group function is desired. **C,** Preferred general location for intercuspal-position contacts when disclusion is desired. Adjacent embrasures will provide space for excursive glide paths.

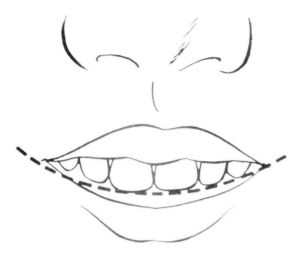

Fig. 15-8. Incisal edges of maxillary anterior teeth form a convex downward curve that tends to follow outline of lower lip in smiling.

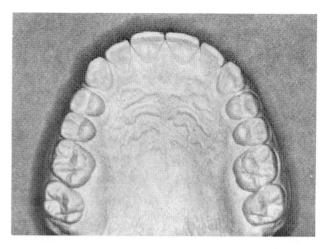

Fig. 15-10. Facial cusp tips of posterior teeth and incisal edges of anterior teeth tend to form a parabolic curve in dentitions that display optimal esthetics and occlusal form.

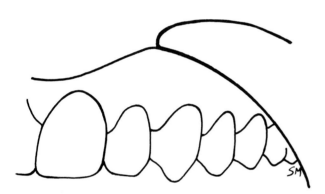

Fig. 15-9. Natural anatomy and arrangement of maxillary anterior teeth form a V-shaped incisal embrasure that gets progressively wider and deeper from central incisors to first premolar. Profiles of facial surfaces of posterior teeth are parallel and similar to those of canines. Geometric shape of incisal embrasures is very important in reestablishing natural esthetics in anterior teeth. Posterior cusp-tip length, its shape, and outline of facial profiles are important in reestablishing proper harmony of these teeth.

1. Mandibular posterior teeth close evenly against the maxillary posterior teeth when the condyles are bilaterally seated in the uppermost articular position.
2. The posterior teeth contact in intercuspal position at a vertical level that permits the jaw-closing muscles to shorten through their power contraction.
3. Each pair of occluding teeth has one support cusp occluding in IP in an opposing fosse.
4. Intercuspal contacts, whenever possible, should be avoided on distal occlusal surfaces of maxillary teeth and mesial-occlusal surfaces of mandibular teeth.

5. Subsummit surfaces of support cusps contact horizontal crests of ridges that surround the opposing occlusal fossae in the intercuspal position. The contacts should occur within 1 to 2 mm of the cusp tip and within 1 mm of the opposing central groove alignment.
6. The intercuspal position is reached as a dead stop with minimal muscular activity.
7. The horizontal overlap of the shearing cusps are enough to keep the cheek and tongue free of the tooth-contact area in the intercuspal position.

Excursive component:
1. Laterotrusive guidance involves a) only the canines or b) one canine and another tooth in the canine segment or c) a pair of teeth in the canine segment while other teeth disclude immediately.
2. Protrusive guidance involves a pair of incisors on each side of the midline. All other teeth should disclude immediately. The protrusive path should be relatively straight forward.
3. A reciprocal arrangement of maxillary and mandibular posterior elevations and depressions occurs in IP and along each diagnostic excursive movement.
4. The optimal clearance of the posterior teeth is 1 mm in all positions when the anterior teeth are in edge-to-edge contact relationships.

The maxillary arch forms the plane of reference and has the following:

Occlusal view:
1. The facial cusp tips, the facial cusp ridges, and the incisal edges are symmetrically aligned to form a parabolic curve (Fig. 15-10).
2. The lingual cusps of molars and premolars are aligned in an anteroposterior direction, resulting in an occlusal table that has the same bucciolingual width.

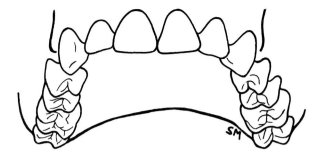

Fig. 15-11. A, Occlusal view of natural dentition Occlusal view of natural dentition displaying optimal occlusal plane. On first premolars, lingual cusps are slightly shorter than facial cusps. On second premolars, lingual and facial cusps are about same length. On first molars, lingual cusps are slightly longer than facial cusps. On second molars, lingual cusps are longer than facial cusps. The difference is more than on first molars.

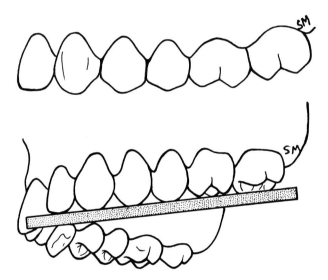

Fig. 15-12. Facial cusp tips of maxillary canine and premolars and first molar fall on same plane. Facial cusp tips of second molar and third molar (when present) are progressively short of this plane.

3. The lingual surfaces of the anterior teeth have distinct concavities from the cingulum to the incisal edges.
4. Posterior and anterior marginal ridges are at the same height.
5. The lingual cusp tips of the first premolars are slightly shorter than the facial cusp tips (Fig. 15-11).
6. The lingual cusp tips of the second premolars are approximately the same length as the facial cusp tips (Fig. 15-11).
7. The mesiolingual cusp tip of the first molar is slightly longer than the facial cusp tips (Fig. 15-11).
8. The mesiolingual lingual cusp tip of the second molar is longer than the facial cusp tips by approximately a millimeter (Fig. 15-11).

Buccal view:
1. The facial cusp tips of the canine, the two premolars, and the first molar lie on the same plane. The facial cusps of the second and third molar become progressively short of the plane (Fig. 15-12).
2. The angulation of inner inclines of maxillary facial and mandibular lingual cusps is relatively flat on second molars but progressively steeper from posterior to anterior. These inclines are associated with laterotrusive movements (Fig. 15-13).
3. The angulation of the inner inclines of maxillary lingual and mandibular facial cusps is relatively steep on second molars and progressively less steep from posterior to anterior. These inclines are associated with mediotrusive movements (Fig. 15-13).
4. The mandibular occlusal plane is a mirror image of the maxillary occlusal plane.
5. The occlusal plane is actually a spiral.

This plan organizes the teeth to permit segmental function and mutual protection. The main load in retruded contact position and intercuspal-position closures is supported by the posterior teeth. The anterior teeth protect the posterior teeth in eccentric empty-mouth closures. The incisors, canines, and posterior teeth function independently without interference from other teeth. Extrusive contact of teeth occurs just outside the normal cyclic jaw movements made during speech and expression. The condyles can reach any position in the joint compartment without guidance from the teeth. A joint-tooth stabilization of the mandible is possible in occluded positions.

This plan encourages a stable neuromuscular functional pattern without strain on the individual units of the stomatognathic system.

OCCLUSAL DIAGNOSIS AND TREATMENT PLANNING

Occlusal therapy is dictated by the functional state of the mandibular system, existing dental conditions, possible alterations, and the occlusal involvement necessitated by restorative needs.

The restorations of patients in orthofunction involving one segment are fitted to the existing IP and anterior guidance. In patients whose restorations involve all three segments in the same arch (including changes in the vertical dimension of occlusion), the occlusion is usually adjusted before beginning restoration. Restorations involving two adjacent segments may be managed with a one-segment restoration or with a three-segment restoration.

Patients with dysfunction should have an initial treatment that is simple in order to solve their prob-

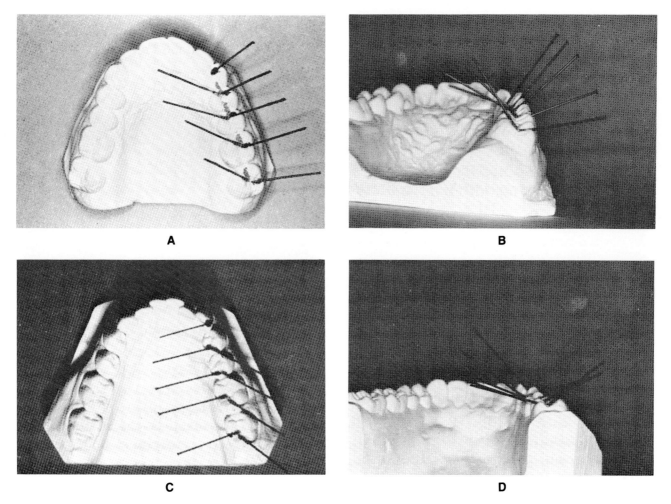

Fig. 15-13. A, and **C,** Plastic rods are attached to cusp inclines of casts from an unworn natural dentition. Rods represent cusp paths of opposing support cusps in laterotrusive and mediotrusive movements. **B** and **D,** Angle of cusp inclines involved in laterotrusive movements get progressively steeper from most posterior tooth to most anterior tooth. Angle of cusp inclines involved in mediotrusive movements get progressively less steep from most posterior tooth to most anterior tooth.

lem. Irreversible occlusal changes are delayed until there is satisfactory resolution of the symptoms. Then the framework for an optimal occlusal scheme is created. Occlusal adjustment by selective grinding may be sufficient; orthodontics, orthognathic surgery, provisional restorations, or a combination of procedures may be required. Once an acceptable framework for the final occlusion has been established, the final restorations can then be fabricated into the treatment.

GUIDELINES FOR OCCLUSAL ADJUSTMENT AND OCCLUSAL THERAPY

Occlusal adjustment by selective grinding is the initial phase of irreversible occlusal therapy. The following factors should be included in the adjustment:

1. A precise and stable IP between the posterior teeth.
2. IP contacts are within 2 mm of the support cusp tips, within 1 mm of the central groove align-

ment, occur between opposing convex surfaces, are pinpoint in size, and avoid incline plane action.
3. The anterior teeth are coupled to establish satisfactory anterior guidance.
4. The mandibular musculature and TMJs are relatively symptom free.
5. The occlusal adjustment performed is within the limitations of existing tooth structure and restorations without sacrificing esthetics.

OCCLUSAL ADJUSTMENT BY SELECTIVE GRINDING

The grinding procedure should consist of grooving, spheroiding, and pointing.[15]

Grooving is the basic step of selective grinding and the way to reestablish normal anatomy.

Spheroiding is used to recreate ridges on the area of the interference not being grooved. The procedure is integrated with the grooving technique to develop a ridge lateral to each groove. A reciprocal arrangement of elevations and depressions is created between the opposing tooth surfaces (Fig. 15-14).

The *doming* phase consists of reshaping the support cusp tip to a normal form to provide a position for the contact of intercuspal position. The cusp tip may be ground to reposition the tip up to 1 mm in any direction. The tip of the cusp is made to migrate toward the opposing central groove alignment and toward mesial surfaces of maxillary teeth and distal surfaces of mandibular teeth. The cusp tip is out of contact when positioned in an opposing fossa.

The three steps are combined into one smooth operation when performed clinically. When the IP is altered by selected grinding, two procedures follow. First, support (centric) cusps are ground. This is necessary to realign the cusps with the opposing central grooves. Many techniques caution against grinding on support cusps and perform all grinding in the opposing fossae. This generally prevents the reestablishment of normal tooth form, natural anatomy, and small IP contacts. Second, the vertical dimension of occlusion is closed sufficiently to permit erasure of the former IP. Otherwise, two IPs or an area IP exist and most function terminates at the more anterior locations, since functional tooth movements are infraborder.

Grinding of fossae definitely changes the vertical dimension of occlusion. The initial phase of occlusal therapy is to align the support cusps with the opposing central groove. In removable prosthodontics, the teeth are positioned in softened wax to establish a satisfactory tooth arrangement in IP. In fixed prosthodontics, the support cusps are waxed to a position for a satisfactory relationship IP. When a total occlusal adjustment is performed, the support cusps must be ground initially to establish a suitable IP arrangement between the cusps and the countersurfaces.

STEPS OF AN OCCLUSAL ADJUSTMENT

Before occlusal adjustment, the musculature should be asymptomatic. If it is not, the activity is reduced with a splint or other appropriate therapy before the adjustment.[11,17-22]

Intercuspal Position Adjustment

1. Idealize the facio-occlusal part of the maxillary arch within the limitations of coronal reshaping.
2. Verify that the incisal edge facets are rounded over on the maxillary canines.
3. Creating a new IP:
   a. Deprogram the musculature. Determine the number of leaves on a "leaf gauge"[23,24] necessary to *just* separate the teeth from contact

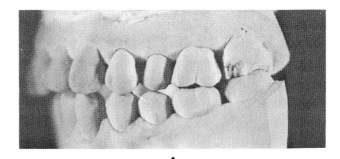

A

B

Fig. 15-14. A, Diagnostic casts where laterotrusive interferences occur between central parts of facial cusps in a Class II relationship. **B,** Diagnostic casts after an occlusal adjustment by selective grinding. Main part of correction was done on mandibular teeth so that esthetics of maxillary cusps is maintained, yet a reciprocal arrangement of elevations and depressions is established.

when the mandible is in terminal hinge position (THP). Place the leaf gauge between the central incisors and centered with the midsagittal plane. Guide the mandible into THP and closure against the leaf gauge. Verify that the patient does not protrude during closure or during the remainder of the procedure. With the mandible secured against the leaf gauge in THP, ask the patient to "try to squeeze your back teeth together, then relax your jaw muscles." Have the patient continue this in five second cycles. Make sure the posterior part of the temporalis muscles is active during the clenching phase. Each time the patient feels tooth contact, add another leaf. Continue the procedure until the patient can go about one minute without further tooth contact. The patient is now ready for occlusal adjustment.

   b. Marking the interference. Reduce two or three leaves from the gauge until there is positive tooth contact. Mark the interference with articulating ribbon as the patient clenches on the leaf gauge. (Make sure THP is maintained). Eliminate the interference following the appropriate rule. After correction, reduce another one or two leaves and mark and eliminate the interference. Continue the process until about three leaves remain. The final phases of the IP adjustment are performed with manual manipulation. Manual manipulation may be used throughout.

c. Initially evaluate each supracontact to determine if either or both of the interfering areas are out of harmony (excessive) with the same elements in the segment and factors of ideal archform. Correct the area that is obtuse.

d. When all interfering occlusal elements are in harmony, reshape interfering maxillary and mandibular support (centric) (stamp) cusps (incisor edges) to sharpen the cusp and to relocate the IP contact within 1 mm of the opposing central groove alignment and near the cusp summit. Also reshape these cusps to eliminate (avoid) any contact in the occlusal surface on distal parts (molar third and premolar halves) of maxillary teeth and mesial parts of mandibular teeth.

e. When interfering occlusal contacts are between opposing ridges that are in harmony with the occlusal elements, and IP contacts are aligned, make a reciprocal groove in the mandibular ridge.

f. When the occlusal elements are aligned and additional adjustment is necessary, reduce the occlusal elements (support cusp, opposing fossa, or marginal ridge) that are incongruent with the other elements.

g. When the occlusal elements are suitably aligned, the occlusal elements are in harmony, and additional adjustment is necessary, divide the grinding between the maxillary and mandibular segments, or concentrate the grinding on the elements that can afford the removal (grinding).

4. Continue the adjustment until the slide has been eliminated between THP and IP. Then:

a. Determine the number and type of anterior teeth contact in IP. If short of the desired plan . . .

b. Continue the adjustment until anterior contact is accomplished.

Laterotrusive Adjustment

1. When a mandibular cusp has an interceptive contact on the inner incline of a maxillary tooth, make, widen, or deepen a transverse groove on the maxillary inner incline.

2. When a maxillary facial cusp (or its triangular ridge) has an interceptive contact on the outer incline of a mandibular tooth, make, widen, or deepen a transverse groove on the mandibular outer incline.

3. When a maxillary cusp (its triangular ridge) and a mandibular cusp (its facial ridge) have an interceptive contact, make a transverse groove in the mandibular cusp (its facial ridge).

4. When a maxillary inner incline has an interceptive contact against a mandibular outer incline, make, widen, or deepen a transverse groove in the maxillary incline in the anterior half of the interference and make, widen, or deepen a transverse groove in the mandibular incline in the posterior half of the interference.

5. When a maxillary lingual cusp has an interceptive contact against a mandibular cuspal element or elements, shorten, reshape, or move the mandibular cuspal element.

Mediotrusive Adjustment

When maxillary and mandibular support cuspal elements have an interceptive contact:

1. Make a mesiolingual groove in the anterior half of the interference on the maxillary cuspal element.

2. Make a distofacial groove in the posterior half of the interference on the mandibular cuspal element.

Protrusive Adjustment

1. The incising edge-to-edge relationship should be as straightforward as possible. If it deviates significantly to one side, level the maxillary incisal edges or non-IP mandibular surfaces (when possible) to attain a straighter incising edge-to-edge position.

2. Eliminate all unnecessary protrusive contact and reshape incisal contact that causes a midline deviation to the edge-to-edge position by:

a. Shortening posterior shear cusps

b. Reshaping maxillary anterior guiding surfaces

c. Reshaping non-IP areas on mandibular teeth

Final Refinement of an Occlusal Adjustment

1. Functional adjustment. The mandible flexes during function. Clinically, one should finalize for functional movements. Ideally, it is done 7 to 30 days after the last corrective adjustment. Have the patient chew on one side on a ¼ to ½-inch square of rubber dam material or chamois skin. Ask the patient to "chew like it is a tough piece of meat." If the patient senses any tooth contact, repeat while marking ribbon (blue or green) is held between the involved teeth. Mark IP contacts in red. Remove all nonred marks and con-

tinue until no teeth touch. Repeat for the opposite side.
2. Supine position. Balance and minimize all IP contacts. Use ribbon, mylar tape, and patient's sensation. One segment should not contact harder. The contacts should feel the same, whether loading the mandible or free swinging. As the contacts are being balanced, make the contacting areas as small as possible and on basically horizontal surfaces.
3. Upright position. Have the patient close into IP. If teeth touch hard, mark with blue or green ribbon. Mark IP in red. Return the patient to supine position and reduce any nonred spots. Continue until upright and supine closures feel the same.

POSTINSERTION GOALS

The essential occlusal scheme is established before fixed prosthodontics and maintained during adjustment of the new restorations. The restorations are checked to ensure that they are complementary to the existing occlusal scheme.

Before inserting a new restoration, the other teeth are checked in the intercuspal position to determine the teeth providing tooth guidance. Insert the restoration and verify the relationships of the other teeth. If the relationships change, then the new restorations need adjustment. In addition, the restorations should:
1. Maintain an appropriate intercuspal position.
2. Provide a joint-tooth stabilization of the mandible in intercuspal position and retruded contact position.
3. Avoid unilateral retrusive interferences.
4. Avoid mediotrusive interferences.
5. Not restrict intercuspal position for eccentric contact movements.
6. Not curtail condylar movement against the articular eminence.

Sustain the occlusal scheme that encourages orthofunction. Occlusal disharmonies do not have to be monumental to cause functional disturbances; low-level chronic microtrauma can precipitate dysfunction.

Occlusal management requires a thorough diagnosis based on a complete history after a comprehensive physical examination of the functional parts. Any change in the occluding surface of a tooth, whether by movement, decay, or restorations has the potential to modify sensory input for muscle response. The ability of the sensory system to detect change is more accurate than clinical diagnosis, so every effort is made to avoid occlusal disharmony.

SELECTED REFERENCES

1. Schwartz, L., and Chayes, C.M.: Facial Pain and Mandibular Dysfunction, 1968. Philadelphia, W.B. Saunders Co.
2. Beyron, H.: Optimal occlusion, Dent. Clin. North Am. 13:537, July 1969.
3. Dawson, P.E.: Temporomandibular joint pain-dysfunction problems can be solved, J. Prosthet. Dent. 29:100-112, 1973.
4. Owens, S.E., Lehr, R.P., and Biggs, N.L.: The functional significance of centric relation as demonstrated by electromyography of the lateral pterygoid muscles, J. Prosthet. Dent. 33:5-9, 1975.
5. Moffett, B.: The morphogenesis of the temporomandibular joint, Am. J. Orthodont. 52:401-415, 1966.
6. Boucher, C.O., ed.: Current Clinical Dental Terminology, St. Louis, 1963. The C.V. Mosby Co.
7. Lundeen, Harry C., and Gibbs, Charles H.: Advances in Occlusion, Boston, 1982. John Wright.
7a. Gibbs, Charles H., and Lundeen, Harry C.: University of Florida, personal communication, 1987.
8. Weinberg, L.A.: Anterior condylar displacement: its diagnosis and treatment, J. Prosthet. Dent. 34:195-207, 1975.
9. Hodge, L.C., and Mahan, P.E.: A study of mandibular movement from centric occlusion to maximum intercuspation, J. Prosthet. Dent. 18:19-30, 1967.
10. Williamson, E.H., Steinke, R.M., Morse, P.K., and Swift, T.R.: Centric relation: a comparison of muscle-determined position and operator guidance, Am. J. Orthod. 77:133, 1980.
11. Williamson, E.H.: Occlusion and TMJ dysfunction. I. J. Clin Orthod. 15:333, 1982.
12. Williamson, E.H.: Occlusion and TMJ dysfunction. II. J. Clin Orthod. 15, 393, 1981.
13. Williamson, E.H., and Lundquist, D.O.: Anterior guidance: its effect on electromyographic activity of the temporal and masseter muscles, J. Prosthet. Dent. 49:816-824, 1983.
14. McAdams, D.B.: Tooth loading and cuspal guidance in canine and group function occlusion, J. Prosthet. Dent. 35:283-290, 1976.
15. Bell, Welden E.: Orofacial Pains: Classification, Diagnosis, Management, Chicago, 1985. Year Book Medical Publisher.
16. Bell, Welden E.: Temporomandibular Disorders: Classification, Diagnosis, Management, Chicago, 1986. Year Book Medical Publishers.
17. Gelb, Harold: Clinical Managements of Head, Neck and TMJ Pain and Dysfunction, Philadelphia, 1985. W.B. Saunders Co.
18. Morgan, Douglas H., House, Leland R., Hall, William P., and Vamvas, S. James: Diseases of the Temporomandibular Apparatus, A Multidisciplinary Approach, St. Louis, 1985. The C.V. Mosby Co.
19. Okeson, Jeffrey P.: Fundamentals of Occlusion and Temporomandibular Disorders, St. Louis, 1985. The C.V. Mosby Co.
20. Ramfjord, Sigurd, and Ash, Major M.: Occlusion, Philadelphia, 1983. W.B. Saunders Co.
21. Travell, Janet G., and Simons, David G.: Myofascial Pain and Dysfunction, The Trigger Point Manual, Baltimore, 1983. Williams & Wilkins.
22. Kantor, M.E., Silverman, S.E., and Garfinkel, L.: Centric-relation recording techniques-a comparative investigation, J. Prosthet. Dent. 28:593-600, 1972.
23. Long, J.H.: Occlusal adjustment, J. Prosthet. Dent. 30:706-714, 1973.
24. Long, J.H.: Locating centric relation with a leaf gauge, J. Prosthet. Dent. 29:608-610, 1973.

16   ARTICULATORS

J. Marvin Reynolds

Articulators are essential in the practice of prosthodontics. They are useful 1) in the diagnosis of dental occlusal and tooth-joint interactions; 2) in planning dental restorations involving replacements, positions, contours, esthetics, and occlusion; and 3) for indirectly fabricated dental restorations. Articulators are also helpful in the teaching of occlusion, condylar movements, and the interactions of both.

Many articulators have been introduced over the years. They were designed to meet the needs of their inventors and/or to correlate with the current knowledge and understanding of mandibular movement. Today, the dental profession has a large selection of articulators from a number of manufacturers. The effectiveness of the articulator depends upon 1) the specific use, 2) the type of the restoration, 3) the dental conditions, 4) the dentist's comprehension, 5) how well the dentist understands condyle and tooth movements and their modifying factors, 6) the procedure to attach the casts, 7) the design of the instrument, and 8) the enthusiasm of the user for the particular instrument system.

CLASSIFICATION

Many classifications have been suggested, but the most popular terms are nonadjustable, semiadjustable, and fully adjustable. Semiadjustable, and to some degree fully adjustable, is a meaningless term. Most instruments are completely adjustable within a design capability. Fully adjustable implies an articulator that duplicates all mandibular movements. This is false.

A more scientific classification would be nonadjustable and adjustable with subdivisions.

Nonadjustable

Denar automark
Hanau gnatus ortoflex
Hanau LTD
Hanau-mate 165-1
Hanau-twin stage occluder
Trubyte simplex

Adjustable

1. Rectilinear guidances
   Denar Mark II
   Denar Omni
   Denar Track II
   Dentatus
   Hanau 183 Wide-vue
   Hanau 184 Wide-vue II
   Hanau 145
   Hanau 158
   Hanau 96H2
   Hanau 181-101
   Quick perfect
   TMJ Deluxe with mechanical fossae
   TMJ Mini with mechanical fossae
   SAM
   Whip Mix 8500
   Whip Mix 8800
   Whip Mix 9000
   Whip Mix 9800
2. Curvilinear guidances
   a. Mechanical adjustments
      Hanau 166-1 radial shift
      Whip Mix 8300
      Whip Mix 8340
      Whip Mix 2000
      Whip Mix DB 2200

  b. Preformed fossae
     Denar Anamark
     Panadent PCL
     Panadent PSL
     Panadent SL
     TMJ Deluxe
     TMJ Mini
  c. Custom created
     Denar D5A
     Denar SE
     Stuart Gnathologic Computer
     TMJ Sterographic

The majority of the articulators manufactured today are arcon types that incorporate the condylar guidances into the upper member of the articulator. The nonarcon type design incorporates the condylar guidances into the lower member. The arcon types are better for teaching mandibular movements and the dynamic relationship between condylar movement patterns and dental articulation.

DESIGN FEATURES OF ARTICULATORS
Denar Articulators

The Denar system offers great versatility with a wide range of accessories.

Automark. The Automark is a non-adjustable articulator. The horizontal condylar guide angle is 25 degrees, and the mediotrusive guide angle is 7 degrees (Bennett angle). It has a positive centric latch and accepts a facebow transfer.

Mark II. The Mark II articulator was introduced in 1975. It has open fossae incorporating a positive centric locking mechanism to hold the two members together and permits 85 degrees of hinge opening. The horizontal condylar inclination is adjustable from 0 to 60 degrees. The mediotrusive guidance has an immediate side shift adjustment of 0 to 4 mm, plus a progressive adjustment of 0 to 15 degrees. The rear walls are straight, but a wall is available that is inclined posteriorly to allow for a backward movement of the rotating condylar element as it moves outward during a lateral side shift. The condylar elements are fixed at 110 mm intercondylar distance.

Anamark. The Anamark model uses three sets of interchangeable premolded fossa analogs for the condylar guidances. The superior surface has a ¾ inch curvature, and its horizontal inclination can be adjusted from 0 to 60 degrees. The medial walls have 0.5 mm, 1.0 mm, or 1.5 mm curved lateral shift (precurrent shift) in the first 3 mm of the surface followed with a 7 degree straight surface (progressive shift) in the remainder of the wall. The remaining features are similar to those of the Mark II.

Omni. The Omni articulator was introduced in 1984. The design allows one to easily exchange closed track-

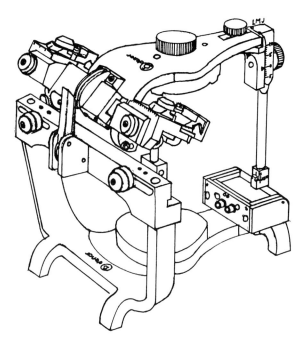

Fig. 16-1. Eccentric fully adjustable Denar Model 5A articulator (Denar Corporation, Anaheim, Calif.).

ing fossa for open fossa. The purpose of this model is to meet the requirements for complete removable and fixed prosthodontics in one articulator. The tracking fossa allows for horizontal condylar inclination adjustments from 0 to 90 degrees, a progressive medial condylar inclination from 0 to 30 degrees. The articulator has a 180 degree hinge opening. There is a CR-CO adjustment from 0 to 4 mm in 0.5 mm increments. With the open fossa, the Omni has a horizontal condylar inclination adjustment of 0 to 60 degrees, a progressive medial wall adjustment of 5 to 15 degrees with 0 to 4 mm immediate side shift adjustment, and a 25 degree posterior inclination to the rear wall. It has a 110 degree hinge opening. The condylar elements are fixed at 110 mm.

D5A. The D5A is a modified version of the articulator Niles Guichet introduced in 1968. The condylar guidances are adjustable in three planes. The medial wall also has an immediate side shift adjustment. A series of curved superior and medial wall inserts is available that can be custom ground or modified as necessary. The intercondylar elements are adjusted from 90 to 150 mm.

SE. The SE model has essentially the same features of the D5A. It does not require tools to remove the inserts and has a removable locking pin that allows for locking of the upper member in the upright position. The D5A and SE models are designed with stereographic records. A pantronic recorder is available with an electronic readout of the settings.

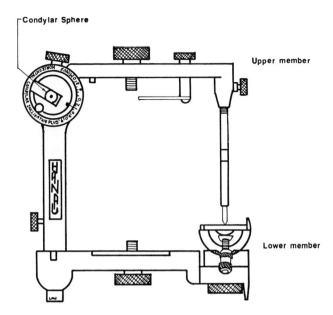

Fig. 16-2. Eccentric semiadjustable nonarcon articulator by Telegyne Hanau (Teledyne Hanau, Buffalo, N.Y.). Condylar sphere is attached to the upper member of the articulator, while the mechanical fossa is part of the lower member of the articulator.

Hanau Articulators

Hanau brand articulators were first introduced to the dental profession in 1921; but since that time a number of models have been manufactured for the changing needs of the profession.

The series 96H2 model is a nonarcon axle articulator that maintains many of the features of the original H-2, which was very popular for many years. It has enclosed track guidances. The horizontal condylar inclinations adjust from 0 to 75 degrees and progressive lateral adjustments adjust from 0 to 30 degrees. The condylar elements are fixed at 110 mm. There is a hinge opening capability at 240 degrees.

The series 145 comes in two models that differ only in the incisal guide pin and table. They maintain all the features of the H-2 model, but have ¾ inch less space between the upper and lower frames.

The 158 series has similar features to the H-2 series. It is of arcon type in design and the horizontal condylar inclination adjustment is 0 to 60 degrees.

The 183 and 184 series have identical features, with one exception. The 183 is a one-piece model, while the 184 has separation capability. These are arcon type articulators and the vertical uprights are designed with unobstructed posterior visibility. The horizontal condylar inclination can be adjusted from −20 to +60 degrees, with a progressive lateral adjustment of 0 to 30 degrees. The condylar elements are fixed at 110 mm and function in a tracking fossa.

The series 166-1 has curvilinear condylar guidances. The superior walls have a ¾ inch curved surface and these walls can be adjusted from 0 to 60 degrees.

The series 166 radial shift model is an arcon instrument with curvilinear guidances. The horizontal guidance has a 3/4 inch curvature that is adjustable in inclination from 0 to 60 degrees. The lateral condylar guidance has a radial curve (precurrent shift) that is adjustable from 0 to 3 mm and is combined with a progressive shift that is adjustable from 0 to 30 degrees. It has a hinge-locking mechanism. The condylar elements are fixed at 110 mm. The design creates generous space in the posterior that permits excellent lingual visibility.

The 165 (Hanau-mate) is an articulator with nonadjustable guidances. The lateral shift is progressive and fixed at 15 degrees; the horizontal guidance is fixed at 30 degrees. The incisal guide table is fixed with 10 degree protrusive and lateral angles. It not only functions with both frames hinged together, but is easily unlocked to separate the upper member from the lower member. It has facebow capabilities also.

The 147 series was designed primarily as a laboratory instrument. It permits progressive lateral excursions of 15 degrees and rectilinear protrusive movement of 20 degrees. It does not have an incisal guide pin or table. Instead, there is a vertical control screw on the posterior part of the frame. The upper member can be easily disengaged from the lower member. It uses disposable mounting inserts instead of mounting plates.

The 181-101 model is a special instrument designed primarily for the fabrication of TMJ and occlusal splints. It has rectilinear track guidances that are calibrated for adjustments in 360 degrees of rotation for each type of splint. Nine calibrated lines spaced 1 mm apart, combined with a protrusive-retrusive adjustment screw, will permit full upward, downward, protrusive, or retrusive positioning of the condylar element to an accuracy of ⅛ mm.

A wide range of accessories and facebows is available.

Panadent Articulators

The molded fossa concept in articulators originated with Panadent. This was an outgrowth of research on condylar movement characteristics by Lee, Lundeen, and others. Their studies revealed the following:

1. The curvatures of all axis paths were similar.
2. The variability in the condylar paths in the vertical plane was in the angle, not the character.
3. The condylar paths in the horizontal plane on the orbiting side were also quite similar, except for the amount of shift in the first 3 mm of movement.

The molded fossa concept of articulators is based on these findings. A predetermined curvilinear superior guidance surface is combined with a medial guidance surface that varies the mount of precurrent shift in the first 2 or 3 mm of mediotrusive movement.

The Panadent System is composed of a series of five statistically determined three-dimensional analogs. The analog fossa feature curvilinear superior surfaces of approximately ½ inch radius. Each set varies slightly, being based on the average from the recordings of each side shift grouping. The five pairs have precurrent side shift of 0.5, 1.0, 1.5, 2.0, and 2.5 mm.

The Panadent Articulator System was introduced in 1978, and the current models introduced in 1983.

In addition to the molded fossa features, these articulators have a hinged centric latch mechanism that holds the two members together, permitting a 180 degree range of opening movement. The latch is easily disengaged to permit lateral movements. The articulators have dynalinks. These are elastic elements attached to the lateral aspects of the upper and lower frames that prevent separation of the two frames, maintain the orbiting condylar element against the superior and medial walls of the analogs during lateral excursive movements, and help return the condylar elements to centric relation afterwards.

The articulators use ¼ inch condylar elements instead of the usual ½ inch size. The elements are fixed at an intercondylar distance of 110 mm. There are three models: SL, PSL, and PCL. The latter two models are machined to 0.01 mm accuracy, which permits interchangeability of casts between different articulators. The SL and PSL have straight incisal guide pins, and the PCL has a curved incisal pin.

The system was designed to select the proper analog and to determine the horizontal condylar guide angle with an extraoral axis path recording device called the Quick Analyzer. Other systems have copied this principle: Denar Mini Recorder and TMJ Mandibular Movement Indicator. An accessory is available that permits analog selection with positional records (check-bites).

The Panadent System is designed to start with a basic setup and the capacity for gradually adding accessories for a complete system.

Stuart Articulator

The Stuart Gnathologic Computer was designed by Dr. C. E. Stuart. Individual guidances are selected and customized to permit curvilinear and/or rectilinear controls along border movements in all three planes from extraoral stereographic recordings. Stuart's teachings and writings have had a major influence on dental articulators.

TMJ Articulators

The TMJ approach to articulators was the design of Kenneth Swanson and was introduced in 1965. The guidances were originally composed of individually customized fossa that were made in autopolyzing acrylic resin from an intraoral horizontal envelope of motion resin tracing molds. The technique requires specific custom resin trays with horizontal recording platforms that fit over the teeth and arches. With the use of a central bearing pin and four studs, the rhomboid envelope of motion molds is generated in resin and then used to generate custom fossae on the articulator.

A mechanical fossa became available in 1970 that could be substituted for the custom fossa. The mechanical fossa allows condylar inclination adjustment from 10 to 55 degrees and a progressive side shift adjustment of 0 to 35 degrees. The superior surface of the fossa has a 3 degree slant, making the mediotrusive path steeper than the protrusive path by that amount.

A series of five premade fossa analogs is also available. These are made with curvilinear surfaces based on averages from an analysis of a large number of custom analogs by Drs. Swanson and Wipf. All the analog sets have a 0.5 mm precurrent side shift with a 7 degree progressive angle. Each set of analogs has a different angulation to the superior surface. The inclinations are 28, 35, 40, 45, and 50 degrees. Additional side shift is possible by offsetting the position of the condylar elements. However, any side shift by this method will be immediate.

There are two articulators, the original or deluxe model and the mini model. Features common to both are a hinge-locking device that permits an opening of 115 degrees, a spring-loaded centric centering lever, a fossa box that will accept all three types of guidance systems available, and plastic or mechanical incisal guide tables.

The deluxe model is larger, and the intercondylar distance is adjustable from 80 to 160 mm and has a curved incisal pin.

The minimodel is smaller and more compact. The intercondylar distance is adjustable from 110 to 150 mm, and the incisal pin is straight. There are a number of accessories, including the Mandibular Movement Recorder.

Whip Mix Articulators

The original Whip Mix articulator and Quick Mount Facebow were introduced in 1963. They were designed by Dr. Charles Stuart to serve as a simplified instrument system to aid in the teaching of occlusion, in occlusal diagnosis, treatment planning, and in the fabrication of uncomplicated prosthodontic restorations. Available articulators can be divided into three general groupings.

The original model is designated as the 8500. The

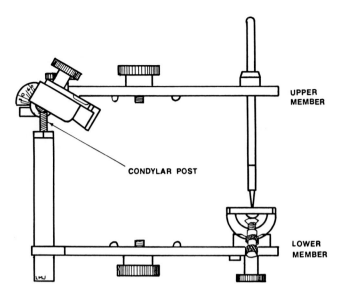

CONDYLAR POST

UPPER MEMBER

LOWER MEMBER

Fig. 16-3. Eccentric semiadjustable arcon articulator by Whip Mix (Whip Mix Corporation, Louisville, Ky.). Condylar sphere is attached to the lower member of the articulator, while the mechanical fossa is part of the upper member (similar to the anatomy of the human skull).

condylar elements on the lower frame are adjustable to three positions having intercondylar distances of 96 mm, 110 mm, and 124 mm. The condylar guides in the upper frame are kept aligned with the condylar elements by removable spacer washers. The condylar guides have rectilinear surfaces. The horizontal condylar inclination is adjustable from 0 to 70 degrees. The medial walls are adjustable from 0 to 45 degrees. The other models in this grouping have identical features except for frame height. The lower frame of model 9000 is ½ inch taller, which allows additional space to mount the mandibular cast. The model 8800 is redesigned to allow ½ inch additional space for mounting the maxillary cast. The model 9800 uses the lower frame from the 9000 and the upper frame from the 8800 to increase the interframe distance by 1 inch over the 8500. All of these models can be ordered with condylar locking screws, which prevent separation of the two frames and will permit a hinge opening up to 45 degrees. Models with this feature are designated 8500A, 8800A, 9000A, and 9800A.

The next grouping is the model 8300 and model 8340. The horizontal condylar guides are curvilinear with a ¾ inch radius, and the medial guide is rectilinear with a fixed progressive angle of 7½ degrees. The medial wall can also be adjusted for immediate side shift from 0 to 4 mm. There is a centric guide pin that can be activated with a thumb pressure that will accurately center the frames in centric position when the side shift guides are set with immediate shift. Condylar locking screws are a standard feature. The 8340 has the same features as the 8300, but has

the "accumount" mounting system on the lower frame. During manufacture, each 8340 model has a special table precisely attached to the lower frame to receive the lower mounting plate. This is done individually and is checked to make sure the tolerance is no greater than 0.001 inch. This assures that casts mounted on one 8340 model are interchangeable with other 8340 models without loss of accuracy.

The third group and newest additions to the Whip Mix line are model 2200 and model DB 2000. The frames are completely redesigned with curved surfaces, rounded edges, and a ¾ inch increased distance between the upper and lower frames. The new design provides for increased visibility and access to casts from the rear of the articulators. Bilateral elastics running from the posts on the lower frame to the lateral aspects of the condylar guides help return the condylar elements from excursive movements. There is a differently designed centric lock mechanism that is an improvement over the one for the 8300 series and 8500 series. The lock will allow for a 70 degree hinged opening and can be easily disengaged to allow for excursive movements or to separate the upper frame. All the other features are identical to those of the 8300. There is also a 2240 model that incorporates the "accumount" like the 8340 model.

The major difference in the DB 2200 model from the 2000 model relates to the side shift guide. The posterior wall of the condylar guide has been machined out somewhat to allow for an elongated medial wall side shift guide that has a curvilinear surface on the extension. There are two pairs of shims. One pair is 1 mm thick and the other pair is 2 mm thick. These can be inserted between the anterior wall of the condylar guide and medial guide anterior wall. Once inserted, the corresponding position of the curved side shift guide is brought into play. This will result in a precurrent medial shift in the first 1 or 2 mm of lateral movement. This feature mechanically creates the same type of guidance in the condylar guides that molded fossa analogs provide. This model also has a curved incisal pin (the only model in the Whip Mix series that does), and the medial guide wall is adjusted with allen screws and a hex screw instead of thumb screws. The side shift adjustments on the 2200 model are identical to those of the 8300 model.

The Quick Mount Facebow permits a convenient, quick, and surprisingly accurate method of using an average axis transfer to any of the Whip Mix articulators. Each articulator has a lug on the outer wall of the condylar guide for attaching the facebow to the articulator during the transfer procedure.

There is a Quick Set Recorder and True Axis Recorder for determining the axis path inclination and the amount of side shift.

Others

A variety of laboratory type instruments is available. The Dentalus is imported from Sweden, and its features are similar to the Hanau H-2. A Quick Perfect articulator that is available from France has a closed fossa guidance with many features similar to those of the Hanau H-2. A SAM articulator is available from Germany. It has a variety of features that are similar to USA models.

THE FACEBOW

A facebow record will record the location of the maxillary teeth and/or arch to predetermined points in the area of both condyles and a horizontal reference plane. The condylar points are assumed to be on the opening-closing axis of the mandible. These points may be located kinematically or estimated from landmarks or from an arbitrary point. The reference plane is created by the axis points and orbitale or some other landmark in the general area.

All movements of the teeth are the result of rotations around and slidings of the axes of the condyles. The more closely these distances are duplicated between casts and the condylar elements of the articulator, the less potential for articulator-produced errors of motion. A facebow record is used to transfer the relative distances from the patient to the articulator. If the location of the centers of rotation in relation to tooth (cusp) differs between the patient and the articulator very much, an error will exist as movement occurs. The differences can affect cusp placement, ridge or groove direction, and other features of the occlusal elements.

A facebow record is not needed to develop an accurate IP in a restoration, provided the restoration is fabricated at the same vertical dimension of occlusion used to mount the working casts. Casts mounted on a small hinge-type articulator will produce a distinct difference in the lateral excursive paths of the casts and those of the teeth. However, these errors may not be significant or come into play when fabricating single restorations for premolars, and perhaps first molars, on dentitions that have excellent canine (incisor) guidance. Consider a vertical overlap of 3 to 5 mm to be excellent.

A facebow record is recommended when fabricating 1) single or multiple posterior restorations where an open anterior bite or end to end anterior relationship exists, 2) single restorations on second molars, 3) segment restorations, (4) anterior restorations that will function as the prime guidance factor in an excursive movement, and 5) restorations involving an entire quadrant or arch.

There are two forms of facebows, the kinematic and estimated (sometimes called arbitrary). The estimated facebows come in two types—the ear bow and facia bow.

Hanau makes two types of earbows, the 164-2 twirl bow and the 153. They also offer two facia bows, the 132-25M and 132-2C. The C type does not have a third reference pointer.

Denar offers a facebow that can be used as an earbow or facia bow. They also make a "slidematic" earbow that comes with a transfer jig that permits cast mounting to the articulator without the need to use the facebow frame. This feature permits multiple mounting with only one facebow frame. There is also a kinematic facebow that comes with the D5A articulator pantograph setup.

The Panadent facebow was designed to be used as an earbow, but accessory arms are available to make it usable with a facia estimated or kinematic axis. Its design is similar to the Whip Mix, from which it was probably copied. The nasion relator has a thumb-locking screw which is an improvement over the Whip Mix. An infraorbital pointer is also available as an accessory. A transfer mounting accessory is available and is similar to the one with the Denar Slidematic that permits multiple mountings with one frame.

The TMJ Company makes only one facebow. It is of the kinematic type, but it can be used with an estimated axis. This facebow is probably the best kinematic type available to the profession.

The Whip Mix Quick Mount bow was the original earbow. It comes in two models; one is constructed entirely of metal and the other has arms of injection molded resin. A special Nasion Relator Assembly accessory has recently become available that locks to the facebow frame. An infraorbital pointer may also be added to the facebow. For routine fixed prosthodontics, the earbows by Panadent and Whip Mix are recommended.

Condylar Guidances

A majority of available articulators have some form of adjustable condylar guidances. The horizontal condylar inclination affects the angulation of cuspal inclines on posterior teeth. If the condylar inclination on an articulator is set at an angle steeper than that which exists on a patient, the finished restoration may have surfaces that will interfere during excursive movements. If the articulator has inclines less steep than the patient's, the finished restoration will have more clearance during excursive movements than planned. An error of this nature has no effect clinically when disclusion exists. The error may have clinical significance when group function or balanced articulation is desired. A flat superior surface will most likely still produce a negative error even when the inclination is correct, since nearly all condylar pathways are convex. A convex surface will initially cause a more rapid condylar descent than a flat surface, with the same inclination until the point of angle determination is reached. A curvilinear guidance path has the potential for less error than a flat path.

Most lateral movements have some degree of side shift to the movement. The medial condylar guidance on the articulator allows for a lateral shift to the rotating condylar element and a medial shift to the orbiting condylar element. If the guide surface is flat, little error occurs on the working side. However, a significant error occurs on the balancing side, certainly in the first 2 or 3 mm of movement. If the guide surface is flat and is adjustable for immediate side shift, an error of a different type is created. The orbiting condylar element will move straight medially before advancing or descending. This makes it impossible to create a precise intercuspal position because the mechanics of the guidance will cause a centric position as wide as the immediate shift settings. Ideally, the side shift control on the articulator should be concave in the horizontal plane and convex in the vertical plane.

Articulator condylar guides can be arbitrarily set by means of positional records (check bites) and with the use of axis path recordings (Denar Mini-Graph, Panadent Quick Analyzer, TMJ Mandibular Movement Indicator, Whip Mix True Axis Recorder, and Quickset Recorder). The axis path recorders were designed to be used to select and align the molded analog fossae.

Condyle Path Movement Characteristics

Recent research has shown that mandibular axis movement patterns have the following characteristics:

1. The center of motion for each condyle is located 55 mm (± 5 mm) from the median plane. The concept of fixed condylar elements with an intercondylar distance of 110 mm now has supportive data.
2. The curvature of all condylar axis pathways on protrusion and mediotrusion have similar curvature. The curvature has a radius of ½ to ¾ inch.
3. The pitch of the curvature of the axis path varies from about 25 to 75 degrees. The average protrusive path is about 40 degrees, and the mediotrusive path is about 45 degrees.
4. Immediate side shift is rarely present. The few that show an immediate shift may be an artifact resulting from starting the recording without the condyle-disc assembly being completely seated.
5. Most lateral movements have a lateral shift (Bennett movement) incorporated into the pathway. The shift on the rotating side is primarily straight lateral. The shift on the mediotrusive side is pre-

current; all the shift is curvilinear and occurs in the initial 2 to 3 mm of movement. The remainder of the mediotrusive path is progressive. Extraoral axis recordings result in a progressive angle of about 7 degrees. Computer projections of center of motion paths within the condyle result in a progressive path of about 12 degrees.

6. The amount of lateral shift ranges from a fraction up to 4 mm. The average is about 0.75 mm with 80 percent of the recording showing 1.5 mm or less.

Articulator Selection

Articulators do not duplicate condylar movement patterns. The condylar elements of articulators function as cams to simulate border tooth movements in the first 3 to 5 mm of motion.

One need not use too complex an instrument for a simple procedure and should not use too simple an instrument for a complex procedure. An articulator will perform no better than its design features or the precision of the adjustment settings. The articulator must be within the understanding and capabilities of the user.

An articulator that can be adjusted to a stereographic recording (pantograph) is no panacea. It still only simulates movements along border pathways. Preciseness and extent of duplication is the best of all instruments available. Articulators are excellent teaching devices in advanced prosthodontic training programs. They may have an advantage in situations of complete reconstruction of at least one arch in combination with one or more of the following factors: 1) flat or no anterior guidance, 2) more than 1.5 mm of side shift, 3) condylar guide angle less than 30 degrees, and 4) restoring lost vertical dimension.

A nonadjustable articulator is acceptable for most single restorations. A simple hinge instrument can even be used in some selected cases.

When larger parts of the segments are involved with multiple restorations and/or fixed partical dentures, an adjustable articulator is preferred. Use of a facebow is recommended. The condylar guidances should be set with positional records or determined by axis recorders. Using the average values of 40 degrees horizontal condylar inclination and 1 mm of side shift may be suitable for selective situations.

Recent models with molded fossae are the best all-round articulators. The next best are those with immediate side shift mechanical adjustments. The Whip Mix DB2000 may prove to be superior in this grouping, since it has precurrent capabilities. It has not been available long enough for its use to be recommended. Articulators with immediate side shift capabilities need precise and convenient centering devices. The instruments having only adjustable progressive side shift capabilities are next and those with fixed controls are least desirable.

The curved superior surfaces are more anatomically correct, but are not necessary unless balanced articulation is desired in part or all of the excursive movements. Fixed condylar elements at 110 mm are quite satisfactory. The only plus for intercondylar distance adjustments of the condylar elements is to simplify the setting of the condylar guidance using positional records. For fixed prosthodontics, open fossa design is very convenient for waxing and porcelain stacking. The closed fossa design may have an advantage when fabricating complete dentures. The final decision between open and closed fossa is more of a personal preference for restoration fabrications if all other features are similar. The open fossa design is preferred as a diagnostic instrument in diagnosing joint-tooth disharmonies.

BIBLIOGRAPHY

Anthony, L.P.: The American Text Book of Prosthetic Dentistry, ed. 7, Philadelphia, 1942, Lea & Febiger, p. 233.

Beck, H.O.: A clinical evaluation of the arcon articulator, J. Prosthet. Dent. 6:359, 1956.

Beck, H.O.: A clinical evaluation of the arcon concept of articulation, J. Prosthet. Dent. 9:409, 1959.

Beck, H.O.: Choosing the articulator, J.A.D.A. 64:468, 1962.

Bell, L.J., and Matich, J.A.: Study of acceptability of lateral records by the whip-mix articulator, J. Prosth. Dent. 38:22, 1977.

Bellanti, N.D.: The significance of articulator capabilities, J. Prosth. Dent. 29:269, 1973.

Boucher, C.O.: Methods of recording functional movements of full denture bases in three dimensions, J. Dent. Res. 14:39, 1934.

Boucher, L.J., et al.: Occlusal articulator, Dent. Clin. North Am. 23:155, 1979.

Gillis, R.R.: Articulator development and the importance of observing the condyle paths in full denture prosthesis, J.A.D.A. 13:3, 1926.

Granger, E.A.: The function of the rotating condyle path of the aderer simulator, Long Island City, N.Y., J. Anderer, Inc.

Heartwell, Charles M., Jr., and Rahn, Arthur O.: Syllabus of Complete Dentures, ed. 4, Philadelphia, 1986, Lea & Febiger, p. 51.

Hickey, J.C., Lundeen, H.C., and Bohannon, H.M.: A new articulator for use in teaching and general dentistry, J. Prosth. Dent. 18:435, 1967.

Hobo, S.: Kinematic investigation of mandibular border movement by means of electronic measuring system, II. Rotational center of lateral movement, J. Prosthet. Dent. 52:66, 1984.

Hobo, S., Shillingbur, H.T., and Whitsett, L.D.: Articulator selection for restorative dentistry, J. Prosthet. Dent. 36:35, 1976.

International Prosthodontic Workshop on Complete Denture Occlusion, Ann Arbor, The University of Michigan, p. 100, 1973.

Lee, Robert L.: Jaw movements engraved in solid plastic for articulator controls, I. Recording apparatus, J. Prosthet. Dent. 22:209, 1969.

Lee, Robert L.: Jaw movements engraved in solid plastic for articulator controls, II. Transfer apparatus, J. Prosthet. Dent. 22:513, 1969.

Lundeen, Harry C., and Wirth, Carl G.: Condylar movement patterns engraved in plastic blocks, J. Prosthet. Dent. 30:866, 1973.

Lundeen, Harry C., Shyrock, Edwin F., and Gibbs, Charles H.: An evaluation of mandibular border movements: their character and significance, J. Prosthet. Dent. 40:422, 1978.

Lundeen, Harry C.: Mandibular movement recordings and articulator adjustments simplified, Dent. Clin. North Am. 23(2):231, 1979.

Lundeen, Harry C., and Gibbs, Charles H.: Advances in Occlusion, Boston, 1982, John Wright PSG Inc.

McCoy, Richard B., and Shyrock, Edwin F.: A method of transferring mandibular movement data to computer storage, J. Prosthet. Dent. 36:510, 1976.

Messerman, T.: A means of studying mandibular movements, J. Prosth. Dent. 17:36, 1956.

Messerman, T., et al.: Investigation of functional mandibular movements, Dent. Clin. North Am. 13:629, 1969.

Mitchell, D.L., and Wilkie, N.D.: Articulator through the years. II. J. Prosthet. Dent. 39:451, 1978.

Mohamed, S.E., Schmidt, J.F., and Harrison, J.D.: Articulators in dental education and practice, J. Prosthet. Dent. 36:319, 1976.

Posselt, U.: Physiology of Occlusion, ed. 2, Oxford, 1968, Blackwell Scientific Publishing, p. 108.

Rilanti, Awni: Classification of articulators, J. Prosthet. Dent. 43-344, 1980.

Rosenblatt, J.: Discussion of "A means of studying mandibular movements," J. Prosthet. Dent. 17-44, 1967.

Sharry, J.J.: Complete Denture Prosthodontics, ed. 3, New York, 1974, McGraw-Hill Book Co., p. 224.

Tanaka, H., and Beu, R.A.: A new semi-adjustable articulator. I. Concept behind the new articulator, J. Prosthet. Dent. 33:10, 1975.

Tanaka, H., and Finger, J.M.: A new semi-adjustable articulator. IV. J. Prosthet. Dent. 40:288, 1978.

Villa, A.H.: Requirements of articulators for protrusive movements, J. Prosth. Dent. 9:409, 1959.

Weinberg, L.A.: An evaluation of basic articulators and their concepts, II. J. Prosthet. Dent. 13:645, 1963.

Weinberg, L.A.: An evaluation of articulators and their concepts. III. J. Prosthet. Dent. 13:873, 1963.

Weinberg, L.A.: The transverse hinge axis: real or imaginary, J. Prosthet. Dent. 9:775, 1959.

Weinberg, L.A.: An evaluation of the face-bow mounting, J. Prosthet. Dent. 11:32, 1961.

Weinberg, L.A.: An evaluation of basic articulators and their concepts. II. Arbitrary, positional, semiadjustable articulators, J. Prosthet. Dent. 24:645, 1963.

Weinberg, L.A.: Arcon principle in the condylar mechanism of adjustable articulators, J. Prosthet. Dent. 13:263, 1963.

Winkler, Sheldon: Complete Denture Prosthodontics, Philadelphia, 1979, W.B. Saunders Co., Chapter 11.

17

Gordon J. Christensen

CEMENTS, LINERS, AND BASES IN FIXED PROSTHODONTICS

For over 150 years, cements resembling those currently in use have been available in dentistry. Weston's insoluble cement was introduced in approximatley 1880[1], and the Ostermann formula of 1832[2] was the forerunner of zinc phosphate cement. Weston's cement contained about 81 percent zinc oxide, 19 percent aluminum silicate, and, as today, included phosphoric acid. Since the introduction of the zinc phosphate cement, significant scientific and technologic advances have been accomplished in all areas of endeavor, but is is *inconceivable* that dental cements have remained relatively unchanged. Nevertheless, there have been specific advancements in dental cements recently verified by longitudinal clinical studies.

Today there are five major categories of dental cements for luting ceramic or cast restorations. They are: 1) zinc phosphate, 2) zinc polycarboxylate, 3) glass ionomer, 4) zinc oxide-eugenol, and 5) resin. Three cements contain zinc oxide as one ingredient; glass ionomer and resin cements are significantly different.

The retention of restorations has been achieved primarily by mechanical interlocking of the cement into irregularities on the internal surfaces of the fabricated restorations and the tooth preparation. Polycarboxylate and glass ionomer cements adhere directly to calcified tissues by chemical attraction to calcium ions in addition to mechanical interlocking. The introduction of polycarboxylate cements marked the first distinct improvement in the attaching mechanism of cements to teeth. True adhesion is desirable because of the potential to reduce microleakage between the tooth and the restoration.

Polycarboxylate cement is currently used about as often as zinc phosphate cements, while glass ionomers are used somewhat less.[3] Resin cements are in an embryonic state, but enjoying increased useage for porcelain veneers and inlays. The frequency of specific cement usage by dentists is an indication of their popularity and perceived value. Polycarboxylate cements have achieved significant popularity, while glass ionomers have exhibited appreciable growth in the past five years. Despite this popularity, dentists have also expressed concern about these cements.

There are genuine, unfilled needs in the area of dental cements. Dentists have made exhaustive efforts to construct well-fitting cast and porcelain restorations to lessen the cement line exposed to oral fluids. However, dentists realize that a perfect seal of a cemented restoration to enamel is impossible, and they achieve only biocompatibility, not perfection, at the margins. Tooth preparations are designed to possess nearly parallel walls to lessen dislodgment, but dentists are actually unaware of the exact magnitude of retention needed. Stronger, more adhesive, and less soluble cements could partially alleviate the quest for nearly perfect margins and parallel preparations. Meanwhile, dentistry is faced with five less than perfect cements.

Bases, or "build-ups", for compromised teeth prior to artificial crowns have become popular over the past 10 years. Before that time, placement of a crown over whatever remained of the tooth was common. Formerly, cast pins on the restoration assisted in retention of the crown. Currently, dentists replace most or all of the missing dental tooth structure with composite, amalgam, glass ionomer cement, and/or a casting. The first three materials may be retained to the remaining tooth structure with nickel-chrome or titanium pins of various sizes, slot preparation, or both. (See Chapter Caries Management)

Liners are placed in deep tooth defects close to the dental pulp before the reconstructive materials are added. These liners accomplish various goals: 1) stimulation of the dental pulp to form more "internal" dentin, 2) insulation of the pulp from thermal changes, and 3) seal of the dental canals and dental pulp from dental materials.

This chapter briefly discusses the physical characteristics of cements, bases, and liners as they relate to clinical applications, and emphasizes their daily use in fixed prosthodontics.

PROPERTIES OF CEMENTS
Zinc Phosphate (Fig. 17-1)

The major advantage of zinc phosphate cement is the prolonged success rate. Dentists have become accustomed to its predictable characteristics in clinical circumstances. These expectations are documented scientifically and empirically,[4,5] and have guided the development of various concepts about tooth preparations, length of F.P.D.s, margin placement, and other factors in fixed prosthodontics.

Zinc phosphate cements contain zinc oxide and magnesium oxide in the approximate ratio of 9 to 1.[6] The water content is about 33 percent. The liquid is approximately 50 percent phosphoric acid buffered by aluminum, with traces of zinc salts. When set, the cement can be described as particles sustained by phosphates. It is commonly believed that the more powder and the less phosphate present in a given mix of zinc phosphate cement, the stronger the set cement will be.[7]

With experience, zinc phosphate cement is relatively easy to manipulate. The assistant cools a thick glass slab and incorporates small increments of powder into the cement liquid by mixing powder and liquid together with a wide circular motion on about one-half of the glass slab. When the mixture follows the spatula about ½ to ¾ inch from the glass slab, it is ready for use as a luting medium (Fig. 17-2).

Two undesirable characteristics are generally attributed to zinc-phosphate cement, pulp irritation and solubility. While adverse effects on the dental pulp have been observed,[8] investigations[9] have indicated that the irritation may be caused by a "residual film of grinding debris containing bacteria and/or a poor seal between the cement filling and the dentin, resulting in leakage of bacteria from the oral cavity into a space between the cement and the cavity walls." This study further stated that "zinc phosphate cement per se does not irritate the pulp." Dentists and patients have observed the immediate pain associated with the cementation of restorations with zinc phosphate cement without anesthesia. However, the true, long-term clinical significance of alleged pulpal irritation is not well documented. Zinc phosphate has been in use for over 100 years, so logic indicates that

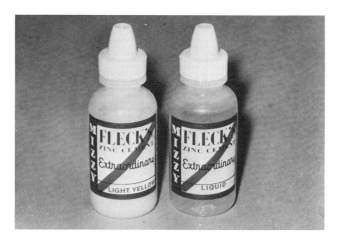

Fig. 17-1. Zinc phosphate cement and its characteristics are well known to dentists and dental assistants. This cement is mixed slowly on a cool glass slab for optimal incorporation of powder and liquid.

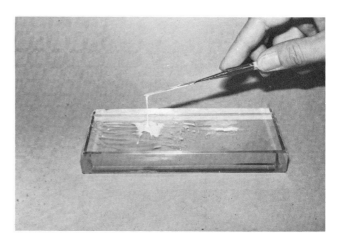

Fig. 17-2. Optimal thickness of zinc phosphate cement has been used as a guide when mixing certain other cements. Typical ½- to ¾-inch string of cement following spatula is shown.

dentists do not observe the routine death of dental pulps or they would discontinue its use. Elimination of pain on cementation and unpredictable long-term pulpal damage after cementation would be welcomed by the profession. Solubility has also been claimed to be a problem with zinc phosphate cement.[10] Certainly an insoluble cement in mouth fluids is desirable, but other dental cements also have poor solubility characteristics. Zinc phosphate is not considered cariostatic; however, certain forms of the cement have added fluoride compounds.

Why does zinc phosphate cement enjoy continued usage? One reason is its compressive strength, which ranges from 9,000 to 20,000 p.s.i., with an average value of about 13,000 p.s.i.[11] This wide variation in strength is related to the quantity of powder added to the liquid. Tensile strength of about 720 p.s.i. is an

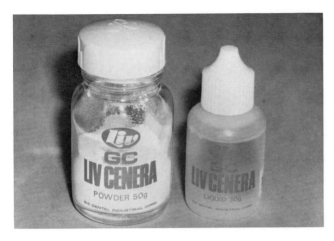

Fig. 17-3. One example of polycarboxylate cements is shown. The preference of one brand is usually personal.

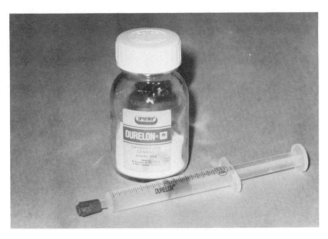

Fig. 17-4. Dentists using polycarboxylate cement have had a problem with the relatively uncontrolled thickness of mixed cement. This liquid-dispensing device introduced by manufacturers of Durelon has allowed easier proportioning of powder and liquid.

even more impressive characteristic.[12] However, there is sparse evidence about needed strength. Gibson and Myers[13] have stated that a compressive strength of 8,000 p.s.i. is suitable for retention of cast restorations, but each dentist designs tooth preparations differently. There are many acceptable preparations with different retentive characteristics. Zinc phosphate cement has survived despite its described weaknesses. Because of its acknowledged effectiveness, newer cements are usually compared to it. This chapter contains comparisons of zinc phosphate with other cements.

Zinc Polycarboxylate (Fig. 17-3)

Polycarboxylate cement has become increasingly popular since its introduction in 1968.[14] Continued use and acceptance of polycarboxylate cement is evidence

of its application. Ample evidence about specific characteristics is available.[15,16] The compressive strength is at least one-half that of zinc phosphate cement, whereas the tensile strength is similar to zinc phosphate cement. Solubility of carboxylate cements is about the same as zinc phosphate, but neither is ideal. The film thickness of the polycarboxylate cements when mixed appropriately is approximately ±20 um, and comparable to zinc phosphate.

This cement has two advantages over zinc phosphate. First, the cement has been demonstrated to be nonirritating to the dental pulp histologically.[17,18] Dentists have also acclaimed the bland nature of the cement clinically. Although the pH of polycarboxylate is similar to that of zinc phosphate cement at the time of cementation,[15] the cement does <u>not</u> initiate pain during cementation without anesthesia. Second, this cement bonds to tooth structure. Although the actual adhesion of carboxylates to enamel, and in a lesser way to dentin, has been demonstrated,[14,19] the clinical significance of this bonding has not been established. The forces required to remove inlays cemented with carboxylates are no greater than the forces required for zinc phosphate cement; however, the nature of the breaking of the cement seal is different. Polycarboxylate cement commonly adheres to the tooth, and the fracture occurs most commonly at the cement-metal junction or within the cement itself. The retention of restorations is <u>not</u> superior to zinc phosphate, but comparable.

Cleaning the surfaces of metal with an airborne abrasive increases the adhesion of polycarboxylate cement to the metal.[20] This appears to have clinical significance when using this cement.

Some dentists have objected to the thick "rubber-like" nature of polycarboxylates when mixed to the manufacturer's specifications. Further, the viscosity of polycarboxylate liquids increases with time, so it is difficult to determine the thickness of the mix attributed to additional powder. Measuring devices have assisted in controlling the thickness of the mix (Fig. 17-4). Mixes that are too thick or thin are thus avoided. A desirable mix of polycarboxylate cement should resemble the previously described and established mix of zinc phosphate cements. The cement should follow the cement spatula about ½ to ¾ inch when the spatula is rapidly moved upward. However, incorporating the powder and liquid slowly and on a glass slab is unnecessary, since the reaction deviates from the zinc phosphate reaction. The working time with the cements is short–2 to 3 minutes. Therefore, polycarboxylate cement for long-span F.P.D.s requires that the dentist and dental assistant be coordinated and efficient.

Polycarboxylate cement has been well accepted,

and when carefully manipulated has the described advantages. Specific uses are described later.

Glass Ionomer (Fig. 17-5)

Glass ionomer cements combine glass particles and polyacrylic or polymaleic acid. Glass ionomer cements have been used increasingly in the past several years, but acceptance has been accompanied by disagreement. These cements have had a slow but growing acceptance since their introduction.[21] Reasons for slow acceptance have been postoperative sensitivity[22] and difficult manipulation characteristics because of high initial solubility.

Glass ionomer cements have a versatile profile and are capable of placement for bases or liners, as a luting agent, or as a restorative material. They are adhesive dental materials that bond to enamel and dentin, while releasing fluoride.

Glass ionomer restorations are recommended for Class V caries and erosion, or Class III lesions that are invisible. The longer the time lapse between preparation and exposure of most glass ionomers to moisture, the higher the (strength) hardness. Varnishes are indicated to protect the margins, but are cement-specific.

In vivo disintegration investigations and other tests have demonstrated that glass ionomer cements are comparable to traditional luting agents, with the added advantage of fluoride release.[23-26] Godoy et al. in Chapter 21 discusses in detail the imaginative aspects of glass iomer, including etching the material and veneering with a microfilled resin. The tensile strength of glass ionomer is relatively low, so crown reconstruction with glass ionomer must be selective.

To reduce the incidence of belated sensitivity with glass ionomer cements, the following procedures are suggested: 1) rapid incorporation of powder and liquid (10-20 seconds) on a sealed surface paper pad until a mix is achieved that strings ½ inch from the mixing pad; 2) slight hydration of the tooth before cementation by placing a drop of water on the tooth during mixing, this is gently blown off just before placing the prosthesis on the tooth; 3) allowing the cement to set hard to the touch, plus 1 minute before removing the excess; and 4) placing glass ionomer cement varnish on the margins of the restoration after removing the excess cement.

Glass ionomers have been constantly improved since their introduction, and their desirable characteristics will encourage continual and increased useage.

Zinc Oxide Eugenol (Fig. 17-6)

Zinc oxide cements do <u>not</u> irritate the pulp, but possess limited strength; there has been a concerted

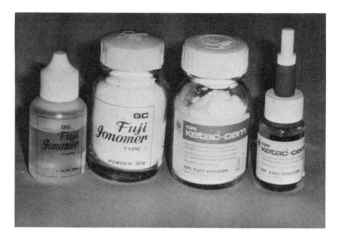

Fig. 17-5. Two widely used brands of glass ionomer cement.

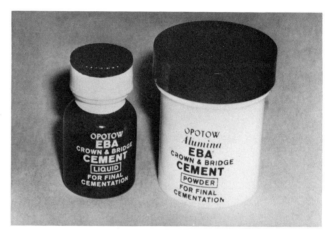

Fig. 17-6. Various brands of reinforced zinc oxide-eugenol cements are available. They offer modernate strength lack of pulpal irritation without water contamination.

effort to reinforce the formula to qualify as final cements. Polymers have been added,[13] and ortho ethoxybenzoic acid (EBA), quartz, and alumina[27] have also been substituted in the mix. The result has been that the strength of these cements[12] is now acceptable for specific cementations. The compressive strength of the reinforced zinc oxide eugenol cements is approximately one-half that of zinc phosphate, whereas the tensile strength is nearly identical to zinc phosphate. The values are similar to the averages for polycarboxylate cements.

The solubility of the reinforced zinc oxide eugenol cements has been reported within the range of zinc phosphate cement[12]; however, continual leakage of eugenol from the cements has been questioned.[28]

Two advantages of reinforced zinc oxide eugenol cements for final cementation are: 1) the palliative effect on the dental pulp and 2) ease of placement in a moist environment. Nevertheless, moisture accelerates the set, and these cements appear to possess no other advantages. Although these cements are not widely used for final cementation, some dentists prefer them routinely as interim luting agents.

Resin (Fig. 17-7)

Many restorations are now cement bonded onto etched enamel surfaces with resin cement. Additionally, the popularity of composite resin use in Class 2 tooth preparations has forced dentists to refine bases and liners to prevent pulpal irritation previously produced by resins placed on dentin surfaces. These clinical techniques have been incorporated into the cementing process for some types of restorations. Current restorations in which resin cement is commonly used are porcelain veneers, porcelain inlays and onlays, resin bonded prostheses, and post and core reinforcements. Most of these cements are thinned versions of composite resins or microfill restorative materials. However, announcements by manufacturers about the availability of "nonpulpal irritating" cements are in the process of being validated, and time is required for proof of this claim.

Porcelain veneers and resin retained prostheses are bonded over acid-etched enamel surfaces without concern for pulp irritation,[30] nor is there concern about pulpal irritation in post and core cementation. However, cementation of porcelain inlays or onlays is accomplished over dentin surfaces. Calcium hydroxide is usually placed over the deepest dentinal penetration and is followed by a thin (0.5 mm) layer of etched glass ionomer liner, described later.

Resin cement possesses some unique characteristics and is insoluble in oral fluids. It also has strength properties that exceed those of other cements in all areas and is relatively easy to use.

However, resin cement does <u>not</u> bond to tooth structure, is not cariostatic, and leaks at dentinal margins. When porcelain inlays are cemented over glass ionomer liners, postoperative tooth sensitivity is occasionally reported. Lack of thorough removal of excess cement leads to serious periodontal problems. Film thickness of resin cements is usually greater than ADA standards, but the significance is questionable since the cement is insoluble.

Use of resin cements will increase as these cements continue to develope improved pulpal tolerance properties, less water sorption, lower expansion and contraction, and molecular attachment to tooth structure.

Other Cements

Numerous other cements have been used over the years, but few have remained popular. Red and black copper cements are examples. These cements were commonly used in the past, primarily because of the

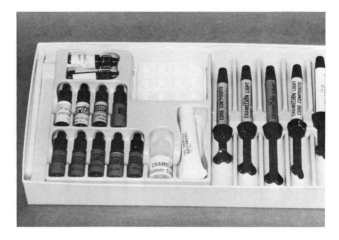

Fig. 17-7. Composite resin cement is extremely strong but irritates the pulp. It is used predominately for porcelain veneer and porcelain inlay cementation.

antibacterial nature of their constituents. However, they have been shown to be excessively irritating to the pulp.

Certain types of zinc phosphate cement that are mixed by adding water have been developed, but these cements are generally weaker and more soluble than conventional cements.[31]

Cyanoacrylate cements have been developed and used to a limited degree, and some reports have been optimistic about retention.[32,33] However, the A.D.A. Council on Dental Materials and Devices has stated that, "the Council believes that cyanoacrylates, on the basis of current knowledge, cannot be recommended for routine use in dentistry."[34] Dentists should monitor the research literature on these cements.

Silicophosphate cement combined the properties of zinc phosphate and silicate cements. It was more translucent than zinc phosphate and cariostatic; however, its popularity has declined steadily, and the current generation of cariostatic glass ionomer cements has replaced it.

CLINICAL APPLICATIONS FOR CEMENTS

Each dentist must decide which cement to use based on available research, clinical application, and specific patient needs. Table 17-1 summarizes the information presented in this chapter.

CATEGORIES OF CEMENTS FOR APPRAISAL

An analysis of Table 17-1 clearly demonstrates that none of the cements is superior in all categories. Therefore, each cement is based on the patient's needs in specific instances. Suggestions for choice of cement follow. These recommendations are based on available research and clinical experience.

Table 17-1. Comparison of popular dental cements

	Glass ionomer	Polycarboxylate	Resin	Zinc oxide eugenol-EBA	Zinc phosphate
Compressive strength	Good-excellent	Fair-good	Excellent	Fair-good	Good
Tensile strength	Poor*	Poor*	Fair*	Poor*	Poor*
Modulus of elasticity (rigidity)	Good	Good	Excellent	Fair	Good
Film thickness	Good	Good	Poor	Good	Good
Solubility (early)	High (extremely soluble)	Low	None	Very low	Moderate
Solubility (when set)	Very low	Low	None	Low-moderate	Low
Flow	Excellent	Fair-good	Poor-fair	Good	Good
Pulp reaction	None (if used properly)	None	Extreme	None	Moderate
Setting time	Fast	Moderate	Variable	Moderate	Slow
Ease of use	Fair (critical mixing)	Good	Good	Fair (messy)	Good
Color (matches tooth)	Fair	Fair	Excellent (tooth colors)	Poor (white)	Good (multiple colors)
Current clinical use	Moderate	Moderate	Low, but increasing	Very low	Moderate
Main advantages	Carlostatic High flow	Low pulp reaction	Matches tooth color	Can be used in moist field	Historical perspective positive
Main disadvantages	Occasional tooth sensitivity	Thixotropic*	Pulp irritation- High film	Solubility	Pulp irritation Slow setting time

Christensen G.J., Christensen R.; Clin. Res. Assoc. Newsletter, (10):3, 1986.
*William F.P. Malone.

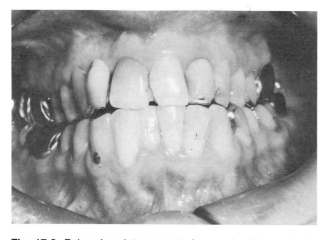

Fig. 17-8. Polycarboxylate cements have gained in popularity over the past few years. Research has supported the use of polycarboxylate cement. The dentist may confidently use polycarboxylate cement for routine single-unit restorations or short-span FPDs.

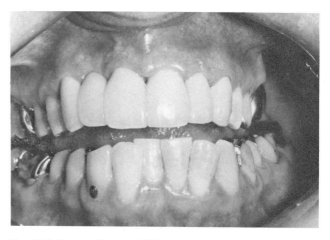

Fig. 17-9. Two- or three-unit FPD shown. Zinc phosphate or glass ionomer are also acceptable.

Retentive Small Single-tooth Castings or Three-unit FPDs (Figs. 17-8 and 17-9)

Polycarboxylate cement is recommended for routine clinical use. Its minimal pulpal irritation, lack of postoperative sensitivity, and moderate strength render it acceptable for these situations. Fresh cement batches and disciplined mixing are mandatory. Zinc phosphate, glass ionomer, or reinforced zinc oxide eugenol are also indicated for routine cementation.

Long-span FPDs (Figs. 17-10 to 17-12)

Polycarboxylate cements have extremely short working times, which makes the seating of long-span FPDs difficult. Further, polycarboxylate and reinforced zinc oxide eugenol have slightly less strength than zinc phosphate. Therefore, zinc phosphate or glass ionomer are recommended for long-span FPDs. Glass ionomer also requires a rapid procedure because of a short working time.

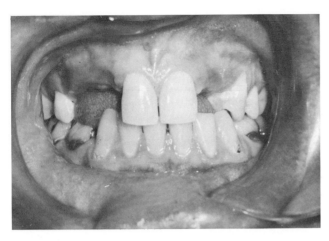

Fig. 17-10. Zinc phosphate cement provides a long historical perspective to observe failure and success. Because it has more compressive and tensile strength than does polycarboxylate or reinforced zinc oxide eugenol cement, it is one of the cements of choice for long-span FPD or those that the dentist has concern about retention. Glass ionomer is also useful in long term if it is mixed properly with moisture control.

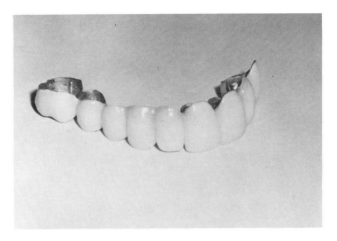

Fig. 17-11. Long span prosthesis with auxillary grooves.

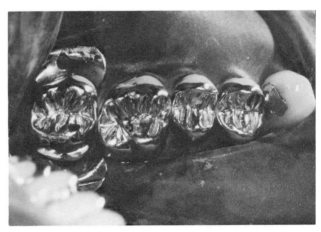

Fig. 17-13. Certain patients have sensitive teeth, and it is difficult to anesthetize them adequately during treatment. Such teeth are better treated with cements that do not irritate dental pulp. Reinforced zinc oxide eugenol or ortho ethoxybenzoic acid (EBA) cements are excellent choices for these patients. Patient shown had sensitive teeth during treatment. However, teeth were not sensitive after restorations were placed with EBA cement.

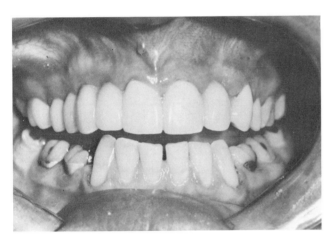

Fig. 17-12. FPD in place.

Sensitive Teeth Receiving Cast Restorations
(Fig. 17-13)

Reinforced zinc oxide eugenol or polycarboxylate should be used. The bland nature of these cements is well known clinically and documented in the research literature.

Cast Restorations in Extremely Caries-Active Patients (Figs. 17-14 and 17-15)

The fluoride content of glass ionomer cement makes it desirable for caries-active patients. Postoperative sensitivity has been a problem; close attention to the points described under glass ionomers in this chapter is recommended.

Porcelain Veneers or Porcelain Inlays
(Figs. 17-16 to 17-19)

Resin cements are excellent for these restorations because of their high strength, impregnation into etched enamel areas, and color-matching capabilities. Appropriate bases or liners are used when dentin is exposed.

Porcelain Jacket Crowns or Cast Glass Crowns
(Dicor) (Figs. 17-20 and 17-21)

Zinc phosphate or resin which is nonirritating to the pulp is the cement of choice because of the various

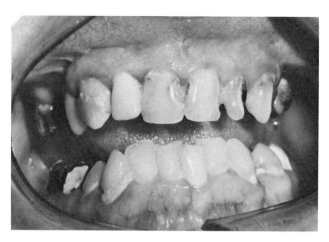

Fig. 17-14. Some mouths have a high caries rate despite attempts to decrease this activity. Cementation of cast restorations in such mouths with a cement containing fluorides may decrease the possibility of recurrent caries around margins.

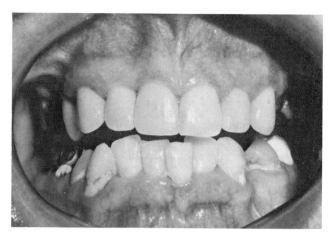

Fig. 17-15. Crowns were cemented with glass ionomer.

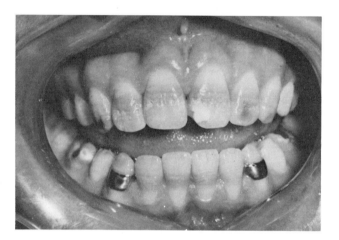

Fig. 17-16. Tetracycline stains of adolescent.

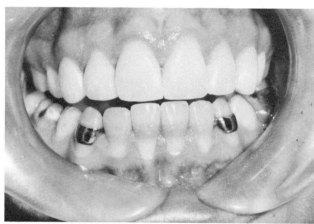

Fig. 17-17. Porcelain veneers in service for 1 year cemented with resin cement over acid etched enamel.

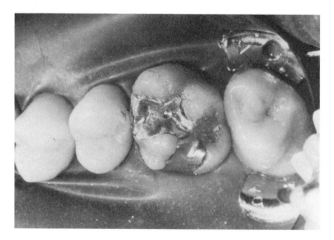

Fig. 17-18. Fractured amalgam on maxillary 1st molar.

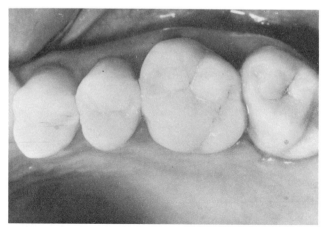

Fig. 17-19. A porcelain inlay cemented over a glass ionomer liner (0.5 mm thick) with resin cement.

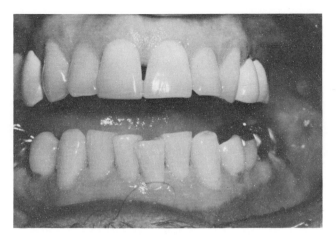

Fig. 17-20. Prerestorative view.

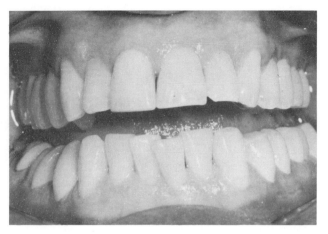

Fig. 17-21. Mouth rehabilitation with DICOR crowns (Dentsply) cemented with zinc phosphate cement. Glass ionomer would be desirable also.

colors and the strength. However, new cements are being developed to provide nonirritating resins in various colors.

Post and Core Cementation

All cements described are used *currently* for post and core cementation. However, a logical choice is glass ionomer, which provides high strength, cariostatic activity, and high flow for ease of post cementation. Thinned resins now available are also excellent if a thicker film thickness is not a liability. Resin cement provides immediate strength and contiguous bond with a subsequent resin core placement.

Continually Dislodged Castings

Occasionally, cast restorations have served for years and become loose, but are still serviceable. In such cases, an extremely strong cement is required. Resin cement may be used with pulp protection over deep dentinal areas. However, glass ionomer is the cement of choice if high caries activity is present.

Castings Cemented in a Wet Field

Reinforced ZOE is the cement of choice because of its lack of sensitivity to moisture.

LINERS IN FIXED PROSTHODONTICS

Liners are used routinely in Restorative dentistry, but they are used in fixed prosthodontics mainly in areas of dentin close to the pulp or with patients having porcelain or glass restorations cemented with resin cement. Two major categories are common: calcium hydroxide (chemical and light cured) and glass ionomer.

Calcium Hydroxide Liners

An extremely popular brand, Dycal (L.D. Caulk) (Fig. 17-22), is used by most dentists. Calcium hy-

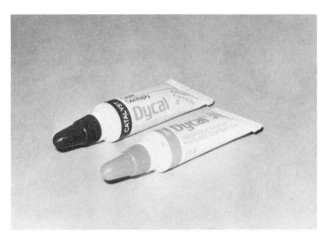

Fig. 17-22. Dycal (Caulk) and Life (Kerr) share the major current use for calcium hydroxide chemical setting liners.

droxide liners should be used only in locations where the dentist believes that the tooth preparation is 0.5 mm or less from the pulp. In fixed prosthodontics, a base or buildup is suggested over the calcium hydroxide liner to prevent displacement by the impression material. Tooth reconstructive procedures are discussed later in this chapter. Light-cured calcium hydroxide liner (VLC Dycal, L.D. Caulk) (Fig. 17-23) is much stronger and less soluble than chemical-cure liner, but neither bonds to tooth structure.

Glass Ionomer Liners

A thin layer (0.5 mm) of glass ionomer liner (Fig. 17-24) is suggested over all dentin in tooth preparations that are receiving resin-cemented porcelain inlays or onlays. The liner should be mixed for 10 seconds to a thickness that allows a ½ inch string from the mixing pad. This liner may be etched for 15 seconds with standard phosphoric acid etching solution

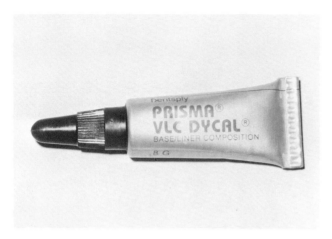

Fig. 17-23. Light-curing calcium hydroxide liners are useful in areas requiring significant strength.

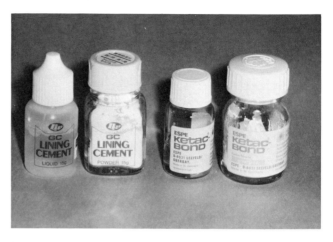

Fig. 17-24. Glass ionomer liners have become extremely popular because of their desirable characteristics, which include cariostatic activity bond to tooth; expansion and contraction similar to tooth strength, and ability to be etched for bond of subsequent cement to the liner.

to provide retention between the resin cement and the glass ionomer liner. These liners have significant molecular bond to tooth structure after 1 day, but they must be manipulated with care to avoid dislodgement during tooth preparation for an inlay.

BASES IN FIXED PROSTHODONTICS

A significant increase in the use of pin-retained bases in fixed prosthodontics has been noted in the past few years. This is encouraging because it allows reduction of the tooth without displacing previous restorative material from the tooth. A suggested technique is the removal of existing restorative materials from teeth that require artificial crowns. The dentist placing the new crown is then convinced that the tooth can support a crown.

Table 17-2 lists a comparison of the four types of bases currently used in dentistry.[35] At this time, composite and glass ionomer with metal reinforcement are the most popular. Amalgam, although popular, often requires a second appointment because it has low strength for several hours. Any of the four types provide adequate base or buildup characteristics, but glass ionomer is indicated in caries-active patients, while composite is indicated where immediate strength is needed. For composite, the margin of the subsequent crown must be at least 1-½ mm gingival to the margin of the composite and the tooth. Further study of the influence of corrosion on composite resin is required before universal application.

Cements, liners, and bases are used daily in dentistry and individual preferences vary. At this time, zinc phosphate, polycarboxylate, and glass ionomer are used equally. Resin cements are being used routinely for porcelain restorations, resin-bonded retainers, and post and core cementation. Currently, cements are the weakest factor in a well-constructed fixed prostheses, and research should be directed to their improvement.

SELECTED REFERENCES

1. Ward, M.L.: American Textbook of Operative Dentistry, ed. 7, Philadelphia, 1940, Lea & Febiger.
2. Flagg, J.F.: Plastics and Plastic Filling, ed. 3, Philadelphia, 1890, Sherman & Co.
3. Christensen, G.J., and Christensen, R.P.: Use survey—1985, Clin. Res. Assoc. Newsletter 9:1, August 1985.
4. Swartz, M.L., Phillips, R.W., Norman, R.D., and Oldham, D. F.: The strength, hardness and abrasion of dental cements, J.A.D.A. 67:367-374, 1963.
5. Paffenbarger, G.C.: Dental cements, direct filling resins, composite and adhesive restorative materials: a resume, J. Biomed. Mater. Res. 6:363-393, 1972.
6. Civjan, S., and Brauer, G.M.: Physical properties of cements based on zinc oxide, hydrogenated resin, o-ethoxybenzoic acid and eugenol, J. Dent. Res. 43:281, March-April 1964.
7. Paffenbarger, G.C., Sweeney, W.T., and Isaacs, A.: A preliminary report on zinc phosphate cements, J.A.D.A. 20:1960-1962, 1933.
8. Massler, M.: Effect of filling materials on the pulp, N.Y.J. Dent. 26:183-198, 1956.
9. Brannstrom, M., and Nyborg, H.: Bacterial growth and pulpal changes under inlays cemented with zinc phosphate cement and Epoxylite CBA 9080, J Prosthet. Dent. 31:556-565, May 1974.
10. Norman, R.D., Swartz, M.L., Phillips, R.W., and Vermani, R.V.: A comparison of the intraoral disintegration of three dental cements, J.A.D.A. 78:777-782, 1969.
11. Phillips, R.W., Swartz, M.L., and Norman, R.D.: Materials for the Practicing Dentist, St. Louis, 1969, The C.V. Mosby Co.
12. Phillips, R.W., Swartz, M.L., Norman, R.D., et. al.: Zinc oxide and eugenol cements for permanent cementation, J. Prosthet. Dent. 19:144-150, February 1968.
13. Gibson, T.D., and Myers, G.E.: Clinical studies of dental cements. IV. A preliminary study of a zinc oxide–eugenol cement for final cementation, J. Dent. Res. 49:75-78, 1970.
14. Smith, D.C.: A new dental cement, Br. Dent. J. 125:381-384, Nov. 5, 1968.
15. Phillips, R.W., Swartz, M.L., and Rhodes, B.: An evaluation of carboxylate adhesive cements, J.A.D.A. 81:1353-1359, December 1970.

Table 17-2. Bases in fixed prosthodontics

	Amalgam		Castings		Composite		Glass ionomer and Silver alloy fillings	
Complexity of use	Fair	(2)*	Poor (In general, above rating is valid, but excellent lab can make significant difference.)	(1)	Excellent	(4)	Good to excellent	(3.5)
Cost to patient	Good	(3)	Poor	(1)	Good	(3)	Good	(3)
Speed of use	Fair	(2)	Poor	(1)	Excellent	(4)	Good	(3)
Cariostatic activity	Fair to good	(2.5)	Poor to fair (Rating is improved by use of glass ionomer cement.)	(1.5)	Poor	(1)	Good	(3)
Adhesion to tooth	Poor	(1)	Poor to fair (Rating can be improved by use of adherent cements such as glass ionomer or polycarboxylate.)	(1.5)	Poor to fair (Rating can be improved by use of dentin adhesive under composite.)	(1.5)	Good	(3)
Strength	Excellent	(4)	Excellent (If fit is acceptable.)	(4)	Good	(3)	(Good	(3)
Radiopacity	Excellent	(4)	Excellent	(4)	Good	(3)	Good (If contains alloy fillins.)	(3)
Years use experience	Excellent (+50 yrs.)	(4)	Excellent (+50 yrs)	(4)	Good (+20 yrs.)	(3)	Fair (+5 yrs.)	(2)
Potential toxicity or lack of biocompatibility	Fair to good (However, currently amalgam is being questioned by some.)	(2.5)	Good (If biocompatible metal used.)	(3)	Good	(3)	Good	(3)
Significant positive characteristics	Strong. Cariostatic. Longevity of use experience. Low cost.		Strong. *If* well done. Longevity of use.		Easy to use. Fast. Low cost.		Easy to use. Fast. Low cost. Cariostatic. Adheres to tooth.	
Significant negative characteristics	Difficult to use. Slow. Alleged lack of biocompatibility. Can cause amalgam tatoos.		Difficult to use. High cost to patient. Technique sensitive.		Not cariostatic		Only few years of experience. Slightly slower to use than composite.	
Current use in profession	Moderate.		Low.		High.		Low, but growing.	

Christensen G.J., Christensen R. Clin. Res. Assoc. Newsletter 7(11):2, 1983.
*Key to number ratings: 4 = Excellent; 3 = Good; 2 = Fair; 1 = Poor.

16. Powers, J.M., Johnson, Z.G., and Craig, R.G.: Physical and mechanical properties of zinc polyacrylate dental cements, J.A.D.A. 88:380-383, February 1974.
17. Truelove, E.L., Mitchell, D.F., and Phillips, R.W.: Biologic evaluation of a carboxylate cement, J. Dent. Res. 50:166, February 1971.
18. el-Kafrawy, A.H., Dickey, D.M., Mitchell, D.F., et al.: Pulp reaction to a polycarboxylate cement in monkeys, J. Dent. Res. 53:15-19, January-February 1974.
19. Smith, D.C.: A review of zinc polycarboxylate cements, J. Can. Dent. Assoc. 37:1-8, 1971.
20. Button, G.L., Barnes, R.F., and Moon, P.C.: Surface preparation and shear strength of the casting-cement interface, J. Prosthet. Dent. 53:34-338, January 1985.
21. Wilson, A.D., and Kent, B.E.: A new translucent cement for dentistry. The glass ionomer cement, Br. Dent. J. 132:133, 1972.
22. Christensen, G.J., and Christensen, R.P.: Sensitivity related to glass ionomer cements, Clin. Res. Assoc. Newsletter 8:2, November 1984.
23. McComb, D., Sirisko, R., and Brown, J.: J. Can. Dent. Assoc. 50:699-701, September 1984.
24. Mitchem, J.C., and Gronas, D.G.: Clinical evaluation of cement-solubility, J. Prosthet. Dent. 40:453-456, 1978.
25. Mitchem, J.C., and Gronas, D.G.: Continued evaluation of the clinical solubility of luting cements, J. Prosthet. Dent. 45:289-291, 1981.
26. Swartz, M.L., Phillips, R.W., and Clark, H.E.: Long-term F release from glass ionomer cements, J. Dent. Res. 63:158-160, February 1984.

27. Brauer, G.M., McLaughlin, R., and Huget, E.F.: Aluminum oxide as a reinforcing agent for zinc oxide–eugenol-o-ethoxybenzoic acid cements, J. Dent. Res. **47**:622-628, 1968.

28. Wilson, A.D., and Batchelor, R.F.: Zinc oxide–eugenol cements. II. Study of erosion and disintegration, J. Dent. Res. **49**:593-598, 1970.

29. Hayes, S.M.: A practical comparison of the three basic types of crown and bridge cements, J. Acad. Gen. Dent. **21**:18-19, September-October 1973.

30. Christensen, G.J., and Christensen, R.P.: Porcelain inlays and onlays, resin-bonded, Clin. Res. Assoc. Newsletter **10**:1-2, May 1986.

31. Paffenbarger, G.C.: New developments in dental materials: a world wide survey, Int. Dent. J. **15**:356, September 1965.

32. Bakland, T., and Baum, L.: Cyanoacrylate in the cementation of threaded retentive pins. J. Ga. Dent. Assoc. **47**:13, Summer 1973.

33. Hanson, E.C., and Caputo, A.A.: Cementing mediums and retentive characteristics of dowels, J. Prosthet. Dent. **32**:551-558, November 1975.

34. American Dental Association Council Report: Polymers used in dentistry. 1. Cyanoacrylates, J.A.D.A. **89**:1386-1388, December 1974.

35. Christensen, G.J., and Christensen, R.P.: Tooth build-up materials and techniques, Clin. Res. Assoc. Newsletter **7**:1-3, November 1983.

18

**Edmund Cavazos, Jr.,
Joseph T. Richardson,
and Richard N. Wells**

PONTICS FOR FIXED PROSTHODONTICS

The pontic is the suspended member of a fixed partial denture. It replaces the lost natural tooth, restores function, and occupies the space of the missing tooth. The pontic is attached to the retainer by a rigid connector such as a solder joint; special cases require a nonrigid connector such as a key and keyway or telescoping retainers.

CLASSIFICATION

Pontics are classified in several ways:
1. The shape of the surface contacting the ridge is used as a classification and includes spheroidal, conical, ridge lap, and modified ridge lap (Fig. 18-1, A to D).
2. The materials used in constructing a pontic are a second method of classification and include all metal, metal and porcelains, and combinations of metal and resins. Research has shown that the porosity of acrylic resins and difficulty in obtaining a highly polished finish makes the material unsatisfactory for a tissue surface.[1] Tissue acceptance is dependent on the finish of the material rather than the material.
3. Another classification is pontics prefabricated by the manufacturer. These designs can be altered by the dentist and reglazed if necessary. Prefabricated facings include flatbacks, trupontics, long-pin facings, pontips, and reverse pin facings (Fig. 18-2, A to E). These facings are protected by an adequate thickness of metal to prevent fracture. In the maxillary arch, where esthetics is important, manufactured facings are used with partial veneer retainers if there is sufficient space. In the mandibular molar area, pontips are used by dentists who desire glazed porcelain in contact with the residual ridge.

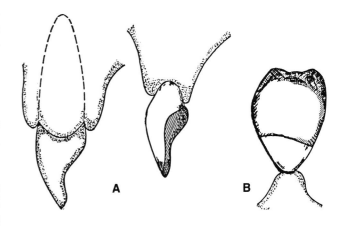

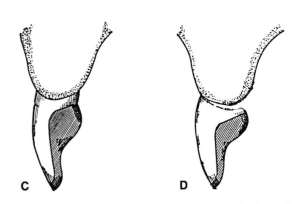

Fig. 18-1. A, Conical pontic; formerly used for anterior immediate replacement. **B,** Spheroidal pontic; used in mandibular posterior region. **C,** Ridge lap; no longer used. **D,** Modified ridge lap to satisfy esthetics and hygiene.

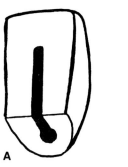 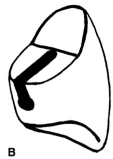 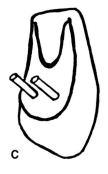 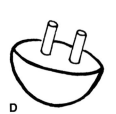 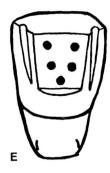

Fig. 18-2. A, Flatback interchangeable facing. **B,** Tru-pontic. **C,** Long-pin facing. **D,** Pontip. **E,** Reverse pin facing.

4. Since the introduction of porcelain fused-to-metal restorations, custom-made pontics have been fabricated in the laboratory. The increased use of porcelain veneer coverage has greatly decreased commercially manufactured facings because construction of pontics and retainers with the same materials is simpler and more esthetically pleasing.

REQUIREMENTS

The requirements of a pontic are to:
1. Restore function.
2. Provide esthetics and comfort.
3. Be biologically acceptable.
4. Permit effective oral hygiene.
5. Preserve underlying residual mucosa.[2]

These requirements form the basis for the design of pontics.

DESIGN

Success of the FPD depends on the pontic design.[3,4] According to Eissmann, the boundaries of the edentulous space are the residual ridge, the opposing occlusal surface, the proximal surfaces of the abutment teeth, and the musculature of the tongue and cheek or lips. The design consists of constructing a substitute tooth that favorably compares in form, function, and appearance with the tooth it replaces[5] (Fig. 18-3, A to C). Changes in the residual ridge, opposing occlusion, and proximal space affect the success of the restoration.

When a tooth is lost, the residual ridge is formed from the gingiva and alveolar mucosa. The pontic is positioned away from movable mucosa to prevent tissue proliferation around the pontic. Irregularities of supporting tissue are recontoured with electrosurgery or periodontal surgery before abutment preparation (Fig. 18-4, A and B). When the vertical height is insufficient, the residual ridge is lowered and reshaped to allow space for a physiologic pontic (Fig. 18-4 C). The practice of scraping the cast is rare. If opposing teeth have supererupted into the edentulous

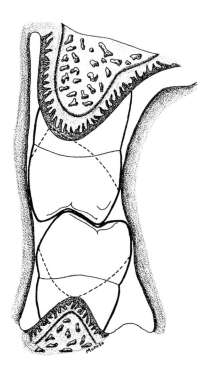

Fig. 18-3. A, Recommended tissue contact for posterior pontics. (Courtesy Dr. Del Maroso, Alton, Ill.)

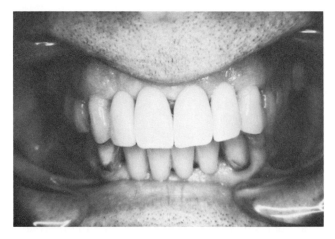

Fig. 18-3. B, Maxillary anterior FPD restoring form, function, and appearance.

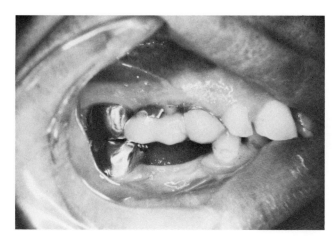

Fig. 18-3. C, Maxillary posterior FPD, which does *not* restore form, function, or appearance.

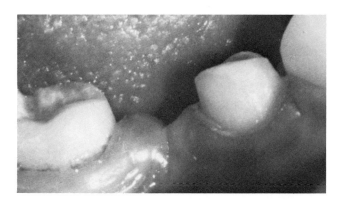

Fig. 18-4. A, Ridge irregularity prior to electrosurgery.

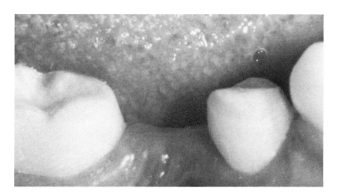

Fig. 18-4. B, recontoured ridge following electrosurgery.

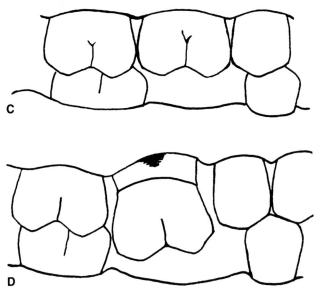

Fig. 18-4. C, Insufficient vertical height requiring residual ridge recontouring. **D,** Gravitated maxillary molar; is corrected for an acceptable occlusal plane prior to FPD construction using a "diagnostic waxup."

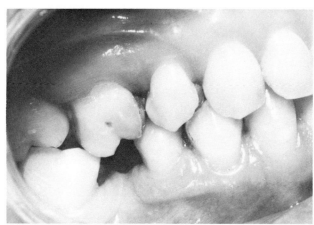

Fig. 18-4. E, Mesial migration of mandibular molar into edentulous space.

Continued

space, occlusal (plane modification) is performed (Fig. 18-4 D). The extent of the procedure is predetermined with a diagnostic waxup on mounted casts. The occlusal plane correction is strongly urged before construction of the FPD. However, concomitant restoration of a supererupted tooth and an FPD is acceptable for an experienced dentist. In most cases, cast restorations are required following the necessary re-

duction. If adjacent teeth have migrated into the edentulous space, then orthodontics may be indicated to encourage appropriate pontic contour and to ensure periodontal health (Fig. 18-4, E to G). Design can be visualized by analyzing each pontic surface individually on the mounted diagnostic casts.

Gingival Surface

The gingival surface is the most interesting aspect of pontic design. The material, the shape, and degree of tissue contact affect the choice of approach. Although dentists have advocated highly glazed porcelain as the material of choice to contact the ridge,

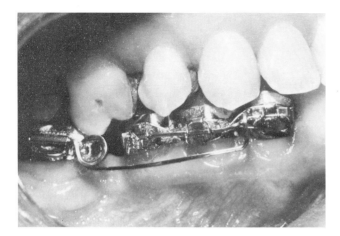

Fig. 18-4. F, Orthodontic movement of mandibular molar.

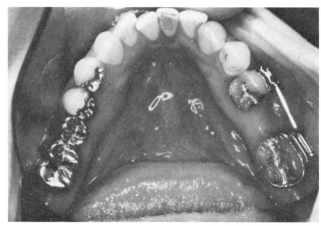

Fig. 18-4. G, Uprighted mandibular molar following orthodontic treatment. (Courtesy Dr. Robert Biggerstaff, San Antonio, Tex.)

studies have revealed that the finish of the material is more important than the material.[1-4] Rough surfaces accumulate plaque and cause irritation. The contour of the gingival surface demands one shape for esthetics and a different shape for hygiene. Therefore, the intraoral location of the pontic determines the shape of the gingival extension.

In the mandibular posterior, esthetics is not a major consideration, so the spheroidal pontic is the design of choice because of its contour (Fig. 18-5). In the maxilla, the modified ridge lap design satisfies both esthetics and hygiene (Fig. 18-6, A to C).

In the mandibular anterior, the bone loss determines the design of the pontic. Where minimal bone loss exists and esthetics are involved, the modified ridge lap is the preferable design. Where extensive bone loss has occurred, Porter recommends the elimination of embrasures between pontics to simplify oral hygiene and curtail expectoration of saliva during conversation[6] (Fig. 18-7).

The ridge lap and conical shape designs are infrequently recommended. The ridge lap design creates an uncleansible concave surface (Fig. 18-8, A to D). The conical shape pontic was designed for insertion into the alveolar socket immediately after extraction. This promotes ridge resorption and an uncleansible area, making it a rare design. A customized ridge lap is fabricated for the patient whose nervous habits cause prolonged irritation on the lingual surface.

When using the spheroidal design, the pontic contacts without pressure the tip of the ridge or the buccal surface, depending upon the relationship of the residual ridge to the opposing occlusion (Fig. 18-9, A and B).

When there is excessive bone loss and the rigidity of the connector is suitable, the pontic is not required to touch the ridge. There should be at least 3 mm of space so the patient can maintain hygiene (Fig. 18-10, A to C). Less than 2 mm space causes food en-

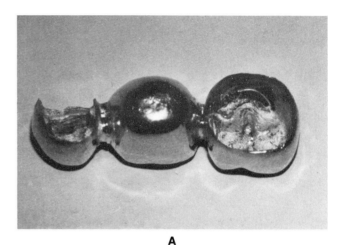

A

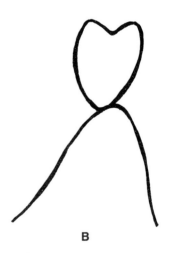

B

Fig. 18-5. A and **B,** Speroidal posterior pontic designed for maintenance of oral hygiene. **A** is a tissue view. **B** is a sagittal view.

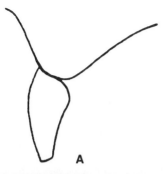

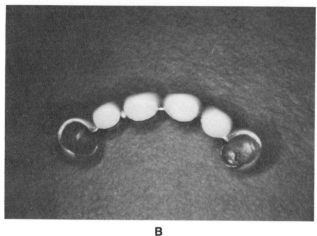

Fig. 18-6. A and **B,** Modified anterior ridge lap pontics designed for esthetic reasons.

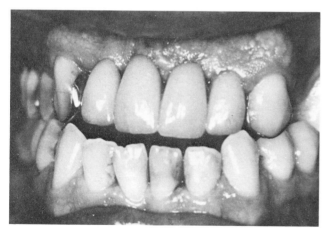

Fig. 18-6. C, A 20-year-old six-unit FPD with reverse pin facings and modified ridge pontics. Open interpontic embrasures and light facial tissue contact ensures hygiene. (Courtesy Dr. W.F.P. Malone, Alton, Ill.)

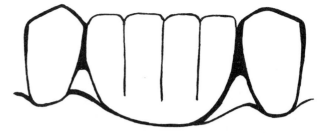

Fig. 18-7. Elective mandibular anterior pontic eliminating interpontic spaces to improve phonetics.

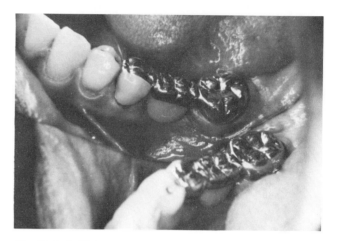

Fig. 18-8. A, Ridge lap pontic showing buccal and lingual tissue contact which renders it uncleansible.

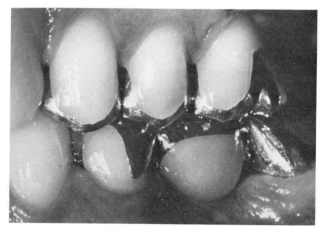

Fig. 18-8. B, Occlusal maxillary plane modification with three-quarter or seven-eighth crowns and mandibular FPD with a cleansible spheroidal pontic. (Courtesy Dr. D.A. Kaiser, San Antonio, Tex.)

trapment. Prototype pontics should be constructed on the treatment FPD to evaluate whether the patient can tolerate the design.

The modified ridge lap pontic contacts the buccal surface of the ridge. A slight buccolingual concavity is usually created that is well tolerated by the tissue if there is a mesiodistal convexity (Fig. 18-11, A to C).

A pontic should have only minimal passive contact with the ridge. Research has confirmed that excessive pressure causes inflammation and proliferation of tissue[1] (Fig. 18-12, A to C). The pontic should not blanch the tissue or be placed on movable mucosa.

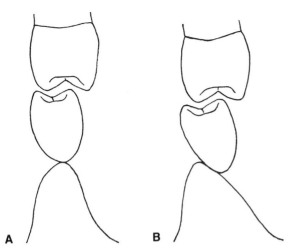

Fig. 18-9. A, Spheroidal pontic contacting crest of ridge. **B,** Spheroidal pontic contacting buccal area.

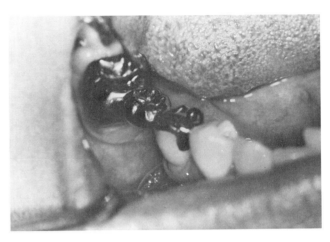

Fig. 18-10. C, Sanitary pontic with appropriate buccolingual dimension for patient's occlusion.

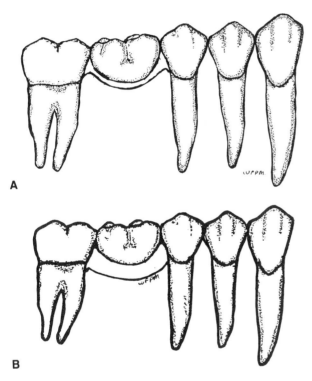

Fig. 18-10. A, Sanitary pontic too close to ridge and thus encouraging redundant tissue. **B,** Sanitary pontic with 3 mm space between tissue, thus encouraging cleanliness.

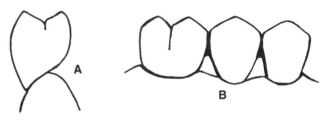

Fig. 18-11. A, Modified ridge lap pontic with slight buccolingual concavity. **B,** Modified ridge lap pontic with mesiodistal covexity.

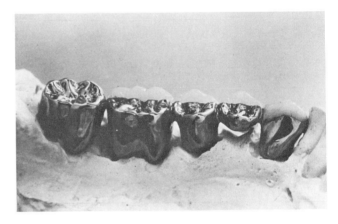

Fig. 18-11. C, Remounted four-unit FPD with broad embrasures and metal contact for lingual stamp cusps of the maxillary arch. (Courtesy F.W. Summers, Westchester Ill.)

Occlusal Surface

The reduction of the occlusal table of the pontic has been suggested for reducing forces exerted on the abutment teeth. Since the proprioceptive mechanism controls occlusal forces, reduction of the table would not diminish the effects on the abutment teeth. It is critical to provide a stable vertical dimension support by suitable placement of the cusps. The positioning of these cusps is dictated by the opposing occlusion, which places the buccal cusps of the mandibular teeth and the lingual cusps of the maxillary teeth into their opposing fossae. Since the maxillary buccal cusps affect esthetics and prevent cheek biting, their positions

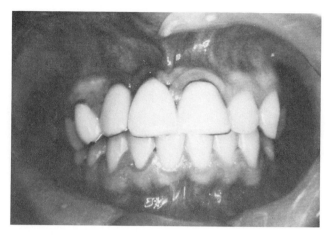

Fig. 18-12. A, Maxillary anterior pontics with excessive tissue pressure.

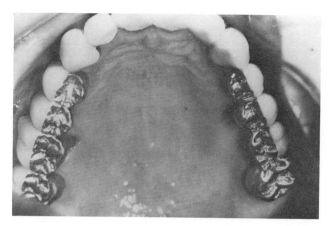

Fig. 18-13. A, Fifteen-year-old completely restored maxillary arch maintaining a narrow anatomic occlusal table.

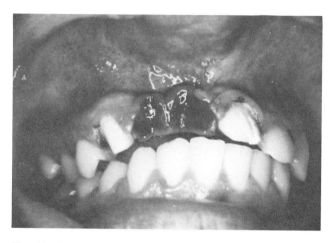

Fig. 18-12. B, Tissue inflammation and proliferation caused by excessive tissue pressure.

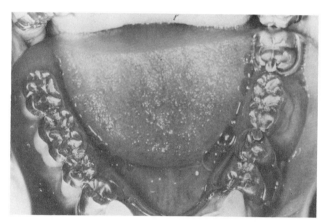

Fig. 18-13. B, Opposing mandibular arch of A showing a RPD with gold occlusals. (Courtesy Dr. W.F.P. Malone, Alton, Ill.)

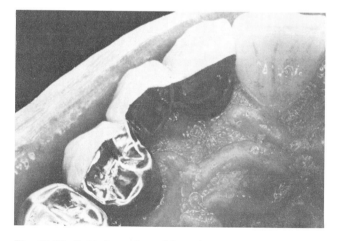

Fig. 18-12. C, Undercontoured lingual cusp to accommodate a mesially drifted canine in the congenitally missing lateral position. Metal to natural tooth aids occlusion and avoids fracture or wear. (Courtesy Dr. W.F.P. Malone, Alton, Ill.)

should not be altered. The mandibular lingual cusps should not be reduced because they protect the tongue and provide anatomic contours to the pontic.

The occlusal table of the pontic is only altered to create a favorable relationship between the pontic and the opposing occlusion or when space has been lost due to drifting (Fig. 18-13, A and B).

Interproximal Surface

Vertical clearance must be sufficient to permit physiologic contour of the pontic and to allow space for the interproximal tissues. Interproximal embrasures are open to permit access for cleaning. The maxillary anterior proximal embrasures are minimal for esthetics but allow sufficient space to prevent papillary impingement (Fig. 18-14, A and B). Moving posteriorly, the size of the embrasures gradually increases. In the mandibular posterior area, wider embrasures are created to facilitate hygiene since esthetics is critical (Fig. 18-15, A and B).

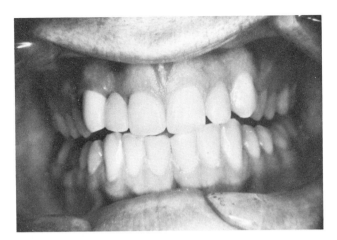

Fig. 18-14. A, Maxillary right lateral pontic satisfying both esthetics and biologic requirements.

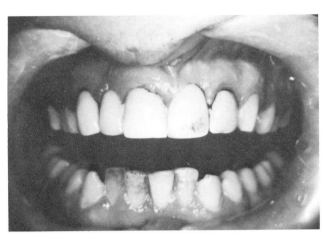

Fig. 18-14. B, Inadequate embrasures of maxillary anterior FPD producing papillary impingement.

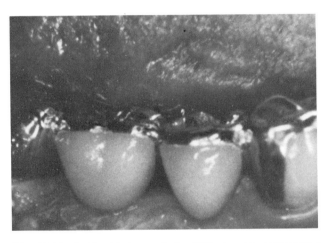

Fig. 18-15. A, Mandibular posterior FPD showing embrasures created to facilitate hygiene and partial converage for anterior retainer.

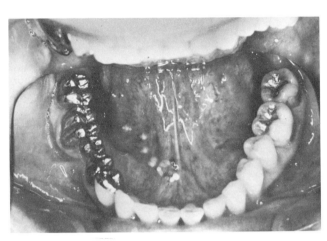

Fig. 18-15. B, Mandibular posterior FPD with narrow occlusal tables, consistent central groove, and fluted molars for cleansible axial contours. (Courtesy Dr. W.F.P. Malone, Alton, Ill.)

Buccal and Lingual Surfaces

The contours of buccal and lingual surfaces of the pontic are determined by esthetic, functional, and hygienic requirements. In the maxilla, esthetics demands maintaining normal facial contour, axial alignment, and length. (Fig. 18-16, A to C).

The lingual contour should harmonize with adjacent teeth from the cusp tip to the height of contour, then sharply recede convexly to the facial or buccal tissue contact area. Embrasures on the lingual are wider than the buccal or facial (Fig. 18-17, A and B).

The same principles apply to the mandibular anterior region. In the mandibular posterior area, the buccal and lingual surfaces follow normal tooth form from the cusp tip to the height of the contour. The spheroidal design results from tapering the buccal and lingual surfaces from the height of contour toward the gingival contact (Fig. 18-18).

PONTIC SELECTION

The design or type of pontic for a specific FPD is determined by:
1. The retainers
2. Esthetics
3. Occlusal gingival height and mesiodistal width of the edentulous area
4. Ridge resorption and contour

When porcelain-bonded-to-metal retainers are used, porcelain-bonded-to-metal pontics are selected in order to coordinate the laboratory procedures and enhance esthetics. When partial veneer retainers are used, prefabricated facings are indicated, using the same metal as the retainer. If complete metal retainers are used, an all metal pontic is appropriate.

In the maxillary anterior segment, esthetics dictates pontic selection. A modified ridge lap is the design of choice, since this is a rational compromise between

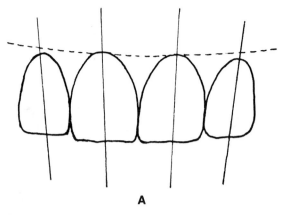

A

Fig. 18-17. A, Maxillary anterior FPD showing wider lingual embrasures.

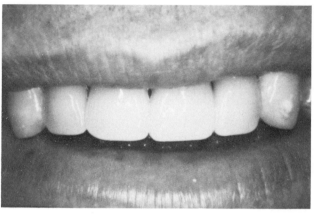

B

Fig. 18-16. A and **B,** Maxillary anterior pontics designed for normal contour, alignment, and length.

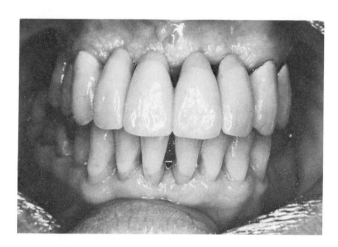

Fig. 18-17. B, Shade characterization of the maxillary seven-unit FPD and open embrasures complement the mandibular teeth. (Courtesy of Dr. Charles B. Porter, San Diego, Calif.)

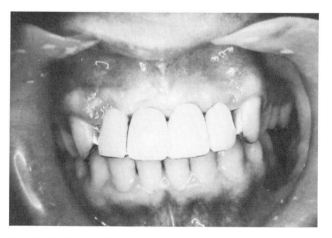

Fig. 18-16. C, Maxillary anterior FPD showing undesirable axial alignment.

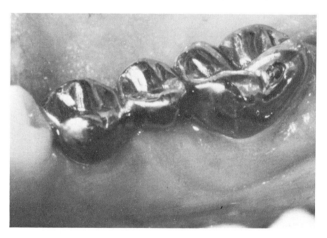

Fig. 18-18. Mandibular posterior FPD with spheroidal pontic.

esthetics and hygiene. When multiple teeth are missing, the interproximal embrasures are minimized on the facial surface to prevent unsightly spaces and to avoid whistling sounds (Fig. 18-19, A and B). The gingival contour of the pontic is usually concave from facial contact to the crest of the ridge and convex in

a mesiodistal direction. In the maxillary posterior area, if esthetics is also a prime consideration, a modified ridge lap design is used. In the mandibular posterior region, esthetics is not as critical, so function and hygiene are emphasised (Fig. 18-20, A and B). A spheroidal pontic is placed without pressure on the ridge

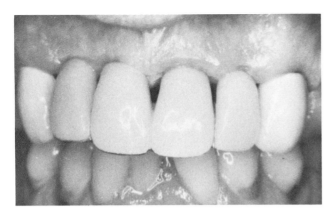

Fig. 18-19. A, Maxillary anterior FPD showing exaggerated embrasures on left.

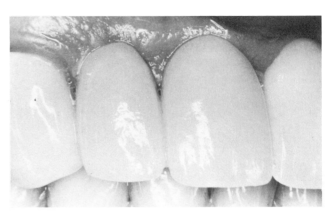

Fig. 18-19. B, An esthetic FPD for a patient with a high lip line; requires continual astringent patient hygiene (Courtesy Dr. W.F.P. Malone, Alton, Ill.)

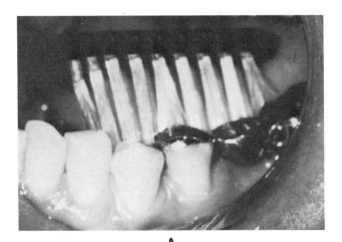

A   B

Fig. 18-20. A and **B,** Mandibular posterior FPD with spheroidal pontic design to facilitate hygiene.

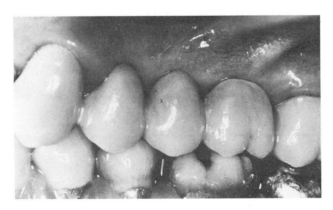

Fig. 18-20. C, Facial adaptation of three modified ridge (Stein) pontics requiring continual oral care.

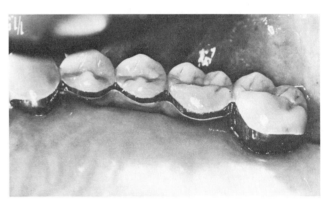

Fig. 18-20. D, Lingual view of five-unit FPD with minimal tissue contact. The splint is temporarily seated with Luralite (Kerr Mfg. Co., Romulus, Mich.) to allow accommodation.

to prevent tissue proliferation. Patients demanding an all ceramic occlusal surface for a posterior FPD require an accommodation period. The prosthesis is inserted with a nonadhesive interim biting agent to allow the dentist to adjust the occlusion (Fig. 18-20, C to F).

The occlusal gingival height and the mesiodistal width of the edentulous space are important determinants of design and materials for FPDs (Fig. 18-21, A to E). Long spans in areas with reduced occlusal gingival height can result in porcelain fracture during

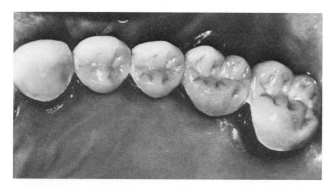

Fig. 18-20. E, Occlusal view of five-unit FPD with a gradual narrowing of the occlusal table from terminal abutment to the canine.

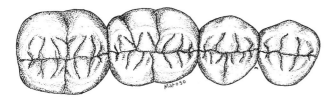

Fig. 18-20. F, Posterior four-unit FPD with gradual anterior reduction of the occlusal table. (**A** and **B,** courtesy Dr. Joseph Cleveland, Charleston, S.C.: **C** to **E,** courtesy Dr. W.F.P. Malone, Alton, Ill., **F,** courtesy Dr. Del Moroso, Alton, Ill.)

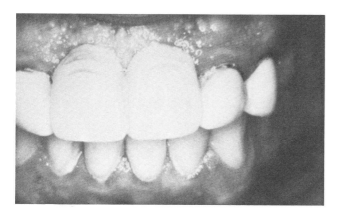

Fig. 18-21. A, Maxillary anterior FPD with overextension of central incisor pontic.

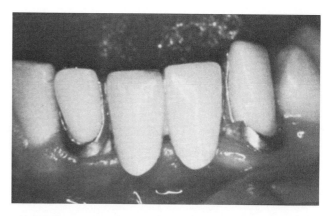

Fig. 18-21. B, Mandibular anterior FPD with overextension of central incisor pontic.

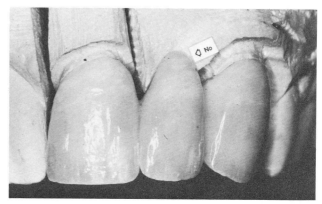

Fig. 18-21. C, Overextension of pontic. The pontic and adjacent abutments should be symmetric.

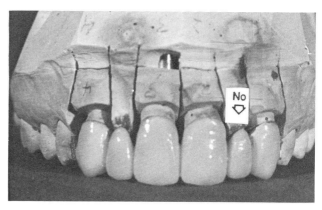

Fig. 18-21. D, Underextended pontics for the maxillary lateral incisors. The gingival should be symmetric to ensure esthetics.
Continued

flexure. Therefore, if esthetics permits, an all metal pontic is preferable; if esthetics is required, porcelain fused to a base metal alloy is more suitable.

The amount of ridge resorption and contour determine tissue contact or tissue clearance. When ridge resorption is extensive, tissue clearance of at least 3 mm is recommended for hygienic reasons. Recontouring and augmentation of the ridge may be indicated in patients when large areas of the ridge are lost; e.g. from trauma (Fig. 18-22, A to D). Exciting designs are being introduced that possess greater strength and use less metal (Fig. 18-23).

The function of the pontic is to replace the missing natural tooth, to restore function and esthetics, and to maintain the stability of the arch.

Pontics are available in many forms and sizes, but there is not a stereotype design. Emphasis should be directed to the surface finish of the material, rather than the choice of the material.

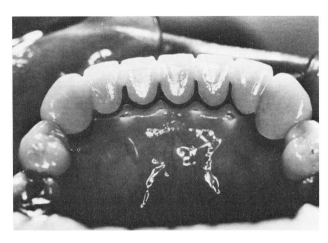

Fig. 18-21. E, Lingual view of "Stein pontics" for nine-unit splint. Note the *five* incisors with light facial contact to encourage hygiene. (Courtesy Dr. W.F.P. Malone, Alton, Ill.)

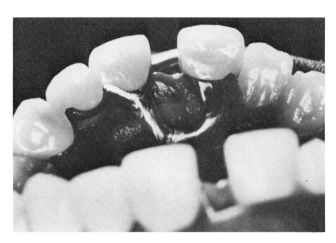

Fig. 18-22. C, Loop connector to preserve anterior diastema on a four-unit FPD. (Courtesy Dr. W.F.P. Malone, Alton, Ill.)

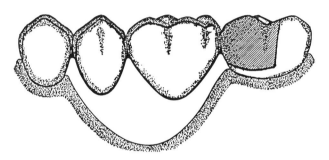

Fig. 18-22. A, Position of mandibular pontics with an excessively resorbed ridge. (courtesy Dr. Donald Smith, Los Angeles, Calif.

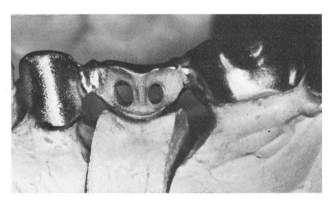

Fig. 18-23. The innovative, revolutionary Inzoma pontic. (Courtesy Dr. W.F.P. Malone, Alton, Ill.) Shoher, I., Whitman, A.E.: Reinforced porcelain system: a new concept in ceramomental restorations. J. Prosthet. Dent. 50:489 1983.

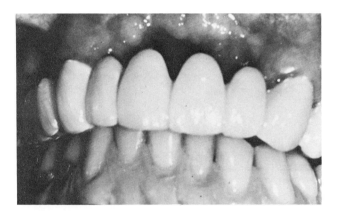

Fig. 18-22. B, gold and acrylic fixed splint to provide esthetics and function after 20 odd years of an RPD. These patients are currently treated with surgical ridge augmentation.

The design of the pontic is probably the most important factor in determining the success of the restoration. If the patient is unable to effectively clean and maintain the pontic, the restoration will be unsuccessful. Some compromises are necessary when esthetics is involved.

Without suitable mechanical and biologic design of the connectors, the FPD will be a biologic compromise. Mechanical requirements include strength, smooth and rounded surfaces, and acceptable esthetics. Biologic requirements suggest that the connector should occupy the normal proximal contact areas to ensure cleansible embrasures. It is commonly necessary to recontour soft tissue to develop biologic pontics.

SELECTED REFERENCES
1. Cavazos, E., Jr.: Tissue response to fixed partial denture pontics, J. Prosth. Dent. **20**(2):143-153, August 1968.
2. Tylman, S.D., and Malone, W.F.P.: Theory and Practice of Fixed Prosthodontics, ed. 7, St. Louis, 1978, The C.V. Mosby Co.
3. Shillingburg, H.T., Jr., Hobo, S., and Whitsett, L.D.: Fundamentals of Fixed Prosthodontics, ed. 2, Chicago, Ill. 1981, Quintessence Publishing Co..

4. Stein, R.S.: Pontic-residual ridge relationship-a research report, J. Prosth. Dent. **16**:251-285, March 1966.
5. Eissmann, H.F., Rudd, K.D., and Morrow, R.W.: Dental Laboratory Procedures, Fixed Partial Dentures, St. Louis, Mo., 1980, The C.V. Mosby Co.
6. Porter, P.D., Jr.: Anterior pontic design: a logical progression, J. Prosth. Dent. **51**:774-776, 1986.
7. Tjan, Antony H.L.: Biologic pontic designs, Gen. Dent. **31**:42, 1983.
8. Maroso, D.J., and Schmidt, J.R.: Fixed prosthodontics manual, Alton, Ill., Southern Illinois University School of Dental Medicine, 1979.

BIBLIOGRAPHY

Beaudreau, D.E.: Atlas of fixed Partial Prostheses, Springfield, Ill., 1975, Charles C Thomas, Publisher.

Beke, A.L.: The biomechanics of pontic width reduction for fixed partial dentures, J. Acad. Gen. Dent. **22**(6):28-32, 1974.

Bruce, R.W.: Clinical applications of multiple unit castings for fixed prostheses, J. Prosth. Dent. **18**(4):359, 1967.

Clayton, J.A.: Roughness of pontic materials and dental plaque, J. Prosth. Dent. **23**:407, 1970.

Crispin, B.J.: Tissue response to posterior denture base-type pontics, J. Prosth. Dent. **42**:259, 1979.

Ewing, J.E.: Reevaluation of the cantilever principle, J. Prosth. Dent. **7**:78, 1957.

Gratton, D.R.: Pontics in fixed prosthesis-status report, J.A.D.A. 91-613, September 1975.

Harmon, C.B.: Pontic design, J. Prosth. Dent. **8**:496, 1985.

Henry, P.J.: Pontic form in fixed partial denture, Aust. Dent. J. **16**:1, 1971.

Hirsberg, S.M.: The relationship of oral hygiene to embrasure and pontic design, J. Prosth. Dent. **27**:26, 1972.

Hood, J.A., Farah, J.W., and Craig, R.G.: Stress and deflection of three different pontic designs. J. Prosth. Dent. **33**:54, 1975.

Johnston, J.F., Phillips, R.W., and Dykema, R.W.: Modern Practice in Crown and Bridge Prosthodontics, ed. 3, Philadelphia, 1971, The W.B. Saunders Co.

Legett, L.J.: Bridge pontics, Int. Dent. J. **8**:45, 1985.

Linkow, L.I.: Contact areas in natural dentitions and fixed prosthodontics, J. Prosth. Dent. **12**:132, 1962.

Malone, W.F.P., and Sarlas, C.H.: Prosthodontic considerations in ephedodontics, Dent. Clin. North Am. **13**:461, April 1969.

Perel, M.L.: A modified sanitary pontic, J. Prosth. Dent. **28**:589, 1972.

Podshadley, A.G.: Gingival response to pontic, J. Prosth. Dent. **19**(1):51-57, 1968.

Podshadley, A.G., and Harrison, J.D.: Rat connective tissue response to pontic materials, J. Prosth. Dent. **16**:110-118, 1966.

Ruhlman, D.C., and Richter, W.A.: A method for pontic stabilization in fixed partial denture construction, J. Prosth. Dent. **17**(4):401-405, 1967.

Schield, H.W.: The influence of bridge pontics on oral health, J. Mich. Dent. Assoc. **50**(4):143, 1968.

Shoher, I., and Whiteman, A.E.: Reinformed porcelain system: a new concept in ceramo-metal restorations, J. Prosth. Dent. **50**:489-496, October 1983.

Schweitzer, J.M., Schweitzer, R.D., and Schweitzer, J.: Free-end pontics used on fixed partial dentures, J. Prosth. Dent. **20**(2):120-138, 1968.

Silverglate, L.: A simplified reverse-pin procelain facing technique, J. Prosth. Dent. **18**:54, 1967.

Staffanou, R.S., and Thayer, K.E.: Reverse pin-porcelain veneer and pontic technique, J. Prosth. Dent. **12**:1138, 1962.

Stein, R.S.: Residual pontic, J. Prosth. Dent. March-April, 1966.

Tjan, A.H.L.: Biologic pontic designs, Gen. Dent. January-February, 1983.

Tylman, S.D.: Anatomic form and function as registered and related to restorative dentistry, Ill. Dent. J. **25**:221, 1956.

Whiteside, W.D.: Practical mandibular anterior pontic, J. Prosth. Dent. **9**:119, 1959.

Zarb, G.A., Bergaman, B., Clayton, J.A., and McKay, H.F.: Prosthodontic Treatment for Partial Edentulous Patients, St. Louis, 1978, The C.V. Mosby Co.

19

Steven M. Morgano and Robert J. Crum

FIXED REMOVABLE PROSTHODONTICS

This chapter concerns two common clinical situations when fixed and removable prosthodontics are integrated: the crowned abutment for a removable partial denture and the overdenture.

CROWNED ABUTMENT FOR A REMOVABLE PARTIAL DENTURE

Diagnosis and Treatment Planning

Successful treatment is the result of a logical diagnosis and a rational sequence to the treatment plan. A comprehensive oral examination, distinct radiographs, and well-defined diagnostic casts are essential.

Treatment planning includes the use of the dental surveyor to locate the most favorable path of insertion on the diagnostic cast for the removable partial denture. The framework is then designed and <u>completely</u> outlined on the diagnostic cast. Lines are scribed parallel to the analyzing rod of the surveyor on the base of the cast to serve as a record of the path of insertion. The crown restorations are then planned to fit the predetermined RPD design.

Clinical Procedures

The diagnostic cast with the outlined framework serves as a fundamental guide during tooth preparation, and it should be present in the operatory. Prior to tooth preparation for cast restorations, guiding planes are developed on the abutment teeth <u>not</u> receiving cast restorations.

Tooth reduction is initiated with the traditional occlusal tooth preparation, followed by axial reduction. Additional axial reduction is performed where guiding planes are planned, and space is provided within the tooth preparation for rest seats of desired contour and depth (Figs. 19-1 to 19-4). Perceptive tooth preparation can eliminate lingual undercuts on mandibular posterior teeth and improve the placement of lingual

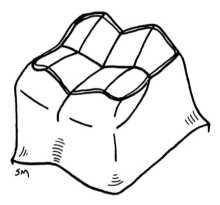

Fig. 19-1. A classic conservative preparation for a complete metal veneer crown with a circumferential chamfer finish line on a mandibular right second molar.

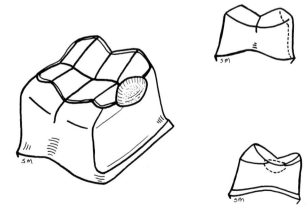

Fig. 19-2. A round-end tapered diamond is used to prepare a shallow 0.5 mm shoulder for the guiding plane. A large round diamond is directed to place a recess for the planned rest seat.

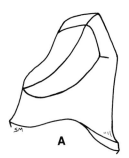
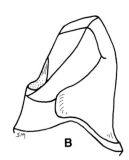

Fig. 19-3. A, A classic conservative preparation for a porcelain-fused-to-metal crown on a maxillary left canine. **B,** Note the modifications to the preparation for the contour of an artificial crown receiving an RPI clasp. The facial shoulder is carried lingually with an axial depth of 0.5 mm to the distolingual line angle. A recess is developed on the mesial surface of the cingulum for placement of a mesial rest seat.

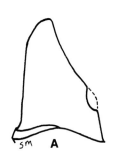
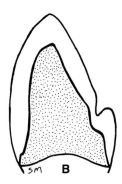

Fig. 19-4. A, The modification required for in inverted v-shaped cingulum rest seat on a mandibular canine. A large round-end tapered diamond is used to prepare a ledge in the cingulum. **B,** Silhouette of the preparation super imposed on an outline of the completed restoration. The cingulum has not been overcontoured.

bracing arms and the lingual bar major connector (See section on the all metal complete veneer crown, Step 3, and accompanying Fig. 19-7 B).

Laboratory Procedures

The technician must have sufficient information, including the diagnostic casts with the removable framework completely outlined and a comprehensive work authorization. The technician must know exactly where the dentist has planned rests, guiding planes, bracing surfaces, and undercuts. Clear communication is essential and prevents future problems.

All metal complete veneer crown. A mandibular right second molar is used for demonstration (Figs. 19-6 to 19-10). The following steps outline the procedure:

1. Wax the crown to obtain normal complete contours and occlusion (Fig. 19-5).
2. Place the master cast on the surveying table, and align the cast consistent with the planned path of insertion and guiding planes prepared on other natural teeth.
3. Cut a guiding plane in the wax pattern that is flat occlusogingivally and parallel to the path of insertion (Fig. 19-6). The original faciolingual contour of the tooth is maintained. A planned lingual bracing surface can be created that is flat occlusogingivally and follows normal tooth curvatures. A lingual ledge is not recommended, since hypercontour of the gingival third of the crown results (Fig. 19-7). A flat lingual bracing surface, especially on mandibular premolars, will also facilitate placement of a lingual bar major connector (Fig. 19-7 B).
4. Wax the facial surface to form an ideal survey line (Fig. 19-8) and a 0.015 to 0.02 inch retentive undercut. This undercut will later be reduced

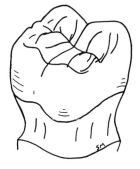

Fig. 19-5. The mandibular right second molar is waxed to normal contours and occlusion.

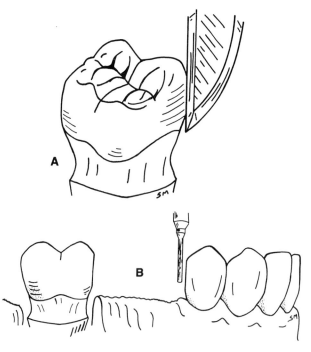

Fig. 19-6. A, A guiding plane is cut in the wax pattern that is flat occlusogingivally and parallel to the planned path of insertion. **B,** The guiding plane must also be parallel to all guiding planes on other natural teeth.

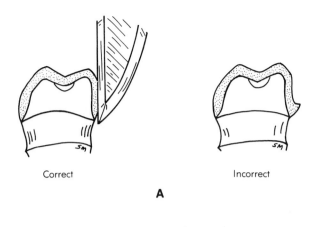

Correct   Incorrect

A

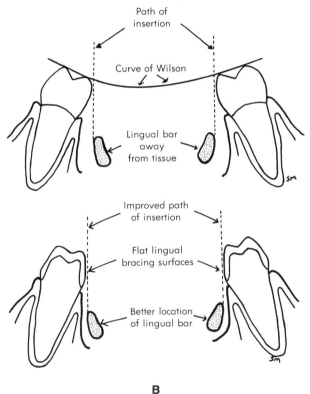

Path of
insertion

Curve of Wilson

Lingual bar
away
from tissue

Improved path
of insertion

Flat lingual
bracing surfaces

Better location
of lingual bar

B

Fig. 19-7. A, A lingual bracing surface can be developed that is parallel to the path of insertion. Capricious placement of a lingual ledge results in overcontour of the gingival third of the crown. Significant overreduction of the lingual surface is required to avoid hypercontour. **B,** The curve of Wilson produces lingual undercuts in the mandible. A lingual bracing surface, as shown here on mandibular premolars, improves the location of the lingual bar major connector and the bracing arms.

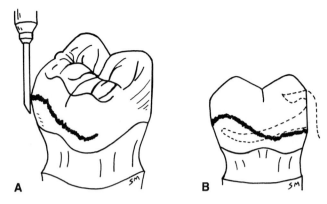

A   **B**

Fig. 19-8. A, The facial surface is waxed to form the desired survey line. **B,** Ideal contour of the survey line permits suitable clasp contour and placement.

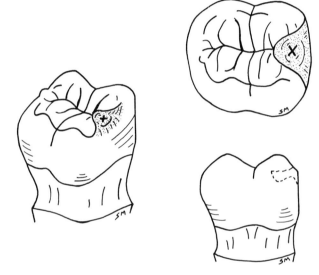

Fig. 19-9. The occlusal rest seat developed in the wax pattern! The deepest portion is at its center (marked with an X). The guiding plane is flat occlusogingivally and follows normal tooth contour faciolingually.

to 0.01 inch during finishing and polishing procedures.

5. Develop the occlusal rest preparation. Wax is removed using a hand-held No. 8 round carbide bur. The contour is then refined with a cleoid-discoid carver.

The occlusal rest preparation is at least one-fourth the mesiodistal width of the crown and one-third the buccolingual width—or one-half the distance between the cusp tips. The depth of the rest seat is at least 1.5 mm in the deepest portion. The rest seat is spoon-shaped when viewed in cross-section with the deepest point at its center. The rest preparation is designed slightly shallower as it crosses the marginal ridge, so that the rest seat will incline toward the tooth. When viewed from the occlusal, the rest preparation is a rounded triangle. There are no sharp angles associated with the occlusal rest seat (Fig. 19-9).

The rest seat for a prepared premolar is similar in size and contour, except that the mesiodistal dimension is at least one-third the mesiodistal width of the crown.

6. Invest, cast, and divest the wax pattern. The casting is surveyed again to ensure desired contours. If necessary, the guiding plane is "refined" by milling with a straight fissure bur in a handpiece secured to the surveyor (Fig. 19-10). The casting is finished and polished and then surveyed for the last time. The final casting should have a definite guiding plane, a lingual bracing surface, a suitably contoured facial survey line with a 0.01 inch undercut in the gingival third of the facial surface, and an appropriately designed rest seat of sufficient depth.

Porcelain-fused-to-metal crown. A mandibular left second premolar is used for demonstration. Steps 1 through 5 are followed as for a complete metal veneer crown:

6. After completing the wax pattern, wax is cut away in the areas to receive the ceramic veneer. The occlusal rest seat, guiding plane, and bracing surface are retained <u>in metal</u> (Fig. 19-11). The

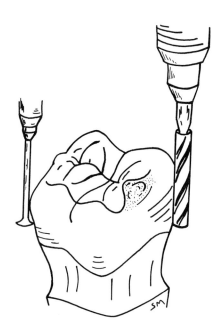

Fig. 19-10. The casting is checked with an undercut gauge for the prescribed undercut. The guiding plane can be "refined" with a straight fissure bur in a handpiece secured to the surveyor.

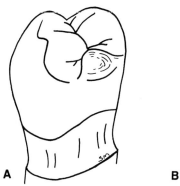 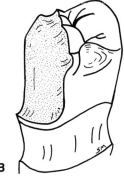

A   **B**

Fig. 19-11. A, The mandibular left second premolar is waxed to complete contours. **B,** Wax is removed from the surfaces receiving the ceramic veneer.

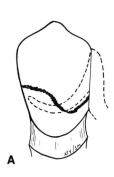 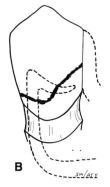

A   **B**

Fig. 19-12. A, An acceptable survey line for a cast or wrought wire circumferential clasp arm. **B,** Desirable survey line for a half-T bar clasp.

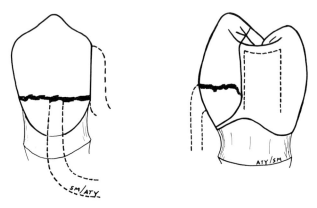

Fig. 19-13. Preferred survey line for an RPI clasp.

retentive arm of the clasp can be successfully placed on glazed porcelain.[1] If occlusal porcelain is planned, the rest seat, guiding plane, and lingual bracing surface are recommended <u>in metal</u>.

7. Invest, cast, and divest the wax pattern. Porcelain is applied, and the crown is surveyed to ensure acceptable contours. The facial porcelain is ground to form an ideal survey line (Figs. 19-12 and 19-13) with a 0.01 inch retentive undercut, and the guiding plane is "refined" if necessary.

8. Characterize and glaze the porcelain. The metal is finished and polished. The crown is then sur-

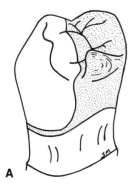 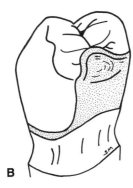

Fig. 19-14. A, Completed porcelain-fused-to-metal crown with a metal occlusal surface. **B,** Completed porcelain-fused-to-metal crown with ceramic occlusal surface.

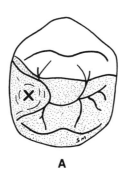 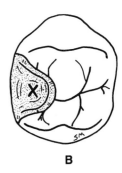

Fig. 19-15. A, Occlusal view of porcelain-fused-to-metal crown with a metal occlusal surface (deepest portion of the rest seat is marked with an X). **B,** Occlusal view of porcelain-fused-to-metal crown with a ceramic occlusal surface (deepest portion of the rest seat is marked with an X).

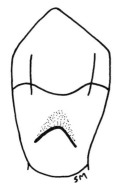 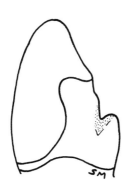

Fig. 19-16. Porcelain-fused-to-metal crown for a mandibular right canine with an inverted v-shaped cingulum rest to support a lingual plate.

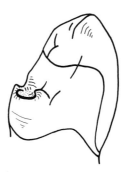 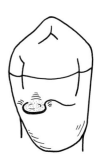

Fig. 19-17. Porcelain-fused-to-metal crown for a maxillary left canine with a mesial rest seat and a distal guiding plane for an RPI clasp assembly.

veyed for the last time. Figs. 19-14 to 19-17 demonstrate completed porcelain-fused-to-metal crowns. Note the contour of the rest seats placed on the anterior teeth (Figs. 19-16 and 19-17).

Problems and Common Errors.

Problems are commonly the result of hasty planning. Often there is insufficient tooth reduction, and this prevents the development of flat guiding surfaces and rest seats of acceptable contour and depth. Frank communication between the dentist and the laboratory technician is essential. Table 19-1 lists common errors associated with the crowned abutment for an RPD and describes the most probable causes of these errors.

Before cementing an artificial crown that serves as an abutment to an RPD, a review with a surveyor for contour and guiding planes is recommended. The occlusal clearance of the rest preparation, especially as it crosses the marginal ridge, should also be carefully evaluated on the mounted casts.

THE OVERDENTURE

The overdenture is a complete or removable partial denture fabricated over retained teeth. It has also been called the tooth-supported denture, overlay denture, telescope denture, or hybrid prosthesis.

Diagnosis and Treatment Planning

Once it has been determined that the remaining teeth are unsuitable for fixed or removable partial dentures, an overdenture should be seriously considered (Table 19-2). A thorough clinical and radiographic examination with diagnostic casts is required for successful diagnosis and treatment planning.

Undercuts and interarch clearance. The diagnostic casts should be carefully evaluated with a dental surveyor for opposing undercuts. The retromylohyoid fossae in the mandible and the tuberosities in the maxillae may oppose the canine eminences. If the treatment plan is designed to retain the canines, the teeth most frequently indicated, the undercuts can

Table 19-1. Common errors associated with the crowned abutment

Error	Cause
1. Guiding plane not parallel with path of insertion.	1. Master cast was not properly oriented on the surveying table, or the surveyor was not used to form the guiding plane, or insufficient proximal reduction. See Figs. 19-2 and 19-3 for correct proximal reduction.
2. Rest seat does not slope toward the tooth.	2. Insufficient tooth reduction, or rest seat was improperly carved in wax. See Figs. 19-2, 19-3, and 19-4 for correct tooth reduction. See Figs. 19-9, 19-11, 19-14, 19-16, and 19-17 for correct contour of rest seats.
3. Rest seat is of inadequate depth.	3. Insufficient tooth reduction, or rest seat was improperly carved. See Figs. 19-2 to 19-4 for correct tooth reduction. See text for proper depth of rest seats.
4. Sharp line angles in rest preparation.	4. Rest seat was improperly carved in wax, or improperly finished and polished. See Figs. 19-9, 19-11, 19-14, 19-16, and 19-17 for correct contour of rest seats.
5. Improperly contoured survey line for retentive arm.	5. Master cast was not properly oriented on the surveying table, or the surveyor was not used when forming the facial surface of the crown. See Figs. 19-8, 19-12, and 19-13 for correct survey line contours.
6. Insufficient or excessive retentive undercut.	6. Surveyor and undercut gauge not used or improperly used. A 0.01 inch undercut in the gingival third of the completed crown is ideal.
7. Hypercontour of the completed crown.	7. Insufficient tooth reduction or improper carving of contours. Lingual ledges predispose to hypercontour; See Fig. 19-7. See Figs. 19-2 to 19-4 for correct tooth reduction.
8. Survey line on the bracing surface is too high.	8. Master cast was not properly oriented on the surveying table, or the surveyor was not used to check the bracing surface, or insufficient tooth reduction. See Fig. 19-7

Table 19-2. Diagnosis and treatment planning flow chart for the overdenture

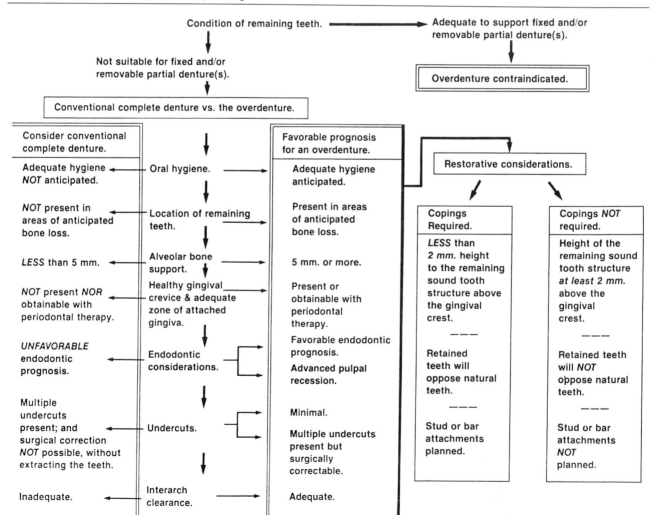

present problems. Undercut maxillary tuberosities are readily corrected surgically. Freidline and Wical have reported a surgical technique for correcting undesirable labial undercuts in the mandible.[2]

Since partial edentulism frequently results in the supraeruption of teeth and alveolar bone, the interarch distance must also be carefully examined. If there is doubt about adequate clearance, the diagnostic casts are mounted on an articulator at an appropriate vertical dimension of occlusion.

Location and number of teeth. Teeth should be retained in areas of anticipated bone loss. Since bone loss is most rapid in the anterior portion of the edentulous mandible,[3-6] priority is given to the retention of the mandibular canines. Ideally, the dentist would plan to retain four mandibular teeth— both canines and one molar on each side of the dental arch. Rarely are more than four teeth retained, but occasionally only one canine is suitable for retention (Fig. 19-18).

Contiguous teeth generally are not retained.[7] The expense of retaining adjacent teeth and the inflammation often associated with the interdental papilla are valid reasons for avoiding retention of contiguous teeth.

Maxillary canines and mandibular molars are commonly retained whenever a maxillary complete denture that will occlude with a mandibular bilateral extension base RPD is anticipated. Since excessive bone loss rarely occurs in the posterior portions of the maxillary residual ridge,[8] there is little justification for retaining maxillary molars. Exceptions include the loss of one tuberosity during extraction and maxillofacial defects.

Periodontal and endodontic considerations. It is important to retain teeth that have a promising prognosis. Teeth possessing only 5 mm of alveolar bone support are still suitable.[9] However, active inflammatory periodontal disease is treated. A healthy gingival crevice and a broad band of attached gingiva (3 to 4 mm of keratinized tissue) must be present or obtainable with periodontal treatment. Slight-to-moderate hypermobility is a minor concern, since dramatic improvement in the crown-to-root ratio usually results in spontaneous remission of the mobility.[10-13]

Since most teeth will require endodontic therapy, the endodontic prognosis must be considered. Teeth with aberrant root canals have a poor prognosis and are not selected when more suitable teeth are available. Teeth that have had previous successful endodontic therapy have priority.

Restorative considerations. It was previously believed that all reduced teeth must be restored with cast gold copings to protect them from dental caries.[14] However, with effective preventive measures, exposed dentin can remain caries free;[13-16] and copings

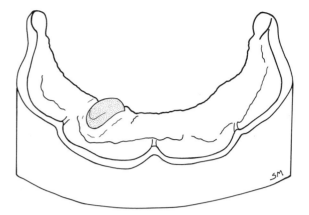

Fig. 19-18. A <u>single</u> canine can support an overdenture.

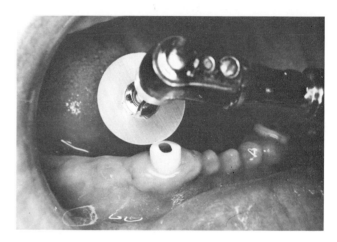

Fig. 19-19. After tooth reduction, silver amalgam is placed in the access to the root canal. The dentin and amalgam are then highly polished.

will not prevent dental caries in the presence of poor oral hygiene.[17]

If adequate tooth structure remains and the tooth can be reduced to a convex contour that extends 2 mm above the gingival crest, a coping is usually not required. After tooth reduction, silver amalgam is placed in the access to the root canal and the dentin and amalgam are highly polished (Fig. 19-19). Covering the exposed dentin with a resin sealant has been recommended.[16] This approach may offer some short-term protection against dental caries, but the sealant would require frequent replacement. A coping is indicated when previous caries or restorations do not provide sufficient tooth structure to create the convex contour 2 mm above the gingival crest.

When natural teeth are present in the opposing arch, severe abrasion and even fracture of the roots of the retained teeth can occur from nocturnal bruxism.[18] Copings encircle the roots and can protect the retained teeth from vertical fractures and abrasion. Copings are also indicated when stud or bar attach-

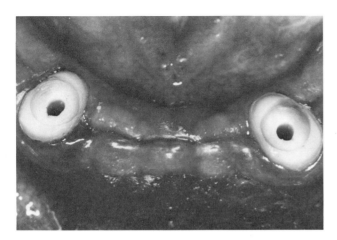

Fig. 19-20. A, Endodontically treated canines prepared for Jackson Rare Earth Magnetic Attachments.

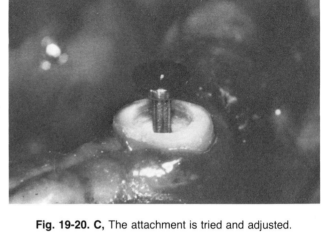

Fig. 19-20. C, The attachment is tried and adjusted.

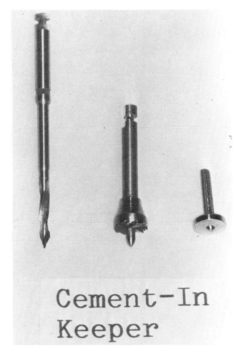

Cement-In Keeper

Fig. 19-20. B, Special rotary instruments were used to prepare a post space 5 to 6 mm deep and countersink the root face to house the attachment, or "keeper."

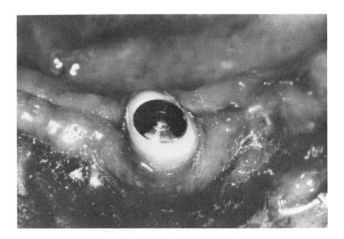

Fig. 19-20. D, The attachment is cemented with a dentin bonding agent and a composite resin luting agent. A coping is not required with sound tooth structure. (Courtesy Thomas R. Jackson, D.D.S., Mt. Airy, N.C.)

ments are planned in conjunction with the overdenture. Various attachments and their use are superbly described by Dr. Raoul H. Boitle in Chapter 22 of Tylman's 7th edition.[19]

Rare earth magnets have been suggested as an alternative to the stud or bar attachment systems.[20,21] Simplicity of design is the primary advantage of these magnetic attachments. There are no mechanical components to wear or break, and copings are often not required (Fig. 19-20). Since the magnets do not depend upon friction to retain the removable prosthesis, there is no loss of retention with repeated insertion and removal of the overdenture (Table 19-3).

Clinical Procedures

Cast overdenture post-copings. An endodontically treated mandibular right canine is used for demonstration (Fig. 19-21).

1. Drill a hole with a No. 4 round bur in the crown of the tooth. A floss threader is used to insert a long piece of dental floss through the hole. The floss is then tied tightly. This floss prevents ingestion or aspiration of the crown. A diamond cylinder is used to amputate the crown 3 mm above the gingival crest (Fig. 19-22).

2. Reduce the tooth with a diamond wheel to a level 1 mm above the gingival crest, and shape the root to reflect the convex contour of the residual ridge (Fig. 19-23).

3. Remove the gutta percha with a Gates Glidden drill. The largest drill size that fits into the canal without binding on the axial walls is selected

Table 19-3. Breakaway retentive force and breakaway cycles were measured using a calibrated SOMFY-TEC gram tension gauge (France) and a precision lathe bed at 0.1 cm/min. Table 3 (Courtesy Thomas R. Jackson, D.D.S., Mt. Airy, N.C.)

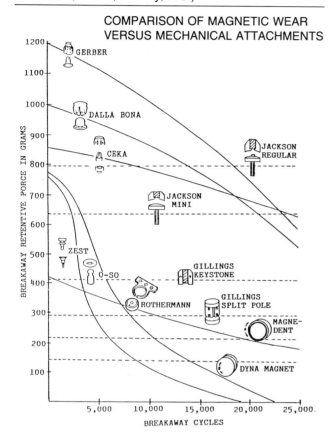

COMPARISON OF MAGNETIC WEAR VERSUS MECHANICAL ATTACHMENTS

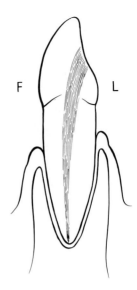

Fig. 19-21. Endodontically treated mandibular right canine.

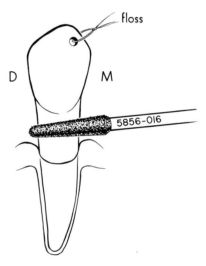

Fig. 19-22. Dental floss is threaded through a hole drilled in the crown, and a diamond cylinder used to amputate the crown 3 mm above the gingival crest.

(Fig. 19-24). An apical seal of 4 mm of gutta percha must be maintained.[22] The adequacy of the preparation and the apical gutta percha can be verified radiographically.

4. Smooth the walls of the post preparation with a Peeso Reamer and eliminate undercuts while removing residual endodontic sealer from the walls of the preparation (Fig. 19-25).
5. Develop an antirotational key with a tapered round-end diamond. This key is placed in the bulkiest area of the root—usually the lingual portion (Fig. 19-26).
6. Place a chamfer finish line with a flame diamond that extends slightly into the gingival crevice. Tooth reduction should be more pronounced on the facial surface to facilitate placement of the artificial tooth and to minimize the bulk of the labial denture flange (Fig. 19-27).
7. Smooth the preparation with a white stone or a fine-grit diamond to eliminate the sharp line angles (Fig. 19-28). The desired tooth preparation allows the placement of a coping that extends 2

mm above the gingival crest, is dome shaped, and free of undercuts[23] (Fig. 19-29). There is a dramatic improvement in the crown-to-root ratio (Fig. 19-30).

Impression procedures. Displacement cord or electrosurgical dilation is used to expose the gingival termination of the tooth preparation without violating the biologic width. Specific procedures for making the impression of the post preparation are outlined in Chapter 22.

Laboratory procedures for cast post-copings. The impression is poured in vacuum-mixed die stone. The dies are sectioned and trimmed. Since the cast post-coping will have an extracoronal and an intracoronal

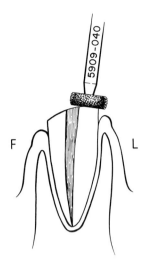

Fig. 19-23. A diamond wheel to reduce the root 1 mm above the gingival crest and shape the root reflecting the convex contour of the residual ridge.

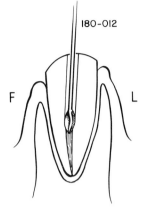

Fig. 19-24. A Gates Glidden drill is guided to remove the gutta percha while maintaining an apical seal of 4 mm of gutta percha.

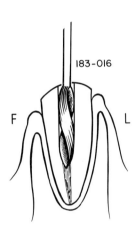

Fig. 19-25. A Peeso Reamer is used to smooth the walls of the post preparation, eliminate undercuts, and remove residual endodontic sealer from the walls of the preparation.

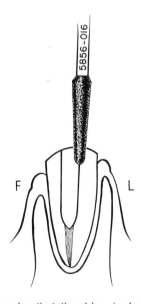

Fig. 19-26. A lingual antirotational key is developed with a tapered round-end diamond.

component, casting expansion must be carefully controlled. To seat without binding, the optimal casting will have a slightly oversized coping and a slightly undersized post.

Die relief can produce an oversized extracoronal casting that seats without binding.[24] A slightly undersized post can be cast by using a quartz investment (Beauty-Cast, Whip-Mix Corp., Louisville, Ky.) and a low-temperature (900° F) burn-out.[25] The combination of die relief and a low-temperature burn-out will control the expansion of the cast post-coping.

When preparing the die, a 50 to 70 μm thickness of die relief is applied to the external surfaces of the die 0.5 mm short of the finish line (Fig. 19-31). Five coats of TRU-FIT (George Taub Products and Fusion Co. Inc., Jersey City, N.J.) will produce a thickness

of approximately 65 μm.[26] This thickness of die relief, twice the 25 to 35 μm thickness often recommended, will compensate for the low-temperature burn-out.

The post-coping is waxed and invested in Beauty-Cast. A single layer of asbestos substitute is used to line the casting ring. If a ring liner is not used in an attempt to "hold back expansion," a distorted casting results due to uneven thermal and setting expansion.

The investment is allowed to bench set. Hygroscopic expansion is <u>not</u> desired; therefore, the ring should <u>not</u> be immersed in water after investing.

After a 45 minute bench set, the ring is placed in a cold oven. The oven is brought to 900° F within 20 minutes. The 900° F burn-out will minimize thermal

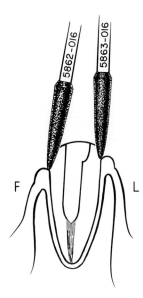

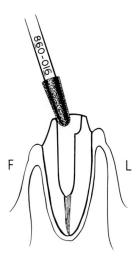

Fig. 19-28. The preparation is smoothed with a white stone or a fine grit diamond.

Fig. 19-27. A flame diamond is used to prepare a chamfer finish line that extends slightly into the gingival crevice. Note that the tooth reduction is more pronounced on the facial surface.

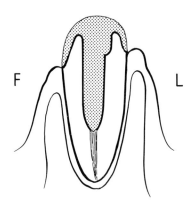

Fig. 19-29. The completed overdenture post-coping.

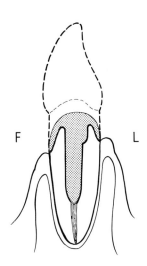

Fig. 19-30. With sufficient tooth reduction and perceptive coping design, a dramatic improvement in the crown-to-root ratio is realized, and there is adequate space for the artificial canine.

expansion of the mold cavity.[25] The ring is held at 900° F for at least 60 minutes and then cast in type III gold. The resultant casting is a slightly undersized post with a slightly oversized coping. Fig. 19-32 illustrates completed cast gold post-copings on mandibular canines.

Overdenture fabrication. Clinical and laboratory techniques for the fabrication of the overdenture do not differ markedly from conventional denture techniques and are detailed in complete denture texts.

Insertion and post insertion care. At the insertion visit, the necessity of maintaining excellent oral hygiene is stressed. All patients are instructed on daily plaque control techniques and on the daily use of a fluoride gel (e.g., 0.4 percent stannous fluoride).[27]

Patients are recalled at 3 month intervals to monitor oral hygiene and to evaluate the condition of the copings, the retained teeth, and the supportive tissues.

Errors

While the procedures involved in the overdenture technique are relatively simple, a disciplined approach to detail is essential.

Overlooked periodontal disease. Gingiva that clinically appears pink may harbor severe infrabony pockets. A careful periodontal examination can reveal hidden disease. If left untreated, periodontitis will progress unabated beneath the denture base, and the diseased tooth will be lost.

Retained teeth left too high. Teeth should be reduced to a convex contour that is 2 mm above the gingival crest. Inordinate height of the retained tooth renders placement of the artificial tooth difficult. Excessive external bulk and/or thin spots in the denture

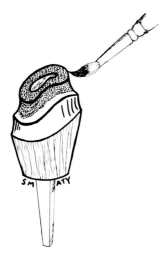

Fig. 19-31. The die for the overdenture post-coping. The external surface of the die is painted with die relief 0.5 mm short of the finish line.

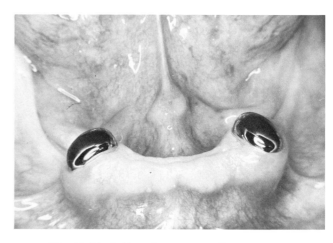

Fig. 19-32. Gold copings on mandibular canines.

base can also occur, and unfavorable lateral stresses are transmitted to the surrounding alveolar bone, accelerating periodontal breakdown.

Overreduction of the retained teeth. The preferred height of the coronal portion of the retained tooth is 2 mm. If the tooth is reduced to less than 1 mm above the soft tissue, or the biologic width is violated, the gingiva will be traumatized and chronically inflamed. If previous caries and/or restorations do not permit preparation of the retained tooth to a convex contour that extends approximately 2 mm above the gingiva, a cast gold coping is fabricated to support the surrounding marginal gingiva.

Multiple undercuts. If numerous undercuts are present at insertion, it may be impossible to seat the overdenture without mutilating the denture base. When planning treatment, the diagnostic cast must be carefully evaluated for undercuts. Perceptive surgical correction of undercuts is usually an option and eliminates the need to over-relieve and/or over-shorten the denture base.

Inadequate interarch clearance. Overdentures with a vertical dimension of occlusion that violates the physiologic rest position of the mandible are not uncommon. If the retained teeth are insufficiently reduced, there may be inadequate space to place the artificial teeth without increasing the vertical dimension of occlusion beyond physiologic tolerance.

The teeth and alveolar bone may have supraerupted and obliterated acceptable interarch clearance, where even overreducing the teeth will <u>not</u> permit placement of the artificial teeth at a physiologic vertical dimension of occlusion. The interarch space must be carefully evaluated during the diagnosis and treatment planning stage.

Problems

Dental caries. The most common problem with the overdenture has been dental caries. Increased awareness of preventive measures has significantly reduced the incidence of caries.[13] Acceptable oral hygiene must be maintained by the patient, and the daily use of a fluoride gel is strongly recommended. Cast gold copings are <u>not</u> the solution to poor oral hygiene <u>nor</u> are submerged roots.

In an attempt to prevent caries, some clinicians have recommended reducing the roots of the teeth below the alveolar crest and covering them with a surgical flap. Initial reaction to this technique was favorable[28-31]; however, a two-year longitudinal study has confirmed a failure rate exceeding 40 percent with submerged roots.[32] This high incidence of failure raises questions about the validity of the submerged root approach.[33]

Periodontal disease. Periodontal disease has been identified as a problem with the retained teeth. Periodontitis will progress rapidly in the presence of poor oral hygiene, and an insidious deterioration of the periodontal tissues is inevitable even in the presence of adequate oral hygiene.[34] Eventually, the zone of attached gingiva may be lost. Surgical correction of the mucogingival defect is usually indicated and should be considered.

Fracture of denture base. Denture base fracture can occur, and is most often associated with thin spots in the base that are the result of incomplete reduction of the retained teeth. The teeth can also create a fulcrum if the denture base is illfitting and not tissue supported, and this will predispose the denture base to fracture.

If the teeth have been sufficiently reduced, the denture base fits well, has adequate thickness, and a high-impact denture base resin (Lucitone 199, The L.D. Caulk Co., Milford, Del.) is used, the incidence of

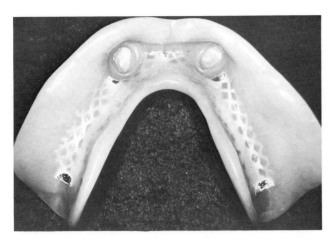

Fig. 19-33. A mandibular overdenture reinforced with a chromium cobalt meshwork.

fracture is significantly reduced. The denture base can also be reinforced with a chromium cobalt meshwork (Fig. 19-33); however, this is not routinely necessary.

Fit of the copings. Inadequate tooth preparation or hasty impression procedures and/or poor laboratory control result in a cast coping that does not fit. Incomplete marginal adaptation of the coping only increases the chances of carious and periodontal breakdown of the retained tooth. The post should not bind on the walls of the post preparation but fit passively, or a vertical fracture of the root results.

Coping retention. Since the teeth are extensively reduced during preparation for copings, a post is commonly indicated to augment the circumferential retention of the coping. The post should be long enough for retention and stabilization without inducing stress, while maintaining 4 mm of gutta percha as an apical seal. Adequate length to the post is more critical when attachments are planned for the overdenture. The post is also vented and sandblasted before cementation, since sandblasting increases the retention of post and cores.[35]

In those instances where advanced pulpal recession has made endodontic therapy unnecessary, long parallel pins are used to retain the coping.

SELECTED REFERENCES

1. Maroso, D.J., Schmidt, J.R., and Blustein, R.: A preliminary study of wear of porcelain when subjected to functional movements of retentive clasp arms, J. Prosthet. Dent. **45**:14-27, 1981.
2. Friedline, C.W., and Wical, K.E.: A method for reducing undesirable labial undercuts for overdenture treatment, J. Prosthet. Dent. **45**:472-473, 1981.
3. Tallgren, A.: The effect of denture wearing on facial morphology, Acta Odontol. Scand. **15**:563-592, 1967.
4. Tallgren, A.: Positional changes in complete dentures—a seven year longitudinal study, Acta Odontol. Scand. **27**:539-561, 1969.
5. Atwood, D.A.: Reduction of residual ridges: a major disease entity, J. Prosthet. Dent. **26**:266-279, 1971.
6. Tallgren, A.: The continuing reduction of the residual alveolar ridges in complete denture wearers: a mixed longitudinal study covering 25 years, J. Prosthet. Dent. **27**:120-132, 1972.
7. Brewer, A.A., and Morrow, R.M.: Overdentures, St. Louis, 1975 The C.V. Mosby Co., p. 34.
8. Kelly, E.: Changes caused by a mandibular removable partial denture opposing a maxillary complete denture, J. Prosthet. Dent. **27**:140-150, 1972.
9. Zamikoff, I.I.: Overdentures-theory and technique, J.A.D.A. **86**:853-857, 1973.
10. Morrow, R.M., Feldman, E.E., Rudd, K.D., and Trovillion, H.M.: Tooth supported complete dentures: an approach to preventive prosthodontics, J. Prosthet. Dent. **21**:513-522, 1969.
11. Brewer, A., and Fenton, A.H.: The overdenture, Dent. Clin. North Am. **17**:723-746, October 1973.
12. Fenton, A.H., and Hahn, N.: Tissue response to overdenture therapy, J. Prosthet. Dent. **40**:492-498, 1978.
13. Toolson, L.B., and Smith, D.E.: A five-year longitudinal study of patients treated with overdentures, J. Prosthet. Dent. **49**:749-756, 1983.
14. Lord, J.L., and Teel, S.: The overdenture: patient selection, use of copings, and follow-up evaluation, J. Prosthet. Dent. **32**:41-51, 1974.
15. Renner, R.P., et al.: Overdenture sequelae: a nine-month report, J. Prosthet. Dent. **48**:377-384, 1982.
16. Renner, R.P., et al.: Periodontal health, prosthodontic factors and microbial ecology of patients treated with overdentures-a 2-½-year report, Quint. In. **15**:645-652, 1984.
17. Becker, C.M., and Kaldahl, W.B.: An overdenture technique designed to protect the remaining periodontium, Int. J. Periodontics Restorative Dent. **4**:28-41, 1984.
18. Bolender, C.L., Smith, D.E., and Toolson, L.B.: Overdentures: their effectiveness and clinical considerations in treating the partially dentate mouth. In Bates, J.F., Neill, D.J., and Preiskel, H.W., Eds: Restoration of the Partially Dentate Mouth, Chicago, 1984, Quintessence Publishing Co., pp. 125-136.
19. Boitel, R.H.: Precision attachments: an overview. In Tylman, S.D., and Malone, W.F.P.: Tylman's Theory and Practice of Fixed Prosthodontics, ed. 7, St. Louis, 1978, The C.V. Mosby Co., pp. 501-568.
20. Gillings, B.R.D.: Magnetic retention for complete and partial overdentures. I, J. Prosthet. Dent. **45**:484-491, 1981.
21. Gillings, B.R.D.: Magnetic retention for overdentures. II, J. Prosthet. Dent. **49**:607-618, 1983.
22. Shillingburg, H.T., and Kessler, J.C.: Restoration of the Endodontically Treated Tooth, Chicago, 1982, Quintessence Publishing Co., p. 21.
23. Warren, A.B., and Caputo, A.A.: Load transfer to alveolar bone as influenced by abutment designs for tooth-supported dentures, J. Prosthet. Dent. **33**:137-148, 1975.
24. Eames, W.B., et al.: Techniques to improve the seating of castings, J.A.D.A. **96**:432-437, 1978.
25. Asgar, K.: Casting restorations. In Clark, J.W., ed.: Clinical Dentistry, Vol. 4, Chap. 7, Philadelphia, 1985, Harper and Row, p. 8.
26. Campagni, W.V., Preston, J.D., and Reisbick, M.H.: Measurements of paint on die spacers used for casting relief, J. Prosthet. Dent. **47**:606-611, 1982.
27. Key, M.C.: Topical fluoride treatment of overdenture abutments, Gen. Dent. **28**:58-60, 1980.
28. Levin, M.P., et al.: Intentional submucosal submergence of non-vital roots, J. Oral Surg. **32**:834-839, 1974.

29. Johnson, D.L., et al.: Histologic evaluation of vital root retention, J. Oral Surg. **32:**829-833, 1974.
30. Guyer, S.E.: Selectively retained vital roots for partial support of overdentures: a patient report, J. Prosthet. Dent. **33:**258-263, 1975.
31. Casey, D.M., and Lauciello, F.R.: A review of the submerged-root concept, J. Prosthet. Dent. **43:**128-132, 1980.
32. MacEntee, M.I., Goldstein, B.M., and Price, C.: Submucosal root retention: A two-year clinical observation, J. Prosthet. Dent. **47:**483-487, 1982.
33. Masterson, M.P.: Retention of vital submerged roots under complete dentures: report of ten patients, J. Prosthet. Dent. **41:**12-15, 1979.
34. Lauciello, F.R., and Ciancio, S.G.: Overdenture therapy: a longitudinal report, Int. J. Periodont. Restor. Dent. **5:**62-71, 1985.
35. Tjan, A.H.L., and Miller, G.D.: Comparison of retentive properties of dowel forms after application of intermittent torsional forces, J. Prosthet. Dent. **52:**238-242, 1984.

BIBLIOGRAPHY

Berg, T., Jr., and Caputo, A.A.: Anterior rests for maxillary removable partial dentures, J. Prosthet. Dent. **39:**139-146, 1978.
Bolouri, A.: Proposed treatment sequence for overdentures, J. Prosthet. Dent. **44:**247-250, 1980.
Crum, R.J.: Tooth supported prostheses (overdentures). In Tylman, S.D., and Malone, W.F.P.: Tylman's Theory and practice of Fixed Prosthodontics, ed. 7, St. Louis, 1978, The C.V. Mosby Co., pp. 569-586.
Crum, R.J., Loiselle, R.J., and Hayes, C.K.: The stud attachment overlay denture and proprioception, J.A.D.A. **82:**583-586, 1971.
Crum, R.J., and Loiselle, R.J.: Oral perception and proprioception: a review of the literature and its significance to prosthodontics, J. Prosthet. Dent. **28:**215-230, 1972.
Crum, R.J., and Rooney, G.E., Jr.: Alveolar bone loss in overdentures: a 5 year study, J. Prosthet. Dent. **40:**610-614, 1978.
Culpepper, W.D., and Moulton, P.: Considerations in fixed prosthodontics, Dent. Clin. North Am. **23:**21-35, January 1979.
Davis, R.K., et al.: A two-year longitudinal study of the periodontal health status of overdenture patients, J. Prosthet. Dent. **45:**358-363, 1981.
Derkson, G.O., and MacEntee, M.M.: Effect of 0.4% stannous fluoride gel on the gingival health of overdenture abutments, J. Prosthet. Dent. **48:**23-26, 1982.
Ettinger, R.L., Taylor, T.D., and Scanddrett, F.R.: Treatment needs of overdenture patients in a longitudinal study: five-year results, J. Prosthet. Dent. **52:**532-537, 1984.
Hammond, R.J., and Beder, O.E.: Increased vertical dimension and speech articulation errors, J. Prosthet. Dent. **52:**401-406, 1984.
Holmes, J.B.: Preparation of abutment teeth for removable partial dentures, J. Prosthet. Dent. **20:**396-406, 1968.
Kay, W.D., and Abes, M.S.: Sensory perception in overdenture patients, J. Prosthet. Dent. **35:**615-619, 1976.
Kratochvil, F.J.: Influence of occlusal rest position and clasp design on movement of abutment teeth, J. Prosthet. Dent. **13:**114-124, 1963.

Levin, A.C., Shifman, A., and Lepley, J.B.: Preservation of occlusal vertical dimension in overdentures, J.A.D.A. **97:**838-839, 1978.
Loiselle, R.J., Crum, R.J., Rooney, G.E., Jr., and Stuever, C.M.: The physiologic basis for the overlay denture, J. Prosthet. Dent. **28:**4-12, 1972.
Malone, W.F.P., Gerhard, R.J., Ensing, H., and Morganelli, J.: Imaginative prosthodontics, J. Acad. Gen. Dent. **18:**21, 1970.
Martin, J.: The overlay denture-treatment planning considerations in cases of advanced periodontal disease with compromised circumstances, Int. J. Periodontics Restorative Dent. **2:**66-79, 1982.
Miller, P.A.: Complete dentures supported by natural teeth, J. Prosthet. Dent. **8:**924-928, 1958.
Morrow, R.M., Powell, J.M., Jameson, W.S., Jewson, L.G., and Rudd, K.D.: Tooth-supported complete dentures: description and clinical evaluation of a simplified technique, J. Prosthet. Dent. 414-424, 1969.
Nagasawa, T., Okane, H., and Tsuru, H.: The role of the periodontal ligament in overdenture treatment, J. Prosthet. Dent. **42:**12-26, 1979.
Parel, S.M.: Overdentures in the maxillofacial prosthetics practice. I. The cancer patient, J. Prosthet. Dent. **50:**522-529, 1983.
Preston, J.D.: Preventing ceramic failures when integrating fixed and removable prostheses, Dent. Clin. North Am. **23:**37-52, January 1979.
Reitz, P.V., Weiner, M.G., and Levin, B.: An overdenture survey: second report, J. Prosthet. Dent. **43:**457-462, 1980.
Renner, R.P., et al.: Four-year longitudinal study of periodontal health status of overdenture patients, J. Prosthet. Dent. **51:**593-598, 1984.
Richard, G.E., et al.: Hemisected molars for additional overdenture support, J. Prosthet. Dent. **38:**16-21, 1977.
Robbins, J.W.: Success of overdentures and prevention of failure, J.A.D.A. **100:**858-862, 1980.
Robbins, J.W.: Periodontal considerations in the overdenture patient, J. Prosthet. Dent. **46:**596-601, 1981.
Rothenberg, L.I.: Overlay dentures for the cleft palate patient, J. Prosthet. Dent. **37:**327-329, 1977.
Strohaver, R.A., and Trovillion, H.M.: Removable partial overdentures, J. Prosthet. Dent. **35:**624-629, 1976.
Thayer, H.H., and Caputo, A.A.: Effects of overdentures upon remaining oral structures, J. Prosthet. Dent. **37:**374-381, 1977.
Toolson, L.B., and Smith, D.E.: A 2-year longitudinal study of overdenture patients. I. Incidence and control of caries on overdenture abutments, J. Prosthet. Dent. **40:**486-491, 1978.
Toolson, L.B., Smith, D.E., and Phillips, C.V.: A 2-year longitudinal study of overdenture patients. II. Assessment of periodontal health of overdenture abutments, J. Prosthet. Dent. **47:**4-11, 1982.
Welker, W.A., and Kramer, D.C.: Waxing tooth copings for overdentures, J. Prosthet. Dent. **32:**668-671, 1974.
White, J.T.: Abutment stress in overdentures, J. Prosthet. Dent. **40:**13-27, 1978.

20

Steven Duke

CROWN AND FIXED PARTIAL DENTURE RESINS

The use of synthetic resins has expanded recently to become an essential part of prosthodontic treatment. Resin materials may be indicated for an individual restoration or as a veneer over a casting. As an esthetic alternative to porcelain, the resin restoration offers the advantages of low cost, convenient repair, ease of fabrication, and no abrasion of opposing dentitions. Whereas acrylic resins have dominated resin applications for years, more refined polymers have emerged and assumed a more extensive role. Current resin materials are not a replacement for dental porcelain, but clinical situations arise when resin is indicated; e.g., function and economics.

TYPES OF SYNTHETIC RESINS

Currently used resins may be classified as:
Type I (acrylic)
Type II (dimethacrylate)
Type III (composite)

The acrylic resins are powder-liquid systems based on methyl methacrylate polymer beads and monomer liquid. They are similar to the self-cured acrylic resins available for custom trays and denture bases. The dimethacrylate resins replaced the methyl methacrylate with higher-molecular-weight dimethacrylate monomers. Because these monomers are high boiling and difunctional, they are cured at higher temperatures and yield cross-linked resins that are wear resistant. The composite resins are similar to composite restorative filling materials. They contain dimethacrylate monomers, usually BIS-GMA or related monomers, or urethane dimethyacrylates and inorganic filler.

Properties

The properties often investigated that are critical to the clinical behavior of resins include wear resistance, color stability, water sorption, coefficient of thermal expansion, hardness, compressive strength, and tensile strength. While direct correlations have not been firmly established between laboratory properties and clinical behavior, they are helpful in understanding the limitations of resins and offer guidance when selecting a material for a patient.

Early resin formulations were low-strength resins with high water sorption and low hardness.[1] As a result, wear resistance, color stability, and deformation were noted.[2,3] A common clinical finding, shown in Fig. 20-1, is an accelerated loss of material, exposing the metal framework. This requires repair with a direct filling resin or fabrication of a new restoration.

The disparity in thermal expansion between the resin and metal framework, including a lack of adhesion of resin to the metal, precipitates the percolation of oral fluids at the resin-metal interface, which contributes to a discoloration of the resin and corrosion of non-noble casting alloys.[4-6]

The low modulus of elasticity and proportional limit associated with the resin veneering materials necessitates a suitably designed metal framework for support during function to prevent plastic deformation.[2] Processing porosity also leads to weakness of the resin, opaque appearance, potential for incubating microorganisms, and tissue irritation due to roughness.[7,8]

The deficiencies of the early resins were obvious, so these materials have been restricted in favor of porcelain for esthetic restorations. Unfortunately, porcelain can be potentially destructive when opposing natural teeth and certain restorative materials (Fig. 20-2). Recommendations focus on avoiding occlusal contacts in porcelain, despite highly glazed surfaces.[9,10]

However, patient demands for anterior esthetics commonly result in compromise. As shown in Fig. 20-

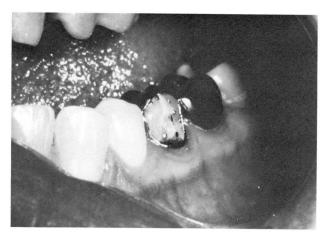

Fig. 20-1. A common clinical result for early acrylic resin veneers was poor wear resistance.

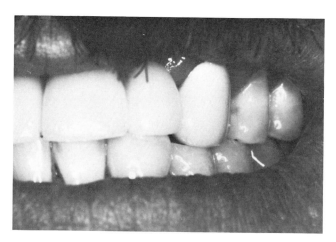

Fig. 20-3. A, A maxillary porcelain fixed partial denture with canine incisal surface in porcelain.

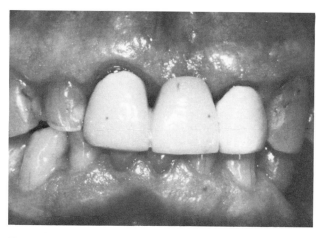

Fig. 20-2. A, Porcelain fixed partial denture with functioning lingual porcelain surfaces.

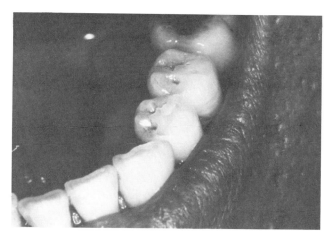

Fig. 20-3. B, Within 5 years patient's occlusion has changed to a group function with abnormal porcelain wear evident on the mandibular canine and premolar.

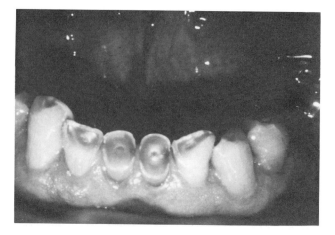

Fig. 20-2. B, Severe wear of opposing teeth.

3, a patient with an anterior protected disclusion developed a group function because of abnormal wear within 5 years. The development of a nondestructive,

wear-resistant resin esthetic material is warranted to meet clinical demands.

A new generation of resin-based veneers for prosthodontics has been introduced as a result of technological advancements with composite filling materials. In contrast to the unfilled acrylic resins, the composite resins contain reinforcing filler particles in the form of silica. Patterned after the "microfilled" restorative composite resins, the silica is routinely introduced in the form of prepolymerized polymer complexes (Fig. 20-4).

Various systems have been developed for the polymerization of these resins, but visible light is the most popular activation and can be used alone or combined with vacuum or heat. One system utilizes high temperature and pressure to accomplish polymerization.

Laboratory testing of these materials has been limited, but initial results are encouraging, with acknowl-

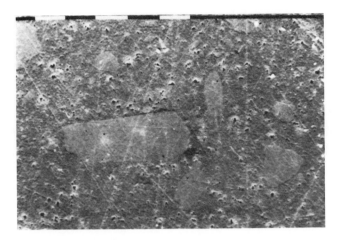

Fig. 20-4. "Microfilled" composite resin with prepolymerized polymer complexes as filler (×1000).

edged improvement in mechanical and physical properties compared to original resin formulations.[11] Table 20-1 lists the laboratory tests of commercial resin materials. Improvements in the physical properties, including better wear resistance, were attained.[12,13] Exceptions have been the low-yield strengths reported in one investigation.[14] Deformation of the resins is possible when they are subjected to functional loads, so the functional forces should be limited.

Clinical evaluations of the new resin materials have not been extensively performed. A one-year investigation demonstrated minimal wear of a material used predominately as a veneer over castings.[15] Until more extensive clinical evaluation has been accomplished, the longevity of the composite veneering resins remains unpredictable.

MANIPULATION AND PROCESSING TECHNIQUES
Acrylic Resins

The use of acrylic resins has recently diminished in crown and FPD procedures. Several techniques for manipulation and processing have been extensively described in the previous edition of this text (see detailed description in Tylman's Theory and Practice of Fixed Prosthodontics, ed. 7).

A technique involving one acrylic resin for the esthetic veneering of castings is still used to a limited extent. The polymer is moistened with a special monomer and applied in small increments to the metal casting (Pyroplast). It is cured directly, exposed to 275° F for 8 minutes. Then the gingival and the incisal colors are applied and blended; curing then follows each lamination. A special curing oven is used that controls the temperature and distance at which the restoration is maintained. After being fully processed, the veneer is finished and polished.

Composite Resins

The first composite resin formulation to be used for crown and FPD work was a chemically activated resin, Isosit. The resin material is supplied in preactivated capsules in various shades. The restoration is formed from the resin dough and placed into a pressure unit that operates a 6 bar pressure with a temperature of 120° C for 5 minutes.

The majority of composite resin materials use visible light to initiate polymerization. The composite resins are supplied as a single paste containing a photoinitiation system. One system uses a diketone, camphoroquinone, and a reducing agent, N, N-dimethylaminoethylmethacrylate. When the material is exposed to visible light at a wavelength of approximately 470 mm, the diketone is transformed to an excited state and combines with the reducing agent to form a complex that is diminished by the free radicals of polymerization.

Composite resins in direct contact with air during polymerization develop unpolymerized surface layers as a result of oxygen being diffused into the resin. One commercial system (Fig. 20-5) provides for light curing under vacuum to overcome air inhibition. The restoration is formulated in small increments with exposure for 5 seconds under an alpha light unit. The final restoration is then cured for 15 minutes in the beta light unit under vacuum. Other commercial systems bulk pack the restoration on the die or casting and process for various times with visible light at room temperature or at elevated temperatures.

Table 20-1. Properties of Prosthodontic Resins

	Compressive strength (MPa)	Diametral tensile strength (MPa)	Hardness (KHN)	Moldulus of elasticity (MPa)	Abrasion resistance (vol. loss, mm³)	% weight inorganic filler
Biolon	55	14	16	2206	2.8	6.7
Dentacolor	331	32	20	2414	0.8	51.8
Isosit-N	310	37	14	1862	1.1	30.7
Visio-Gem	338	30	21	2483	1.0	39.2

From Schelb, E., et. al., J. Prosthet. Dent. **58**:246, 1987.

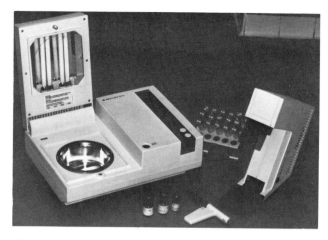

Fig. 20-5. Commercial crown and fixed partial denture resin that utilizes light curing under vacuum (Visio-Gem, ESPE-Premier).

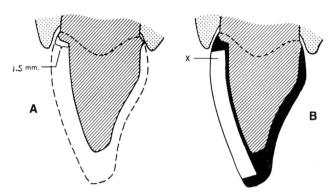

Fig. 20-7. Perceptively prepared tooth. **A,** Dotted line is contour of original tooth. Cervical finishing line on surfaces to be veneered must be a shoulder, at least 1.5 mm wide. **B,** Composite resin veneer crown on tooth; 1.5 mm shoulder permits composite veneer to extend apically to free margin of gingival tissues and to be thick enough at X to effectively mask underlying metal without being overcontoured.

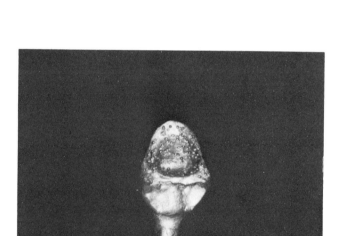

Fig. 20-6. **A,** Example of retentive beads on framework to hold composite.

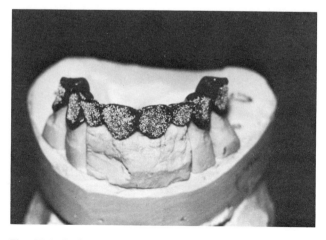

Fig. 20-6. **B,** Glass beads are commonly used on wax pattern to gain required retention.

RESIN RETENTION

The retention of crown and FPD resins to underlying metal frameworks is accomplished with mechanical retention or an intermediary coupling agent. The use of retentive beads, loops, or ladders has been suggested since the introducion of acrylic resins as a veneer material in the early 1940s. There must be sufficient mechanical retention without sacrificing the strength of the metal framework or influencing esthetics (Fig. 20-6). Opaque layers of material are applied so that the retentive patterns are not totally obstructed, thus leaving the opaque layer as the only material locked into the retentive patterns. Failures upon debonding occur at the resin-opaque interface; if the final resin engages the retentive patterns, greater retention results.[16]

The use of adhesive coupling agents to retain crown FPD resins is relatively new. One system based on the principle of flaming silica onto the casting alloy has reported retentive bond strengths comparable to those obtained with conventional retentive methods.[17,18] Alternate commercial preparations are also available, and despite limited research, the results are encouraging.

Another form of retaining resin materials to base metal alloys involves electrolytically etching a microretentive surface. Adapted from the technology of resin-bonded retainers (RBRs), extremely high bond strengths are accomplished with this technique.

The obvious advantages of the new techniques of resin retention over conventional beads are a more conservative preparation, reduced cost, and improved esthetics. A disadvantage to the alternative retention systems is the difficulty in clinical repairs of fracture veneers. If a fracture occurs at the opaque-metal in-

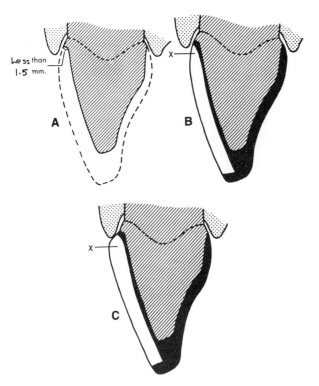

Fig. 20-8. Hastily prepared tooth. **A,** Cervical shoulder on this preparation is less than 1.5 mm wide. **B,** Inadequate shoulder width permits composite veneer to extend apically to free margin of gingival tissues, but veneer is too thin at X to effectively mask underlying metal. **C,** Veneer on this crown is overcontoured at X to mask metal. Resultant restoration does not duplicate size and shape of original tooth, as shown by dotted line in A.

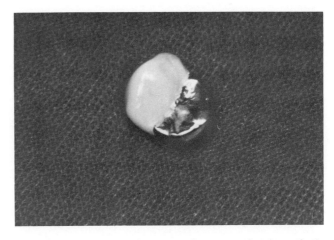

Fig. 20-9. A, Example of a composite veneer that for esthetic reasons was extended onto occlusal table short of holding contacts.

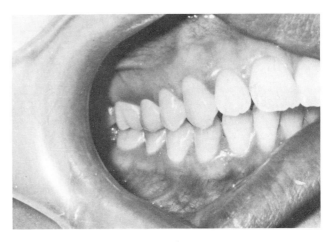

Fig. 20-9. B, Composite veneer on second premolar is protected due to a canine disclusion on this patient.

terface, bonding a resin chairside requires additional mechanical retention.

CLINICAL APPLICATIONS

Crown and FPD resins have numerous clinical applications. If the dentist is familiar with the limitations of these materials and is knowledgeable about clinical techniques, these resins can be a vital adjunct to prosthodontics. Techniques discussed include the partial veneer restoration, complete resin restorations, pontics for resin-bonded retainers, and custom laminate veneers.

Tooth Preparation for Resin Veneer Crowns

The restoration of a tooth with an artificial veneer crown duplicates the morphology of the natural tooth to ensure the health of the dentition. With this goal in mind, adequate tooth preparation is performed to accommodate the demands of function and esthetics. In areas where the resin material provides esthetics, a minimum depth of tooth preparation of 1.5 to 2 mm is required to adequately mask the underlying metal framework, with sufficient space for mechanical retention of the resin (Fig. 20-7). A beveled shoulder is

prepared on the labial surfaces and into the interproximal surfaces to accommodate the veneer. The shoulder blends into a chamfer finish line on surfaces without a veneer. Most tooth surfaces to be veneered possess a vertical convexity. They should exhibit a similar convexity after preparation if the veneer is to have adequate thickness to duplicate original tooth size without overcontouring the restoration (Fig. 20-8).

It is advisable to restrict occlusal function to the casting alloy and protect the veneer resin materials due to weak wear resistance. The occlusal or incisal boundaries of the veneer are extended for esthetics without subjecting the resin to excessive occlusal loading. Identifying the maximum extension of the veneer onto the occlusal of incisal table requires an awareness of the patient's occlusal patterns. For example, if a patient possesses an anterior protected disclusion, a veneer for a premolar can be extended onto the occlusal surface short of the centric holding areas (Fig. 20-9). Conversely, if a patient possesses a group func-

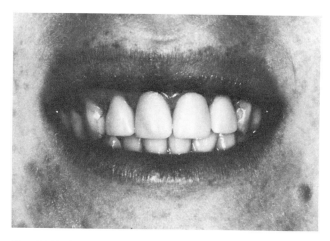

Fig. 20-10. Maxillary incisors are restored with processed treatment composite restorations. Restorations were left in place for 6 months until posterior restorative needs were accomplished.

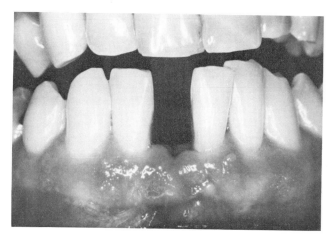

Fig. 20-11. Resin-bonded retainer application. **A,** Prepared teeth for resin-bonded retainer. Minimal occlusal function present to limit stresses to pontic.

tion occlusal relationship, excessive forces can cause premature fracture of the veneer. Therefore, acrylic-veneered gold FPDs are commonly indicated for patients with a reduced interocclusal relationship. Repair of fractured or discolored facings can then be satisfactorily accomplished with light-activated resins.

Complete Crown Restorations

Resin-based materials for complete crowns can only be described realistically as interim restorations, but there are specific clinical situations when they are indicated. Developing esthetic and suitably contoured restorations with mandibular central and lateral incisors is arduous. In most cases, extensive tooth reduction is required to fabricate esthetically pleasing veneered castings. A more conservative preparation is possible when the resin materials are used to minimize the underlying framework. Sufficient preparation is made to allow room for the composite material (1 to 1.5 mm), and a complete crown is fabricated with composite resin. This technique is also helpful in managing a case having a guarded prognosis. When occlusal conditions are favorable, i.e., with minimal function, reasonable success can be anticipated for an otherwise difficult clinical situation.

The composite materials are also indicated for fabricating custom treatment restorations. Teeth requiring a more extensive restorative treatment can be stabilized with heat-processed temporaries for a prolonged period (Fig. 20-10).

Pontics for Resin-Bonded Retainers

The pontic of an acid-etched, resin-bonded retainer has been traditionally fabricated with dental porcelain. The use of porcelain requires that the metal be com-

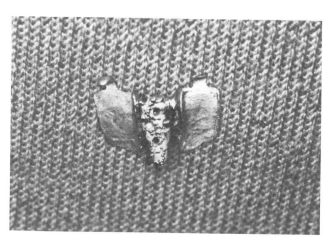

Fig. 20-11. B, Fabricated retainer framework with mechanical retention design. Gingival surface of pontic may be in alloy to facilitate hygiene.

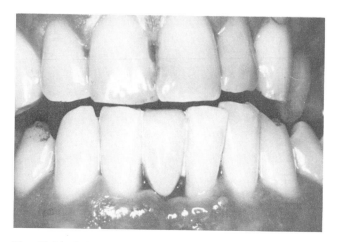

Fig. 20-11. C, Bonded appliance in place with limited function on composite pontic.

patible with porcelain. This restriction, combined with the requirement that the alloy be electrolytically etched, limits the alloys used with this technique. The porcelain pontic also substantially increases the cost of the appliance.

A laboratory heat-cured composite material for an esthetically desirable pontic is a reasonable solution to these concerns. The cost of the prosthesis is less, due to decreased laboratory time and ease of fabrication. Alloy selection is more expensive if the alloy can be electrolytically etched.

The situation shown in Fig. 20-11 is an indication for a resin-bonded retainer. These prostheses are usually designed to have limited function on the pontics. The tissue surface of the pontic can be in alloy, which produces a favorable tissue response with less plaque.

Custom Laminate Veneers

One of the most popular uses for the crown and FPD composite resins has been in the fabrication of custom laminate veneers. The patient's teeth are minimally prepared to allow for resin material and an impression is made. The depth of enamel reduction is normally 0.5 to 1 mm. to ensure attractive results without overcontouring the labial surface of the restoration. The poured casts are used to fabricate the acrylic laminate veneers. Using a composite resin on etched enamel surfaces, the laboratory then fabricates the heat-cured laminates that are to be bonded by the dentist (Fig. 20-12).

Additional Applications

The composite resin veneering materials have recently been considered for use with implant techniques. These materials are believed to be more "forgiving" than porcelain or alloy surfaces and also support the requirements of implant prostheses.

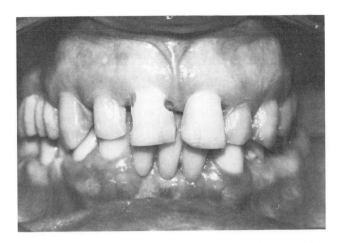

Fig. 20-12. B, Teeth to be veneered are prepared in enamel to a depth of 0.5 mm. Preparation into dentin should be avoided. The preparations are carried cervical to the height of the free gingival margins.

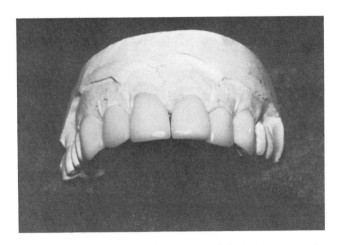

Fig. 20-12. C, Custom laminates are fabricated in composite resin in the laboratory.

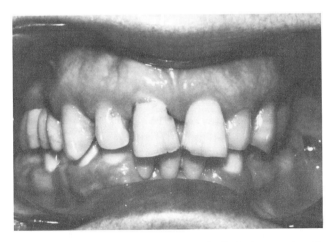

Fig. 20-12. Custom laminate veneers. **A,** Patient presents with compromised anterior esthetics. A conservative treatment is possible due to patient's occlusion.

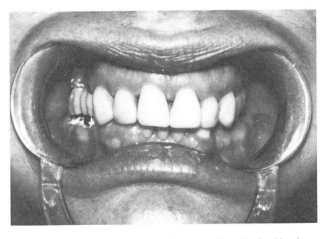

Fig. 20-12. D, The prepared teeth are acid etched with phosphoric acid for 60 seconds. The custom laminates are then bonded to the etched enamel with the use of a light cured composite resin. (Courtesy Dr. T. Girvan. San Antonio, Tex.)

Composite resins have also been used for custom occlusal splint therapy. A diagnostic waxup of the proposed occlusion with mounted casts is created initially. An index of the wax surfaces is then accomplished in a clear matrix material to form the heat-polymerized resin surfaces. This technique commonly requires a cast framework, such as a removable partial, to support the resin material.

Future Research

The use of composite materials for prosthodontic applications has progressed in recent years and ongoing research should unveil additional applications. As composite materials improve, more definitive and diversified uses may be possible.

SELECTED REFERENCES

1. Peyton, F.A., and Craig, R.G.: Current evaluation of plastics in crown and bridge prosthesis, J. Prosthet. Dent. **13:**743-753, 1963.
2. Phillips, R.W.: Skinner's Science of Dental Materials, ed. 8, Philadelphia, 1982, W.F. Saunders Co., pp. 216-247.
3. Craig, R.G.: Restorative Dental Materials, ed. 7, St. Louis, 1985, The C.V. Mosby Co., pp. 225-242.
4. Lamstein, A., and Bleachman, H.: Marginal seepage around acrylic resin veneers in gold crowns, J. Prosthet. Dent. **6:**706-709, 1956.
5. Soremark, R., and Bergman, B.: Studies on the permeability of acrylic facing material in gold crowns, a laboratory investigation using Na 22, Acta Odontol. Scand. **19:**297-305, 1961.
6. Issa, H.: Marginal leakage in crowns with acrylic resin facings, J. Prosthet. Dent. **19:**281-287, 1968.
7. Tylman, S.D.: Theory and Practice of Crown and Fixed Partial Prosthodontics (Bridge), ed. 6, St. Louis, 1970, The C.V. Mosby Co., pp. 837-856.
8. Swartz, M.L., and Phillips, R.W.: A study of adaptation of veneers to cast gold crowns, J. Prosthet. Dent. **7:**817-822, 1957.
9. Mahalick, J.A., Knapp, F.J., and Weiter, E.J.: Occlusal wear in prosthodontics, J.A.D.A. **82:**154-159, 1971.
10. Monasky, G.E., and Taylor, D.F.: Studies on the wear of porcelain enamel, and gold, J. Prosthet. Dent. **25:**299-406, 1971.
11. Jones, R.M., Moore, B.K., Dykema, R.W., and Goodacre, C.J.: Comparison of physical properties of four prosthodontic veneering resins, J. Dent. Res., vol. 65, special issue, abstract no. 1281, 1986.
12. Staffanou, R.S., Hembree, J.H., Rivers, J.A., and Myers, M.L.: Abrasion resistance of three types of esthetic veneering materials, J. Prosthet. Dent. **53:**309-311, 1985.
13. Nathanson, D., Osorio, J., and Chai, T.: In vitro abrasion resistance of new crown and bridge polymers, J. Dent. Rest. **46:**515-518, 1981.
14. Greener, E.H., and Duke, E.S.: Chemistry and physical properties of crown and bridge veneering resins, J. Dent. Res., vol. 65, special issue, abstract no. 530, 1986.
15. Leinfelder, K.F.: Clinical evaluation of crown and bridge composite resin veneering materials, J. Dent. Rest., vol. 65, special issue, abstract no. 531, 1986.
16. Nicholls, J.I., and Nakanishi, D.R.: Tensile bond strengths of veneering resins to opaque systems, Quint. Dent. Technol. **10:**35-38, 1986.
17. Twesme, D.A., Lacefield, W.R., and O'Neal, S.J.: Effect of silicoating and etching on alloy-composite bonding, J. Dent. Res., vol. 65, special issue, abstract no. 1304, 1986.
18. Re. Gerald et al: Various forms of metal retention for resin bonded retainer, J. Prosthet. Dent. in press.

21

**Franklin Garcia-Godoy,
Jerry W. Nicholson,
and John W. McLean**

GLASS IONOMER CEMENTS: CLINICAL APPLICATIONS

Glass ionomer cements were invented by Wilson and Kent[1,2] and developed for clinical use by McLean and Wilson.[3] The glass ionomer cements have strength characteristics similar to those of the silicate cements,[4] but they are more resistant to acid attack like the polycarboxylate cements. They are only mildly irritating to pulpal tissue, and the extent of the inflammatory response is moderated by any residual dentin. The glass ionomer cements have the added advantage of translucency.

Glass ionomer and polycarboxylate cements bond to enamel and dentin because they adhere to substrates by polar and ionic attractions (physicochemical adhesion). They are based on the hardening reaction between ion-leachable glasses and aqueous solutions of homopolymers or copolymers of acrylic acid. Additions of tartaric acid improve the working and setting characteristics. On mixing the two components, hydrated protons from the liquid penetrate the surface layers of the powder particles. Cations (mainly Al and Ca) are displaced and the aluminosilicate network is degraded to a hydrated siliceous gel. Cations of fluoride complexes migrate into the aqueous phase of the cement paste, where metallic salt bridges are formed between the long chains of charged polycarboxylate ions, cross-linking them and causing the aqueous phase to gel and the cement to set. Toxic monomers are not involved. The setting reaction is represented:

$$\text{Glass (base)} + \text{Polyelectrolyte (acid)} =$$
$$\text{Polyhydrogel (salt)} + \text{Silica gel}$$

Calcium ions are more rapidly bound to the polyacrylate chains than aluminum ions and are responsible for the cement's initial set. Later, aluminum salt bridges form and the cement hardens; the high ionic potential of the trivalent aluminum ion ensures a stronger cross-linking than with divalent ions alone.

Water is the reaction medium, and additions of tartaric acid improve working and setting characteristics.

The glass ionomer cements have a double setting reaction that confers interesting rheological properties on the hardening paste. Initially, the cement sets enough to permit carving similar to amalgam (calcium ion-exchange); later it sets hard (aluminum ion-exchange).

The glass ionomers adhere to wet dentin because they are polar polymers that compete with water for the polar enamel surface. Glass ionomer is a highly ionic polymer with a multiplicity of COOH groups that form strong hydrogen bonds to enamel apatite. Wilson[5] also considers that attachment to collagen in dentin via NH_2 or COOH on pendant side chains is possible. Recently, it has been demonstrated that phosphate and calcium ions are displaced from synthetic apatite by sodium polyacrylate solution, forming a calcium phosphate–polyacrylate crystalline structure acting as an interface between tooth enamel and the set cement.[5]

Glass ionomer cements possess impressive compressive strength of 140 to 200 MPa, but are weak in flexural strength (10 to 40 MPa). They are adhesive and, with the fluoride leach, possess cariostatic properties. The matrix of the glass ionomer cements contains sheathed droplets of calcium fluoride,[5] so the hardened cement paste continually releases fluoride ions.[6-9] Because the cement becomes attached via ionic and polar bonds to the enamel and dentin, the intimate molecular contact facilitates fluoride ion exchange with the hydroxyl ions in the apatite of the surrounding enamel. Glass ionomers are also biologically compatible with the tooth structure and pulp if placed over dentin. In deep carious lesions or in direct contact with the pulp, glass ionomers are irritants.[10]

APPLICATIONS OF GLASS IONOMER CEMENTS
Fissure Sealing

The use of glass ionomer cements for fissure sealing and filling was first proposed by McLean and Wilson in 1974.[11] Sparse studies have evaluated the clinical performance of glass ionomers as fissure sealants.

Fast-setting glass ionomer cements such as Ketac-Bond, Ketac-Silver (Espe/Premier), GC Lining (GC International), and Chem-Fil Junior (DeTrey/Dentsply) are capable of fissure sealing. These cements have a bond strength to enamel that exceeds their cohesive strength, and they are resistant to weak acids if the cement is confined to the fissure. Newer metal-reinforced cements such as Ketac-Silver are markedly improved in abrasion resistance compared to the regular materials, and may be used for the more extensive fissure sealing.

Technique for sealing fissures. The tooth is isolated with a rubber dam or cotton rolls. A thorough prophylaxis is performed followed by a 10-second application of 10 to 35 percent polyacrylic acid solution in a cotton pellet and eased into the fissures with a fine dental explorer. The polyacrylic acid solution cleans the surface and removes the smear layer. The polyacrylic acid is rinsed for 30 seconds and the surface dried with compressed air for a few seconds, but not dehydrated. The cement is applied to the fissures with a fine dental explorer or injected. During the initial set (usually 2 to 4 minutes after insertion) the glass ionomer is protected from moisture contamination. This protection is achieved with Burlew's dry foil (that is burnished into position) or with Kerr's green occlusal indicator wax. After the requisite setting time specified by the manufacturer, the glass ionomer is trimmed with a fine round diamond or carbide burs. Strategic removal of the cement is also accomplished by gentle scraping with a sharp spoon excavator.

Fissure Filling

A tooth exhibiting a sticky fissure or minimal fissure caries is considered for fissure filling with glass ionomer. Pit and fissure caries are difficult to diagnose in the early stages, since histologically the white spot lesion forms bilaterally on the walls of the fissure,[12] but the fissure that appears caries-free may histologically exhibit an early lesion. The "sticky fissure" may be caries-free, since a sharp explorer can enter a patient's fissure and bind on the walls, producing the tactile sensation of carious dentin. Visual examination rather than tactile exploration may be a more reliable method.

In addition, the use of bite-wing radiographs is essential. A detailed diagnostic procedure has been presented by Kidd.[13] Where radiographic evidence indicates caries, mechanical preparation is essential.

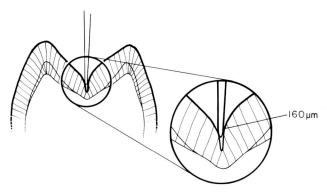

Fig. 21-1. Where the explorer enters to a depth of 1 mm or more, it is likely that the fissure opening is at least 160 μm.

These preparations are minimal and remove only the carious dentin. If there is no radiographic evidence of caries, but the fissure is stained and difficult to clean, a fissure sealant or filling should be placed.

Technique for filling fissures. The tooth is isolated with a rubber dam or cotton rolls, and the fissures inspected with a sharp explorer. If the tip of the explorer enters the fissure, it indicates that the fissure is patent with an opening of at least 80 μm—about the diameter of the explorer tip.[14] If the explorer enters to a depth of 1 mm or more, it is likely that the fissure opening is at least 160 μm (Fig. 21-1). The fissures are difficult to clean, and as Kidd[13] demonstrated, prone to caries in the dentin even when the enamel is enriched with fluoride.

A fissure filling does not involve preparation of an occlusal cavity, but rather widening of the fissure and removing the carious dentin using slow-speed handpieces, preferably with fiberoptics and/or magnification.[13,26]

The procedure is as follows:
1. Enter the fissure using high speed and water spray with a fine diamond and slightly widen the fissure to explore the base. The operation is termed "fissure cleaning."
2. Check with an explorer and fiberoptic light to detect any carious dentin and remove with a small round bur. Pulpal approximation requires lining with calcium hydroxide.
3. Apply a 10 to 35 percent solution of polyacrylic acid for 10 seconds. This cleans the surface and removes the smear layer, but does not open cut dentinal tubules.
4. Clean the debris and acid with air-water spray and dry the tooth with warm air for a few seconds without dehydrating.
5. Inject the glass ionomer cement into the fissure and burnish Burlew's dry foil to position, or use Kerr's green occlusal indicator wax. The following materials could be used as fissure restoratives: Ketac-Fil, Ketac-Silver (Espe/Premier),

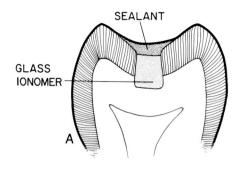

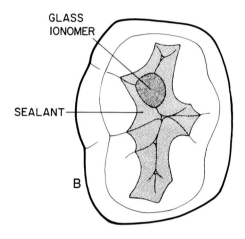

Fig. 21-2. The preventive glass ionomer restoration.

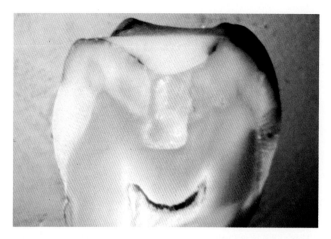

Fig. 21-3. Preventive glass ionomer restoration showing dye penetration short of sealant-glass ionomer junction. (Reprinted with permission from Comp. Cont. Educ. Dent. **9**:88-94, 1988.)

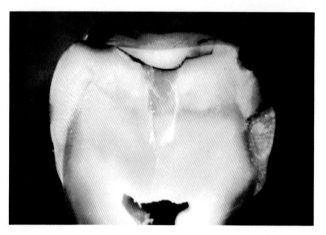

Fig. 21-4. Preventive glass ionomer restoration showing dye penetration to and along the sealant-glass ionomer interface. Dye penetration is not observed along the axial walls. (Reprinted with permission from Comp. Cont. Educ. Dent. **9**:88-94, 1988.)

Fuji II (GC Int. Corp.), Chem-Fil II (DeTrey/Dentsply), and Hy-Bond (Shofu Mfg. Co.).

6. After the setting time specified by the manufacturer, the filling should be trimmed with fine round diamond or carbide burs. A sharp excavator is also an advantage in removing excess without damaging fine edges. Ketac-Silver is fast-setting and could be trimmed under water spray after setting 5 minutes. Other materials may require between 8 and 15 minutes.

7. Immediately after trimming, the cement is coated with varnish or a light-cured bonding resin. The more quickly the protective coating is applied, the better the result. Ketac-Silver does <u>not</u> require protection and can be burnished.

Glass ionomer cements have been used as fissure fillings for the past 14 years. The improved abrasion resistance of Ketac-Silver provides the option of more extensive occlusal usage.[15] More clinical studies are necessary, however, to establish their long-term success.

Preventive Glass Ionomer Restorations

Preventive glass ionomer restorations have been placed in minute occlusal cavities where carious lesions have barely extended into dentin (Fig. 21-2).

The procedure is similar to the preventive resin restoration,[16] but a glass ionomer fills the cavity. The glass ionomer is then covered with a fissure sealant resin that extends into the occlusal fissures. Glass ionomer is indicated as the restoration, based on its adhesive properties to enamel and dentin, and its ability to release fluoride. The latter property enhances cariostatic action if there is microleakage of the fissure sealant.[17,18] Preventive glass ionomer restorations demonstrated less microleakage (8 percent) than preventive resin restorations (16 to 25 percent), and in the cases with leakage, dye penetration stopped at the glass ionomer-enamel interface (Figs. 21-3 and 21-4).

Clinical technique. Local anesthesia is administered to minimize patient discomfort. A rubber dam is used to prevent moisture contamination of the glass ionomer and the etched surfaces. The occlusal surface is cleaned with a slurry of flour of pumice in a rubber

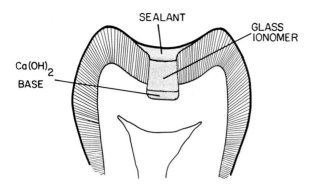

Fig. 21-5. The preventive glass ionomer restoration. If the carious lesion extends deeply into dentin, a thin layer of calcium hydroxide should be carefully placed in the bottom of the preparation. If the preparation is not deep, the calcium hydroxide liner is not necessary. (Reprinted with permission from Quint. Int. **17**:617-619, 1986, published by the Quintessence Publishing Co., Inc., Chicago.)

cup mounted in a slow-speed handpiece. The tooth is then rinsed with water. The procedure is:

1. A small round bur or a No. 330 carbide bur just large enough to remove the caries is used to prepare a small cavity. Retention is not necessary, and a cavosurface bevel can be placed, but is not mandatory.

2. If the carious lesion extends deep into dentin, a thin layer of an acid-resistant calcium hydroxide liner is carefully placed on the floor of the cavity (Fig. 21-5).[16]

3. The cavity is rinsed with water and gently dried with oil-free compressed air followed by a 10-second application of 10 to 35 percent polyacrylic acid impregnated in a cotton pellet. This partially removes the smear layer from the dentin, improving the adhesion of the glass ionomer to the dentin and enamel.[19]

4. After a 10-second application of polyacrylic acid, the tooth is thoroughly rinsed with a gentle stream of water for approximately 30 seconds and then gently dried.

5. A glass ionomer lining cement such as GC Lining or Ketac-Bond is mixed according to the manufacturer's instructions and injected in the preventive cavity or inserted with an applicator or the tip of an explorer. For GC Lining and Ketac-Bond, a powder-to-liquid ratio of 1:1 is adequate for covering the dentin surfaces. Ketac-Silver is also indicated but may produce a gray reflection through the sealant when only thin layers are present.

6. After the glass ionomer has set for approximately 2 to 4 minutes, the remaining pit and fissures and the glass ionomer restoration are etched with 37 to 40 percent phosphoric acid for 30 seconds. An acid gel or solution is suitable because there

is no difference regarding penetration into the fissures.[20]

7. The tooth is rinsed with water for 30 seconds and then gently air-dried. The enamel and glass ionomer should exhibit a frosted appearance; if not, the occlusal surfaces should be re-etched for an additional 20 seconds.

8. A light-cured or autopolymerized sealant is placed on the entire occlusal surface. The sealant is extended over the inclined cuspal planes around the preventive glass ionomer restoration. Fissure sealants are retained mainly by the enamel cuspal inclines.[20-22] The occlusion is then adjusted after the sealant has cured.

The advantages of preventive glass ionomer restorations are:

1. Excellent adhesion to dentin and enamel.[19,23]

2. One-step placement without a bonding agent.

3. Cariostatics by fluoride release.[6-10]

The preventive glass ionomer restoration has one distinct disadvantage; glass ionomers are weaker than posterior composite resins. In the case of a preventive glass ionomer restoration, however, the cement is confined to a pit or a portion of a fissure (low stress-bearing areas) without being exposed to appreciable occlusion forces. The improved adhesion and fluoride release is therefore used to maximum advantage.

Internal Occlusal Fossa Preparation ("Tunnel" Preparation)

Smooth proximal surface caries is an insidious process requiring approximately 4 years to progress through the enamel.[13] The lesion is triangular, with the base on the enamel surface and the apex directed toward the DE junction. The area of enamel penetration on the surface is generally small, but once the lesion reaches dentin, lateral spread is rapid and cavitation occurs. A different approach to treating this lesion concentrates on removing carious dentin, not enamel.[15,24-27] Some authors have suggested glass ionomer tunnel preparations through an already placed analgam restoration.[27a]

Essentially, the internal or tunnel preparation allows for the removal of proximal caries through an occlusal access, with limited tooth preparation preserving an intact marginal ridge. This preparation can be performed on any tooth with interproximal caries and intact marginal ridge. Rubber dam isolation is indicated.

Clinical technique

1. The entry point should be at least 2 mm within the marginal ridge, leaving a strong occlusal rim of enamel (Fig. 21-6).

2. Direct the diamond point diagonally toward the lesion for entry to the soft caries (Fig. 21-7). Extend the entry point at this stage buccolin-

Access channel

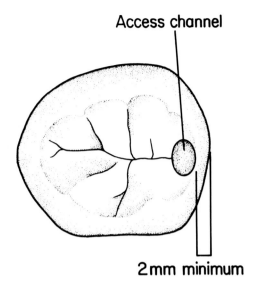

2mm minimum

Fig. 21-6. For internal occlusal fossa cavity preparations, entry point should be at least 2 mm within the marginal ridge, leaving a strong occlusal rim of enamel. (Reprinted with permission from J. Calif. Dent. Assoc. **14:**20-27, 1986.)

Access channel widened bucco-lingually if necessary

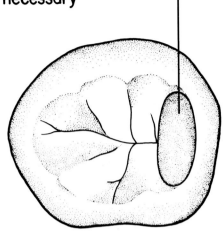

Fig. 21-8. A slow-speed handpiece with a round diamond bur is used to extend the entry point buccolingually while remaining within the fossa area. (Reprinted with permission from J. Calif. Dent. Assoc. **14:**20-27, 1986.)

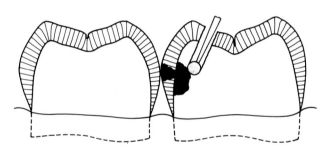

Fig. 21-7. Directing the diamond point diagonally towards the lesion, entry to the soft caries is made. (Reprinted with permission from J. Calif. Dent. Assoc. **14:**20-27, 1986.)

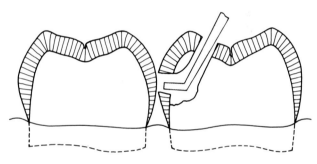

Fig. 21-9. The original enamel wall lesion should be approached with small excavators or chisels. (Reprinted with permission from J. Calif. Dent. Assoc. **14:**20-27, 1986.)

gually, remaining within the fossa area with a slow-speed handpiece and the same round diamond bur (Fig. 21-8). The carious lesion is now visible and generally extends gingivally.

3. Remove the caries using a No. 1 or 2 round tungsten bur, with slow speed and tactile sensation. The lesion will have spread laterally, and the enamel is comparatively intact. A caries-disclosing solution, such as fuchsin staining, and fiberoptic lighting with copious water spray to disperse the debris is useful. Magnification at this stage is desirable.

4. Widen the occlusal access channel internally to facilitate complete removal of carious dentin, but <u>not</u> at the expense of the peripheral enamel. This must be left intact as a strong supporting ring.

5. Smooth the enamel walls with fine-plated diamond stones and clean the original enamel wall lesion. This should <u>not</u> be performed with a

rotating bur in order to avoid damage to the adjoining teeth; use instead small excavators or chisels (Chisel MCI, Cottrell and Co.) similar to those for gold foil preparations (Fig. 21-9).

6. Insert a thin metal matrix band lubricated with silicone grease into the contact area and wedge it tightly so a close fit may be seen through the access channel.

7. Clean the cavity for 10 seconds with a 10 to 35 percent solution of polyacrylic acid; wash and dry. Calcium hydroxide is optional.

8. Fill the floor of the preparation with any glass ionomer. However, Ketac-Silver mixed according to the manufacturer's instructions is less liable to wear or erode with interdental cleaning procedures such as flossing. The glass ionomer cement is injected through the access channel, inserting the nozzle to the maximum depth (Fig. 21-10).

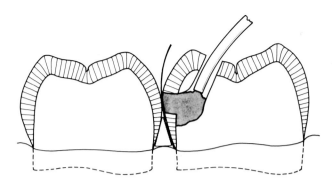

Fig. 21-10. The glass ionomer is injected through the access channel, taking care to insert the syringe to the maximum depth possible. (Reprinted with permission from J. Calif. Dent. Assoc. **14:**20-27, 1986.)

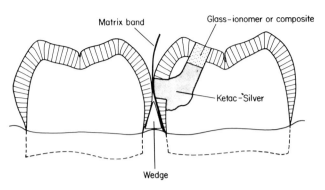

Fig. 21-11. After setting, the glass ionomer may be removed to a depth of 2 mm and the enamel and cement etched for 30 seconds, washed and dried, and a posterior composite inserted by standard technique. (Reprinted with permission from J. Calif. Dent. Assoc. **14:**20-27, 1986.)

9. Force the cement into position with a slightly damp cotton pellet held in tweezers and then covered with Burlew dry foil as described for fissure sealing. Light burnishing ensures occlusal adaptation.

10. After 5 minutes setting, the glass ionomer is contoured with round diamond stones or, preferably, sintered diamonds, and finally trimmed with sharp excavators. When trimming with rotary instruments, water spray is used. Do not trim dry.

11. If preferred, the glass ionomer could be removed to a depth of 2 mm and the enamel and cement etched for 30 seconds, washed and dried, and a posterior composite inserted by standard technique (Fig. 21-11). Posterior composites are more resistant to wear than glass ionomer cements, but the cement ionomers may have overcome this problem.

Restorations

Temporary restorations. In patients with active caries, glass ionomers are used as temporary restorations for caries control. The fluoride release of these cements is of significant preventive value.

Classes I and II. Glass ionomers are not the material of choice for Class I or II restorations because they are not as strong as amalgam or even composite materials. However, in the Class I restoration the cement ionomer Ketac-Silver may show improved properties.

Cavity lining. Glass ionomers have recently been suggested as a liner, or dentin replacement material, under the composite resin restoration. For Class I and II restorations, glass ionomers could be used as a base. The glass ionomers enhance the bond of the entire restoration to the tooth, since glass ionomers bond to enamel and dentin, in addition to composites.[19,23,26-32]

Etched glass ionomer-lined composite restorations are purported to be more resistant to microleakage than the conventional composite restoration,[33] but some studies do not support this.[34,35] The polymerization shrinkage of the composite bonded to the glass ionomer separates the original bond between the glass ionomer and the dentin, allowing microleakage.[35] This is probably due to using a cement lining that is too thin. Glass ionomer-lined composite restorations improve the adhesion of the composite to the enamel and dentin according to studies demonstrating etching capabilities,[36,37] and have excellent cohesive strength with dentin, enamel, and composite resins.[19,31,32,38] Also, the fluoride release of glass ionomers reduces secondary caries.[6-10,29,39-42] Another benefit of lining the cavities with glass ionomers is that they prevent acid etchants from reaching the dentin while etching the enamel.[43]

Clinical technique. Cavity preparation is similar to that for the composite restoration.[44-46] Glass ionomer placement is similar to the preventive glass ionomer restoration. A powder-to-liquid ratio of 1:1 is adequate.

When used as a base for composite restorations, glass ionomers should be applied in maximum bulk and then etched for 30 seconds.[29] When thin layers are used, the cement is easily destroyed. For optimum results, glass ionomer cements should be used to replace the dentin completely.

Gingival Lining (for Class II Restorations)

Amalgam alloy and composite restorations can fail at the gingival margin of the proximal box due to leakage and caries. Glass ionomer cements (Ketac-Silver and Gingiva Seal) have been used for this technique because of their chemical adhesiveness and cariostatic properties. Their clinical success has not been determined, however.

Clinical technique. A matrix band is applied, firmly wedged, and the cement preferably injected into the Class II cavity to restore approximately 2 mm height

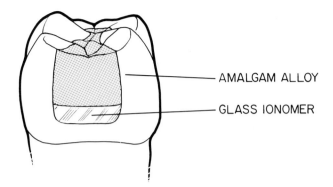

Fig. 21-12. Amalgam alloy packed over silver-containing glass ionomer cement. (Reprinted with permission from J. Calif. Dent. Assoc. **14:**20-27, 1986.)

of the proximal box. The cement is then spread over the pulpal floor and burnished to a thin film over the dentin and enamel walls (Figs. 21-12 and 21-13). At this stage, the gingival floor is restored with the glass ionomer sealing the dentin-matrix band junction. Do not let amalgam or composite material extrude into the gingival sulcus. The amalgam or composite is then placed using conventional techniques.

Classes III and V

Composite resins are considered the most esthetically pleasing restorative material for extensive surfaces of facial enamel, and the acid-etch technique enables attachment to the enamel with well-defined prisms. The effectiveness of the marginal seal is affected by the anatomic position and structural surface conditions of the tooth enamel.[47] Cervical enamel is thinner and more irregular in prism structure, and the surface can be devoid of characteristic prism markings.[48] A marginal seal is established by etching enamel walls in butt and bevel preparations in the incisal and body surfaces of the tooth. However, the Class V cavities and cavities extending into areas of structureless cervical enamel present problems. The use of glass ionomers with composite resin veneers offers an acceptable solution. The cervical dentin or enamel is sealed with glass ionomer and a composite resin is used to restore the enamel structure.

Clinical technique. Standard Class III or V cavities are prepared; after caries removal, the preparation is filled with glass ionomer. The enamel walls are cleansed of cement, the enamel and cement etched with phosphoric acid for 30 seconds, and a composite material inserted. The enamel cavosurface margins are finished with or without a bevel; however, a butt-joint is provided at the dentin or cervical enamel finishing line and the cement chamfered to the edge, allowing attachment of the composite filling material (Figs. 21-14 and 21-15). A calcium hydroxide cement is indicated in deeper excavations.

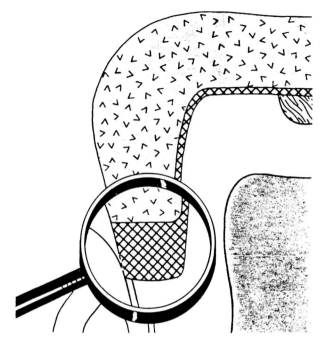

Fig. 21-13. Gingival lining in Class II restorations with a non-silver-containing glass ionomer cement (Gingiva Seal).

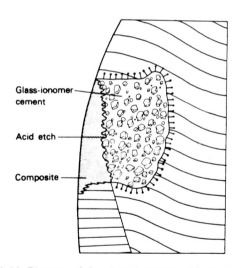

Fig. 21-14. Diagram of the glass ionomer acid-etch technique for a Class V cavity. (Reprinted with permission from Br. Dent. J. **158:**410, 1985.)

Cavity cleansing with polyacrylic acid, acid etching of the glass ionomer base, and application of the bonding agent before insertion of the composite resin is the procedure followed.

For example, a Class V restoration is illustrated, using a light-cured composite resin system (Figs. 21-16 to 21-24). The rubber dam is preferable if the tooth preparation or erosion extends subgingivally. The attachment of composite resins to glass ionomer-coated dentin surfaces is accomplished under dry conditions.

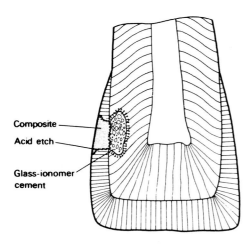

Fig. 21-15. Diagram of the glass ionomer acid etch technique for a Class V cavity. (Reprinted with permission from Br. Dent. J. **158**:410, 1985.)

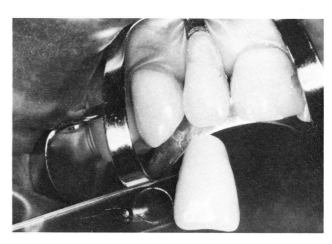

Fig. 21-16. Class V cavity prepared in maxillary right lateral incisor. (Reprinted with permission from Br. Dent. J. **158**:410, 1985.)

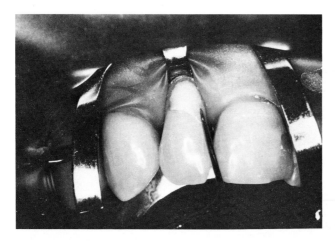

Fig. 21-17. Glass ionomer cement inserted and contoured to enamel and dentin margins. A fine explorer is useful for the final and delicate smoothing of the margins. (Reprinted with permission, Br. Dent. J. **18**:410, 1985.)

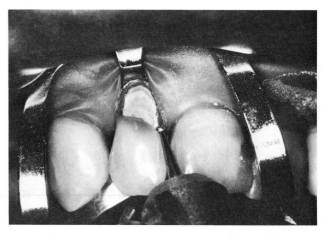

Fig. 21-18. Cement removed from enamel wall with a small, round diamond stone and contoured exactly to the level of the dentition margin. (Reprinted with permission from Br. Dent. J. **158**:410, 1985.)

If the restoration is not veneered with composite, finishing of the glass ionomer cement restoration should be delayed for at least 24 hours after placement.[49,50]

Root Surface Caries

The glass ionomer cements have many advantages in the restoration of root surface caries.[51] They provide an esthetic restoration with adhesion to dentin and release fluoride that is absorbed by the surrounding dentin and cementum.[6,52] They have also demonstrated a resistance to plaque formation, gingival tissue tolerance,[53,54] and prevention of secondary caries formation around the restoration, as well as primary caries in the adjacent sound root surface.[40,42]

The clinical technique is direct because cavity preparation is minimal. Complete removal of caries is man-

datory, and minimal mechanical retention is desirable but not mandatory. Cavity lining with calcium hydroxide is required with less than 1 mm of remaining dentin,[51] and cavity cleansing with polyacrylic acid removes the smear layer.

When restoring root surface caries with glass ionomer cements, complete isolation from the oral environment is necessary for several hours after placement. This can be achieved by applying the commercial varnish or by coating the glass ionomer with a light-cured bonding agent immediately after removal of the matrix.[55] Another common technique is using a glass ionomer base with a microfilled or posterior composite veneer[28] described for the Class III and Class V restorations. If this technique is used, the glass ionomer cement is not completely covered at the gingival margin, and 1 mm of glass ionomer cement re-

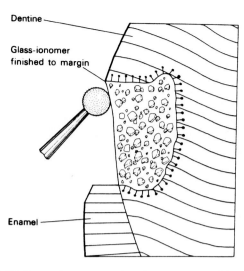

Fig. 21-19. Removing excess glass ionomer cement in order to leave a 0.5 to 1 mm space for the composite resin. It is important that the resin finish exactly at the dentin cavosurface margin, leaving a chamfered edge in the cement providing adequate surface resin bulk. (Reprinted with permission from Br. Dent. J. **158:**410, 1985.)

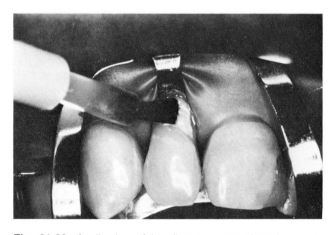

Fig. 21-20. Application of bonding agent to glass ionomer–enamel surfaces. (Reprinted with permission from Br. Dent. J. **158:**410, 1985.)

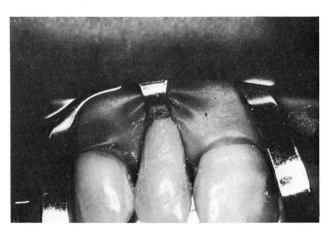

Fig. 21-21. Composite resin contoured to position. (Reprinted with permission from Br. Dent. J. **158:**410, 1985.)

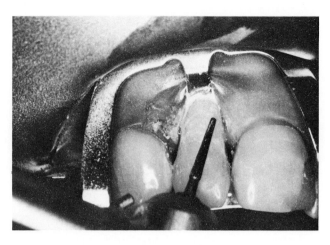

Fig. 21-22. Finishing with white diamond stones or fluted carbide burs. (Reprinted with permission from Br. Dent. J. **158:**410, 1985.)

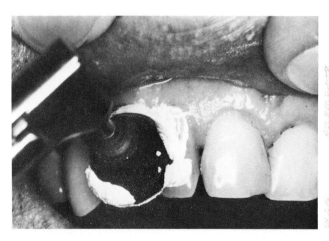

Fig. 21-23. Polishing with abrasive rubber polishing cups and a slurry of aluminum oxide. (Reprinted with permission from Br. Dent. J. **158:**410, 1985.)

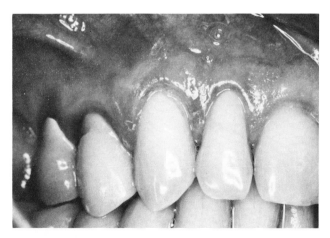

Fig. 21-24. Completed restorations in the maxillary lateral incisor and canine. (Reprinted with permission from Br. Dent. J. **158:**410, 1985.)

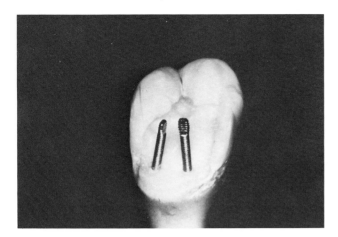

Fig. 21-25. Accessory pins inserted at converging angles and extending beyond the occlusal surface. (Reprinted with permission from Quint. Int. **16:**333-343, 1985, published by Quintessence Publishing Co., Inc., Chicago.)

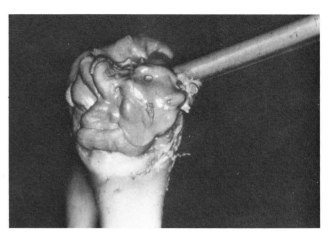

Fig. 21-26. Silver-containing glass ionomer cement injected around the pins and into retention holes and base of tooth. (Reprinted with permission from Quint. Int. **16:**333-343, 1985, published by Quintessence Publishing Co., Inc., Chicago.)

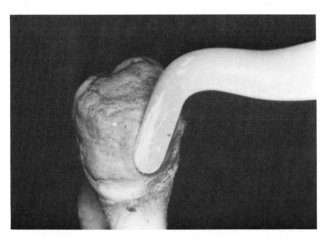

Fig. 21-27. Additional silver-containing glass ionomer cement applied and smoothed in place with a plastic spatula. (Reprinted with permission from Quint. Int. **16:**333-343, 1985, published by Quintessence Publishing Co., Inc., Chicago.)

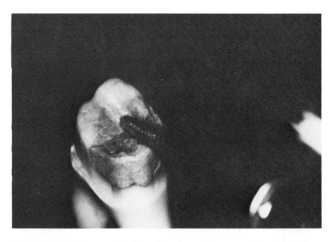

Fig. 21-28. Silver-containing glass ionomer cement core buildup, trimmed. Tooth prepared for full-veneer crown restoration. (Reprinted with permission from Quint. Int. **16:**333-343, 1985, published by Quintessence Publishing Co., Inc., Chicago.)

mains exposed at the margin. This is because the combined properties of dentin adhesion and fluoride release reduce microleakage and recurrent caries if dentin and cementum cavosurface margins adjoin composite resin.[51]

Tooth Buildups Reconstruction

Glass ionomers have been recommended for tooth reconstruction (buildups) with adequate dentin for bonding and space for at least 1 mm thickness of material.[15]

After removal of caries, the deepest penetration in the tooth is covered with a thin layer of calcium hydroxide liner. Whenever possible, the maximum amount of sound tooth structure is preserved and holes drilled in the dentin to retain the cement. In patients

with massive destruction of coronal dentin, accessory pin retention is indicated. Pins are placed at converging angles to a depth of 2 mm in the dentin. The pin length extends right through the core buildup (Fig. 21-25).

The tooth surface is cleansed for 5 to 10 seconds with a 10 to 30 percent polyacrylic acid solution. The glass ionomer cement (Ketac-Silver or Miracle Mix) is injected into the tooth (Fig. 21-26). Additions of cement are made to existing material, and the core buildup smoothed with plastic instruments (Fig. 21-27). After 5 minutes, the core buildup can be trimmed with conventional diamond stones or tungsten carbide burs under water spray with light pressure to avoid overtrimming (Figs. 21-28 to 21-29).

For tooth reconstruction (buildups), silver-contain-

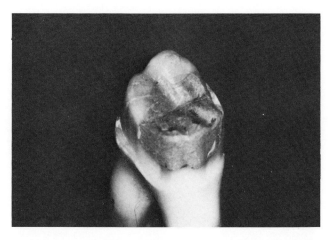

Fig. 21-29. Core buildup finished. (Reprinted with permission from Quint. Int. **16:**333-343, 1985, published by Quintessence Publishing Co., Inc., Chicago.)

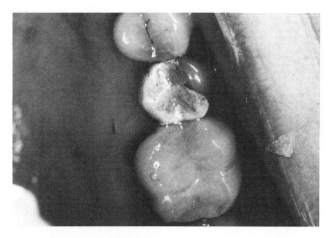

Fig. 21-30. Ketac-Silver restoration inserted in tooth 25 prior to veneer crown preparation. (Reprinted with permission from Quint. Int. **16:**333-343, 1985, published by Quintessence Publishing Co., Inc., Chicago.)

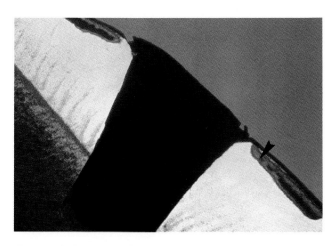

Fig. 21-31. Photomicrograph of specimen cemented with glass ionomer cement after imbibition in water. The inlay is still in place. The cement at the base of the cavity is considerably thicker than on the walls. Outer lesions *(arrows)* have formed at some distance from the cavity walls. (×38) (Courtesy Dr. Edwina Kidd. Reprinted with permission from Br. Dent. J. **147:**39, 1979.)

ing glass ionomer cements are the more suitable. They are particularly suited for restoring teeth prior to oral rehabilitation. Old restorations can be removed while the vitality of the pulp and mechanical weakness in the tooth are determined. Often these restorations remain for a year or more to allow secondary dentin formation (Fig. 21-30), so crowns or FPD can be placed in quadrants.

Repair of Margins of Gold and Ceramic Restorations

Another indication for the glass ionomer cements is repairing the faulty margins of restorations.[56,57] Most dentists have encountered faulty extensive restorative dentistry from gingival erosion or unacceptable marginal fit of metal-ceramic restorations.

Other methods of repair generally involve some form of cavity preparation, with the subsequent insertion of a composite resin or similar material. If the margins are thoroughly cleaned and the microleakage has not extended into the depths of the restoration, the sealing of defective margins with glass ionomer cement is practical.

Generally, a radiograph combined with an examination using a sharp explorer establishes the integrity of the internal surfaces of the tooth preparation. The cement should be firmly packed into the crevice area and covered with a cervical matrix similar to the erosion lesion. It is then convenient to trim the set material with sharp knives to avoid subgingival bleeding, which contaminates the set cement. After the trimming is completed, a light-cured composite resin bonding agent is applied over the glass ionomer to protect the surface from moisture contamination.

Luting Agent for Crown and Bridge Work

Glass ionomer cements have been also used as a luting agent for crown and FPDs. They have also been suggested for cementation of stainless steel crowns in pediatric dentistry and stainless steel bands in orthodontic appliances.[58,59] Cementation of cast gold restorations with glass ionomer cements displayed fewer secondary caries than those cemented with zinc phosphate cement (Figs. 21-31 to 21-33).[39]

Treatment of Enamel Defects

When large areas of facial enamel and dentin are discolored, as with tetracycline staining, the stained dentin that is difficult to mask is removed and filled with glass ionomer cement. The color of the cement provides an excellent background for attachment of a facial composite (Fig. 21-34).[28,56]

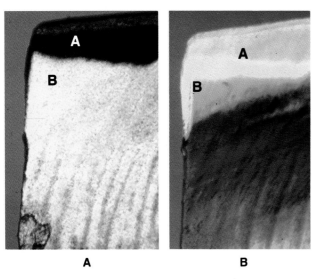

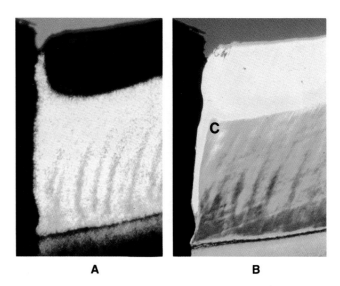

Fig. 21-32. Photomicrographs of occlusal aspect of specimen cemented with zinc phosphate cement after imbibition with water **A** and quinoline **B**. Note outer (A) and wall (B) lesions. (×60) (Courtesy Dr. Edwina Kidd. Reprinted with permission from Br. Dent. J. **147**:39, 1979.)

Fig. 21-33. Photomicrographs of occlusal aspect of specimen cemented with glass ionomer cement after imbibition with water **A** and quinoline **B**. Note in water, the outer lesion at some distance from the cavity wall and in quinoline, the wall lesion (C). (×60) (Courtesy Dr. Edwina Kidd. Reprinted with permission from Br. Dent. J. **147**:39, 1979.)

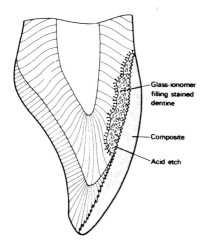

Fig. 21-34. Diagram of method of restoring stained dentin involving extensive areas of labial enamel. (Reprinted with permission from Br. Dent. J. **158**:410, 1985.)

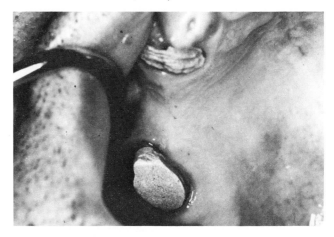

Fig. 21-35. Maxillary molar root capped with Ketac-Silver prior to insertion of an overdenture. (Reprinted with permission from Quint. Int. **16**:333-343, 1985, published by Quintessence Publishing Co., Inc., Chicago.)

Sealing Root Surfaces

When teeth have been endodontically treated and prepared for overdentures, silver-containing glass ionomer cements are particularly suited to sealing the root.[15] Ancillary pin anchorage may be used on a box preparation in the root (Fig. 21-35). This approach is useful in carious mouths where oral hygiene is poor because of the fluoride release from glass ionomers.

SELECTED REFERENCES

1. Wilson, A.D., and Kent, B.E.: The glass-ionomer cement: a new translucent dental filling material, J. Appl. Chem. Biotech. **21**:313, 1971.
2. Wilson, A.D., and Kent, B.E.: A new translucent cement for dentistry. The glass-ionomer cement, Br. Dent. J. **132**:133-135, 1972.
3. Kent, B.E., Lewis, B.G., and Wilson, A.D.: The properties of a glass ionomer cement, Br. Dent. J. **135**:322-326, 1973.
4. McLean, J.W., and Wilson, A.D.: The clinical development of the glass ionomer cements. I. Aust. Dent. J. **22**:31-36, 1977.
5. Wilson, A.D., Prosser, H.J., and Powis, D.M.: Mechanism of adhesion of polyelectrolyte cements to hydroxyapatite, J. Dent. Res. **62**:590-592, 1983.
6. Swartz, M.L., Phillips, R.W., and Clark, H.E.: Long-term F release from glass ionomer cements, J. Dent. Res. **63**:158-160, 1984.
7. Meryon, S.D., and Smith, A.J.: A comparison of fluoride release from three glass ionomer cements and a polycarboxylate cement, Int. Endod. J. **17**:16-24, 1984.
8. Forsten, L.: Fluoride release from a glass ionomer cement, Scand. J. Dent. Res. **85**:503-504, 1977.

9. Garcia-Godoy, F., and Marshall, T.: Fluoride release from glass ionomer cements. Unpublished data.

10. Langeland, K., and Pascon, E.A.: Methodology in, and bio-evaluation of glass ionomers, J. Dent. Res. **65**:772 (Abstract 415), 1986.

11. McLean, J.W., and Wilson, A.D.: Fissure sealing and filling with an adhesive glass ionomer cement, Br. Dent. J. **136**:269-271, 1974.

12. Mortimer, K.V.: Some histological features of fissure caries in enamel, Eur. Org. Caries Res. **2**:85-92, 1964.

13. Kidd, E.A.M.: The diagnosis and management of the "early" carious lesion in permanent teeth, Dent. Update **11**:69-81, 1984.

14. McLean, J.W., and von Fraunhofer, A.: The estimation of cement film thickness by an in vivo technique, Br. Dent. J. **131**:107, 1971.

15. McLean, J.W., and Gasser, O.: Glass-cermet cements, Quint. Int. **16**:333-343, 1985.

16. Garcia-Godoy, F.: The preventive glass ionomer restoration, Quint. Int. **17**:617-619, 1986.

17. Garcia-Godoy, F.: Microleakage of type C preventive resin restorations, Comp. Cont. Educ. Dent. **8**:764-769, 1987.

18. Garcia-Godoy, F.: Microleakage of preventive glass ionomer restorations. Comp. Cont. Educ. Dent. **9**:88-94, 1988.

19. Powis, D.R., Folleras, T., Merson, S.A., and Wilson, A.D.: Improved adhesion of a glass ionomer cement to dentin and enamel, J. Dent. Res. **61**:1416-1422, 1982.

20. Garcia-Godoy, F., and Gwinnett, A.J.: Penetration of acid solution and gel in occlusal fissures, J.A.D.A., **114**:809-810, 1987.

21. Garcia-Godoy, F., and Gwinnett, A.J.: A SEM study of fissure surfaces conditioned with a scraping technique, Clin. Prev. Dent. **9**: 9-13, 1987.

22. Taylor, C.L., and Gwinnett, A.J.: A study of the penetration of sealants into pits and fissures, J.A.D.A. **87**:1181-1188, 1973.

23. Aboush, Y.E.Y., and Jenkins, C.B.G.: An evaluation of the bonding of glass ionomer restoratives to dentine and enamel, Br. Dent. J. **161**:179-184, 1986.

24. Jinks, G.M.: Fluoride-impregnated cements and their effect on the activity of interproximal caries, J. Dent. Child. **30**:87-91, 1963.

25. Hunt, P.R.: A modified Class II cavity preparation for glass-ionomer restorative materials, Quint. Int. **15**:1011, 1984.

26. Knight, G.M.: The use of adhesive materials in the conservative restoration of selected posterior teeth, Aust. Dent. J. **29**:324, 1984.

27. McLean, J.W.: New concepts in cosmetic dentistry using glass ionomer cements and composites, J. Calif. Dent. Assoc. **14**:20-27, 1986.

27a. Garcia-Godoy, F., Marshall, T.D., and Mount, G.J.: Microleakage of glass ionomer tunnel restorations, Am. J. Dent., in press.

28. McLean, J.W., Prosser, H.J., and Wilson, A.D.: The use of glass-ionomer cements in bonding composite resins to dentine, Br. Dent. J. **158**:410-414, 1985.

29. A.D.A. Council on Dental Materials and Devices: Status Report on the Glass Ionomer Cements, J.A.D.A. **99**:221-226, 1979.

30. Wilson, A.D., and Prosser, H.J.: A survey of inorganic and polyelectrolyte cements, Br. Dent. J. **157**:449-454, 1984.

31. Negm, M.M., Beech, D.R., and Grant, A.A.: An evaluation of mechanical and adhesive properties of polycarboxylate and glass ionomer cements, J. Oral Rehabil. **9**:161-167, 1982.

32. Draheim, R.N., Titus, H.W., and Garcia-Godoy, F.: Shear bond strength of posterior composites to base materials, J. Dent. Res. **66**: 209 (Abstr. 821), 1987.

33. Welsh, E.L., and Hembree, J.H.: Microleakage at the gingival wall with four class V anterior restorative materials, J. Prosth. Dent. **54**:370-372, 1985.

34. Gordon, M., Plaschaert, A.J.M., Soelberg, K.B., and Bogdan, M.S.: Microleakage for four composite resins over a glass ionomer cement base in Class V restorations, Quint. Int. **16**:817-820, 1985.

35. Garcia-Godoy, F., and Malone, W.F.P.: Microleakage of posterior composites using glass ionomer cement bases, Quint. Int. **19**:13-17, 1988.

36. Garcia-Godoy, F., and Malone, W.F.P.: The effect of acid etching on two glass ionomer lining cements, Quint. Int. **17**:621-623, 1986.

37. Garcia-Godoy, F., and Malone, W.F.P.: Effect of various etching times on two glass ionomer lining cements, Texas Dent. J. **104**: 12-15, 1987.

38. Sneed, W.D., and Looper, S.W.: Shear bond strength of a composite resin to an etched glass ionomer, Dent. Mater. **1**:127-128, 1985.

39. Kidd, E.A.D., and McLean, J.W.: The cavity sealing ability of cemented cast gold restorations, Br. Dent. J. **147**:39-41, 1979.

40. Wesenberg, G., and Hals, E.: The structure of experimental in vitro lesions around glass ionomer restorations in human teeth, J. Oral Rehabil. **7**:175-184, 1980.

41. Hicks, M.J., Flaitz, C.M., and Silverstone, L.M.: Secondary caries formation in vitro around glass ionomer restorations, Quint. Int. **17**:527-532, 1986.

42. Hicks, M.J.: Artificial lesion formation around glass ionomer restorations in root surfaces: a histologic study, Gerodontics **2**:108-114, 1986.

43. Walker, T.M., Jensen, M.E., and Chan, D.C.N.: Acid penetration through glass ionomer bases, J. Dent. Res. **65**:344 (abstract 1580), 1986.

44. Suzuki, M., Jordan, R.E., and Boksman, L.: Posterior composite resin restoration-clinical considerations. In Vanherle, G., and Smith, D.C.: Posterior Composite Resin Dental Restorative Materials, St. Paul, Minn., 1985, Peter Szulc Publishing Co./3M Co., pp. 455-464.

45. Lutz, F., Imfeld, T., Barbakow, F., and Iselin, W.: Optimizing the marginal adaptation of MOD composite restorations. In Naherle, G., and Smith, D.C.: Posterior Composite Resin Dental Restorative Materials, St. Paul, Minn., 1985, Peter Szulc Publishing Co./3M Co., pp. 405-420.

46. Lutz, F., Krejci, I., and Oldenburg, T.R.: Elimination of polymerization stresses at the margins of posterior composite resin restorations: a new restorative technique, Quint. Int. **17**:777-784, 1986.

47. Van Noort, R.: Controversial aspects of composite resin restorative materials, Br. Dent. J. **155**:383-385, 1983.

48. Gwinnett, A.J.: The ultrastructure of prismless enamel of permanent human teeth, Arch. Oral Biol. **12**:381-389, 1967.

49. Mount, G.J.: Restoration with glass ionomer cements: requirement for clinical success, Oper. Dent. **6**:59-63, 481.

50. Wong, T.C.C., and Bryant, R.W.: Glass ionomer cements: dispensing and strength, Aust. Dent. J. **30**:336-340, 1985.

51. Mount, G.J.: Root surface caries: a recurrent dilemma, Aust. Dent. J. **31**:288-291, 1986.

52. Retief, D.H., Bradley, E.L., Denton, J.C., and Switzer, P.: Enamel and cementum fluoride uptake from a glass ionomer cement, Caries Res. **18**:250-257, 1984.

53. Garcia, R., Caffesse, R.G., and Charbeneau, G.T.: Gingival tissue response to restoration of deficient cervical contours using a glass ionomer material; a 12-month report, J. Prosth. Dent. **46**:393-398, 1981.

54. Knibbs, P.J., and Plant, C.G.: A clinical assessment of a rapid

setting glass ionomer cement, Br. Dent. J. **161**:323-326, 1986.

55. Earl, M.S.A., Hume, W.R., and Mount, G.J.: Effect of varnishes and other surface treatments on water movement across the glass ionomer cement surface, Aust. Dent. J. **30**:298-301, 1985.

56. Mount, G.J.: Glass ionomer cements: clinical considerations, Clin. Dent. **4**:1-23, 1984.

57. McLean, J.W., and Wilson, A.D.: The clinical development of the glass ionomer cement. II. Some clinical applications, Aust. Dent. J. **22**:120-127, 1977.

58. McLean, J.W., Wilson, A.D., and Prosser, H.J.: Development and use of water-hardening glass ionomer luting cements, J. Prosth. Dent. **52**:175-181, 1984.

59. Garcia-Godoy, F., and Bugg, J.L.: Clinical evaluation of glass ionomer cement on stainless steel crown retention, J. Pedod. **11**: 339-344, 1987.

RESTORATION OF ENDODONTICALLY TREATED TEETH

BASIC PRINCIPLES

Endodontically treated teeth present restorative problems because they frequently have insufficient sound coronal tooth structure to retain the restoration. Due to loss of tooth structure and the endodontic treatment, the teeth become brittle and are subject to fracture. Various techniques have been introduced to address specific problems of coronal-radicular stabilization (Figs. 22-1 to 22-4). These techniques use dowels in the roots to provide the necessary retention for the cores and to prevent separation of the crown from the root (Fig. 22-5).

Prior to treatment, an evaluation is performed to determine the restorability of the tooth, the health of the periodontium, and the role of the tooth in the treatment plan. There should be sufficient tooth structure to retain the post and core during mastication. Occasionally, the tooth is so compromised by caries and extensive restorations that the restorability of the tooth is questionable (Fig. 22-6). Additional procedures, such as periodontal crown lengthening or orthodontic extrusion, transform a near-insurmountable problem into a favorable prognosis. These procedures should not injure the periodontium, violate the biologic width, or harm adjacent teeth.

The periodontal evaluation confirms adequate support for the tooth. The level of the bone is considered at a sufficient height when the dowel extends below the alveolar crest.[1] Finally, the role of the tooth in the treatment plan is determined. The strategic position of the tooth and whether its retention appreciably enhances the success of treatment are factors considered before a complex, heroic effort is initiated to retain a tooth with a guarded prognosis (Fig. 22-7).

The reinforcement of the tooth is essential when selecting a dowel and core technique. The procedure

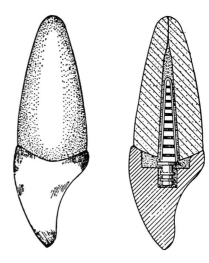

Fig. 22-1. Detached dowel with all porcelain crown. Cross-sections show relative position of dowel in root and in base of crown. Cement unites tooth, dowel, and crown into one rigid unit. This former design, connecting the dowel and core with the crown is currently discouraged.

should not further weaken the tooth or risk the loss of the endodontic seal.[1-4] Excessive canal enlargement or apical extension that leaves less than 4 or 5 mm of gutta percha is avoided. Tilk et al. studied approximately 1,000 extracted teeth and revealed that the mesial-distal width of roots in the apical one-third was often less than 2 mm, especially with maxillary posterior teeth and mandibular teeth other than canines.[5] Dowel preparation in the apical one-third of these teeth increased the risk of perforation.

The cast post and core maintains the integrity of the tooth, with a cervical collar exhibiting the "ferrule effect" that is impossible to obtain with prefabricated dowels. However, a 2 mm cervical collar included in

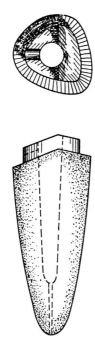

Fig. 22-2. Coronal-radicular stabilization for a maxillary anterior abutment. Note extent of root preparation with shoulder prior to reception of a dowel.

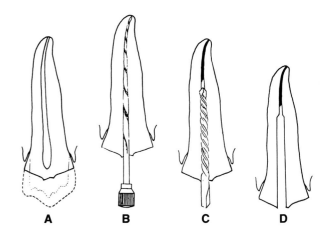

Fig. 22-4. A, Diagram of tooth with loss of tooth structure and internal anatomy of canal. **B,** Entire length of canal with file in place. Note that final shape and size of post room depends on size of file in final preparation. **C,** With increasing diameter of files, internal shape of post core system is achieved. Apical third of canal is endodontic seal. **D,** Internal shape of the diameter and length of prepared post room.

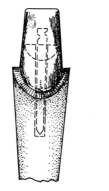

Fig. 22-3. Cast core for porcelain jacket crown encircles plateau portion of preparation and occupies half width of shoulder. Note that some of the coronal portion of tooth is retained when possible.

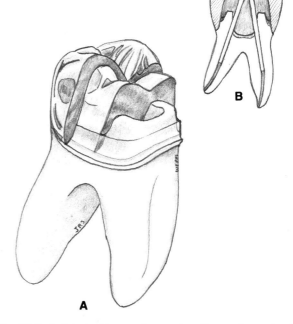

Fig. 22-5. A, Interlocking cast cores for divergent canals of a mandibular molar. **B,** Sound tooth structure is sustained to support the cores.

the final restoration performs a similar function.[6] The preparation of the tooth should extend 2 mm beyond the cervical margin of the dowel and core for strength and to finish the margins of the restoration. Lastly, the dowel should <u>not</u> transmit excessive forces to the root; e.g., threaded posts that require tapping and screwing impart expansive stresses to the roots, which increases the chances of root fracture.[7-9]

ANTERIOR VERSUS POSTERIOR TEETH

Restored endodontically treated anterior teeth routinely require a post to prevent separation of the crown

from the root. There is insufficient sound tooth structure after tooth preparation and that can result in fracture (Fig. 22-8). Anterior teeth with conservative proximal restorations and a minimal endodontic access opening can be stabilized with a preformed dowel. Separation of the crown from the roots in endodontically treated posterior teeth is infrequent.

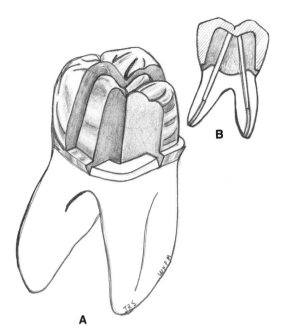

Fig. 22-6. A, Interlocking cores for divergent posts to restore a severely compromised mandibular molar. **B,** Complete core replacing the entire, unsupported coronal portion of the tooth.

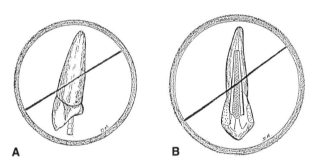

Fig. 22-8. A, Preparation is accomplished before initiation of core pattern. **B,** The use of cast or prefabricated posts to fill the canal space is avoided because without removal of unsupported tooth structure they are prone to fracture and arduous to retreat.

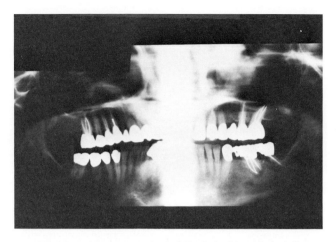

Fig. 22-7. Complete intraoral rehabilitation with periodontal support to justify heroic coronal dentistry. Post crowns are common in extensive restorative dentistry.

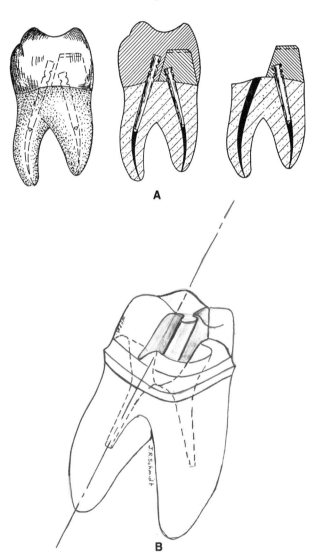

Fig. 22-9. A, Complete cast crowns for molars are usually fabricated in two parts because of root angulation. **B,** Multirooted tooth with divergent roots that require an auxillary post are restored with an interlocking core. *Continued*

Posterior teeth are wider at the cervical area and do not possess the same cervical constriction as anterior teeth. They are also shorter occlusogingivally than anterior teeth, and the occlusal forces are vertical—not tangential as with anterior teeth. Therefore, a dowel in a posterior tooth does not function so much to support and stabilize the tooth as it does to afford a means of retaining the core. If more than 50 percent of the coronal tooth structure remains, placing a core within the coronal pulp chamber for retention is suitable. If there is less than 50 percent of coronal tooth structure, a single post or a dowel with an auxillary post is inserted in the roots to retain the core (Fig. 22-9).

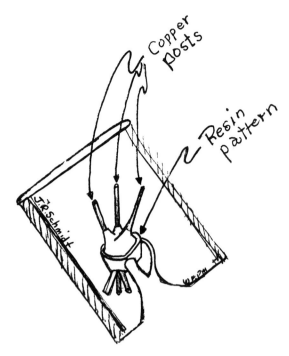

Fig. 22-9. C, Maxillary molar invested for casting with auxillary posts to restore a tooth and maintain arch integrity after prolonged orthodontic retention.

TECHNIQUES
Restorations without Dowels

Posterior teeth with small restorations, sufficient remaining tooth structure, or both, should be restored with cast restorations covering the occlusal surface, e.g., onlay, partial-veneer crown. A heavy reverse bevel is recommended over the cusps for further protection.

For patients with reduced tooth structure, a complete crown is indicated. If a core is needed, it is placed using the coronal pulp chamber for retention. Occasionally, the retention of the core is supplemented with threaded pins. Caution should be exercised when using screw-in threaded pins because of induced stress in these brittle teeth.

Restorations with Dowels

Two types of dowels are used in the restoration of endodontically treated teeth: prefabricated dowels and custom (cast) post and cores. The prefabricated dowels are subdivided into smooth or serrated, parallel-sided or tapered, and tapped and threaded.[10] The cast dowels and cores are indicated for most single-rooted teeth. Prefabricated dowels are more appropriately used in multirooted teeth to support an amalgam or, in rare instances, composite core buildup.

Dowel Space Preparation

Studies have suggested the appropriate size and length of a dowel.[1,2,4,11,12] Generally, dowels smaller than a No. 70 endodontic file are inadequate. Canal preparation that is minimally the size of a No. 80 endodontic file is preferred. However, excessive canal preparation to provide a dowel with maximum strength weakens the root and increases the chances of perforation.[4,5,11]

The recommended length of the dowel preparation is:

1. Equal to the length of the artificial crown of the restoration.
2. Two-third the length of the root.
3. Below the crest of the alveolar bone if periodontally compromised.

It is prudent to fabricate a long post, but without disturbing the apical seal. This infers that the radicular preparation extends to within 4 to 5 mm of the apex. The retentiveness of a dowel is directly related to length. Increasing the length of a dowel from 5 mm to 8 mm has been reported to improve retention from 150 to 225 percent.[13,14]

Custom (Cast) Dowel and Core

Custom cast post and cores can be fabricated for single-rooted teeth as well as multirooted teeth with divergent canals. The technique can be direct or indirect with an impression and stone dies. The advantage to cast post and cores is that they are custom fit to irregularly shaped canals, not cylindrically shaped canals, as are preformed dowels. More important is the fact that the post and core are cast in one unit rather than two separate materials. Therefore, they do not usually require auxiliary retention such as pins to retain the core as in some prefabricated systems. The direct technique is used most frequently because it is efficient. The indirect technique is indicated when there are multiple dowels and cores, and especially when the post and cores are serving as overdenture attachments.

Direct Technique

Single-rooted teeth. The tooth is prepared for a cast restoration (usually a complete crown) after the previous restorations and caries are removed. This will determine the amount of sound dentin that will remain after the preparation. Weakened, thin, and/or undermined tooth structure is removed, since it does not support the post and core. The remaining coronal tooth structure is sloped to the buccal and to the lingual surface to produce a ferrule effect (360 degree collar) with the dowel and core (Fig. 22-10). Specific files, Pesso reamers, or Gates Glidden drills are used to prepare the canal so that it is appropriately long and is approximately the size of a No. 90 file. The coronal end of the canal is funneled, and an antirotational notch is placed with a tapered bur (Fig. 22-11). If the canal is elliptical in shape, an antirotational

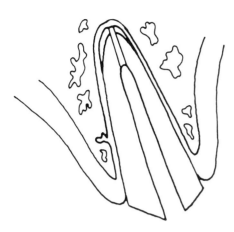

Fig. 22-10. Dowel preparation with buccal and lingual sloping to provide a ferrule effect.

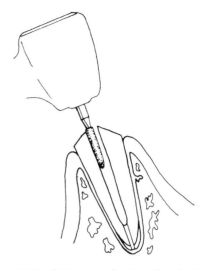

Fig. 22-11. Placement of antirotational notch.

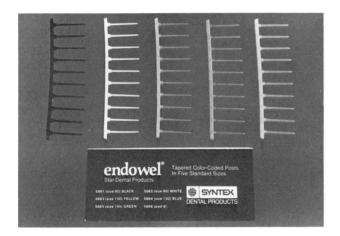

Fig. 22-12. Star Endowels sizes 80, 90, 100, 110.

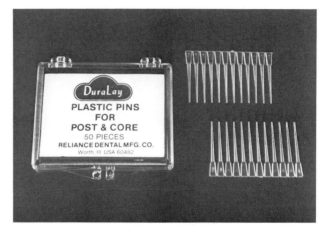

Fig. 22-13. Duralay dowels.

notch is unnecessary. Plastic dowels (Star Endowels) that are sized to match the last file used to prepare the canal or other plastic dowels, e.g., Duralay Dowels, are available to carry acrylic or wax to form the pattern of the canal (Figs. 22-12 and 22-13). Toothpicks, nails, paper clips, and so on have also been recommended to develop the pattern for the canal.[15] A prefabricated gold alloy dowel (Kerr Endo Post, Kerr Dental Mfg.) may also be used for the dowel. It is notched and roughened to facilitate attaching the acrylic or wax that is used for the core portion of the pattern. The pattern is invested, and the gold alloy used for the casting will simply cast to the Kerr Endo Post.

The dowel (post) is checked for fit at the base of the prepared canal. The canal is lubricated. If a smooth plastic dowel is used, it is roughened or slightly notched to facilitate retention of the acrylic. A resin such as Duralay (Reliance Dental Mfg. Co.), Snap or

Relate (Parkell), or Trim (Bosworth) is applied to the dowel. After the resin reaches the doughy stage, the dowel is inserted into the canal. After a few moments, the dowel is pumped up and down in the canal to prevent its being locked in an undercut in the canal. Acrylic resin is added with a brush to reconstruct the coronal aspect. After the resin has set, the pattern is removed. If there are any voids in the acrylic in the dowel, soft beading wax is placed in the voids, and the pattern is reinserted in the tooth. This step is repeated until the dowel pattern is satisfactory. The coronal aspect is next shaped to resemble an ideal tooth preparation (Fig. 22-14). The pattern is then invested and cast in a metal of choice. The investment is mixed thin and measures are instituted to minimize the expansion.

Multirooted teeth. Multirooted teeth frequently provide a challenge in fabricating a custom dowel and core. The canals are usually not parallel, but curved

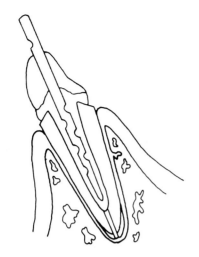

Fig. 22-14. Completed dowel and core pattern.

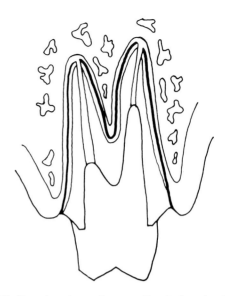

Fig. 22-15. Dowel and core for a multirooted tooth with a long primary dowel and short, parallel secondary dowel.

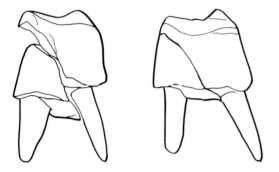

Fig. 22-16. Interlocking dowel and core using maximum length of divergent canals.

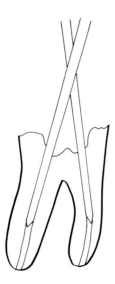

Fig. 22-17. Larger plastic dowel in the distal canal and lubricated stainless steel dowel in the mesial canal.

or short, with one of the canals frequently being small. One technique is to select the larger, longer canal for the primary post, e.g., the palatal canal of maxillary molars or the distal canal of mandibular molars, while the other canal is made parallel to the primary canal with minimum preparation for the secondary post. The secondary post is usually not more than 3 or 4 mm in length. The technique is the same as for single-rooted teeth (Fig. 22-15). A modification of this technique is to make an interlocking post and core for divergent canals. This enables the dentist to incorporate more of the length of the secondary canal[16,17] (Fig. 22-16). This is a rather time consuming and arduous task.

A simpler technique is to use two or even three canals when they are not parallel.[18,19,20] The primary post is positioned in the larger, longer canal, while the other canal or canals are used for the secondary dowel or dowels. The technique for a dowel (post) and core for a mandibular molar is described, but the same technique can be employed for any multirooted, non-parallel endodontically treated tooth.

A plastic dowel is seated in the distal canal, and a lubricated stainless steel dowel of the same size as the last file used is placed in the mesial canal (Fig. 22-17). The plastic dowel is notched, roughened, and coated with resin. After the resin loses its gloss, the dowel is inserted back into the distal canal. Resin is added to reconstruct the coronal aspect of the tooth, embedding the lubricated stainless steel post in the pattern. The core is shaped to resemble an ideal tooth preparation after the resin has set. The stainless steel dowel is removed from the tooth and the pattern with a pliers. The core and the dowel in the distal canal are then removed.

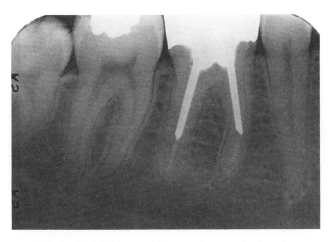

Fig. 22-18. Radiograph of a dowel and core with divergent canals. Cast dowel in the distal canal and a prefabricated stainless steel dowel cemented through the casting into the mesial canal.

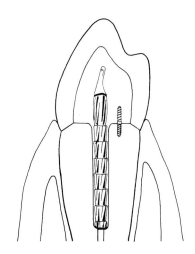

Fig. 22-19. Paraposts with auxillary pin for retention and a composite core.

The stainless steel dowel is heated in a Bunsen burner until it is oxidized, as indicated by its turning cherry red. After it cools, it is reinserted into the pattern from which it had been removed earlier. This maintains the patency of the hole for the post in the mesial canal during casting. The oxidation of the stainless steel dowel prevents it from becoming an integral part of the casting. The pattern is invested and cast with minimal expansion in a metal of choice. After casting, the stainless steel dowel is removed from the casting with a pliers. When fitting the post and core, a new stainless steel dowel of the same size as the original is inserted in the hole in the casting after the casting is seated in the tooth (Fig. 22-18).

A cast dowel for a single-rooted tooth or the primary dowel of a multirooted tooth should be at least the size of a No. 90 endodontic file. A cast post smaller than the size of a No. 90 file may result in a weak casting. In that case, a prefabricated gold alloy dowel, such as Kerr Endopost (Kerr Dental Mfg.), instead of a plastic dowel provides the desirable strength. The gold alloy will cast to the endopost and become a single unit.

Fitting and Cementing Custom Dowel and Cores

The casting must be carefully inspected and any bubbles on the inner surface removed before insertion in the canal. An appropriate size file is used to remove temporary cement or debris from the canal so the casting is not forced, but passively seated. After the casting is seated satisfactorily, it is examined for occlusal clearance and axial contour. These final corrections are accomplished, and the dowel and core are ready for cementation.

The canal is cleaned with a solvent to remove residual lubricant used for the pattern. The canal is then dried with absorbent points. The cement is mixed to a desirable consistency and spun into the canal with a lentulo spiral. The dowel and core is also coated with cement and then placed into the tooth and maintained under finger pressure until the cement sets. Zinc phosphate, resin, and glass ionomer cements are the most commonly used cements for post and cores. The tooth is now ready for the final preparation and impression. It is important to have a minimum of 1 to 2 mm of sound tooth structure apical to the gingival margin of the dowel (post) and core[5].

Prefabricated Dowels

Prefabricated dowels are cylindrical. The majority are designed to be matched with a specific size endodontic file, Pesso reamer, or Gates-Glidden drill. Prefabricated dowels do not resist a rotation because of their cylindrical shape, unless they are threaded or have a serrated surface. The coronal aspect of the prefabricated dowel contains a mechanism for retaining the coronal core material, e.g., amalgam or composite resin. Cements including glass ionomer cement are not recommended as core material because of inadequate strength.[21]

Numerous prefabricated dowel systems are available. It is unnecessary to be familiar with each system; the dentist needs only to understand the characteristics of the various types.[10] The Para-Post is a parallel-sided post that fits passively in the canal with a threaded or spiral fluted surface. The amalgam core is retained by the coronal extension of the Para-Post, often with auxiliary retention provided with screw-in pins (Figs. 22-19 and 22-20).

The Dentatus Screw Post is a tapered, threaded post (Fig. 22-21). It was originally designed as a screw-in post, but because of the incidence of root fracture, the Dentatus Post is now recommended to be passively fitted. The threads in the post simply provide

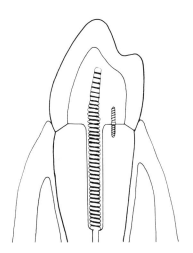

Fig. 22-20. Paraposts with auxillary pin for retention and a composite core.

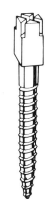

Fig. 22-21. Dentatus screw post.

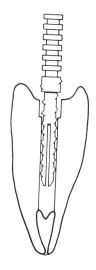

Fig. 22-22. Flexi-post. Note split in the post that reduces stress when tapping and threading.

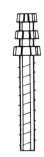

Fig. 22-23. Brasseler/Vlock Post.

retention for the cement. The post has a rectangular head that retains the core.

A unique tapped and threaded screw post was recently introduced to minimize root fracture. The Flexi-Post has a split shank that closes during insertion, absorbing stresses (Fig. 22-22). The manufacturers have reported 750,000 Flexi-Post insertions without a root fracture. When there are maximal retentive demands on a post, the Flexi-Post provides a satisfactory solution.[22]

The Brasseler-Vlock Drill and Post System has a parallel-sided microthreaded post. The post hole is precisely cut with the drill provided to match the microthreaded post, thus reducing stress (Fig. 22-23) and improving retention.

Prefabricated dowels and cores are cemented similarly to the custom post and cores. Virtually all of the prefabricated dowels have an escape (vent) channel for the cement. However, dowels do not closely adapt to the canals because of the irregularities in the internal surface of the canals.[23] The escape channel is, therefore, a minor feature to a dowel design. Cement is spun into the canal with a lentulo spiral, the dowel is coated with cement, and the dowel seated or gently screwed into place. After the cement sets, the core is fabricated with composite resin in incisors and amalgam or composite resin in posterior teeth while retention is frequently supplemented with pins. Some questions have been raised regarding the use of composite resin as a core material because of water sorption.[24] The gingival margin is <u>not</u> to terminate on composite resin or amalgam, without exception.

Indirect Technique

The indirect technique is indicated when there are multiple teeth treated, especially when the dowel and core is a coping for a tooth-supported (overdenture) prosthesis abutment. In the former instance, chair time is reduced by relegating the fabrication of the pattern to the laboratory. In the latter case, fitting of the margin of the coping in the gingival crevice, alignment of the overdenture attachment, and paralleling of the coping are facilitated with an accurate stone cast.

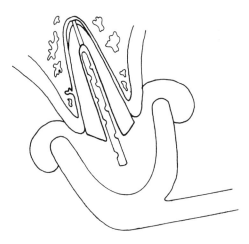

Fig. 22-24. Making an impression for a custom dowel and core.

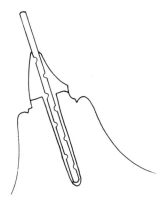

Fig. 22-25. Finished pattern for a dowel and core on the stone die. Soft beading wax is used in the canal, and inlay wax is used for the coronal aspect.

The preparation of the tooth is completed similarly to the direct technique. If the restoration is an overdenture coping, the margins are prepared in the gingival crevice and the tissues retracted to make the impression. Although some dentists state that reversible hydrocolloid can be used, the other elastomeric impression materials, such as rubber base, polyether, and vinyl polysiloxane, are more desirable for the impression within a canal.

A loose-fitting plastic or metal dowel is placed into the canal to the end of the preparation. The coronal end of the plastic or metal dowel is notched or bent to retain it in the impression. The dowel is coated with the proper impression material adhesive. The impression material is injected into the canal or spun into the canal with a lentulo spiral. The dowel is coated with the impression material and placed into the canal to the end of the dowel preparation. Additonal impression material is injected around the tooth and into the gingival crevice, when necessary, and the tray is seated (Fig. 22-24). If the impression is satisfactory, it is poured in die stone. In many instances, it is unnecessary to fabricate removable dies, so a single solid cast is satisfactory.

After the cast has been retrieved from the impression, the dies are trimmed to expose the margins. Care is exercised to prevent debris from falling into the canal. Another loose-fitting dowel is carefully placed into the end of the canal without abrading the internal aspect of the canal. A plastic dowel or a narrow toothpick is suitable. The stone die is lubricated with die lubricant. The dowel pattern is formed by flowing molten soft beading wax over the loose-fitting dowel and inserting it into the canal. The dowel is withdrawn, and more beading wax is added incrementally until a satisfactory pattern is obtained. Because beading wax is a dead soft wax, it can easily be drawn out from any irregularities or undercuts in the canal.

The coronal portion of the pattern is completed with inlay wax (Fig. 22-25). The pattern is sprued and invested as in the direct technique, using minimum expansion of the investment. The retrieved casting is inspected for casting imperfections and carefully fitted onto the die. It is trimmed, smoothed, and prepared for the patient. (See Chapter 19 for placing the attachments and flow chart for coronal-radicular stabilization.)

ENDODONTIC-RESTORATIVE COOPERATION FOR IMPROVED POST AND CORE PLACEMENT

After endodontic shaping of the canal, a gutta percha seal of 4 to 7 mm is established. Instead of filling the entire canal with gutta percha, a precast post is fitted from standard plastic endowels sizes 80 to 120. A radiograph is taken to verify the position of the precast post before the patient returns to the restorative dentist.

Technique of "Pickup" Casting of Core[25,26]

The radiograph and fitted precast post is forwarded to the restorative dentist illustrating the 3 to 5 mm apical seal. The treatment restoration with the lingual stopping is removed, and the coronal tooth reduction initiated (Figs. 22-26, A and B). The unsupported tooth structure and existing restorations are removed and orifice keys placed. A two-planed faciolingual preparation is recommended with a severely compromised tooth (Fig. 22-26 C). The precast post is gently seated, the coronal extension notched, and a limited amount of duralay strategically placed to completely cure, thus stabilizing the post in the canal. Duralay is added in increments free-hand or with plastic core forms[27] to shape the coronal portion of the preparation, establishing a facial to lingual *"cant"* for porcelain bulk and a concave lingual seat to accommodate protrusive movements (Figs. 22-26, D and F).

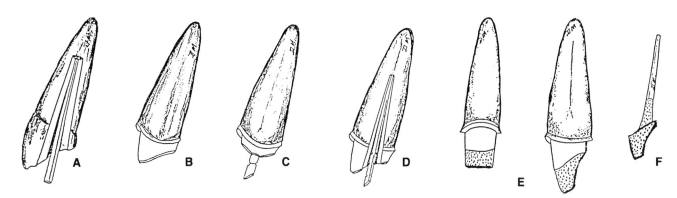

Fig. 22-26. A, Precast post fitted intraorally at the time the 3 to 5 mm special seal is completed after endodontic treatment. **B,** Coronal tooth preparation is initiated. All the existing composite resin or amalgam is removed. A reverse bevel or orifice key is used to prevent torque. **C,** Two-plane preparation is recommended if the coronal structure is severely compromised. **D,** Precast post is shortened to remain within the confines of the core buildup. **E,** Duralay or wax is used to duplicate the coronal portion of the orifice, keys and reverse bevel. The pattern represents the final preparation and the margins of the tooth remain visible. **F,** A "pick-up casting" is accomplished. Although the bond between a precast gold post and custom core is more compatible, different post metals have been successful, i.e., alba cast and etc., but the core and post materials are identical. 22-6 A-E Courtesy Dr. D. J. Maroso, Alton, Il.

Table 22-1. Coronal-radicular stabilization

I. Single-rooted teeth to be restored require dowels. With 80 percent of remaining tooth structure, a preformed stabilization dowel will suffice. (See Section IV.)

II. Restoration without dowels: multirooted teeth only
   A. Seventy-five percent remaining tooth structure—complete crown. Use coronal pulp chamber to retain core. Retention occasionally supplemented with pins.

III. Cast dowels
   A. Single-rooted teeth
      1. Direct technique
      2. Indirect technique
         a. Multiple dowel and cores
         b. Overdenture abutments
   B. Multirooted teeth
      1. Single dowel or multiple parallel dowels
      2. Nonparallel dowels
         a. Interlocking castings
         b. Nonparallel dowel(s) fitted through primary dowel and core casting

IV. Preformed dowels
   A. Smoothsided, tapered, e.g., Unitek, Kerr Endo Post
      1. Minimal retention. Least effective to retain core
      2. Primarily used for stabilization, 90 percent remaining tooth structure
   B. Parallel-sided with serrations or grooves for retention, e.g., Parapost
      1. Stabilization of single-rooted teeth
      2. Core retention in multirooted teeth
   C. Tapered-threaded post, e.g., Dentatus
      1. Threads for retention, post is not screwed in
      2. Core retention in multirooted teeth
   D. Tapered and threaded posts, e.g., Flexi-Post, Brasseler/ Vlock system
      1. Maximum retention
      2. Useful with short roots to retain core
   E. Core retention can be supplemented with pins

V. Precast posts with customized cores including coronal one-eighth of post.
   A. Less perforations.
   B. Saves time

The advantages of this approach are:

1. The intraradicular preparation is concomitantly performed with endodontic treatment by a dentist familiar with the radicular anatomy of the tooth.
2. Prevents inadvertent perforations.
3. Saves time.
4. An ideal introduction to coronal radicular stabilization for the DS III (Table 22-1).
5. Encourages efficient direct patterns that address specific root morphology rather than universal application of one method (as indicated by flow chart).

Inlay wax can be applied to the duralay pattern as the core enters the canal to increase adaptation to radicular walls. The completed pattern should be smooth and resemble the final post and core to reduce chair time at cementation.

The communication between the endodontist and the restorative dentist has become more coordinated, which benefits the patients. There are fewer compromised teeth than 20 years ago, so the "key" teeth are being salvaged to maintain arch integrity. Two or three precast posts can be forwarded to the restorative dentist when an inordinate amount of tooth structure is missing from a multirooted tooth. These teeth are rarely indicated for a terminal abutment of an FPD or an RPD abutment, but are encouraged for maintaining a complete dentition.

SELECTED REFERENCES

1. Stern, N., and Hirshfeld, Z.: Principles of preparing endodontically treated teeth for dowel and core restorations, J. Prosthet. Dent. **30**:162, 1973.
2. Sorensen, J.L., and Martinoff: Clinically significant factors in dowel design, J. Prosthet. Dent. **52**:28, 1984.
3. Camp, L., and Todd, M.: Effect of dowel preparation on apical

seal of three common obturation techniques, J. Prosthet. Dent. **50:**664, 1983.

4. Gutman, J.L.: Preparation of endodontically treated teeth to receive a post-core restoration, J. Prosthet. Dent. **38:**413-419, 1977.
5. Tilk, M.A., Lommel, T.J., and Gerstein, H.: A study of the mandibular and maxillary root widths to determine dowel size, J. Endodont. **5:**79, 1979.
6. Rosen, H., and Partida-Rivera, M.: Iatrogenic fracture of roots reinforced with a cervical collar, Oper. Dent. **11:**46, Spring 1986.
7. Deutsch, A., et al.: Root fracture and the design of prefabricated posts, J. Prosthet. Dent. **53:**637, May 1985.
8. Deutsch, A., et al.: Root fracture during insertion of prefabricated posts related to root size, J. Prosthet. Dent. **53:**786, June 1985.
9. Standlee, J.D., et al.: Analysis of stress distribution of endodontic posts, Oral Surg. **33:**952, 1972.
10. Deutsch, A.S., Musikant, B.L., Cavallari, J., and Lepley, J.B.: Prefabricated dowels: a literature review, J. Prosthet. Dent. **49:**498, 1983.
11. Abou-Rass, M., et al.: Preparation of space for posting: effect on thickness of canal walls and incidence of perforation in molars, J.A.D.A. **104:**834, 1982.
12. Eissman, H.F., and Radke, R.A.: Post endodontic restoration in Cohen, S., and Burns, R.C.: Pathway of the Pulp, St. Louis, 1976, The C.V. Mosby Co., pp. 537-575.
13. Schillingburg, H.T., and Kessler, J.C.: Restoration of the Endodontically Treated Tooth, Chicago, 1982, Quintessence Publishing Co., Inc., pp. 13-44.
14. Standlee, J.P., Caputo, A.A., and Hanson, E.C.: Retention of endodontic dowels: effects of cement, dowel length, diameter and design, J. Prosthet. Dent. **39:**401, 1978.
15. Taleghani, M., and King, B.: New approach to cast post and core fabrication, Compend. Contin. Dent. Educ. **7:**334, May 1986.
16. Welsh, S.L., and Priddy, W.L.: Direct fabrication of interlocking endodontic posts, J. Prosthet. Dent. **39:**115, 1978.
17. Lovdahl, P.E., and Dumont, T.D.: A dowel core technique for multirooted teeth, J. Prosthet. Dent. **27:**44, 1972.
18. Said-Jabil, S.: Direct pattern technique for fabrication of the cast post-core for divergent root teeth, Quint. Int. **16:**519, 1985.
19. Ziebert, G.J., and Johnson, R.S.: A cast dowel-core technique for multirooted teeth with divergent canals, J. Prosthet. Dent. **49:**207, 1983.
20. Spector, M.: Cast core system with interlocking posts, J. Prosthet. Dent. **56:**16, July 1986.
21. Chaine, J., Dhuru, V., McGivney, G., and Ziebert, G.: Diametral tensile strength of glass ionomer-silver amalgam mixtures for core build-ups, J. Dent. Res., vol. 64, special issue, abstract 552, March 1985.
22. Deutsch, A.S., et al.: Retentive properties of a new post and core system, J. Prosthet. Dent. **53:**12, 1985.
23. Goldman, M., DeVitre, R., and Tenca, J.: A fresh look at the anatomy of the prepared post space, Comp. Contin. Educ. Dent. **6:**628, 1985.
24. Oliva, R.A., and Lowe, J.A.: Dimensional stability of composite used as a core material, J. Prosthet. Dent. **56:**554, November 1986.
25. Hatton, J., Maroso, D.J., and Malone, W.F.P.: Pick-up casting for improved coronal radicular stabilization, submitted for publication 1988.
26. Watson, Philip: Cast Restorations in operative dentistry. In Current Treatment in Dental Practice, Philadelphia, 1986, W.B. Saunders Co., pp. 118-119.
27. Kahn, Henry, Fishman, I., and Malone, W.F.P.: A simplified method for constructing a core following endodontic treatment, J. Prosthet. Dent. **37:**32, 1977.

BIBLIOGRAPHY

Abou-Rass, M., Jann, J.M., Jobe, D., and Tsutsui, F.: Preparation of space for posting: effect on thickness of canal walls and incidence of perforation in molars, J.A.D.A. **104:**834-837, 1982.

Christian, G.W., Button, G.L., Moon, P.C., et al.: Post and core restoration in endodontically treated posterior teeth, J. Endodont. **7:**182-185, 1981.

Deutsch, A.S., Cavallari, J., Musikant, B.L., et al.: Root fractures and design of prefabricated post. J. Prosthet. Dent. **53:**637-640, 1985.

Deutsch, A.S., Musikant, B.L., Cavallari, J., and Bernardi, S.: Retentive properties of the new flexi-post system, J. Prosthet. Dent. **53:**12-14, 1985.

Deutsch, A.S., Musikant, B.L., Cavallari, John, and Lipley, J.B.: Prefabricated dowels: a literature review, J. Prosthet. Dent. **49:**498-503, 1983.

Greenfeld, R.S., and Marshall, F.J.: Factors affecting dowel (post) selection and use in endodontically treated teeth. J. Can. Dent. Assoc. **11:**777-783, 1983.

Greenfeld, R.S., and Weldman, Steven: An in vitro post removal study—a comparison of zinc phosphate cement, glass ionomer cement and composite resin when used as luting agents for post, University of British Columbia, Vancouver, B.C. School of Dentistry, 1986 (unpublished).

Guzy, G., and Nicholls, J.I.: In vitro comparison of intact endodontically treated teeth with and without endo-post reinforcement, J. Prosthet. Dent. **42:**39-44, 1979.

Halle, Enborg, B., Nicholls, Jack I., and Van Hassle, H.J.: An in vitro comparison of retention between a hollow post and core and a custom hollow post and core, J. Endodont. **10:**96, 1984.

Hertle, H., Nicholls, J.I., and Van Hassle, H.J.: The effect of crimping on the retention of hollow posts, J. Endodont. **10:**135, 1984.

Kurer, Grant: Factors influencing dowel retention, J. Prosthet. Dent. **38:**515-24, 1977.

Miller Amp W., III: Post and core systems: Which one is best? J. Prosthet. Dent. **48:**27-38, 1982

Peters, M.C.R.B., Poort, H.W., Farah, J.W., and Craig, R.G.: Stress analysis of a tooth restored with a post and core, J. Dent. Res. **62:**760-763, 1983.

Ross, I.F.: Fracture susceptibility of endodontically treated teeth, J. Endodont. **6:**560-565, 1980.

Sorenson, John A., and Martunoff, James T.: Clinically significant factors in dowel design, J. Prosthet. Dent. **52:**28-35, 1984.

Sorenson, John A., and Martinoff, James T.: Intracoronal reinforcement and coronal coverage: a study of endodontically treated teeth, J. Prosthet. Dent. **52:**780, 1984.

Standlee, J.P., Caputo, A.A., and Hanson, E.C.: Retention of endodontic dowels: effects of cement, dowel length, diameter and design, J. Prosthet. Dent. **39:**401-405, 1978.

Tjan, A.H.L., and Whang, Sung B.: Resistance to root fracture of dowel channels with various thicknesses of buccal dentin walls, J. Prosthet. Dent. **53:**496-500, 1985.

Trope, Martin, Maltx, David O., and Tronstad, Leif: Resistance to fracture of restored endodontically treated teeth, Endodont. Dent. Traumatol. **1:**108-111, 1985.

Wood, W.W.: Retention of posts in teeth with non-vital pulps, J. Prosthet. Dent. **49:**504-6, 1983.

23

Elwood H. Stade and Earl L. Woerner

STOMATOGNATHIC DYSFUNCTION

Present-day dentists must be astute diagnosticians. With ever increasing refinement in treatment modalities and greater financial commitment by patients, simple-to-complex oral reconstruction must be evaluated in light of the pathologic conditions that make them necessary. This chapter provides the dentist with various concepts to assess, treat and/or refer the dysfunctional patient before definitive reconstruction.

The patient with mandibular dysfunction is not always aware of a problem. The symptoms can be subclinical and patient perception totally absent. Conversely, the patient may periodically perceive dysfunction in daily activities but dismiss the discomfort as a tolerable, intermittent distraction not requiring treatment.

Agerberg and Carlsson[1] have reported that over half of their adult population had experienced some signs or symptoms of dysfunction; however, in most instances these people have become asymptomatic without treatment. Some patients with severe symptoms, after examination but without treatment, have been asymptomatic for years, which indicates the problem is cyclical.

At the other extreme is the patient with prolonged acute pain who may have been seeking medical treatment without finding relief. The pain threshold for perception of pain does not vary greatly among individuals; however, the threshold for reaction to pain varies greatly among individuals and for the same individual under varying circumstances.[2] Psychogenic pain can tremendously complicate pain perception and reaction.

In 1956, Schwartz coined the phrase "temporomandibular joint pain-dysfunction syndrome" to describe a group of associated symptoms.[3] Dull pain, dysfunction, and reduced mandibular movements were the symptoms most frequently reported in hundreds of cases. The initial symptoms often appeared after sudden or prolonged stretching and proprioceptive changes following rapid or extensive occlusal changes in patients predisposed by constitution and temperment to this disorder. The syndrome was commonly manifested as a functional disorder of the mandibular musculature and an associated constant dull pain and limited mandibular movement. Malocclusion was believed to be only a contributing factor; the incidence of organic disease was low, and the incidence in female patients was four times more than in male patients.

Campbell also conducted an excellent 11-year study involving 899 cases.[4] He discovered a similar incidence of the female-to-male patient occurences. The pain was concentrated at the origins and insertions of the muscles of mastication, with the joint as the most common pain site. The patient's pain was constant and dull in locations away from the joints. Areas of the neck and shoulders were also involved (Fig. 23-1). The treatment instituted was insertion of acrylic splints to recreate an optimal jaw-joint relationship, followed by occlusal reconstruction. Treatment by altering occlusion and repositioning of the mandible was reported to be successful in more than 75 percent of cases.[5]

Laskin further expanded the psychophysiology as a causative agent. His studies support the role of muscle fatigue as related to psychologically motivated oral habits with resultant muscle spasms. He further termed the condition "myofascial-pain dysfunction syndrome (MPD)."[6]

Travell and Rinzler have also shown that in the pain-dysfunction syndrome the involved musculature may refer pain to remote areas of the head and neck.[7] This complicates the diagnosis and treatment of the disorder.

Internal joint derangements can occur concurrently or independently of muscle symptoms; these frequently are discs displaced in relationship to the condyle head. The displacement, associated with trauma, can produce an anterior displacement of the disc and perforation of the posterior ligamentous attachment that causes the jaw to click with jerky movements.[8] Autopsy reports have demonstrated that anterior displacements of the disc are evident.[9] Trauma to the TMJ ligament can also lead to a malrelation of the condyle-disc complex. Other theories of disc displacement are vertical dimension and/or occlusal disharmonies that alter the disc condylar relationship, resulting in a physical displacement of the condyle off the central portion of the disc.

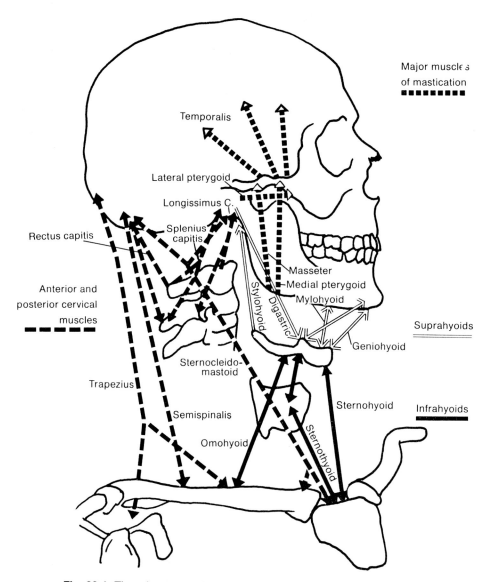

Fig. 23-1. The primary muscles of the craniocervical-mandibular complex.

Failure of the posterior teeth to attain full eruption, or loss of the posterior teeth that maintain the physiologic vertical dimension of occlusion can lead to posterosuperior condylar displacement off the disc. The unilateral loss of posterior teeth can also encourage a torquing or rocking of the jaw about the remaining posterior teeth in an arch. This establishes a Class I lever system with an injurious effect on the joints and musculature. Normal muscle function may be proprioceptively altered, which is exhibited as increased tensional states predisposing a patient to muscle spasms and dysfunction.

The lateral pterygoid muscle is a critical muscle in mandibular movements. The superior head is inserted into the anterior border of the disc, whereas the inferior head inserts into the neck of the condyle. Un-

coordinated contraction of the two heads of the lateral pterygoid muscle produces unsynchronized movements between the condyle and disc, with a resultant click sound heard in the affected joint.[10,11] The click sound is due to collision of the condylar head with the anterior or posterior edge of the disc. Recently, patients have exhibited conditions with the condyle totally off the disc, with disc deformation anteriorly blocking normal condyle movements.[12] This results in restricted openings or the closed lock symptom.

Hypermobility can indicate internal joint derangements. Uncoordinated muscle activity and associated muscle spasms can luxate or dislocate the mandible into a position anterior to the articular tuberculum and sustain this position due to spasms of the masseter, temporal, and internal pterygoid muscles. Occasion-

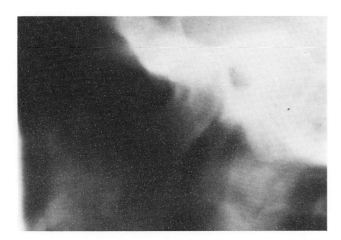

Fig. 23-2. Tomogram of the left temporomandibular joint of patient O.B. with the jaw in centric occlusion.

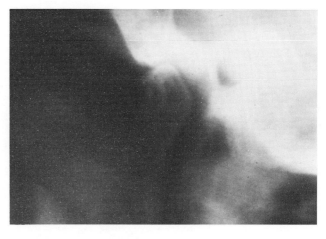

Fig. 23-3. Tomogram of the left temporomandibular joint of patient O.B. with maximum opening. Note the anterior spur on the condyle and the limited condylar movement.

ally, the combination of lidocaine injections and manipulation reduces the dislocation. Recurrent dislocations appear to be related to psychic tension and may need surgery, i.e., eminectomies, to prevent chronic reoccurrences. Subluxation is the term used to describe a mandible that is temporarily stuck or locked in a certain position. Anatomically, the condylar head does not ride over the articular tubercle as in dislocations. The patient experiences a partial or incomplete dislocation, and the teeth do not articulate. This is due to incoordination resulting from muscle spasm and occurs during or after prolonged opening. Subluxations normally disappear upon successful treatment of the muscle spasm. Both luxation and subluxation can be symptoms of the myofascial-pain dysfunction syndrome (MPD).

Joint dysfunction and pain may be involved in temporomandibular joint arthritis. The arthritic condition can be rheumatoid, pyogenic, or osteodegenerative. The joint arthralgia is usually described as a dull, depressing, poorly localized discomfort of varying intensity aggravated by movement and pressure.

Rheumatoid arthritis is a chronic disease of the joints characterized by inflammatory changes in the synovial membrane and periarticular structures with atrophy of the bones.[13] Joint inflammation is usually evident, as are systemic symptoms. Patients with long-standing rheumatoid arthritis can deteriorate into severe joint destruction, anterior open bites, and ankylosis. Since other joints of the body usually are also involved, it is a medically managed and confirmed disease.

Osteoarthritis is the common arthropathy of the joint. It is commonly observed in elderly patients and is a degenerative noninflammatory disturbance of the joints. The symptoms are:

1. Crepitation, cracking, or clicking of a joint.
2. Pain and tenderness in a joint on movement.
3. Luxation and subluxation.
4. Difficulty in opening, and possibly locking of a joint at certain positions.
5. Joint pain on heavy biting.
6. Ear pain and dizziness.
7. Strain, stiffness, or tiredness in neck or back of head.
8. Strain or tiredness in the joint.
9. Mandibular deviation upon jaw movements.[13]

Arthrosis, or noninflammatory degenerative joint change, has been confirmed in 80 to 90 percent of the population over 60 years of age.[14] Many of these cases result from years of microtrauma to the joint; however, the patient history may reveal a prior joint injury. Radiographic techniques are useful in assessing the extent of the joint changes, and functional comfort can be restored to selected patients by occlusal therapy (Figs. 23-2 to 23-9). Mongini has shown that the degenerative bony changes can be arrested and that constructive remodeling occurs following occlusal therapy.[15]

In the normal joint, the articular disc and synovial fluid perform as a separating structure, forming a hydrocushion between the condylar head and the slope of the articular eminence. Disc perforations lead to bone-on-bone contact, producing crepitus and the bony contour changes seen radiographically in the condyle head. Bruxism can be the cause, as tensional habits are one of the major causative factors.[15] Unfortunately, the disc is avascular and has limited potential for repair, so condylar degenerative changes are a natural sequel.

Infectious arthritides of the temporomandibular joint are rare. It may occur from injection penetrations or direct extensions, especially from the ear or hema-

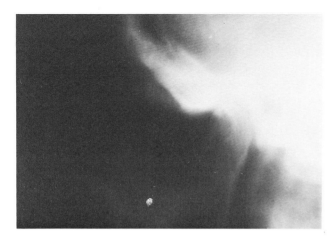

Fig. 23-4. Tomogram of the right temporomandibular joint of patient O.B. with the jaw in centric occlusion.

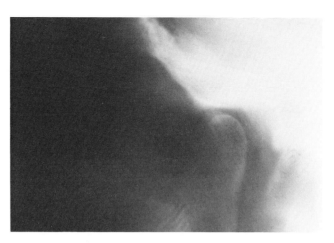

Fig. 23-5. Tomogram of the right temporomandibular joint of patient O.B. with maximum opening. Note the more regular, smooth condylar form and the greater amount of translation as compared to left joint in Fig. 23-3.

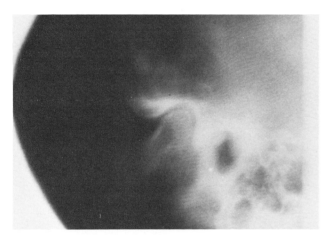

Fig. 23-6. Tomogram of the left temporomandibular joint of patient G.U. with the jaw in centric occlusion.

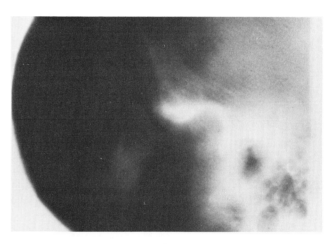

Fig. 23-7. Tomogram of the left temporomandibular joint of patient G.U. with maximum opening.

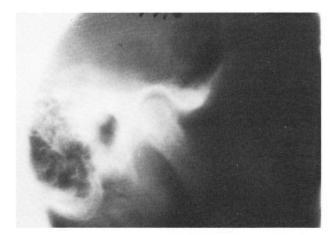

Fig. 23-8. Tomogram of the right temporomandibular joint of patient G.U. with the jaw in centric occlusion.

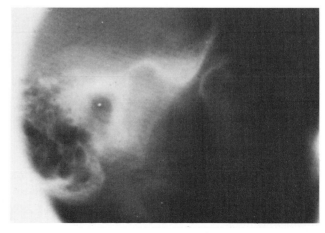

Fig. 23-9. Tomogram of the right temporomandibular joint of patient G.U. with maximum opening. Note the unusually large degree of translation of the condyle.

togenously.[14] Gonorrheal, streptococcal, and staphylococcal infections of this joint have been reported, but systemic disease symptoms can be elicited in the patient history. The infected joint displays an inflammatory process of pain, heat, and swelling with marked restriction of movement and tissue destruction.

When these joint diseases become painful, the somatic pain induces central excitatory effects, causing referred pains, secondary hyperalgesias, and spreading painful muscle spasms.[16] These symptoms resemble an acute mandibular pain dysfunction syndrome; knowledge and skill in diagnosing the arthralgias is crucial for rendering a diagnosis and treatment regime.

Anomalies of growth and development, neoplasms, and condylar hyperplasia occur, but are commonly observed as facial asymmetries. Their diagnosis and treatment is beyond the scope of this chapter.

A brief comment should be made about the neuralgias. The symptom is pain that follows the course or distribution of a nerve. It is severe, throbbing, or stabbing in character. Trigeminal neuralgia, or tic douloureux, is the most frequent and excruciating neuralgia seen by a dentist. It is differentiated from joint or muscle pain by its distribution, which follows the branches of the fifth cranial nerve, and is also diagnosed by hypersensitive areas called "trigger zones." Patients develop guarded jaw movements to avoid triggering the pain. This leads to functional muscle fatigue and increased tensional states which sponsor associated masticatory muscle pain and tenderness.[17] The unique symptoms, and the ability to block the trigger zones anesthetically, distinguish this affliction from a temporomandibular joint disturbance.[18]

With this brief historical background of the muscle and joint disturbances, a review of anatomy is needed to understand the words of Irby: "the temporomandibular articulation is a delicately balanced mechanism functioning under neuromuscular dictation. The TMJ is subject to many extrinsic influences, including occlusal disharmony. Through hypertonicity and spasm, the muscles of mastication must certainly reflect the impact of emotional or psychogenic disturbances: i.e., especially recently induced. Aside from this circumstance, the dentist must be aware that the joint is subject to both pathologic and functional disturbances similar to any other human joint. This serves as the focus of pain that initiates muscle spasm. Therefore, when the entire spectrum of etiological factors is reviewed, the dentist must consider both extrinsic and intrinsic factors."[19]

Before the clinical examination and evaluation of the patient, a thorough medical, dental, and psychological history is necessary. The psychological history should include periods of personal stress in the life of patients and how they dealt with these problems. It is an indicator of the patient's past and present emotional status. Another indicator of psychological significance is when the symptom complex is inconsistent with anatomic and physiologic findings, so the focus shifts to the extent of psychogenic pain. Consultation with the family physician for a psychological evaluation may be advisable.

When considering a complaint of pain, Bell has listed the following[17]:

1. Intensity of the pain—mild vs. severe
2. Mode of onset—spontaneous vs. induced
3. Manner of flow of the pain—flowing vs. paroxysmal
4. Quality of the pain—dull, aching, burning, pricking, itching, pulsing
5. Temporal behavior—intermittent vs. continuous
6. Duration of individual pains—time
7. Localization behavior—local vs. diffuse
8. Effect of functional activities—initiates pain, trigger zones
9. Concomitant neurologic signs—sensations, changes
10. Anatomic description where the pain is felt—muscle or bone

CLINICAL EXAMINATION

The initial examination of a patient to exclude the presence of muscle and/or joint dysfunction can be performed efficiently by a dentist. A written checklist for a patient to answer concerning symptoms and history of mandibular dysfunction can initially be helpful for screening purposes (See occlusal screening form.) It involves minimal effort by a dentist to review. However, a patient's subjective perceptions are a crucial but not sole ingredient for diagnosis and only augment an objective clinical examination.

Bell has listed four clinical symptoms[20]:

1. Pain of masticatory origin emanating from the muscles of mastication and/or the temporomandibular joints.
2. Restricted mandibular movements that originate in muscle and/or the joint.
3. Interferences during mandibular movements identified as abnormal joint sounds, sensations, and/or movements occurring during normal function.
4. Acute malocclusions seen as changes in occlusal relationships secondary to a temporomandibular disorder and perceived as abnormal by the patient.

Pain of masticatory origin can possibly be identified by the patient. However, the pain may be present but with subclinical symptoms that the patient consciously perceives and responds to only during muscle and joint palpation (Fig. 23-1). Therefore, the clinician must be trained in the appropriate techniques of muscle and joint palpation described by Schwartz and Chayes.[2] The use of the Myotronics EM$_2$, a portable electromyograph, is one proven method for assessing the tensional state of the muscles of mastication. It readily records and prints, by the use of a microcomputer, numerical values representative of resting and functional states of the anterior and posterior temporalis, masseter, and anterior digastric muscles. The dentist can also compare the state of balance between left- and right-side muscle groups, as well as the effect of treatment on the musculature.

Crispin has demonstrated that the pantograph is another means for identification and evaluation of muscle dysfunction.[21]

Functional tests such as maximal jaw opening measurements, deviational opening and closing movements, and inhibited eccentric movements help establish the presence and degree of dysfunction. The mandible will be seen to deviate on opening movements to the affected side. This normally can be correlated to symptomatic musculature and/or joint dysfunction. Auscultation of the joints can locate a click that usually indicates internal disc derangement. Crepitus, or grating sounds, will be indicative of degenerative joint changes. Degenerative joint diseases can usually be documented and evaluated with tomography techniques or CAT scan radiography (Fig. 23-3). Internal derangements are evaluated with arthrography and magnetic resonance imaging.

Oral examination of the patient's occlusion often reveals traumatic occlusion. Occlusal disharmony is evidenced by premature occlusal contacts, deflective interfering tooth contacts in eccentric movements, faceting of tooth surfaces, thermal sensitivity, tooth mobility, or fremitus and fractured cusps (see occlusal analysis forms I and II).

For a less obstructive evaluation of the occlusion and its relationship to the joints, diagnostic casts are mounted on a semiadjustable articulator in the centric relation position. Following this procedure, the casts are positioned into the patient's centric occlusion position, and the condyle-fossa relationship is evaluated. The degree of disharmony between the teeth and the temporomandibular condyle fossa relationship in the horizontal plane becomes evident. In many instances, the dentist can then correlate the prior documented muscle symptoms (spasms) to a malrelated, tooth-dictated jaw position. Thus, total comprehension of the series of events occurring occlusally explains how the symptomology relates to the malfunction.

A disharmonious relationship between the occlusion and the temporomandibular joint can be manifested by disease and/or dysfunction in the joint, teeth, or musculature. It is observed in one or all of the components that compose this triad, and the weaker components of the triad usually manifest the symptoms first.

The purpose of this chapter is to develop an appreciation by the dentist of the signs and symptoms of stomatognathic dysfunction. Definitive treatment schemes are beyond its scope; however, the dentist should not consider customary dental treatment beyond his or her capability. Many pain dysfunction patients require normal treatment procedures that restore lost vertical dimension to the occlusion and the physiologic postural positions to the jaw-joint complex. The use of easily fabricated acrylic occlusal splints can produce successful results[22-25] (Figs. 23-10 to 23-13).

Properly fabricated splints are usually reversible treatment procedures. This statement by no means insinuates that all dentists should fabricate an occlusal splint for treating all symptomatic patients. This is an area of dentistry that demands highly developed diagnostic and treatment skills. Since we deal with a multifactorial problem, the dentist must realize treatment limitations as a dentist and refer the patient for additional medical and human behavior evaluation. The dentist as a member of a health care team can benefit by seeking consensus on treatment direction. Dental treatment may at times totally restore function and eliminate pain, but conversely, it may only decrease the patient's suffering to tolerable levels. In rare cases, it produces no effect, in which situation the patient is aided by elimination of the questionable dental component in a quest for relief and successful treatment.

SELECTED REFERENCES

1. Agerberg, G., and Carlsson, G.E.: Symptoms of functional disturbances of the masticatory system. A comparison of frequencies in a population sample and in a group of patients, Acta Odont. Scandinav. **33**:183, 1975.
2. Schwartz, L., and Chayes, C.: Facial Pain and Mandibular Dysfunction, Philadelphia, 1968, W.B. Saunders Co.
3. Schwartz, L.: A temporomandibular joint pain-dysfunction syndrome, J. Chron. Dis. **3**:284, 1956.
4. Campbell, J.: Distribution and treatment of pain in temporomandibular arthroses, Br. Dent. J. **205**:393, 1958.
5. Lindblom, G.: Disorders of the temporomandibular joint. Causal factors and the value of temporomandibular joint radiographs in diagnosis and therapy, Acta Odont. Scandinav. **11**:61, 1953.
6. Laskin, D.M., Etiology of the pain-dysfunction syndrome, J.A.D.A. **79**:147-153, 1969.
7. Travell, J., and Rinzler, S.H.: The myofascial genesis of pain, Postgrad. Med. **11**:425, 1952.
8. Farrar, W.: Diagnosis and treatment of anterior dislocation of the articular disc, N.Y.J. Dent. **41**:348, 1971.

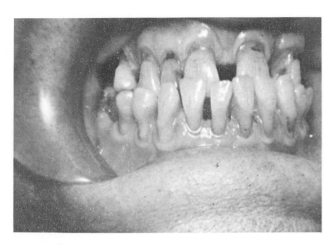

Fig. 23-10. Patient P.G. in centric occlusion. He has history of myofascial-pain dysfunction syndrome exhibited by facial pain, bilateral T.M.J. clicking, excessive occlusal wear, deflection into an acquired Class III malocclusion, and muscular hypertonicity.

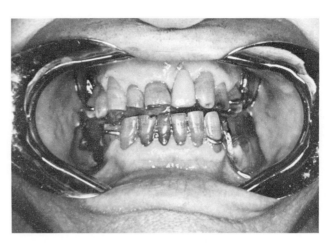

Fig. 23-12. Orthotics in place showing restoration of vertical dimension and correction of Class III malocclusion.

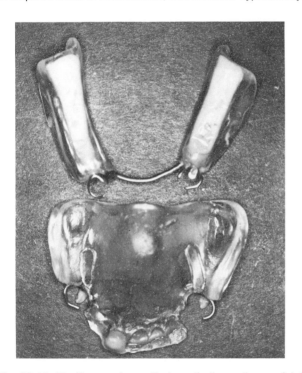

Fig. 23-11. Maxillary and mandibular orthotic appliances fabricated for patient P.G. in centric relation at a restored vertical dimension of occlusion. Note flat occlusal planes in posterior areas and incisal guidance on maxillary orthotic. Tooth No. 9 was extracted and temporarily replaced in the orthotic appliance.

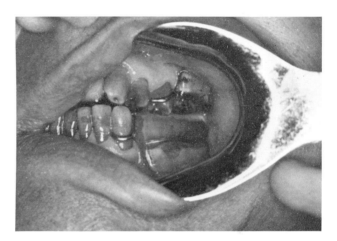

Fig. 23-13. Lateral view of orthotics in place. Note capability to alter posterior occlusion with new autopolymerizing acrylic overlay.

9. Hanson, T.L., Solberg, W.K., and Tenn, M.O.: Temporomandibular joint changes in young adults, J. Dent. Res. (Abstract No. 700), 1979.
10. Rees, L.A.: Structure and function of the mandibular joint, Br. Dent. J. **96**:125, 1954.
11. Sicher, H.: Structural and functional basis for disorders of the temporomandibular articulation, J. Oral Surg. **13**:175, 1955.
12. McCarty, W.L., Jr., and Farrar, W.F.: Surgery for internal derangements of the temporomandibular joint, J. Prosthet. Dent. **42**:191, 1979.
13. Beeson, P., and McDermott, W., eds.: Cecil-Loeb Textbook of Medicine, ed. 13, Philadelphia, 1971, W.B. Saunders Co.
14. Morgan, D., House, L., Hall, W., and Vamvas, S.: Diseases of the Temporomandibular Apparatus, ed. 2, St. Louis, 1982, The C.V. Mosby Co..
15. Mongini, F.: Condylar remodeling after occlusal therapy, J. Prosthet. Dent. **43**:568, 1980.
16. Irby, W.B., and Baldwin, K.H.: Emergencies and Urgent Complications in Dentistry, St. Louis, 1965, The C.V. Mosby Co.
17. Bell, W.E.: Orofacial Pains, Differential Diagnosis, Dallas, 1973, Denedco of Dallas.
18. Laskin, D., Greenfield, W., Gale, E., et al.: The President's Conference on the examination diagnosis and management of temporomandibular disorders, Chicago, American Dental Assoc., 1983.
19. Irby, W.B.: Surgery of the temporomandibular joint. In Irby, W.B., ed.: Current advances in Oral Surgery, St. Louis, 1974, The C.V. Mosby Co.
20. Bell, W.E.: The President's Conference on the examination, diagnosis, and management of temporomandibular disorders, Chicago, American Dental Assoc., 1983.

21. Crispin, B.J., Myers, G.E., and Clayton, J.A.: Effects of occlusal therapy on pantographic reproducibility of mandibular border movements, J. Prosthet. Dent. **40**:29-32, 1978.

22. Shore, N.A.: A mandibular autorepositioning appliance, J.A.D.A. **75**:908-911, 1967.

23. Schulman, J.: A technique for bite plane construction, J. Prosthet. Dent. **29**:334-339, 1973.

24. Krammer, Von R.: Constructing occlusal splints, J. Prosthet. Dent. **41**:105-108, 1979.

25. Stade, Elwood, and Malone, W.: The prosthetic treatment of pain—dysfunction syndrome case, Ill. State Dent. J., December, 1969.

METAL/CERAMIC CROWNS: PORCELAIN FUSED TO METAL

Although the complete metal crown is a biologic restoration, it is generally confined to the posterior quadrants of the oral cavity. For esthetic reasons, anterior complete crowns are modified with a porcelain veneer. This modification is commonplace with the anterior 10 maxillary teeth, 8 mandibular teeth, and occasionally the maxillary first molar.

When the porcelain veneer is selected, the tooth preparation is modified by increased reduction on the surfaces. This modification allows additional space for the thickness of porcelain.

Historically, the porcelain veneer facing was a customized porcelain denture tooth adapted to fit a specific preparation. After the facing was adapted with lateral recesses, it was waxed (Fig. 24-1) into a prepared crown. The facing was removed from the wax and luted with cement after the casting was finished. The assembled two-part crown was then cemented to the patient's tooth.

PORCELAIN-FUSED-T0-METAL VENEER CROWNS

Woolson presented an early effort to overcome the difficulty that arises when porcelain is fired to metal.[1] Porcelain fired directly to gold alloys developed cracks after firing because of the different coefficients of expansion of the two materials. The problem was partially resolved when a slip plane was interposed, allowing each material to manifest its own physical laws of contraction and expansion. Since the early 1940's, metallurgic research has provided many advancements, such as vacuum firing and superior ceramic mixtures, to enhance the use of complete porcelain-fused-to-metal crowns. Until the late 1950's, porcelain-fused-to-metal crowns lacked natural color and vitality when used as a restoration for the maxillary four incisors.

Improvements in the bonding of the porcelain to the metal and the properties of the porcelain have made this restoration popular. Porcelain-fused-to-metal complete crowns are used extensively as individual restorations and as FPD retainers. Fig. 24-2 shows the labial view of the tooth preparation for a

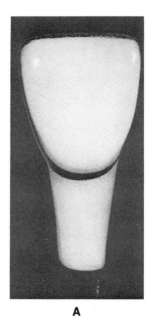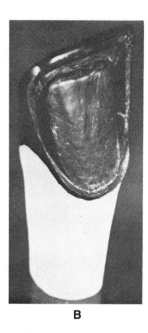

A　　　　　　　　**B**

Fig. 24-1. A, Porcelain denture tooth formed and waxed to a model of the prepared tooth. **B,** With the facing removed to show recesses in the wax into which lateral extensions of porcelain facing extend.

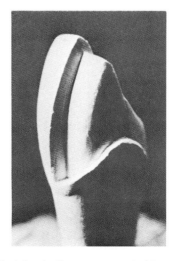

Fig. 24-2. Facial reduction recommended for veneer crown.

porcelain-fused-to-metal crown for a maxillary central incisor, indicating the recommended facial reduction. Fig. 24-3 displays the proximal surfaces for a porcelain-fused-to-metal crown preparation.

Indications

The primary reasons for using complete porcelain-fused-to-metal crowns are similar to indications for the complete porcelain crown. However, the metal/ceramic crown is more versatile because of its common employment as an FPD retainer. It can also be placed as a single posterior restoration where esthetics is a consideration.[4,5] In addition to the indications for the complete porcelain crown, the porcelain-fused-to-metal veneer crown is also suitable for:

1. Single and multiple restorations for both anterior and posterior teeth.
2. Retainers for a RPD.
3. FPDs.
4. Superstructures for splinted periodontal prostheses.
5. Mandibular anterior teeth where full shoulder preparations are prohibitive.
6. Peg-shaped laterals or teeth with similar morphologic deviations.
7. Patients with a reduced interocclusal clearance or a strong masticatory musculature.

Disadvantages

Although the application of porcelain veneer crowns is diverse, there are disadvantages incident to their use, namely:

1. The porcelain-fused-to-metal veneers are susceptible to fracture.
2. Facial reduction and margins for porcelain veneer crowns subject the pulp and investing tissue to trauma.
3. Esthetic considerations that accommodate tissue tolerance may be difficult because of overcontouring.
4. The longevity of these restorations is related to veneer durability.

Along with the disadvantages, there are clinical conditions that limit the use of porcelain veneer crowns:

1. Younger patients with larger pulps dictate modification of the facial shoulder preparation.
2. Establishment of satisfactory occlusal relationships is exacting.
3. Patients with poor hygiene restrict the latitude of the dentist in the placement of the gingival margin.

The limitations of any restoration are placed in the relative order of importance. The dentist, with the permission of the patient, may elect to place complete veneer crowns despite clinical difficulty. Belated peri-

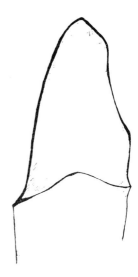

Fig. 24-3. Proximal surface of porcelain-fused-to-metal veneer crown preparation.

odontal complications are common. The rough, overcontoured margins of crowns within the gingival sulcus cause inflammation. Whenever the gingival sulcus is involved, the material selected should be compatible with tissue, and the preparation performed with minimal trauma.[9,10] However, recent research has demonstrated that some inflammation of the periodontal tissue is inherent with all subgingival crowns.

Requirements

Pulpal considerations. The facial reduction is usually responsible for pulpal involvement; however, few individual crowns are placed on healthy teeth. The prepared teeth usually have previously received a carious, periodontal, or traumatic insult. Belated pulpal responses after preparation and crown placement are realistic components on all fixed prosthodontics. Preparation of a healthy tooth as an abutment for a fixed prosthesis is an exception. The opportunity of creating an ideal preparation without the modifications associated with fixed prosthodontics is a rare occurrence. Nevertheless, near-ideal preparations are possible if regimented caries-control programs with amalgam restorations are performed prior to cast restorations.

Restoration of function and anatomy. The complete metal veneer crown meets nearly all the requirements of a successful dental restoration if placed where indicated and satisfactorily prepared. It is possible not only to simulate the natural tooth but also to restore esthetics and function. In addition, the complete metal veneer crown allows the dentist more latitude in restoring a tooth to innocuous occlusal relationships.

The use of porcelain-fused-to-metal veneer crowns

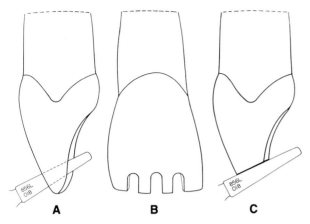

Fig. 24-4. A, The incisal depth grooves are 1.5 to 2.5 mm deep and oriented parallel to the terminal protrusive functional pathway. **B,** Incisal depth cuts placed at the midincisal and the junction of the proximal and middle third of the incisal edge. **C,** Final reduction is accomplished by connecting initial depth cuts while maintaining a protrusive pathway.

with total occlusal coverage of porcelain for an entire quadrant presents a problem. Gold is used as a restorative material, in addition to its noble-metal attributes, because the attrition rate is similar to tooth structure. When porcelain is placed on opposing teeth, on maxillary to mandibular molars, and/or used in key occlusal relationships, a bisque-baked try-in is necessary. The use of full porcelain coverage on posterior teeth warrants more longitudinal studies. Patients with an immediate canine-guided disclusion who require maximum esthetics can be given full porcelain occlusal coverage posteriorly. Patients with a group-function occlusion with maximum intercuspal articulation during lateral excursions present overwhelming complications. Some of the problems noted immediately by the dentist are porcelain fractures or opposing tooth wear; the belated problems are supportive bone loss.

Adjustment of porcelain-to-porcelain surfaces is difficult without additional porcelain firing. Contact areas on porcelain-fused-to-metal crowns can be bulky compared to original tooth contours unless laboratory support is precise.

Investing tissues. Porcelain-fused-to-metal crowns restore the entire coronal portion of the tooth. Optimum contours for facial surfaces of crowns are still being closely reviewed by dentists and scrutinized by researchers.[11]

Overcontoured crowns, misplaced proximal contacts, and poorly designed occlusal relationships sponsor adverse gingival tissue responses. The concept of splinting crowns to obtain a more favorable supportive tissue response is also controversial. Splinting may add support to a tooth or teeth, but it limits the patient's oral hygiene. Additional studies are needed to determine when splinting is appropriate.[12] Presently, the disadvantages outweigh the advantages unless the restorative measures are a terminal attempt to avoid a removable prosthesis. Single units are more conducive to positive tissue health.

Uniformity of tooth reduction. Diagnostic aids in the form of radiographs and diagnostic casts enhance uniformity of tooth reduction. Crowns placed on the posterior teeth present a formidable problem from the standpoint of access and visibility. Modifications of traditional preparation designs are made for a myriad of reasons, but mainly because of extensive caries, which is routine during preparation for complete metal veneer crowns. Periodontally involved teeth require profound fluting, and possibly supragingival margins.

Instrumentation

Ultra high-speed cutting instruments have made extremely arduous procedures easier. The selection of diamonds and carbide burs is a matter of preference. Four-handed dentistry also affects the manipulation of the instruments.

Sequence of Preparation

The porcelain-fused-to-metal restoration is a combination of metal and porcelain; therefore, the preparation is likewise a combination of preparations. The facial and proximal reductions are sufficient to provide space for a metal coping and porcelain to achieve the desired esthetic result. Generally this requires 1.2 to 1.5 mm of facial reduction. The lingual surface requires enough reduction for adequate metal thickness (generally 1.0 mm), but more if it is to be covered with porcelain.

The preparation is divided into two distinct portions, the "initial preparation" and "margination." The initial portion is intended to create a gingival ledge around the tooth; if carried subgingivally, this ledge terminates at the gingival crest. If the final preparation does not terminate subgingivally, this ledge should terminate 0.1 mm occlusal or incisal to the intended gingival extension. The second portion of the preparation is to prepare the margin.

Step 1—incisal reduction. The incisal plane is reduced from 1.5 to 2.5 mm (Fig. 24-4) so that there is suitable thickness of gold and porcelain. Incisal reduction should be adequate to ensure clearance in protrusive movements of the mandible, encourage esthetics, and enhance function.

Depth cuts gauge and facilitate preparation, and identify the dimensions of the reduction. Generally, initial preparation is conservative; a depth of 1.5 mm is appropriate for these depth cuts. Their orientation is parallel to the terminal protrusive functional path-

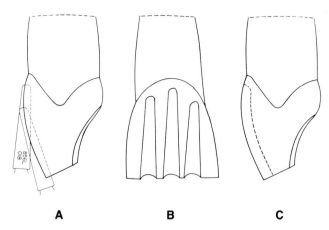

Fig. 24-5. A, Depth cut placed at gingival termination identifying path of draw and extension incisally to follow original contour of facial surface. **B,** Depth cuts in midfacial, mesial, and distal halves of facial surface. **C,** The final facial reduction closely follows the original tooth contour.

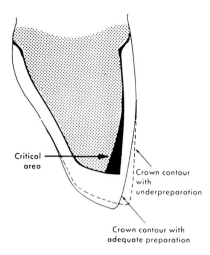

Fig. 24-6. A common problem is insufficient labial reduction in the incisal one-third. (From Fisher, W.F., ed. Hosp. Dent. Serv. Bull., R.D.A., October 1969. Walter Reed Army Hospital, Washington, D.C.)

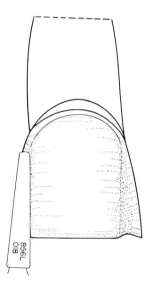

Fig. 24-7. The instrument is aligned over the profile of the proximal reduction, oriented parallel to the line of draw and with the tip positioned to create a gingival ledge with the same dimension as the facial.

way. Depth cuts are normally placed one each at midincisal and at the junction of each proximal. For efficiency, these depth cuts are accomplished with the same diamond used for facial reduction.

The occlusal reduction for a posterior veneer crown is similar to that of the complete metal crown, except the occlusal reduction is a minimum of 2 mm over the surface veneered with porcelain.

Step 2—facial reduction. The initial step in axial wall reduction is to determine the path of draw. This takes into account the anatomy and contour of the tooth (or teeth if an FPD preparation); the relationship of the prepared tooth to the adjacent teeth and op-

posing teeth; and the relationship with other teeth in the prosthesis. Ideally, this path of draw is along the long axis of the crown. However, there are modifications to this guideline.

A depth cut identifying the path of draw after a reduction of 1.5 to 2 mm reduction at the height of contour is placed in the midfacial (Fig. 24-5). Additional depth cuts may be placed in the mesial and distal halves of the facial surface. These depth cuts generally follow the original contour of the facial surface.

After placement of the depth grooves, the ribs of unprepared tooth structure remaining are removed. This reduction is continued around the line angles to establish the profile of the proximal reduction. The gingival extent of this reduction results in a uniform ledge that maintains a suitable axial depth.

The facial reduction closely follows the original facial tooth contours. Failure to observe this operative procedure results in a protrusive veneer (Fig. 24-6) with lack of space at the incisal plane. This is called "biomechanical reduction."

Step 3—proximal reduction. Proximal reduction is accomplished to maintain parallelism with the line of draw without damaging an adjacent tooth (Fig. 24-7). Occasionally, because of the alignment of adjacent teeth, this can be difficult; if necessary, parallelism along this wall is compromised to protect the adjacent tooth.

To prepare the proximal surface, align the instrument used for facial reduction over the profile of the proximal reduction and with the orientation parallel to the line of draw; position the tip to create a gingival ledge the same dimension as the facial. Check to en-

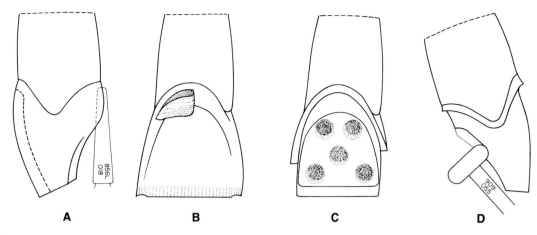

Fig. 24-8. A, Reduction of the cingulum wall to maintain parallelism with the facial wall. **B,** One-half of the cingulum wall reduced, illustrating a definite wall. **C,** Depth divots placed for lingual fossa reduction. **D,** Final lingual fossa reduction with a wheel-shaped diamond.

sure that the instrument passes through without damaging the adjacent tooth. If the diamond does not clear the adjacent tooth, move it bodily toward the center of the prepared tooth to create clearance between the diamond and the adjacent tooth. In this position, observe the dimension of gingival ledge created by the diamond tip. If not excessive, continue the proximal reduction with this orientation. If the gingival ledge is too broad, tip the diamond to maintain clearance with the adjacent tooth while creating a gingival ledge the same dimension of the facial, forfeiting a degree of parallelism.

Step 4—lingual reduction. All the enamel is not removed from the lingual surface of complete metal veneer crowns. Adequate reduction for strength to withstand the forces of occlusion is the normal guideline. The porcelain-fused-to-metal veneer requires more reduction than the resin veneer. Anatomically, the lingual surface of the anterior tooth has two distinct components—the cingulum and the lingual fossa. Accordingly, preparation of this surface is also divided into two component stages.

Cingulum Wall Reduction

The cingulum axial wall is the only portion of the lingual surface to provide parallelism with the axis of draw. Depending on anatomy of the tooth and position of the gingival tissue, it may be possible to produce a short axial wall that is relatively parallel to the axis of draw (Fig. 24-8). Examine the contour of the cingulum wall and extend the reduction of this wall to join the proximal reduction.

This reduction is accomplished with the same diamond used for the facial and proximal reduction, but with less diameter, since this area is merely reduced for metal coverage.

Lingual Fossa Reduction

The reduction of the lingual fossa depends on the design of the restoration. If the lingual surface of the restoration is metal, the reduction requires only 1 mm. However, if the design is full porcelain coverage, reduction must be 1.25 mm to 1.5 mm throughout the surfaces of porcelain coverage.

The dimension of reduction is gauged by depth cut grooves or divots (Fig. 24-8). The groove can be made with the tip of the diamond used for facial proximal and cingulum wall reduction to extend from the crest of the cingulum through the linguoincisal. In lieu of this groove, depth divots are made with a round bur. The No. 2 round bur is 1 mm in diameter and is used where metal coverage is planned. The No. 4 round bur is 1.5 mm in diameter and is indicated where porcelain coverage is planned. Round burs have a propensity to abruptly "dig in" as enamel is perforated. Accordingly, rather than trying to cut a "hole" of given depth, a divot generated by a pendulum cut is more controllable. The final reduction of the lingual fossa is accomplished with a wheel-shaped or football-shaped diamond instrument.

Step 5—gingival margin preparation. For a complete description of margin configuration, the reader is referred to other sources.[13] Common margin configurations taught in dental schools are probably the shoulder, the beveled shoulder, and heavy chamfer (Fig. 24-9). The heavy chamfer offers several advantages and provides acceptable marginal adaptation provided a dimension of metal at the collar area is maintained. If esthetics is paramount, the metal collar may be thinned, with a compromise in marginal fit. An alternative to thinning the metal collar is a porcelain butt shoulder. This chapter illustrates the heavy chamfer as the margin configuration of choice.

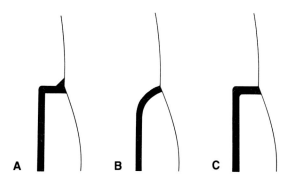

Fig. 24-9. A, A shoulder margin configuration. **B,** A heavy chamfer margin configuration. **C,** A beveled shoulder margin configuration.

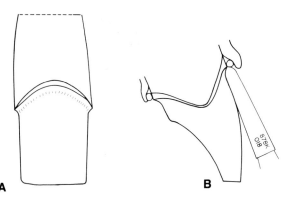

Fig. 24-10. A, Chamfer-forming instrument placed so that one-half of diameter at tip is cutting; the rest of the instrument should just touch gingival portion of the initial preparation. **B,** The final margin should follow the contour of the gingiva and be uniform in width.

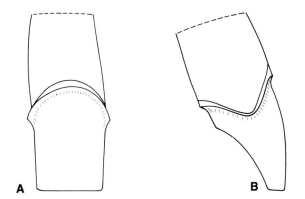

Fig. 24-11. A, Facial view of finished preparation. **B,** Proximal view of finished preparation.

Tissue management to secure gingival margins is reviewed elsewhere in Chapter 9. Cords and electrosurgical techniques are both advocated.

The cervical margin is normally placed slightly below the crest of the soft tissue facially. More latitude can be exercised during preparation of the lingual surface. Placement of the facial margin subgingivally usually enhances esthetics. If the smile lip line of the patient terminates below the gingival crest or below the cervical third of the clinical crown, this procedure is not critical. Posteriorly, the facial margin on the premolars is subject to the same rules as the incisors, but the gingival margins on the molar can terminate at a position more supragingivally to promote the health of the soft tissue if there is sufficient vertical length for retention. This is particularly true in periodontally treated patients.

With the gingiva retracted, a chamfer-forming diamond—generally 3 mm at the tip—is used to prepare the subgingival margin (Fig. 24-10). Embed the tip of the instrument through the initial preparation ledge until it extends to the desired gingival level and po-

sition it into the tooth to the desired depth. The instrument is secured parallel to the axis of draw and moved through the tooth structure in a back-and-forth motion to create a smooth chamfer. The tissue contour is followed carefully while the tip of the instrument is cutting in order to minimize trauma to the tissue (half of the diameter of the diamond is outside the contour of the tooth). The contour of the tooth is followed at the level of the margin so that the margin is uniform in width. The marginal dimension is reduced on the lingual surface and the lingual portion of the interproximal areas.

Step 6—finishing the preparation. Gross scratches are removed and the line angles and corners are rounded. Fig. 24-11 illustrates a finished porcelain-fused-to-metal preparation.

CONCLUSIONS

The finished preparations are a miniature reproduction of the original teeth with margin modification.

There are limited contraindications for the use of porcelain veneer crowns. Porcelain-fused-to-metal crowns presently enjoy unparalleled popularity among restorative dentists; however, one must remember that the longevity of a veneer crown is directly proportional to the durability of its veneer. Veneers placed on molar teeth are rare, as in situations of exceptionally demanding esthetics.

Improvements in porcelain-fused-to-metal veneer crowns are forthcoming and will be welcomed by the entire profession.

NOTE: A color display illustrating the strength and esthetics of PFM crowns is available in the back of the text (24-12, A to E).

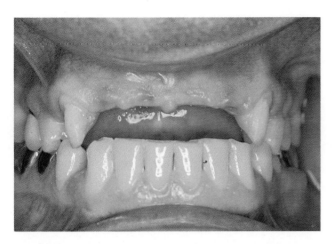

Fig. 24-12. A, Tooth preparation with beveled shoulders for a six unit anterior FPD of PFM. Note the erosion approximating the gingival tissue.

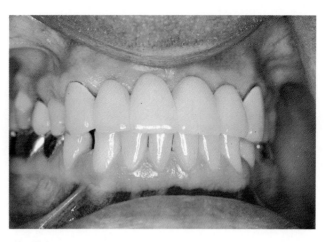

Fig. 24-12. B, Six unit porcelain fused to metal prosthesis with a metal collar to avoid over contouring.

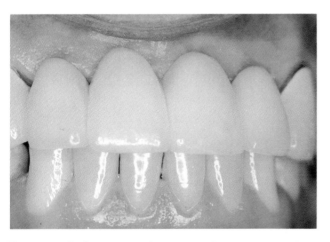

Fig. 24-12. C, Closer view of PFM with characterization of the gingival porcelain and metal collars to cover erosion.

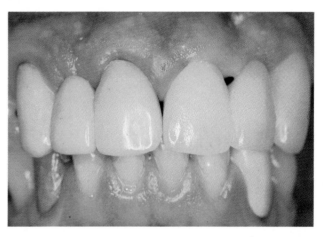

Fig. 24-12. D, Two three unit maxillary PFM, FPDs demonstrating the difference between a collarless crown and a metal collar for the gingival finish.

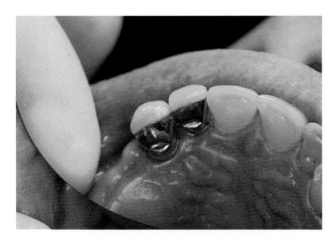

Fig. 24-12. E, Splinted PFM crowns with lingual rests for abutment of a RPD. (Courtesy W.F.P. Malone, Alton, Ill.

SELECTED REFERENCES

1. Woolson, A.H.: Restorations made of porcelain backed on gold, J. Prosthet. Dent. **5**:65, 1955.
2. Dawson, P.E.: Evaluation, Diagnosis and Treatment of Occlusal Problems, St. Louis, 1974, The C.V. Mosby Co.
3. Guyer, S.E.: Multiple preparations for fixed prosthodontics, J. Prosthet. Dent. **23**:529-553, 1970.
4. Breaker, S.C.: Porcelain fused to gold, J. Calif. Dent. Assoc. and Nevada Dent. Soc. **36**:425-429, 1960.
5. Johnston, J.F., Mumford, G., and Dykema, R.W.: Porcelain veneers bonded to metal castings, Practical Dent. Monogr., March 1963, pp. 3-32.
6. Shell, J.S., and Neisen, J.P.: Study of bond between gold alloys and porcelain, J. Dent. Res. **41**:1427-1437, 1962.
7. Shillingburg, H.T., Hobo, S., and Fisher, D.W.: Preparation design and margin distortion in porcelain fused to metal restorations, J. Prosthet. Dent. **30**:28-36, 1973.
8. Hobo, S., and Shillingburg, H.T.: Porcelain fused to metal: tooth prepartion and coping design, J. Prosthet. Dent. **30**:28-36, 1973.

9. Myers, G.E.: Textbook of Crown and Bridge Prosthodontics, St. Louis, 1969, The C.V. Mosby Co., pp. 68-92.

10. Weinberg, L.A.: Esthetics and the gingiva in full coverage, J. Prosthet. Dent. **10**:737, 1960.

11. Kahn, A.E.: Partial vs. full coverage, J. Prosthet. Dent. **10**:167, 1960.

12. Lorey, R.E., and Myers, G.E.: The retentive qualities of bridge retainers, J.A.D.A. **76**:568, 1968.

13. McLean, J.W.: The Science and Art of Dental Ceramics, Vol. II, Chicago, 1980, Quintessence Publishing Co., Inc.

BIBLIOGRAPHY

Baker, C.R.: Banded-cast metal crowns, J.A.D.A. **56**:522, 1958.

Caputo, A.A., and Stanlee, J.P.: Biomaterials in Clinical Dentistry, Chicago-Tokyo, 1987, Quintessence Publishing Co.

Craig, R.C., el-Ebrashi, M.K., and Peyton, F.A.: Experimental stress analysis of dental restorations. I. Two-dimensional photoelastic stress analysis of dental restorations. II. Two-dimensional photoelastic stress analysis of crowns, J. Prosthet. Dent. **17**(3):292-302, 1967.

Ewing, J.E., and Bentman, D.: Porcelain veneered full crown restorations made with cadmium patterns, J. Prosthet. Dent. **18**(2):140-150, 1967.

Gordon, T.: Telescopic reconstruction: an approach to rehabilitation, J.A.D.A. **72**:97-105, 1966.

Herrick, P.W., Shell, J., Timmermans, J., and Turpin, D.: Investigation of hygroscopic investment (control water added) for casting multiunit bridges, J. Dent. Res. **40**:744, 1961.

Isaacson, G.O.: Telescopic crown retainers for removable partial dentures, J. Prosthet. Dent. **21**:458-465, 1969.

Jameson, L.M.: Comparison of crevicular fluid volumes between restored and non-restored teeth (master's thesis), Maywood, Ill., Loyola University Dental School, 1976.

Leff, A.: Evaluation of high speed in full coverage preparations, J. Prosthet. Dent. **10**:314, 1960.

Lyon, D.M., Cowger, G.T., Woycheshin, F.F., and Miller, C.B.: Porcelain fused to gold—evaluation and esthetics, J. Prosthet. Dent. **10**:319, 1960.

Marcum, J.S.: The effect of crown marginal depth upon gingival tissue, J. Prosthet. Dent. **17**:479, 1967.

Miller, I.F., and Feinberg, E.: Full coverage restorations, J. Prosthet. Dent. **12**:317-325, 1961.

Miller, Lloyd L.: Framework design in ceramo-metal restorations, Dent. Clin. North Am. **21**:699, 1977.

Preston, J.D.: Rational approach to tooth preparation for ceramo-metal restorations, Dent. Clin. North Am. **21**:683, 1977.

Schweitzer, J.M.: Gold copings for problematic teeth, J. Prosthet. Dent. **10**:163, 1960.

Stein, R.S., Kuwata, M.: A dentist and a dental technologist analyze current ceramo-metal procedures, Dent. Clin. North Am. **21**:729, 1977.

Swartz, M.L., and Phillips, R.W.: Study of adaptation of veneers to cast gold crowns, J. Prosthet. Dent. **7**:817, 1957.

Wagman, S.S.: Tissue management for full cast veneer crowns, J. Prosthet. Dent. **15**:106-117, 1965.

Weinberg, I.A.: Double casting of metal to metal in full coverage, J.A.D.A. **63**:821, 1961.

Weiss, Peter: New design parameters: utilizing the properties of nickel-chromium superalloys, Dent. Clin. North Am. **21**:769, 1977.

25 CERESTORE

Edwin J. Riley

SHRINK-FREE CERAMIC CROWN: CERESTORE SYSTEM*

Dentistry has long recognized the esthetic advantages of an "all-ceramic crown." Land used feldspathic porcelains and platinum foil matrices to fabricate porcelain jacket crowns,[1] but this approach was limited by the lack of precision and strength of the porcelain material (Fig. 25-1). During the past 80 years, numerous investigators have improved the fabrication technique and strength.[2-6] Most notably, the process of dispersion strengthening[7] has resulted in substantial improvement in the porcelain, but has not overcome problems related to firing shrinkage that potentially lead to distortion of the matrix, marginal inaccuracy, and inadequate functional strength.

The advent of new ceramic technologies in restorative dentistry has expanded the application of all-ceramic crowns. The development of nonshrinking ceramics such as the Cerestore System has provided an alternate treatment.[8] Using transfer molding, it is now possible to fabricate nonmetallic ceramic crowns directly on the master die with excellent marginal fit.[9] To realize the potential of shrink-free ceramics, it is important to understand the material chemistry, the fabrication technique, and the recommended clinical procedures.

CHEMISTRY

The innovative feature of the Cerestore system is the dimensional stability of the core material in the molded (unfired) and fired states. Conventional ceramic materials shrink 10 to 20 percent during firing.

*Cerestore System, Johnson and Johnson Dental Products Company, East Windsor, N.J.

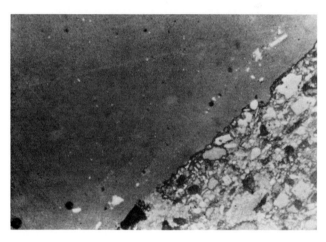

Fig. 25-1. Cross-section Cerestore crown microstructure. Note: polycrystalline nature of core (left) and wetting at junction by veneer (right).

The Cerestore core material offsets conventional ceramic shrinkage by a combination of chemical and crystalline transformations.

Chemical Transformation—Oxidation of Silicone

The silicone resin used as the binder during transfer molding compensates for shrinkage of the core material by conversion of SiO to SiO_2 during firing from 160°C to 800°C. Thus, instead of eliminating the binder during firing as in conventional systems, the silicone organic binder is converted to silica and is taken into the glass constituent of the fired state.

Crystalline Transformation

Compensation for the firing shinkage in ceramics involves combining constituents so that the transformation during firing (Table 25-1) results in the fired ceramic components occupying a greater volume than the raw ingredients. Although the interaction of the various raw materials in the Cerestore core material is complex, the primary inorganic reactions involve MgO, Al_2O_3, and glass frit. As shown in Table 25-2, the MgO and Al_2O_3 (<10 mm) react to form spinel ($MgAl_2O_4$), thereby offsetting shrinkage. This reaction is further enhanced by the glass frit that takes MgO and Al_2O_3 into solution and subsequently precipitates the spinel phase during firing from 900°C to 1300°C.

Table 25-1. Unfired composition Cerestore core material

Component	Weight (%)
Al_2O_3 (less than 10 mm)	43
Al_2O_3 (less than 45 mm)	17
MgO	9
Glass frit	13
Kaolin clay	4
Silicone resin	12
Calcium stearate	1
Steryl amide wax	1

It is the spinel phase in conjunction with the coarser Al_2O_3 that acts as strengthening agents in the fired core.[10] Alpha-Al_2O_3 is a known strength enhancer, as evidenced by the aluminous porcelain jacket crown. However, spinel is also among the mechanically strongest oxide ceramic materials.[11,12] A typical fired Cerestore coping composition is listed in Table 25-3.

The microstructure of the core material consists of a multiphased mixed oxide system of aluminates. Aluminum oxide (Al_2O_3) is the primary component of the chemical composition. In addition, alpha-aluminum oxide (corundum) is the dominant phase in the microstructure. The basic ratio of crystalline to glass phase is comparable to industrial high-strength 85 percent alumina ceramics.[10] The representative fired Cerestore crown microstructure shown in Fig. 25-1

Table 25-3. Fired composition Cerestore core material

Plase	Weight (%)
Al_2O_3 (corundum)	60
$MgAl_2O_4$ (spinel)	22
$BaMg_2Al_3$ ($Si_9Al_2O_{30}$)	10
Glass phase	8

demonstrates the high polycrystalline nature of the core material and the excellent wetting by the veneer glass.

STRENGTH

Success with Cerestore depends on a combination of fit, coping design, and mechanical properties of the core material.[13,14,15] Table 25-4 lists the mechanical properties of the standard core material.

The crucial physical property of an all-ceramic dental restoration is flexural strength. Substantial improvement in the flexural strength of the Cerestore core material has been reported.[16] Flexural strengths with nonshrink ceramics in excess of 225 Mn/m^2 (32,000 psi) has been accomplished by further recrystallization of the residual glass and consolidation of the enclosed porosity (Fig. 25-1). Increases in flexural strength provide an increase in the safety factor of single-unit restorations and expand the clinical capabilities to multiple units.

Table 25-5 shows physical properties other than high flexural strength that are advantageous in the second-generation Cerestore core ceramic.

Table 25-4. Physical properties of first-generation Cerestore core material

Compressive strength	1048 MN/m^2
Modulus of elasticity	1.23×10^5 MN/m^2
Flexural strength	120 MN/m^2
Piosson's ratio	0.23
Linear coefficient of thermal expansion	$5.6 \times 10^{-6}/°C$
Density	2.9 gm/cm^3

Table 25-2. Phase change mechanism for offsetting shrinkage

Spinel ($MgAl_2O_4$)		Alumina (Al_2O_3)	+	Magnesia (MgO)	$\longrightarrow$	
	Density (g/cm³)	3.97		3.58	$\longrightarrow$	3.60
	Mol. wt. (g)	101.96	+	40.31	$\longrightarrow$	142.27
	Vol. $\left(\dfrac{Mol.\ wt.}{Density}\right)$	25.72 cm³	+	11.26 cm³	$\longrightarrow$	39.52 cm³
		36.98 cm³			$\longrightarrow$	39.52 cm³
	Net vol. increase	=	2.54 cm³			
	Net % vol. expansion	=	6.87%			
	Net % linear expansion	=	2.35%			

Table 25-5. Advantages of second-generation Cerestore core material

Recrystallization of residual glass	→	Flexural strength > 225 MN/m² (32,000 psi)
High polycrystalline content	→	↓ Static fatigue potential compared to high glass content systems
Same relative thermal conductivity of core and veneer porcelain	→	↓ Interfacial stress compared to ceramometal systems
Low coefficient of thermal expansion	→	↑ Thermal shock resistance
		↓ Interfacial stress
		↓ Solubility as a result of
		↓ alkali components
High modulus of elasticity	→	↓ Stress on cement[17]

TECHNIQUE

Perceptive tooth preparation is critical to success. In general, the tooth reduction for a successful Cerestore crown is similar to that recommended by many authors[18,19] for the metal-ceramic restoration: labial, lingual, and interproximal, reduction of 1.25 mm to 1.5 mm; incisal and occlusal, reduction of 1.5 mm to 2.0 mm.

The preferred marginal design is a 90 degree full shoulder with a rounded gingivalaxial line angle (width 1.0 mm to 1.5 mm). Featheredge and beveled preparations are contraindicated. The internal line angles are rounded (e.g., occlusoaxial line angles) as sharp edges, and points act as stress concentrators in the ceramic coping.

Regardless of strength levels achieved in all-ceramic crowns, they are inherently less forgiving than metallic restorations and as such require systematic preparation to ensure suitable reduction and avoidance of stress. The following approach to preparation is suggested:

1. Isolate the tooth using a round-end tapered diamond. Note: the preparation of the proximal shoulder is critical. The preparation does not encroach on the epithelial attachment. The dentist must watch the contour of the gingival crest and see that the preparation rises in harmony with the anatomy of the tooth. This is achieved with a round-ended stone (Fig. 25-2).

2. A necked, round diamond or carbide is selected to complete uniform depth grooves. The depth grooves are prepared at the height of the gingival crest and segmenting the facial and lingual surfaces (Fig. 25-3). Note: The large round stone will control the depth of each groove by allowing the stone to penetrate only to the shank. This provides uniform depth without excessive penetration. Another advantage of a round stone is that it prepares the desired shoulder regardless of the angle of the handpiece.

On the incisal and occlusal surfaces, penetration is approximately one-half to two-thirds the

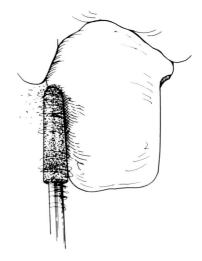

Fig. 25-2. Interproximal reduction and isolation of tooth.

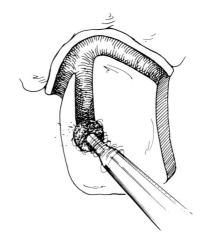

Fig. 25-3. Preparation of depth grooves.

diameter of the stone (Fig. 25-4). The exact penetration depends on the diameter of the stone. The diameter of all diamonds used in preparation is measured to ensure predictable tooth reduction. As a general rule, a cut performed to the shank is slightly less than half the measured di-

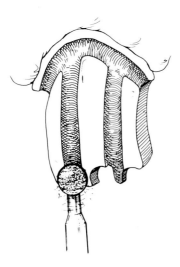

Fig. 25-4. Incisal depth cut.

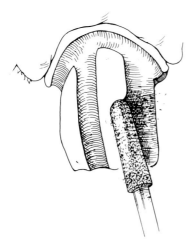

Fig. 25-5. Removing islands of tooth structure created by depth grooves.

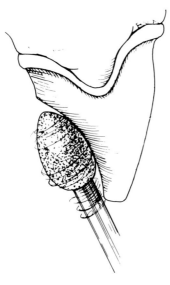

Fig. 25-6. Lingual reduction.

ameter of the stone. A round stone measuring 2.2 mm produces a penetration of about 1 mm.

3. Gross reduction is performed with a coarse, round-end, tapered diamond. The islands of tooth structure created by the depth cuts are eliminated. The round-end diamond is useful in defining the interproximal rounded shoulder and preserving the previously established rounded gingival-axial line angle on the labial and lingual surfaces (Fig. 25-5).

4. The lingual (occlusal) surface is prepared using a football-shaped diamond stone. Use of a thickness gauge (Flexible Clearance Guide, Belle de St. Claire, 16147 Valerio St., Van Nuys, Calif. 91406) in checking reduction is also helpful (Figs. 25-6 and 25-7).

5. Smooth and refine the preparation using a fine diamond the same shape as used for gross reduction. There should be no sharp angles or undercuts, and maximum parallelism at the cervical axial walls, allowing only one path of insertion. This is commonly accomplished using slow speed.

6. After placing the retraction cord, redefine the labial finish line to ensure the desired relation to the gingival crest. Note: it is important to avoid any peripheral lip on the preparation. This is usually accomplished by using a round-end, tapered diamond slightly larger than the developed rounded shoulder (Fig. 25-8).

IMPRESSIONS

Impression-making procedures for the Cerestore crowns are similar to those for conventional restorations. Traditional impression materials are acceptable.

LABORATORY TECHNIQUE

The nonshrink property of the core material encourages a direct approach rather than indirect cast-

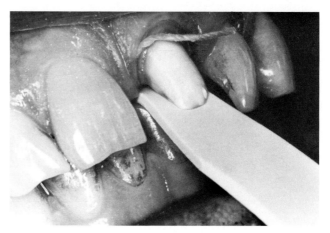

Fig. 25-7. Use of preparation thickness guide to ensure proper reduction.

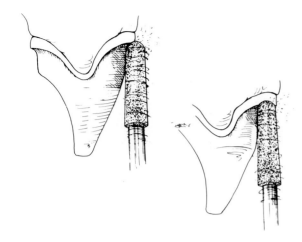

Fig. 25-8. Refining finish line. Left, correct. Right, incorrect.

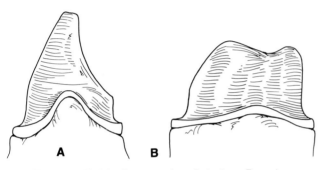

Fig. 25-9. Finished preparation. **A,** incisor. **B,** molar.

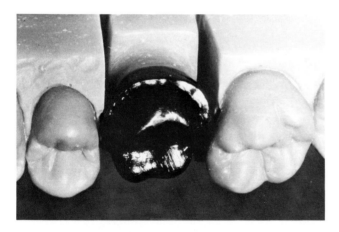

Fig. 25-10. Coping waxed on epoxy.

ing. There is no solidification shrinkage, nor the need to control investment expansion.

Copings are formed by transfer molding the ceramic directly onto nonshrinking, heat-stable epoxy master dies. Transfer molding is unique to dental ceramics but is identical to the injection molding of acrylic resin denture bases (Fig. 25-9).

The ceramic is supplied as a dense pellet of the compacted shrink-free formulation. The pellet is heated until the silicone resin carrier in the ceramic is flowable (160°C) and then transferred by pressure into the plaster mold directly on the master die. The silicone resin is thermoplastic and thermosetting, so after the material is injected into the mold and around the master die, it sets. The substrate is then removed from the die, refined with conventional stones, and sintered.

The coping is fired in a microprocessor-controlled furnace to approximately 1300°C. By controlling the firing schedule, the chemical and crystalline transformations are generated, and the ceramic achieves the physical properties with zero shrinkage. Once fired, the coping is ready to be veneered.

Flowchart 25-1 and Figs. 25-10 to 25-16 summarize the procedures for fabricating a Cerestore crown:

COPING DESIGN

A successful restorative system is a function of rational design and favorable physical properties. Maximal advantage is taken of the core material in high-stress areas. Paper-thin copings do not significantly strengthen the restoration. Optimal coping design should capitalize on core thickness, anticipating shade development with 0.8 mm of veneer porcelain. This provides a minimum of 0.5 mm of core material on the facial and lingual and 0.7 mm on the occlusal surface. The strength increases exponentially with core thickness.

Flowchart 25-1

Prepare tooth with rounded shoulder
↓
Obtain impression
↓
Prepare Cerestore epoxy die and apply cement spacer
↓
Waxup and sprue coping on epoxy die
↓
Invest waxup with epoxy master die in flask
with dental stone and plaster
↓
Boil out wax
↓
Heat flask to 180°C
↓
Transfer mold ceramic into lost wax cavity
directly on the master die
↓
Retrieve master die with formed coping from plaster
↓
Trim sprue and refine coping
↓
Fire coping in programmable furnace
↓
Add transition and veneer porcelains
in conventional fashion

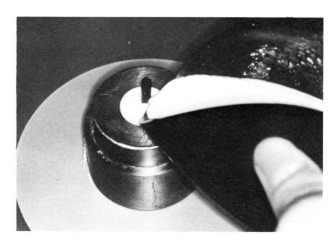

Fig. 25-11. Investing wax up on die with plaster.

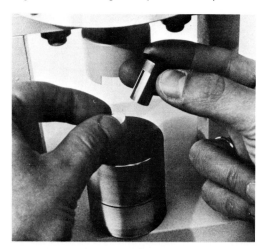

Fig. 25-12. Placing ceramic pellet in flask for pressing.

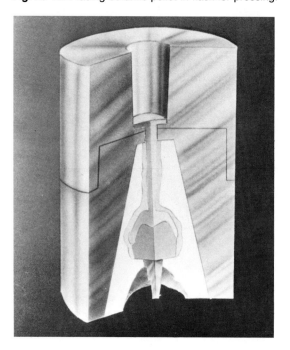

Fig. 25-13. Cross-sectional diagram of ceramic injected into mold.

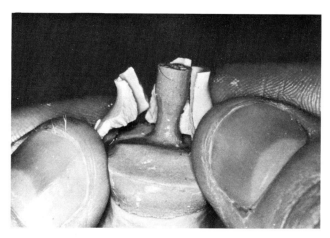

Fig. 25-14. Plaster removal from pressed coping and master die.

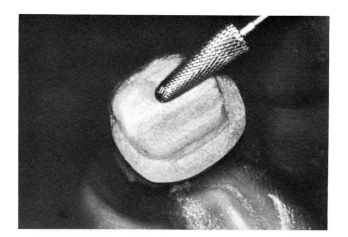

Fig. 25-15. Refining green state (unfired) coping.

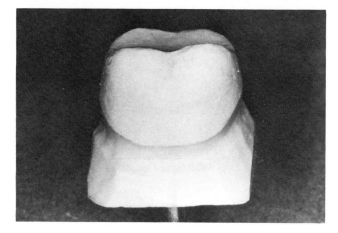

Fig. 25-16. A, Pressed coping (unfired) on master die.

The optimal design of copings for an anterior and posterior restoration is exhibited in Figs. 25-17 and 25-18. The design is a miniaturization of the final shape and provides an easy veneer placement with excellent support. Because the core and veneer have similar

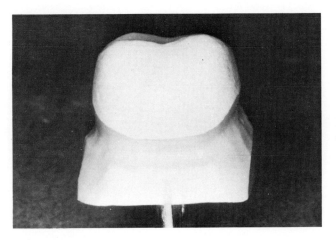

Fig. 25-16. B, Fired state coping on master die.

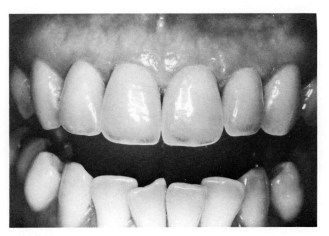

Fig. 25-19. All ceramic crowns maxillary central and lateral incisors. Note gradation of translucency.

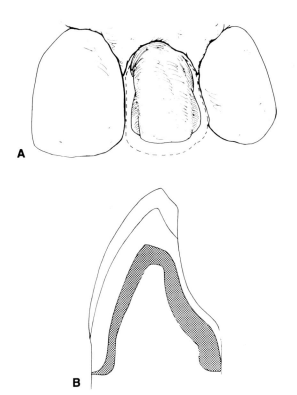

Fig. 25-17. A, Optimal coping design anterior. **B,** Cross-sectional diagram of anterior restoration.

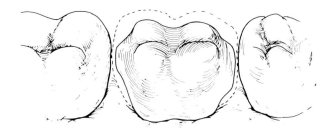

Fig. 25-18. Optimal coping design posterior.

thermal conductivities and matched coefficients of thermal expansion, uniform veneer thickness is not critical as in metal ceramics.

VENEER

Optional shade development in Cerestore restorations is accomplished by using internal color placement with translucent enamel overlay.[20,21,22] The available veneer porcelain system demonstrates a gradation in chroma and translucency. The innermost dentinal layer has the greatest chroma and least translucence. Chroma decreases and translucency increases during progression externally through the body, enamel, and finally, clear porcelain. This arrangement mimics the natural tooth and creates the color depth necessary for esthetics (Fig. 25-19).

INSERTION: CLINICAL CONSIDERATIONS
Fit

The fit of ceramic crowns is passive. It should not bind on insertion because of tensile forces. However, a passive fit does not infer grossly oversized. A restoration should not rotate on the die, but have a positive seat with one path of insertion.

Transfer-molded crowns should exhibit exceptional fit[9,24] (Fig. 25-20) because of the direct molding process, the stable dimensions of the epoxy die, and the expansion of the fired core material by adjustment of firing temperature.

For uneventful cementation, the following are recommended:

1. Be certain preparation is clear of temporary cement.
2. Seat crown with finger pressure and check proximal contacts before seating.
3. Simulate the cementing media by inserting the restoration with a low-viscosity silicone ("wash").

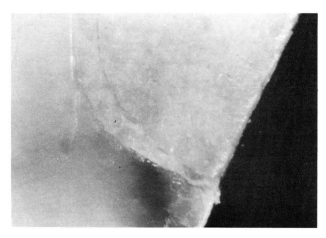

Fig. 25-20. Cross-section cemented restoration. Thickness of zinc phosphate cement at margin, 20 microns.

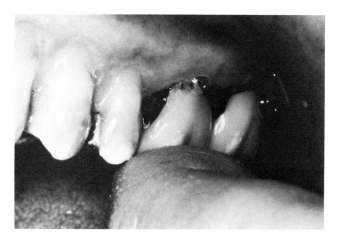

Fig. 25-21. A, Trial insertion with silicone.

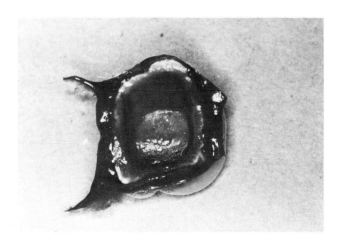

Fig. 25-21. B, Visual examination of cement space and marginal seal.

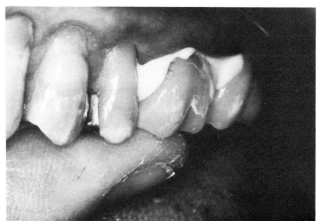

Fig. 25-21. C, Actual cementation with finger pressure.

This allows radiographic evaluation and occlusal adjustment in the "cemented" position. In addition, visual examination of the cement space is feasible with identification of binding spots (Fig. 25-21).

4. After chairside adjustments of occlusion or contour, the restoration is reglazed and/or polished.
5. Cementation. Any "permanent" cement is used with manufacturer's directions for a low-viscosity FPD mix. The color of the cement is not critical, since the core material prevents the cement or root discoloration, buildups, or cores from affecting the overall shade (Fig. 25-22). Because passive fit has been established, a bite stick is unnecessary. The crown is seated with finger pressure only.

Radiographic Appearance

Because of the presence of the barium osumilite phase ($BaMg_2Al_3[Si_9Al_2O_3]$) in the fired core material,

the radiodensity of the shrink-free ceramic is similar to that of enamel. This allows radiographic examination of marginal adaptation and visualization under the crown; i.e., pulp, bases, pins, posts, and caries (Fig. 25-23).

Biocompatibility

Animal and in vitro testing of the shrink-free alumina ceramic used in the Cerestore system has demonstrated the biocompatibility of the material.[27,28] Observations during in vivo studies in dogs[29] supported the findings that plaque accumulation on glazed porcelain surfaces is appreciably less than on other restorative surfaces and less than on homogeneous uncrowned teeth.[30,31]

Advantages of Shrink-Free Ceramic Crown

1. Marginal integrity generated by direct molding without distortion during veneer applications.
2. Esthetics—depth of color without metal.

3. Biocompatibility—totally inert core with glazed porcelain veneer that is more resistant to plaque formation.
4. Low thermal conductivity—reduced thermal sensitivity.
5. Low coefficient of thermal expansion and high modulus of elasticity; protection of cement seal.
6. Radiodensity similar to that of natural enamel.

Disadvantages of Shrink-Free Ceramic Crown

1. Specialized laboratory equipment needed.
2. Tooth preparation requires close attention to detail.
3. Not recommended in patients with heavy bruxism or inadequate clearance.
4. Contraindicated in long-span FPD.

COMMON CAUSES OF FAILURE OF A CERESTORE CROWN

Laboratory

1. Inadequate coping design. Thin copings (less than 0.5 mm), especially on occlusal surface of posterior teeth.
2. Failure to dye check copings for flaws before veneering.
3. Poor technique in veneer placement, leaving porcelain inside of coping.
4. Inappropriate firing temperatures, creating overexpansion of epoxy die or ceramic coping, leading to a loose fit. The adaptation is passive and loose!

Clinical

1. Unsuitable preparation. Insufficient tooth reduction (less than 1.5 mm on posterior occlusal surface), sharp angles causing stress, large undercuts resulting in large blockouts on master die.
2. Forcing a binding crown to seat, as when using a bite stick.
3. Malocclusions prior to placement.

FUTURE DEVELOPMENTS

The evolution of shrink-free alumina will continue with research in core material equipment and technique. Because metal substructures are unesthetic and costly, considerable interest in all-ceramic systems will continue. The goal remains to replace metals with ceramics that have flexural strengths comparable to those of precious alloys. The development of ceramic crowns and FPDs that compare with the metal-ceramic systems that resist tensile stress would then become a reality. Color demonstrations of Cerestore crowns are available in the back of the text (Figs. 25-24 to 28).

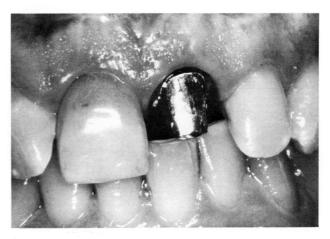

Fig. 25-22. A, Preop maxillary left central incisor.

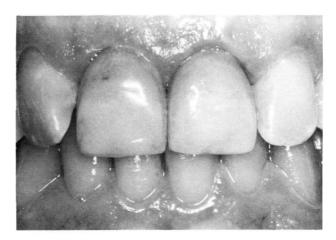

Fig. 25-22. B, Postop maxillary left central incisor.

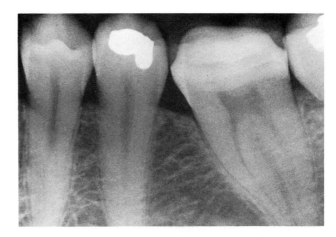

Fig. 25-23. Radiograph Cerestore crown mandibular first molar.

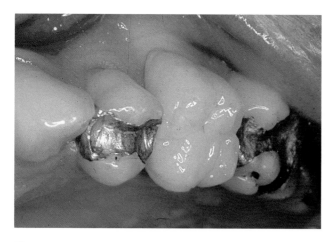

Fig. 25-24. A, Cerestore crown maxillary 1st molar.

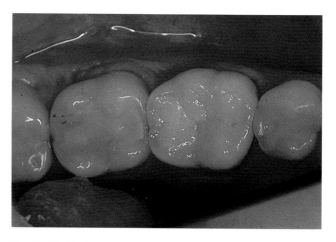

Fig. 25-24. B, Cerestore crown mandibular 1st molar.

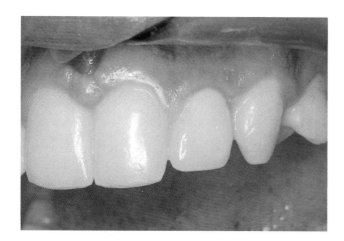

Fig. 25-24. C, Cerestore crown maxillary left lateral.

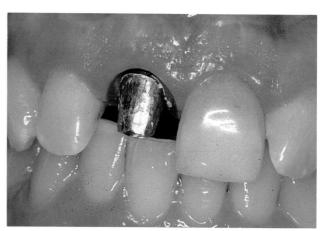

Fig. 25-25. A, Preoperative endodontically treated central incisor.

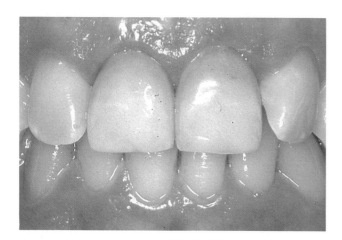

Fig. 25-25. B, Postoperative view of Cerestore crown.

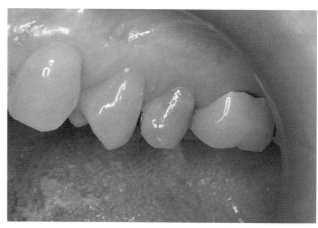

Fig. 25-26. A, Preoperative of discolored maxillary 2nd premolar.

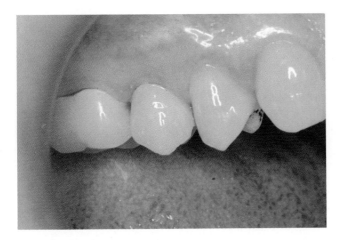

Fig. 25-26. B, Postoperative facial view of Cerestore crown.

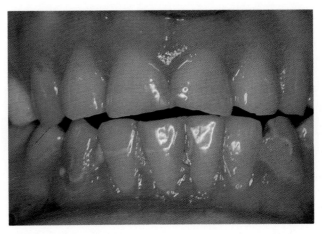

Fig. 25-27. A, Preoperative fractured anterior—maxillary and mandibular incisors.

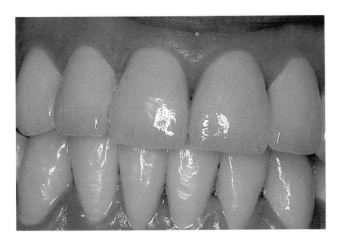

Fig. 25-27. B, Postoperative facial view.

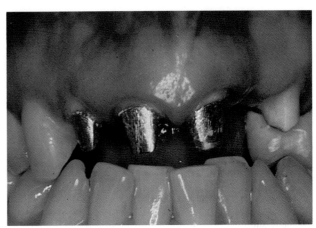

Fig. 25-28. A, Preoperative view of three endodontically treated teeth and missing lateral incisor.

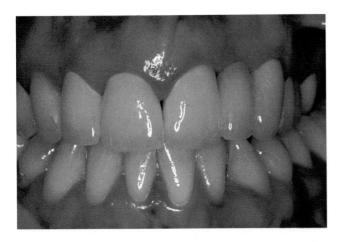

Fig. 25-28. B, Postoperative view including FPD. (Fig. 25-24 to 25-28. courtesy Dr. Edwin J. Riley, Boston, Mass.)

SELECTED REFERENCES

1. Land, C.: Porcelain dental arts, Dent. Cosmos. **45**:615, 1903.
2. Southan, D.E., and Jorgensen, K.D.: Precise porcelain jacket crowns, Aust. Dent. J. **17**:269, 1972.
3. Riley, E.J., et al.: Precision porcelain jacket crown technique, J. Prosthet. Dent. **34**:346, 1975.
4. McLean, J.W., and Sced, I.R.: The bonded alumina crown. I. The bonding of platinum to aluminous dental porcelain using tin oxide coatings, Aust. Dent. J. **21**:2, 1976.
5. McLean, J.W., et al.: The bonded alumina crown. II. Construction using the twin foil technique, Aust. Dent. J. **21**:262, 1976.
6. Faull, T.W., et al.: Marginal opening of single and twin platinum foil-bonded aluminous porcelain crowns, J. Prosthet. Dent. **53**:30, 1985.
7. McLean, J.W., and Hughes, T.H.: The reinforcement of dental porcelain with ceramic oxides, Br. Dent. J. **119**:251, 1965.
8. Sozio, R.B., and Riley, E.J.: The shrink-free ceramic crown, J. Prosthet. Dent. **49**:182, 1983.

9. Sato, T., Wohlwend, A., and Scharer, P.: Marginal fit in a "shrink-free" ceramic crown system, Int. J. Perio. Rest. Dent. **3**:9, 1986.

10. Starling, L.B.: Transfer molded "all ceramic crowns": the Cerestore System, presented at W.K. Kellogg Foundation Institute, University of Michigan, Oct. 12, 1983.

11. Ryshkewitch, E.: Oxide Ceramics, New York, 1970, Academic Press, p. 269.

12. Hague, W.F., et al.: Refractory ceramics for aerospace, Columbus, Ohio, American Ceramic Society, 1964, p. 277.

13. Davis, D.: Clinical efficacy of all ceramic crowns: the experience of a general practitioner, Compend. Cont. Ed. **6**(10):742, 1985.

14. Philip, G.K., and Burke, C.E.: Compressive strengths of conventional, twin foil and all ceramic crowns, J. Prosthet. Dent. **2**:215, 1985.

15. Josephson, B.A., et al.: A compressive strength study of an all ceramic crown. J. Prosthet. Dent. **53**:301, 1985.

16. Sozio, R.B., and Riley, E.J.: Shrink-free ceramic, Dent. Clin. North Am. **29**(4):205, 1985.

17. Starling, L.B., and Cook, S.D.: An evaluation of stress within ceramic tooth reconstructive materials, Assoc. Dent. Res. Annual Meeting, presentation 336, 1983.

18. McLean, J.W.: The Science and Art of Dental Ceramics, Chicago, 1979, Quintessence Publishing Co., Inc.

19. Shillingburg, H.T., Hobo, H., and Fisher, D.W.: Preparation for Cast Gold Restorations, Chicago, 1974, Quintessence Publishing Co., Inc.

20. Muia, P.J.: The Four Dimensional Tooth Color System, Chicago, 1982, Quintessence Publishing Co., Inc.

21. Kuwata, M.: Theory and Practice of Ceramometal Restorations, Chicago, 1980, Quintessence Publishing Co., Inc.

22. Yamamoto, M.: The Metal Ceramics, Chicago, 1985, Quintessence Publishing Co., Inc.

23. Sozio, R.B., and Riley, E.J.: Esthetic considerations of the all ceramic crown, Calif. Dent. Assoc. J. **12**(4):117-121, 1984.

24. Burke, C.E., and Philip, G.K.: The fit of Cerestore, twin foil and conventional ceramic crowns, IADR Program and Abstracts No. 1689, 1985.

25. Sato, T., Wohlwend, A., and Sharer, P.: Shrink-free ceramic crown system: factors influencing the core margin fit, Quintessence J. of Dent. Technol. 10(2), 1986.

26. Campbell, S.D., Riley, E.J., and Sozio, R.B.: Evaluation of a new epoxy resin die material, J. Prosthet. Dent. **54**:136-140, 1985.

27. Autian, J.: Toxilogical evaluation of biomaterials: primary acute toxicity screening program, Artif. Organs **1**:53, 1977.

28. Primary acute toxicity screen, Project No. PT01747, Materials Science Toxicology Laboratories, University of Tennessee, Center for the Health Sciences, Memphis, Tenn.

29. Riley, E.J., Sozio, R.B., and Krech, K.: Shrink-free ceramic crown versus ceramo-metal: a comparative study in dogs, J. Prosthet. Dent. **39**:766, 1983.

30. Newcomb, G.: The relationship between the location of subgingival crown margins and gingival inflammation, J. Periodontol. **45**:151, 1974.

31. Kaquelar, J.C., and Weiss, M.B.: Plaque accumulation on dental restorative materials, I.A.D.R. Abstract No. 615, 1970.

26

William D. Sulik

THE DICOR CASTABLE GLASS-CERAMIC SYSTEM

Restorative dentistry is constantly pursuing the ideal artificial material to replace missing tooth structure. While no such material exists, dentistry has made tremendous strides with the introduction of the castable glass-ceramic, or Dicor, system. This system has been specifically designed to allow the fabrication of accurate restorations with outstanding esthetics. The unique properties of this dental material are unprecedented in any one dental restorative material, and these properties are responsible for the unique advantages of this system. Presently, the cast glass-ceramic is used to fabricate single-tooth, complete veneer crowns, inlays, onlays, three-quarter crowns, and laminate veneers; research is in progress for short-span FPDs.

Castable glass-ceramic, or Dicor, restorations were introduced to dentistry in the fall of 1984 after more than 7 years of intensive research. The present system represents the cumulative efforts of Peter Adair of Biocor, Inc., David Grossman, Ph.D., of The Corning Glass Works, and Dentsply International.

This chapter provides information about the material, its development, and laboratory procedures. The major emphasis is on the advantages that this system offers over more conventional alternatives, including clinical recommendations.

MATERIAL

The ancestry of Dicor cast glass-ceramic restorations dates back to the early 1930s. Frederick Carter, the founder of the Steuben Division of The Corning Glass Works, perfected fabricating objects in glass with the lost wax-casting process. Although delicate objects were cast accurately, the mechanical properties of glass restricted its use to artistic applications. In the 1950s, with the evolution of glass-ceramic systems conceived by Stookey of The Corning Glass Works, functional applications became possible. Glass ceramics represented a major achievement because a whole family of materials with endless potential was realized. Glass-ceramics are composite materials of a glassy matrix phase and a crystal phase. After the glass article is formed, nucleation and crystal growth are created during a controlled heat treatment, or "ceramming process."[1] The physical and mechanical properties of glass-ceramic materials depend upon the type of crystalline form concentration within the glass. The Dicor cast glass-ceramic is comprised of SiO_2, K_2O, and MgO, a fluoride (MgF_2), small amounts of AlO_3 and ZrO_2, and a fluorescing agent.[2] It is technically described as a tetrasilicic fluoromica glass-ceramic. Tetrasilicic fluoromica crystals comprise 55 percent by volume of the material, the remaining 45 percent is glass. These crystals, which are pennylike in shape, are approximately 1 μm thick and 5 to 6 mm in diameter (Fig. 26-1). This unique composition of glass and crystals is responsible for the advantages of Dicor as a dental restorative material.

ADVANTAGES

Strength

No restorative material may be deemed acceptable by dentists or patients unless it possesses sufficient strength to survive the oral environment. Feldspathic porcelains, used in metal-ceramic restorations, and some all-porcelain restorations, are glasses. Consequently, they are subject to the inherent frailties of glass. Although glasses look and behave like solid objects, they are in fact supercooled liquids or noncrystalline solids. Their microstructure is amorphous, with minimal crystalline form for strength. A scanning electron micrographic comparison between a fused feldspathic porcelain and the Dicor glass-ceramic reveals the difference between the two materials (Fig. 26-2). There are limited crystals remaining in the feldspathic porcelain (12 to 15 percent by volume), and most of the mass is amorphous glass. The interlocking network of mica crystals that reinforces the glass is readily observed in the glass ceramic. Flaws (Griffith's flaws) develop on the surface of any glass during its fabrication process (Fig. 26-3), and these flaws have a propensity to self-propagate, so the role of the mica crystals is critical for enhancing the strength of the glass-ceramic. In effect, the crystals stop the propagation of the Griffith's flaws. Since feldspathic porcelains have sparse crystalline form, they require strength-

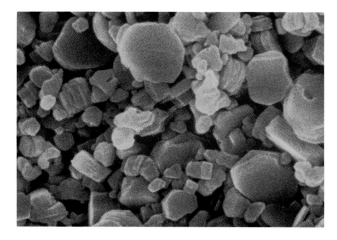

Fig. 26-1. SEM of etched castable ceramic specimen revealing mica crystal morphology. (X5000.)

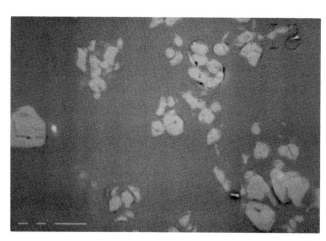

Fig. 26-2. SEM of fused feldspathic porcelain revealing a minimal amount of crystal-line phase (12 to 14 by volume). (Courtesy Dentsply International.)

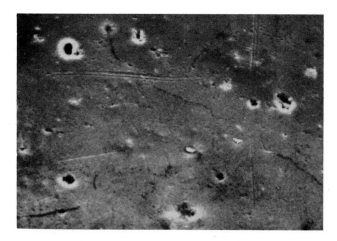

Fig. 26-3. SEM of the surface of glazed feldspathic porcelain revealing surface cracks (Griffith's flaws).

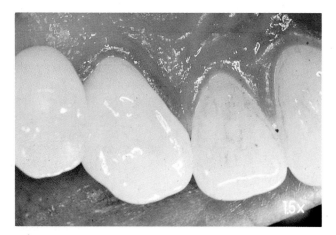

PHYSICAL PROPERTY DATA   TABLE 1

REFERENCE	CAST CERAMIC (1)	ENAMEL (2)	DENTINE (2)	POR-CELAIN (2)	COM-POSITE (2)	GOLD ALLOY (2)	AMAL GAM (2)
COEFFICIENT OF EXPANSION x10⁻⁶/°C	7.2	<11.4>	–	8.0	26-40	14.4	22-26
M.D.R. - PSI / MPa	22000 / 152	1500 / 10.3	7500 / 51	11000 / 75.9	6600 / 12.1	6500 / 132	10000 / 69
COMP. STRENGTH PSI / MPa	120000 / 828	58000 / 400	43000 / 297	25000 / 172	35000 / 194	– / –	55000 / 379
MODULUS OF ELASTICITY PSIx10⁶ / GPa	10.2 / 70.3	12.2 / 84.1	2.65 / 18.3	12.0 / 82.8	2.41 / 16.3	13.0 / 90	9.0 / 62
MICROHARDNESS KHN	362	343	68	460	30	90-220	110

(1) Internal Measurements, Physical Prop. Dept., Corning Glass Works, Corning, NY
(2) Restorative Dental Materials, Ed. By R.G.Craig, C.V. Mosby Co. 1980

Fig. 26-4. Comparative flexural strengths of dental porcelains. (Courtesy Dentsply International.)

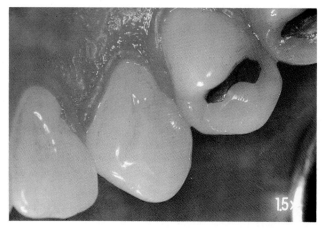

Fig. 26-5. A, Gingival tissue response around castable ceramic restoration.

Fig. 26-5. B, Gingival tissue response around contralateral control tooth.

ening from an underlying substructure. If the coefficients of expansion of the porcelain and a metal are matched, and if proper framework design parameters are employed, porcelain-fused-to-metal is a versatile restorative material.

Through dispensive strengthening techniques or, in effect, by increasing the crystalline content in the glass, McLean developed aluminous porcelains that are stronger than feldspathic porcelains and that can be used to fabricate cores for all-ceramic restorations.[3] This represented a major technologic advancement in restorative dentistry, although its application is restricted because of limited strength, especially in posterior restorations. Fig. 26-4 compares the flexural strength of feldspathic, aluminous, and glass-ceramic materials. The increased strength afforded by the glass-ceramic microstructure accounts for its success as a single-tooth restorative material.

Marginal Adaptation (Fit)

The marginal adaptation of Dicor glass-ceramic, full-veneer crowns has been documented by several authors.[4,5] These investigations have substantiated that Dicor crowns can be fabricated with marginal integrity. Holmes et al. compared the cemented absolute marginal discrepancy (which is defined as the combined vertical and horizontal discrepancies between the cavosurface angle of the preparation and the margin of the restoration) of Dicor crowns and type III gold crowns.[6] The average absolute marginal discrepancy for 10 Dicor crowns measured at four locations around the margin was 48 ± 7 μm compared to 57 ± 19 μm for the gold crowns. According to a Randomized Block Analysis of Variance (ANOVA) at the $P = 0.01$ level of confidence, this difference was not statistically significant. The Dicor castings were statistically more consistent in terms of "fit" than were the gold crowns, according to an unpaired t-test. These results support the empirical judgment of experienced clinicians who feel that glass-ceramic margins compare favorably to metal margins.

Biocompatibility

It has been observed by dentists that the soft tissue response to glass-ceramic restorations is similar to that of unrestored control teeth (Fig. 26-5). There appears to be less plaque accumulation on Dicor restorations than on other restorative materials or on natural teeth. A recently completed clinical research project reports that "seven fold fewer viable bacteria colonized Dicor cast glass-ceramic restorations as compared to that found on natural contralateral teeth."[7] These authors also determined that there was statistically less plaque accumulation around Dicor crowns.

There are several possible reasons for these findings. As previously discussed, 1) the marginal adaptation is exceptional, 2) the fluoride content of the material somehow inhibits bacterial colonization, and 3) the surface of the restoration is smooth and nonporous. Whatever the reason, the phenomena cited represent a major tissue health benefit to patients and an improvement over existing restorative materials.

Wear Potential

A goal of restorative dentistry is to replace that which is missing and to maintain healthy dentition. The potential for accelerated wear of enamel opposing conventional porcelains, especially where functional or rubbing contacts exist, represents a major drawback to those materials. A comparison of microhardness displayed in Figure 26-6 reveals that the Dicor glass-ceramic has a microhardness closely matched to that of enamel, while the microhardness of feldspathic porcelains is one-third greater. Wear does not relate to hardness values alone. The surface of the Dicor can be polished to a very smooth, nonporous finish. This surface is as smooth as, if not smoother than, the glazed feldspathic porcelain. Lingual contours that represent a physiologic anterior guidance are also a crucial factor in minimizing wear. Everything else being equal, it seems logical that a material with a more compatible hardness value would induce less wear in an opposing natural dentition. Unfortunately, there are no longitudinal studies to document the wear of Dicor. Clinical evaluation of restorations in place for four years reveals no detectable wear. Laboratory evaluations simulating wear are in progress, but have not yet been reported. Nonetheless, the compatability of the hardness value of Dicor with enamel represents an improvement.

Thermal Conductivity

This material has a low thermal conductivity that insulates the underlying tooth from changes in temperature. Any all-ceramic restoration has a low coefficient of thermal expansion with insulation.

Simplicity

The technical aspects of fabricating castable ceramic restorations are relatively uncomplicated. The concept is based on the lost wax-casting technique with which dental laboratory technicians are familiar. Consequently, it is relatively easy for the technician to develop the expertise required to fabricate these restorations.

Esthetics

The most significant advantage of the castable ceramic restoration is its lifelike vitality. The translucency inherent in the Dicor material makes it possible

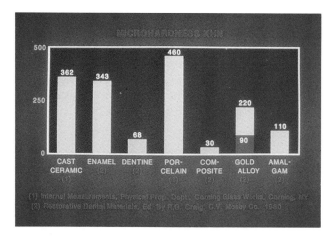

Fig. 26-6. Microhardness of dental porcelains. (Courtesy Dentsply International.)

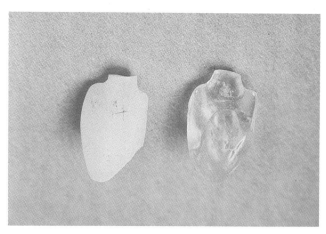

Fig. 26-9. Dicor crowns before and after ceramming. (Courtesy Dentsply International.)

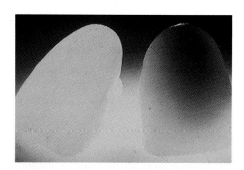

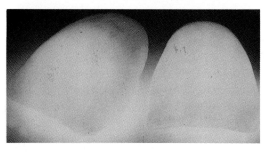

Fig. 26-7. *Top,* Light interaction comparison between Dicor and feldspathic porcelain. *Bottom,* Light interaction comparison between Dicor and natural tooth structure.

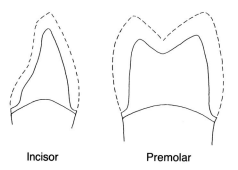

Incisor   Premolar

Fig. 26-8. Full-veneer crown preparation form.

with the castable ceramic identically to the way it reacts with enamel (Fig. 26-7). Because the material appears like enamel, it is possible for technicians and clinicians of modest artistic abilities to create restorations with remarkable realism.

INDICATIONS

Although the castable ceramic is ideally suited for complete veneer crowns on anterior teeth because of esthetics, it is also well suited for complete veneer crowns on posterior teeth. It can be used for single restorations or extensive reconstruction not involving FPDs. Inlays, onlays, three-quarter crowns, and other partial veneer restorations can also be fabricated; laminate veneers are a recent application of the castable ceramic. It is especially indicated in periodontally compromised patients because of plaque resistance and excellent periodontal response.

CONTRAINDICATIONS

The most significant contraindication is if the clinical crown length of the tooth is exceptionally short. In such cases, tooth reduction would compromise resistance and retention of the preparation. In such pa-

to fabricate single-tooth restorations that bear a remarkable resemblance to natural teeth. Grossman, Adair, and Pameijer compared the color in natural teeth to the metal ceramic and castable ceramic restorations.[8] They reported that the hue and chroma levels found in natural teeth could be duplicated with metal ceramic or castable ceramic restorations; however, the value level and translucency observed in natural teeth could only be duplicated by the castable ceramic material.

The mica crystals within the castable ceramic cause incident light to scatter similarly to the light scattered by the enamel rods within a natural tooth. Light reacts tients another material, crown extension surgery, or elective endodontics should be considered.

TOOTH PREPARATION

The recommended tooth reduction for complete veneer castable ceramic crowns differs only slightly from that for metal-ceramic crowns. That difference is in the cervical third of the lingual surface. For a metal-ceramic restoration, the tooth reduction is slightly less because this surface will have no porcelain. Uniform reduction is maintained, however, around the entire marginal circumference of a tooth to receive a castable ceramic crown. The margin design may be a heavy chamfer or a shoulder. A heavy chamfer can be established with a diamond instrument (e.g., Brasseler 878K.018). Knife-edged, feather-edged, sliced, light chamfered, or beveled margins are contraindicated because thin margins fracture. The recommended reduction at the axiogingival angle of the finish line is 0.5 to 1.0 mm. All line and point angles are rounded to minimize stress concentration in these areas. The recommended preparation form is depicted in Fig. 26-8.

IMPRESSIONS

Any impression material or technique used to fabricate working models for metal castings is acceptable.

LABORATORY PHASE

Two coats of a colored die spacer are applied to the dies and serve the same purpose as for other castings.[9] The die spacers are colored to match the various shades of cement used for final cementation. This allows the technician to visualize on the die the effect the cement has on the shade of the restoration. A full contour waxing is then developed to the exact configuration required for function and esthetics. The waxing is invested in a specially formulated phosphate-bonded investment. After setting, the investment is heated first to 450°F and held for ½ hour and then heated to 1750°F and held for ½ hour. A 4 g ingot of glass is placed in a Zirconia crucible and heated to 2600°F in the motor-driven, centrifugal casting machine. The molten glass is quite viscous. Consequently, to ensure a complete and dense casting, the machine remains spinning for 4½ minutes. The glass casting is allowed to cool and is carefully removed from the investment with finger pressure. The final remnants of investment are removed with 25 μm aluminum oxide abrasive at a pressure not exceeding 40 psi. The sprue is removed and the casting is embedded in a gypsum-bonded investment and subjected to a controlled heat treatment or "ceramming" process. This process causes the mica crystals to precipitate in the glass matrix, thus realizing the glass-ceramic. The ceramming process converts the clear glass casting into

an achromatic with a Munsell value level of 6 (Fig. 26-9). The cycle runs from room temperature to 1900°F in 1½ hours and is sustained for 6 hours.

The restoration is now ready for shading. Several layers of a specially formulated veneering porcelain are applied to the external surface to develop the appropriate shade. There is a specific shading porcelain to match each tab on the Bioform and Vita shade guides. The shading porcelains are not traditional ceramic stains but rather low-fusing, highly enameled, feldspathic porcelains with metallic oxide pigments incorporated for the color. A thin, uniform layer of thickly mixed shading porcelain is painted over the exterior of the restoration. The medium is then volatized, and the restoration is fired in air from 1300°F to 1725°F and held for 1 minute. The restoration is allowed to cool, and the shading process is repeated until the appropriate shade is developed. Three layers of shading porcelain are required to develop most shades. Characterization for decalcified areas can be created with conventional ceramic stains. The final shade is achieved by the combined influence of the surface shading and the underlying colored cement.

TRY-IN

The restoration or restorations are normally returned from the laboratory ready for cementation. All-ceramic restorations are seated on the preparation with light finger pressure to avoid fractures. Consequently, the proximal contacts are checked carefully and adjusted. A low-viscosity impression material of contrasting color is used to evaluate the internal adaptation of the casting. Once the fit is established, the impression material can stabilize the casting on the tooth during occlusal adjustment. Occlusal adjustments are performed with a fine diamond in a high-speed handpiece with light pressure. These areas should be polished with a hard rubber wheel and a diamond-impregnated polishing paste.

CEMENTATION

Cementation is accomplished with any "permanent" cement. However, a colored zinc phosphate or light-activated, chemically cured urethane resin cement specifically designed for castable ceramic restorations are recommended because the color of the cement influences the shade of the restoration. If zinc phosphate is used, the zinc oxide powder of the appropriate shade is mixed with water to evaluate the color of the cement. If the resin cement is selected, the try-in paste of the appropriate shade is used for the same purpose. If the cement is too light, a darker one is selected. Finger pressure only is required to seat the restoration during cementation, since a passive fit has been created by the die spacer. There is evidence that

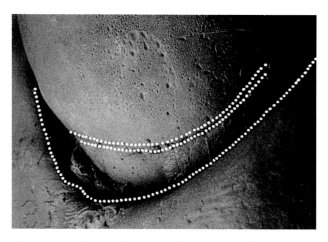

Fig. 26-10. SEM depicting fit of a Dicor veneer with a cemented marginal discrepancy of 25 um.

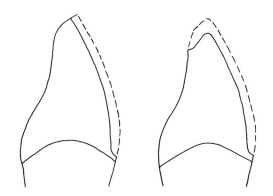

Fig. 26-11. Dicor laminate veneer preparation form.

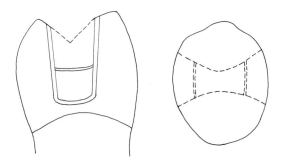

Fig. 26-12. Dicor inlay preparation form.

the effective strength of Dicor restorations was increased substantially by etching (described later) and cementing with the Dicor urethane resin cement.[10,11,12]

ACID-ETCH

Since the castable ceramic material is biphasic and composed of fluoromica crystals within a glass matrix, it can be etched to create micromechanical retention similar to etching enamel with phosphoric acid. The

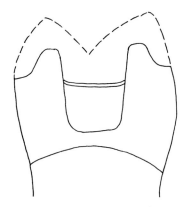

Fig. 26-13. Dicor onlay preparation form.

bond strengths between the castable ceramic material and the resin cement are constantly in the 2500 to 3000 psi range rather than the 1400 to 1600 for resin bonded to enamel. This bonding, coupled with inherent strength and outstanding esthetics, renders the castable ceramic material ideal for laminate veneers, inlays, onlays, and other types of partial veneer retainers.

LAMINATE VENEERS

Veneers can be cast so accurately that they can be made to fit with as little as a 25 μm marginal discrepancy when cemented with the light-activated chemically cured urethane resin (Fig. 26-10). This virtually eliminates excessive finishing of the margins or sealing the margins with unfilled resins, common with other ceramic veneers.

Teeth that are to receive a veneer are prepared within the enamel. The recommended preparation form is presented in Fig. 26-11. The Dicor resin cement is opaque and has unique optical properties due to the presence of mica crystals, which impart reflective properties that enhance the color, translucency, and vitality of the castable ceramic veneers. Before cementation, the veneers are etched for 1 minute with a 10 percent solution of ammonium bifluoride. The etched surface is then treated with a silane coupling agent that chemically bonds the restoration to the resin cement. The appropriate color of try-in paste is used to evaluate the shade. The tooth is then etched in the usual manner, and a layer of bonding agent is cured to the etched enamel. The selected color of resin cement is placed on the veneer and seated with finger pressure. The excess resin is removed, and curing is accomplished for 1 minute with a curing light.

INLAYS AND ONLAYS

Inlays and onlays with lifelike esthetics, excellent marginal adaptation, and physiologic wear can also be fabricated with the castable ceramic material. Inlay

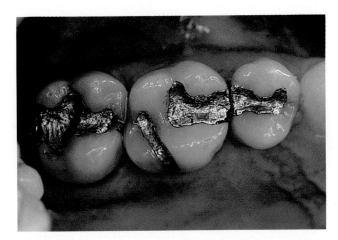

Fig. 26-14. A, Pretreatment view of a quadrant of amalgam restorations.

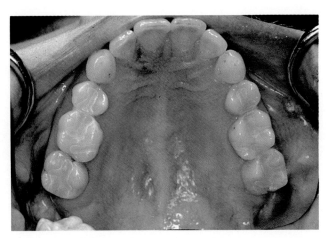

Fig. 26-14. B, Post treatment illustrating Dicor injectable porcelain inlays replacing the amalgam restoration.

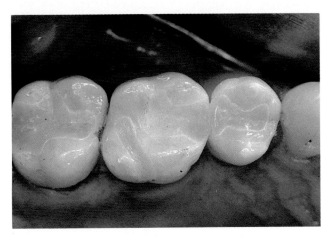

Fig. 26-14. C, Post treatment of Dicor injectable porcelain inlays replacing amalgam restorations.

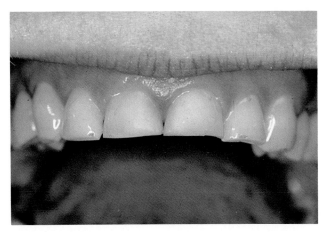

Fig. 26-15. A, Pretreatment of patient with abraded incisors.
Continued

cavity preparation is uncomplicated. A No. 271 carbide bur with a rounded cutting end is used to develop the cavity preparation without sharp axiopulpal or axiogingival line angles. There are no occlusal or proximal bevels. The gingival floor is a heavy chamfer or a shoulder finish line. Fig. 26-12 shows the ideal preparation form for castable ceramic inlays.

Onlay cavity preparations are accomplished with the No. 271 carbide bur for the intracoronal portion. The isthmus and proximal box forms are the same as for inlay preparations. Cusps that are onlayed are reduced 1.5 mm. A heavy chamfer finish line is established on the facial and lingual surfaces of the reduced cusps. The gingival floor is either a shoulder or a heavy chamfer. The ideal preparation form for castable ceramic onlays is shown in Fig. 26-13.

Cementation of inlays and onlays is accomplished with the Dicor light-activated, chemically cured urethane resin or a glass ionomer cement. The teeth are isolated, preferably with a rubber dam. If the resin cement is used, the enamel is etched and the castings

are etched and treated with the silane coupling agent. If glass ionomer cement is used, the casting is etched, only without silane. Cementation with either cement can then be accomplished in the usual manner.

The excitement generated by this material is contagious, but must be tempered by familiarization, with a eye to future research. Additional color illustrations (26-14 to 16) are available at the end of the chapter comparing porcelain laminates, esthetic bonding, porcelain fused to metal crowns, Cerestore crowns, and Dicor crowns.

SELECTED REFERENCES

1. Grossman, D.G.: Processing a dental ceramic by casting methods. Presented at conference on recent developments in ceramic and ceramic-metal systems for crown and bridge, Ann Arbor, Mich., Oct. 10-12, 1983. Pamphlet published May 1985.
2. Adair, P.J., and Grossman, D.G.: The castable ceramic crown, Int. J. Periodontal. Restor. Dent. 4:33, 1984.
3. McLean, J.W.: The science and art of dental ceramics, Vol. 1, Chicago, Quintessence Publishing Co., 1979.

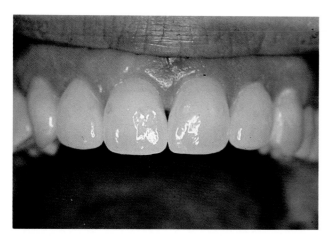

Fig. 26-15. B, Posttreatment with Dicor laminates on the lateral incisors, Dicor complete veneer crowns on the maxillary centrals, and esthetic bonding on the canines. Note tissue health.

4. Adair, P.J., and Hoekstra, K.E.: Fit evaluation of a castable ceramic. J. Dent. Res. **61**:345, 1981, Abstract No. 1500.

5. Fit of Dicor castable ceramic crowns. Dicor Research Report, York, Pa., Dentsply International, February 1986.

6. Holmes, J.R., Bayne, S.C., Sulik, W.D., and Holland, G.A.: Marginal fit of castable ceramic (Dicor) crowns, J. Dent. Res. **66**:283, 1987, Abstract No. 1413.

7. Savitt, E., Socransky, S., Melcer, J., et al.: Effects on colonization of oral micobiota by Dicor glass ceramic, Boston, Mass., Forsythe Institute, February 1986.

8. Grossman, D.G., Adair, P.J., and Pameijer, C.H.: Evaluation of the color of a cast ceramic restorative material, J. Dent. Res. **59**:542, 1980, Abstract No. 1094.

9. Eames, W.B., O'Neal, S.J., Montiero, J., et al.: Techniques to improve seating of castings, J.A.D.A. **96**:432, 1978.

10. Grossman, D.G., and Nelson, J.W.: The bonded Dicor crown, J. Dent. Res. **66**:206, 1987, Abstract No. 800.

11. Eden, G.T., and Kacicz, J.M.: Dicor crown strength improvement due to bonding, **66**:207, 1987, Abstract No. 801.

12. McInnes-LeDoux, P.M., LeDoux, W.R., Weinberg, R., and Rappold, A.: Luting castable ceramic restorations—a bond strength study, I.A.D.R. **66**:207, 1987, Abstract No. 802.

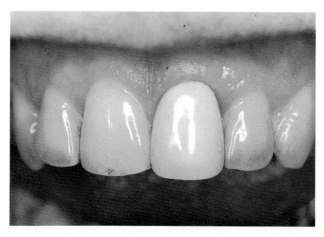

Fig. 26-16. A, Pretreatment of central incisor with PFM crown.

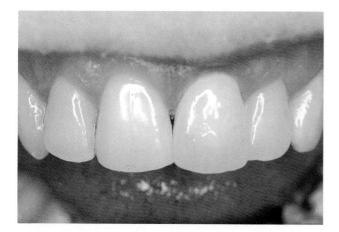

Fig. 26-16. B, Posttreatment after placement of Dicor injectable porcelain crown after removal of existing crown. (Courtesy of Dr. William D. Sulik, Chapel Hill, N.C. Figs. 26-14 to 26-16.)

INDEX